DENTAL PUBLIC HEALTH & RESEARCH
Contemporary Practice for the Dental Hygienist

Fourth Edition

Christine Nielsen Nathe, *RDH, MS*
Professor and Director
Division of Dental Hygiene
Vice Chair
Department of Dental Medicine
University of New Mexico
Albuquerque, NM

PEARSON

Boston   Columbus   Indianapolis   New York   San Francisco
Amsterdam   Cape Town   Dubai   London   Madrid   Milan   Munich   Paris   Montreal   Toronto
Delhi   Mexico City   São Paulo   Sydney   Hong Kong   Seoul   Singapore   Taipei   Tokyo

Publisher: Julie Levin Alexander
Publisher's Assistant: Sarah Henrich
Executive Editor: John Goucher
Program Manager: Nicole Ragonese
Editorial Assistant: Amanda Losonsky
Director of Marketing: David Gesell
Marketing Manager: Brittany Hammond
Marketing Specialist: Michael Sirinides
Project Management Lead: Cynthia Zonneveld
Project Manager: Patricia Gutierrez
Operations Specialist: MaryAnn Gloriande

Art Director: Maria Guglielmo Walsh
Text & Cover Designer: STUDIO MONTAGE
Cover Art: Kasto/Fotolia
Media Director: Amy Peltier
Lead Media Project Manager: Lorena Cerisano
Full-Service Project Management: Cenveo® Publisher Services
Composition: Cenveo® Publisher Services
Printer/Binder: R.R Donnelley/Roanoke
Cover Printer: Phoenix Color/Hagerstown
Text Font: Times Roman

Credits and acknowledgments for content borrowed from other sources and reproduced, with permission, in this textbook appear on the appropriate page within the text.

Notice: The author and the publisher of this book have taken care to make certain that the information given is correct and compatible with the standards generally accepted at the time of publication. Nevertheless, as new information becomes available, changes in treatment and in the use of equipment and procedures become necessary. The reader is advised to carefully consult the instruction and information material included in each piece of equipment or device before administration. Students are warned that the use of any techniques must be authorized by their medical advisor, where appropriate, in accordance with local laws and regulations. The publisher disclaims any liability, loss, injury, or damage incurred as a consequence, directly or indirectly, of the use and application of any of the contents of this book.

Many of the designations by manufacturers and seller to distinguish their products are claimed as trademarks. Where those designations appear in this book, and the publisher was aware of a trademark claim, the designations have been printed in initial caps or all caps.

Library of Congress Cataloging-in-Publication Data

Names: Nathe, Christine Nielsen, author.
Title: Dental public health & research: contemporary practice for the dental
    hygienist / Christine Nielsen Nathe.
Other titles: Dental public health and research
Description: Fourth edition. | Boston : Pearson, [2017] | Preceded by Dental
    public health and research / Christine Nielsen Nathe. 3rd ed. c2011. |
    Includes bibliographical references and index.
Identifiers: LCCN 2015043542| ISBN 9780134255460 | ISBN 0134255461
Subjects: | MESH: Dental Care—United States. | Dental Hygienists—United
    States. | Delivery of Health Care—United States. | Education,
    Dental—United States. | Public Health Dentistry—United States.
Classification: LCC RK60.7 | NLM WU 90 | DDC 617.6/01—dc23
LC record available at http://lccn.loc.gov/2015043542

10 9 8 7 6 5 4 3 2 1

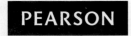

ISBN 10: 0134255461
ISBN 13: 9780134255460

This book is dedicated to my husband, Chris Nathe,
and our children, Rhen, Marissa and Chad Nathe,
who make every day of my life a joy,
and to my parents, John Nielsen and Susan Nielsen, RDH,
for their support and example.

Brief Contents

Contents

UNIT III DENTAL HYGIENE RESEARCH 179

UNIT IV PRACTICAL STRATEGIES FOR DENTAL PUBLIC HEALTH 293

Foreword

When Alfred Civilion Fones followed his dream to create within the dental staff a dental therapist whose focus would be the prevention of dental disease, his intention was not merely to have this person perform in dental offices. He recognized from the start that the most effective way to "spread the word" was to provide direct services, educational and clinical, to groups of people—to the masses. Ideally, those groups would be composed of children who would be taught at an early age the importance of dental health and prevention of dental disease. Where better to interface with children than in grammar schools? And so in time, what was known as the Bridgeport, Connecticut, School Dental Hygiene Corps was established, composed of members of Dr. Fones' classes of 1914, 1915, and 1916. Ergo the first dental hygiene public health program.

I will fast-forward to the early 1950s when thirtythree young women and I were enrolled at the University of Bridgeport's Fones School of Dental Hygiene. As part of our fieldwork rotation, we traveled to longestablished dental clinics throughout the city's schools. I remember being extremely fond of that assignment because I liked interacting with the children. But the real thrill of those trips was coming face-to-face with members of those first classes who were still in charge of the various clinics. These women knew Dr. Fones personally. During lunch hours, they had a captive audience and would relate to us how it all began: the first school in the carriage house adjacent to Dr. Fones' and his father's dental building; his perseverance and determination in convincing city fathers, the board of education, and the dental society to allow the early dental hygienists to conduct programs within the schools.

I know how proud and delighted they would be— Dr. Fones and "the pioneers"—to see how dental hygienists have positioned themselves today in various public health settings, and how impressed they would be with Christine Nathe's *Dental Public Health and Research: Contemporary Practice for the Dental Hygienist.* It is a remarkable testimony to the premise that public health dental hygienists have the ability to play a valuable and critical role in the dental health of people everywhere.

Janet Carroll Memoli, RDH, MS
Retired Director, Fones School of Dental Hygiene
Professor Emeritus, University of Bridgeport,
Bridgeport, CT

Preface

The guiding principles that served as the impetus for the first three editions of *Dental Public Health and Research* remain consistent with an added emphasis on the dental hygienist's understanding of research principles. The twenty-first century mandates a change in the practice and understanding of dental public health concepts. The dental hygiene practitioners who will be practicing in this century need information on how to effectively practice and conduct dental hygiene research in the dental public health setting.

The fourth edition expands on public health science from its inception and further explains the essence of dental public health. The chapter on dental care funding is expanded to focus on the current issues in dental care financing and the government's role in this area. Moreover, a chapter on the importance of collaboration in dental care, building coalitions to help advocate for the oral health of all people, and an introductory discussion on grant writing are included.

The second unit focuses on learning theories, populations, and programs. The cultural diversity chapter emphasizes the effect culture has on dental health, and the chapter on target populations has been expanded and diversified. This focus is necessary in a public health book because it helps future providers understand how cultures, populations, and health relate. The program planning chapter is significantly updated and expanded with regard to benchmarks and effective programs presently in place.

The research unit is greatly expanded to provide detailed information on the study of dental hygiene research. The focus of this unit is to comprehensively discuss the reasons research is necessary in dental hygiene and how research impacts the practicing dental hygienist. Areas of expansion include discussions on the pivotal role research plays in dental hygiene, ethics in research, evidenced-based principles of practice, the roles of government and private entities in dental research, oral epidemiology, and the measurement of oral diseases and conditions. Expansion of this unit should help colleges that teach research within the community dental/public health courses. Additionally, this unit may be useful in conjunction with other materials in stand-alone research courses.

Teaching and Learning Package

Additional student resources can be found at www.pearsonhighered.com/healthprofessionsrecources.

Follow this URL and select Dental Hygiene as your discipline. Click on this title to view extra practice questions and information for students to use outside of class to test their knowledge or for additional review of topics covered in each chapter.

Instructor's Resource Manual

The Instructor's Resource Manual contains a wealth of material to help faculty plan and manage their course. This manual includes:

- A test bank of more than 550 questions
- Discussion items to provide ideas for classroom discussion
- Laboratory or field experiences with process evaluations for student and faculty member use
- Laboratory exercises

This Instructor's Resource Manual is available for download from www.pearsonhighered.com from the Instructor's Resource Center. Instructors should register at the site to obtain a username and password.

Instructor Resources

Additional instructor resources are available at www.pearsonhighered.com. These include the complete test bank that allows instructors to design customized quizzes and exams. The TestGen wizard guides instructors through the steps in creating a simple test with drag-and-drop or point-and-click transfer. Faculty members can select test questions either manually or randomly and use online spell checking and other tools to quickly polish the test content and presentation. The question formats include multiple choice, fill in the blank, true/false, and essay. Tests can be saved in a variety of formats both locally and on a network, organized in as many as twenty-five variations of a single test, and published in an online format. For more information, please visit www.pearsonhighered.com/testgen.

The Instructor Resources also include a PowerPoint lecture package that contains key discussion points for each chapter. This feature provides dynamic, fully designed, integrated lectures that are ready to use and allows instructors to customize the materials to meet their specific course needs.

Acknowledgments

The author wishes to acknowledge the contributing authors for their work to enhance the fourth edition. Important academic support was provided by Demetra Logothetis, Professor Emeritus, and Cynthia Guillen, Supervisor, Administrative Support, Division of Dental Hygiene, University of New Mexico. And, of course, editorial support and advice from John Goucher, Executive Editor, and Nicole Ragonese, Program Manager, Pearson. Also, the copyeditor, Michael Rossa, and Susan McNally, the production editor at Cenveo® Publisher Services. The book would not be possible without support from these individuals.

Reviewers

Susan Barnard, DHSc, RDH
Bergen Community College
Paramus, NJ

Julie Bencosme, RDH
Hostos Community College
Bronx, NY

Peg Boyce, RDH, MA
Parkland College
Champaign, IL

April Catlett, RDH, BHSA, MDH, PhD
Central Georgia Technical College
Macon, GA

Kathy Conrad, RDH, BS
Columbia Basin College
Pasco, WA

Brenda Fisher, RDH, BSDH
AB Tech Community College
Asheville, NC

Beverly Hardee, RDH
Cape Fear Community College
Wilmington, NC

Joanna Harris, RDH, MSDH
Clayton State University
Morrow, GA

Joyce Hudson, RDH, MS
Ivy Tech Community College
Anderson, IN

Mindy Jay, RDH, AAS, BHS, Med
Pensacola State College
Pensacola, FL

Susan Kass, EdD
Miami Dade College
Miami, FL

Amy Krueger, CRDH, BSDH, MS
St. Petersburg College
St. Petersburg, FL

Previous Editions

Sheila Bannister, Vermont Technical College

Eugenia B. Bearden, Clayton College and State University

Maryellen Beaulieu, University of New England

Lynn Ann Bethel, Mount Ida College

Jacqueline N. Brian, Indiana University–Purdue University

Fort Wayne

Janice Brinson, BSDH, MS, Tennessee State University

Diane L. Bourque, Community College of Rhode Island

Sandra George Burns, Ferris State University

Valerie L. Carter, St. Petersburg College

Kenneth A. Eaton, University College London

Michele M. Edwards, Tallahassee Community College

Kerry Flynn, Palm Beach Community College

Jacque Freudenthal, Idaho State University

Theresa M. Grady, Community College of Philadelphia

Beverly H. Hardee, Cape Fear Community College

Sheranita Hemphill, Sinclair Community College

Jamar M. Jackson, Hostos Community College

Tara L. Johnson, Idaho State University

Mary E. Jorstad, Lake Land College

Nancy K. Mann, Indiana University–Purdue University Fort Wayne

Patricia Mannie, St. Cloud Technical College

Jill Mason, Oregon Health Sciences University

Aamna Nayyar, Santa Fe Community College

Robert F. Nelson, University of South Dakota

Marian Williams Patton, Tennessee State University

Mary S. Pelletier, Indian River State College

Connie M. E. Preiser, Catawba Valley Community College

Barbara Ringle, Cuyahoga Community College

Martha H. Roberson, Virginia Western Community College

Judith Romano, Hudson Valley Community College

Kari Steinbock, Mt. Hood Community College

Edith Tynan, Northern Virginia Community College

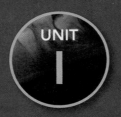

UNIT I

Introduction to Dental Public Health

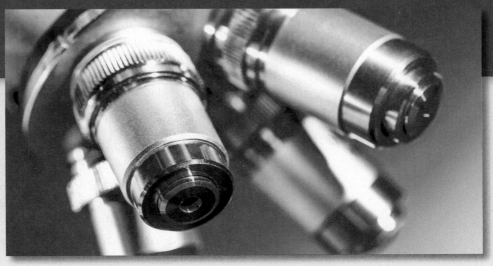

Science photo/Shutterstock

The following excerpt eloquently states the need for educating dental hygienists about the need for dental public health:

> Children live for months with pain that grown-ups would find unendurable. The gradual attrition of accepted pain erodes their energy and aspirations. I have seen children in New York with teeth that look like brownish, broken sticks. I have also seen teenagers who were missing half their teeth. But, to me, most shocking is to see a child with an abscess that has been inflamed for weeks and that he has simply lived with and accepts as part of the routine of life.*

* Kozol J. *Savage Inequalities: Children in America's Schools.* New York, NY: Crown Publishers; 1991.

Unfortunately, this statement reflects a problem that exists throughout the world. Dental problems cause pain, infection, disease, and disability and can easily be prevented. And, although this paragraph was written over twenty years ago, it is still paramount to the overall goal of the dental hygiene discipline. For over one hundred years, dental hygienists have had the skills necessary to help alleviate this problem. This introductory unit focuses on the definition of public health, its historical development as a true public health profession, and evidence-based preventive health modalities that are practiced in public health. This unit also discusses the current status of dental care delivery in the United States and abroad with an emphasis on government structures, financing, laws and initiatives affecting dental hygiene care.

Dental Public Health: An Overview

OBJECTIVES

After studying this chapter, the dental hygiene student should be able to:

- Define public health
- Describe the evolution of public health science and practice
- Define dental public health
- Describe factors affecting dental public health

COMPETENCIES

After studying this chapter and participating in accompanying course activities, the dental hygiene student should be competent to do the following:

- Promote positive values of oral and general health and wellness to the public and organizations within and outside the profession
- Evaluate factors that can be used to promote patient adherence to disease prevention and/or health maintenance strategies
- Evaluate and utilize methods to ensure the health and safety of the patient and the dental hygienists in the delivery of dental hygiene
- Pursue career options within the health care industry, education research and other roles as they evolve for the dental hygienist.
- Access professional and social networks to pursue professional goals

KEY TERMS

Assessment 4
Assurance 4
Community dental health 9
Dental public health 9
Malpractice 14
Policy development 4
Primary prevention 3
Public health 3
Public health goals 5
Public health services 5
Secondary prevention 3
Serving all functions 4
Socioeconomic status
  (SES) 13
Tertiary prevention 3

Science photo/Shutterstock

Public health is concerned with the health care of all people. It focuses on the health of a population as a whole rather than on the treatment of an individual. The goal of public health is to protect and promote the health of the public across three essential domains: health protection, disease prevention, and health promotion.[1] Health protection is protecting society from disease, illness, and accidents, whereas disease prevention is actually preventing disease from occurring. Promoting health is the work that is accomplished when healthy ideas and concepts are encouraged.

Public health has become an essential component of developed societies. Many of the major improvements in the health of populations have resulted from public health measures such as ensuring safe food and water, controlling epidemics, and protecting workers from injury.[2] Most people, however, do not give much thought to the public health until a crisis occurs or the system fails.[2] Infectious disease outbreaks, the incidence of cancer, and the increasing number of working people unable to afford health care services draw attention to the infrastructure that protects the health of the public.[2]

Public health initially involved caring for a population with a disease, but the focus shifted to controlling the disease itself. It has subsequently evolved to emphasize disease prevention (Figure 1-1 ■), which enhances quality of life, helps deter illness or outbreaks, and is cost effective. **Primary prevention** is the employment of strategies and agents to forestall the onset of disease, reverse its progress, or arrest its process before treatment becomes necessary. An example of primary prevention would be the provision of immunizations to children. Dental hygiene is a form of primary dental prevention as is the use of fluoride to prevent tooth demineralization.

Most people recognize the efficacy of primary levels of prevention, but they are less likely to think of secondary prevention as being effective at preventing disease. **Secondary prevention** employs routine treatment methods to terminate the disease process and/or restore tissues to as nearly normal as possible; this can also be called *restorative care*. Setting a broken arm so that the bone heals correctly is an example of secondary prevention. One dental example of secondary prevention is the use of fluoride to remineralize tooth surfaces that have been demineralized.

Did You Know?

Fluoride can be a primary preventive agent or a secondary preventive agent depending on the use of fluoride.

Another dental example is periodontal debridement to reduce periodontal pocketing. **Tertiary prevention** employs strategies to replace lost tissues through rehabilitation. The use of prosthetics to replace missing limbs is an example. Using dental materials to restore demineralized tooth surfaces to stop an infection and prevent the loss of a tooth due to tooth decay is an example of tertiary dental prevention. See Table 1-1 ■ for more examples of the levels of dental prevention.

Dental public health is only one component of public health. An understanding of the foundation of *public health* is important when discussing the topic of dental public health.

Public Health Defined

The World Health Organization (WHO) defines health as a state of complete physical, mental, and social well-being and not merely the absence of disease or infirmity.[3]

Table 1–1 Levels of Dental Preventive Care

Levels of Prevention	Therapies and Services
Primary prevention	Oral evaluation
	Dental prophylaxis
	Fluoride as a preventive agent
	Dental sealants
	Health education
	Health promotion
Secondary prevention	Dental restorations
	Periodontal debridement
	Fluoride use on incipient caries
	Dental sealants on incipient caries
	ART, alternative restorative treatment
	Endodontics
Tertiary prevention	Prosthodontics
	Implants
	Oromaxillofacial surgery

Source: Based on Harris, NO, Garcia-Godoy, F and Nathe, CN. Primary Preventive Dentistry, 8th edition. Upper Saddle River, NJ: Pearson, 2013, page 6.

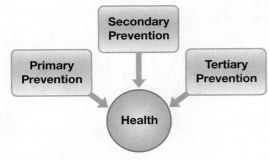

FIGURE 1–1 Disease Prevention Levels

Source: © Pearson Education, Inc.

Further, the WHO and others have defined *public health* as the effort to promote physical and mental health and prevent disease, injury, and disability at the population level. This involves a wide range of products, activities, and services aimed at the entire population although it is sometimes delivered to the individual.[3,4] Many postulate that public health is the approach to health care that concerns the health of the community as a whole. The first dentist to be president of the American Public Health Association, John W. Knutson, originally defined public health as:

> Public health is people's health. It is concerned with the aggregate health of a group, a community, a state, or a nation. Public health in accordance with this broad definition is not limited to the health of the poor, or to rendering health services or to the nature of the health problems. Nor is it defined by the method of payment for health services or by the type of agency responsible for supplying those services. It is simply a concern for and activity directed toward the improvement and protection of the health of a population group and the aggregate.[5]

This definition appropriately places value on the description of public health to address the public's health, regardless of financial resources, the provision of clinical, educational or social services nor the particular health issue. Public health in totality addresses all aspects of *the* public's health. Examples of public health could be clinical care provided in a government-funding or private clinic, research conducted to treat disease, data collected to monitor health or social services provided to access care.

In the report *The Future of the Public's Health in the 21st Century,* the Institute of Medicine (IOM) defined public health as "what we, as a society, do collectively to assure the conditions in which people can be healthy." The IOM identified core functions that were to be conducted by government public health agencies: assessment, policy development, assurance, and serving all functions.[6]

- **Assessment** involves monitoring the health of communities and populations to identify health problems and priorities. It includes activities such as performing public health surveillance, collecting and interpreting data, finding case applications, and evaluating outcomes of programs and policies.
- **Policy development** is the process by which society makes decisions about problems, chooses goals and strategies to address the problems, and allocates resources to reach them. Formulation of public policies usually occurs through collaboration among community, private sector, and government leaders.
- **Assurance** involves making certain that all populations have access to appropriate and cost-effective services to reach agreed-on public health goals. In addition to treatment services for individuals, assurance activities include health promotion and disease-prevention services.

- **Serving all functions** is the research for new insights and innovative solutions to health problems.[6]

These functions can facilitate public health policy and decision making and further enhance planning public health programs (Figure 1-2 ■). As stated, these functions ensure that the public's health should be assessed, so that policies can be developed to address needs and mechanisms can be enacted to ensure that these policies are meeting the needs. Researching new innovations, titled serving all functions, ensures that this cycle of needs assessments, policy development, and assurance is constantly and consistently occurring.

The IOM subsequently published *For the Public's Health: Investing in a Healthier Future,* which addressed three topics related to population health in the United States: measurement, law and policy, and funding in the context of health care changes.[7]

Did You Know?

Population health means the health of the population, or the public's health and focuses on public health efforts. Many times, public health is thought of as health care for those without financial means, but public health is much broader, essentially encompassing the public's health in totality.

Data collection, reporting, and action—including public policy and laws informed by data and quality metrics—were felt needed to support activities that will alter the physical and social environment for better health.[7] The report cited failure of the health system, including both

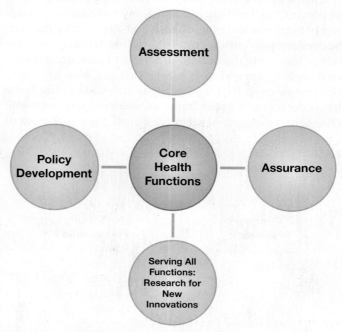

FIGURE 1–2 Core Functions of Public Health

medical care and governmental public health, as evidenced in the poor performance of the United States in life expectancy and other major health outcomes and the increasing financial issues associated with medical care. Solutions proposed included controlling administrative waste; remedying sources of excess cost and other inefficiencies in the clinical care, while improving quality; achieving universal coverage; and implementing population-based health improvement strategies.[7] This report focused on the areas that could be improved in health care delivery.

Goals and Challenges

The American Public Health Association states that the practice of public health should reduce human suffering, help children thrive, improve the quality of life, and save money.[8] They emphasize that public health is prevention, policy development, and population health surveillance. Policy development should continually be developing and amending infrastructure so that prevention is practiced and public health is easily accessed. Surveillance is continually needed to adequately assess the public's health and needs, which interventions are deemed successful or not successful, and cost effectiveness of prevention and/or interventions.

Did You Know?

Former US Surgeon General C. Everett Koop once stated that health care matters to all of us some of the time; however, public health matters to all of us all of the time.

Public health goals are goals that guide all public health activities. They dictate the services needed to ensure the promotion of health and prevention of disease and injury (see Boxes 1-1 ■ and 1-2 ■). An example of a public health goal that promotes healthy behaviors is the distribution of mouth guards to student athletes. Screening for dental decay illustrates the monitoring of health status to identify community health problems.

Public health services are those interventions that help attain public health goals. Preventing illness and promoting health through the delivery of efficient and effective public health services lie at the core of society's ability to create an exemplary circle of better health, more productive citizens, and affordable health care.[1] At a time of renewed concern about communicable diseases, such as Ebola virus disease, tuberculosis, and HIV, as well as new anxieties about events such as bioterrorism, people in many countries also face the challenges of lifestyle-related diseases, such as obesity, diabetes, cancer, and cardiovascular disease, which are significantly influenced by diet, physical activity, tobacco use, and alcohol abuse.[1] Public health services aid in educating the public about preventive measures to decrease the risk of some diseases.

With health care services placing more and more pressures on budgets as well as a financial burden for

Box 1–1 Public Health Goals

- Prevent epidemics and the spread of disease
- Protect against environmental hazards
- Prevent injuries
- Promote and encourage healthy behaviors
- Respond to disasters and assist communities in recovery
- Ensure the quality and accessibility of health services

Source: Based on Public Health Functions Steering Committee, Members (July 1995): American Public Health Association; Association of Schools of Public Health; Association of State and Territorial Health Officials; Environmental Council of the States; National Association of County and City Health Officials; National Association of State Alcohol and Drug Abuse Directors; National Association of State Mental Health Program Directors; Public Health Foundation; US Public Health Service—*Agency for Health Care Policy and Research; Centers for Disease Control and Prevention; Food and Drug Administration; Health Resources and Services Administration; Indian Health Service; National Institutes of Health; Office of the Assistant Secretary for Health; Substance Abuse and Mental Health Services Administration,* http://www.health .gov/phfunctions/public.htm

Box 1–2 Public Health Services

- Monitor health status to identify community health problems
- Diagnose and investigate health problems and health hazards in the community
- Inform, educate, and empower people about health issues
- Mobilize community partnerships to identify and solve health problems
- Develop policies and plans that support individual and community health efforts
- Enforce laws and regulations that protect health and ensure safety
- Link people to needed personal health services and ensure the provision of health care when otherwise unavailable
- Ensure a competent public health and personal health care workforce
- Evaluate effectiveness, accessibility, and quality of personal and population-based health services
- Research for new insights and innovative solutions to health problems

Source: Based on Fall 1994. Public Health Functions Steering Committee. Public Health Functions Steering Committee, Members (July 1995): American Public Health Association; Association of Schools of Public Health; Association of State and Territorial Health Officials; Environmental Council of the States; National Association of County and City Health Officials; National Association of State Alcohol and Drug Abuse Directors; National Association of State Mental Health Program Directors; Public Health Foundation; US Public Health Service—*Agency for Health Care Policy and Research; Centers for Disease Control and Prevention; Food and Drug Administration; Health Resources and Services Administration; Indian Health Service; National Institutes of Health; Office of the Assistant Secretary for Health; Substance Abuse and Mental Health Services Administration.* http://www.health .gov/phfunctions/public.htm

individuals and families, the practice of public health has become a cause of great concern for governments and health systems. The World Health Organization (WHO) operates in an increasingly complex and rapidly changing landscape, and the boundaries of public health action extend into other sectors that influence health opportunities and outcomes.[1] WHO responds to these challenges using a six-point agenda to help navigate the health of the public (see Box 1-3 ■).

Historical Perspective of Public Health

Learning from history cannot be underestimated when developing effective solutions to current public health issues. Widespread outbreaks of communicable disease can be traced back to the plague, including the infamous Black Death, which had devastating effects on populations in many nations and continents for decades (Figure 1-3 ■). Public health activities such as quarantines, mass burials, and ship inspections were subsequently developed to prevent such horrendous epidemics.

Public health preventive measures have been seen in tribal customs of primitive societies.[9] These measures were probably developed to serve as a survival mechanism. These measures included hygiene and cleanliness customs. This is, of course, interesting since dental hygienists hope that the current population feels the same way about hygiene and cleanliness of the oral cavity.

The first significant recording of public health measures in the United States occurred in South Carolina in 1671 when a water protection measure was enacted to prevent diseases caused by water supplies.[10] Specifically, it stated:

> Should any person cause to flow into or be cast into any of the creeks, streams or inland waters of this State any impurities that are poisonous to fish or destructive to their spawn, such person shall, upon conviction, be punished.10

In England in 1777, a Gloucestershire milkmaid told her physician, Dr. Edward Jenner, that she was fortunate to have contracted cowpox because it conferred protection against smallpox. Dr. Jenner, in turn, collaborated with other providers to study the relationship and establish the scientific principle of immunization that eventually resulted in eliminating smallpox.[11]

In 1798, the United States passed an act that provided for the relief of sick and disabled seamen, which established a federal network of hospitals for the care of merchant seaman, the precursor of the US Public Health Service, which was initiated in 1902.[12] Recall that many times communicable diseases were spread country to country by seamen. In today's world intercontinental travel is common, and many people travel to many countries, as opposed to a century earlier when seamen were often the only international travelers. Interestingly, the first supervising surgeon of this network was the predecessor to today's US Surgeon General.

The identification of a polluted public water well as the source of an 1854 cholera outbreak in London resulted in a major advancement in public health.[13] Dr. John Snow used a logical, epidemiological approach to study the outbreak. At the time, many suspected pollution as the cause of the cholera, but by studying the geographical relation of the sick to a water pump, he was able to help control the outbreak.

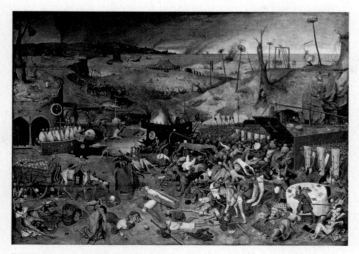

FIGURE 1–3 Triumph of Death: Black Death

Source: Scala/Art Resource, NY

Box 1–3 World Health Organization's Six-Point Agenda

1. **Promoting development** The ethical principle of equity directs health development: Access to life-saving or health-promoting interventions should not be denied for unfair reasons, including those with economic or social roots.
2. **Fostering health security** One of the greatest threats to international health security is from outbreaks of emerging and epidemic-prone diseases.
3. **Strengthening health systems** For health improvement to operate as a poverty-reduction strategy, health services must reach poor and underserved populations.
4. **Harnessing research, information, and evidence** Evidence provides the foundation for setting priorities, defining strategies, and measuring results.
5. **Enhancing partnerships** WHO carries out its work with the support and collaboration of many partners, including UN agencies and other international organizations, donors, civil society, and the private sector.
6. **Improving performance** WHO participates in ongoing reforms to improve its efficiency and effectiveness at both the international level and within countries.

Retrieved September 23, 2014 from http://www.who.int.

Did You Know?

Epidemiology is the study of the amount, distribution, determinant, and control of disease and health conditions among a given population.

The first one-room laboratory for public health was opened in 1887 on Staten Island, New York, and was the forerunner to the National Institutes of Health, which still is the main health care research institution in the United States.[12]

During the first years of the 1900s, Dr. Sara Baker, a physician, led teams of nurses into the crowded neighborhoods of Hell's Kitchen in New York City and taught mothers how to dress, feed, and bathe their babies. Baker established many programs to help the poor in that city keep their infants healthy. After World War I, many states and countries followed her example to lower infant mortality rates.[14]

Did You Know?

Archeologists reported that two molar teeth about 63,400 years old show that the presence of grooves on the teeth formed by the passage of a pointed object, thought to be a small stick, indicates that Neanderthals may have cleaned their teeth.[15]

Pickett and Hanlon described the historical evolution of public health as a science and practice and the role of the medical profession in public health from past to present. History recorded the gross inadequacies of medical care in the early 1800s. Physicians were not educated in academic institutions as they are today. In fact, back then, the prestige of the medical profession was at its lowest and medical practice lacked uniform educational and practice standards. Medical education was largely proprietary in nature or based on apprenticeships, resulting in physicians who were poorly prepared, and the services they provided were frequently of poor quality, not uniform, and cheap.[9]

Although there were public health laws enacted to ensure basic sanitation and prevention of communicable diseases, there were no mechanisms to recognize noncompliance with requirements. Further, because of the greatly expanded population and subsequent issues this created, public health measures were not a priority, so that other seemingly more pressing problems could be addressed. Adding to this mix was the low public expectation of medical care and the lack of a unified voice for physicians to advocate for solutions aimed at essential public health issues.[9]

Did You Know?

In 1914, New York City Health Commissioner Herman M. Bigges remarked that "public health is purchasable," adding that "within natural limitations, a community can determine its own death rate."[16]

With the advent of accredited medical academic institutions, advanced education, and documented clinical standards, the country now places a socially accepted respect and prestige for physicians and a much higher expectation for medical care than in the past. Additionally, when public health issues arise, there now are professional physician associations that are the voice for the science and practice of medicine. Physicians' opinions and recommendations have significant credibility and are a powerful influence in dealing with public health issues in today's America.

The dramatic increase in the average life span during the 1900s is widely credited to public health achievements, such as vaccination programs and control of infectious diseases; effective policies such as motor vehicle and occupational safety; improved family planning; antismoking measures; and programs designed to decrease chronic disease. The US Department of Health and Human Services (HHS) has incorporated dental public health into many of the more than 300 programs it offers (see Box 1-4 ■). Actually, a dental public health preventive effort, community water fluoridation, is one of the ten great public health measures adopted during the past century (see Box 1-5 ■).

More recent public health efforts include the response to crises such as the September 11, 2001, terrorist attacks and the aftermath of recent hurricanes, tsunamis, tornadoes, mudslides, and wildfires. The emergence of diseases of the past, in part as a result of the public's resistance to prevention through vaccinations, is being witnessed throughout the world. Public health is now being focused on violence witnessed in all areas of society, which seems to be increasingly common, as is the intentional acts of terror witnessed throughout the world.

Campaigns to promote healthy habits, such as exercising, and decrease unhealthy habits such as chewing smokeless tobacco are routinely used to improve the public's health. Specific to oral health are innovative public health preventive efforts including the increased utilization of dental hygienists in school settings to reduce dental decay. See Box 1-6 ■ for historic events involving the US Public Health Service.

Dental Public Health Defined

Dental health is a wide-reaching field of study, but it is grounded in distinct concepts within public health. The American Board of Dental Public Health (ABDPH) defines dental public health as:

the science and art of preventing and controlling dental diseases and promoting dental health through organized

Box 1–4 Historical Highlights

The roots of the US Department of Health and Human Services go back to the early days of the nation:

1798: An act for the relief of sick and disabled seamen was passed, establishing a federal network of hospitals for the care of merchant seamen; forerunner of today's US Public Health Service.

1871: The first supervising surgeon (later called Surgeon General) was appointed for the Marine Hospital Service, which had been organized the prior year.

1887: The federal government opened a one-room laboratory on Staten Island for research on disease, thereby planting the seed that was to grow into the National Institutes of Health.

1906: Congress passed the Pure Food and Drugs Act, authorizing the government to monitor the purity of foods and the safety of medicines, now the responsibility of the Food and Drug Administration.

1921: The Bureau of Indian Affairs Health Division, the forerunner to the Indian Health Service, was created.

1946: The Communicable Disease Center, forerunner of the Centers for Disease Control and Prevention, was established.

1955: The Salk polio vaccine was licensed.

1961: The First White House Conference on Aging was held.

1964: The first Surgeon General's Report on Smoking and Health was released.

1965: The Medicare and Medicaid programs were created, making comprehensive health care available to millions of Americans. In addition, the Older Americans Act created the nutritional and social programs administered by HHS Administration on Aging, and the Head Start program was created.

1966: The International Smallpox Eradication program led by the US Public Health Service was established; the worldwide eradication of smallpox was accomplished in 1977.

1970: The National Health Service Corps was established.

1990: The Human Genome Project was established, and the Nutrition Labeling and Education Act was passed to authorize nutritional labeling of food.

1993: The Vaccines for Children Program was established, providing free immunizations to all children in low-income families.

1995: The Social Security Administration became an independent agency.

1996: The Health Insurance Portability and Accountability Act (HIPAA) was enacted.

1997: The State Children's Health Insurance Program (SCHIP) was created, which enables states to extend health coverage to more uninsured children.

1999: The initiative on combating bioterrorism was launched.

2002: The Office of Public Health Emergency Preparedness was created to coordinate efforts against bioterrorism and other emergency health threats.

2003: The Medicare Prescription Drug Improvement and Modernization Act of 2003 was enacted—the most significant expansion of Medicare since its enactment, including a prescription drug benefit.

2010: The Affordable Care Act was signed into law, putting in place comprehensive US health insurance reforms.

Source: Historical Highlights: US Department of Health and Human Services. http://www.hhs.gov/about/hhshist.html. Accessed September 16, 2014.

community efforts. It is that form of dental practice that serves the community as a patient rather than the individual. It is concerned with the dental health education of the public, with applied dental research, and with the administration of group dental care programs, as well as the prevention and control of dental diseases on a community basis. Implicit in this definition is the requirement that the specialist have broad knowledge and skills in public health administration, research methodology, the prevention and control of oral diseases, and the delivery and financing of oral health care.[17]

Box 1–5 Great Public Health Achievements of the Twentieth Century

- Vaccination
- Motor vehicle safety
- Workplace safety
- Control of infectious diseases
- Decline in deaths from coronary heart disease and stroke
- Safer and healthier food
- Healthier mothers and babies
- Family planning
- Community water fluoridation
- Recognition of tobacco as a hazard

Source: Ten Great Public Health Achievements—United States, 1900–1999. *MMWR Morb Mortal Wkly Rpt.* 1999;8(12):241–243.

Box 1–6 US Public Health Service Commissioned Corps Timeline

1798: President John Adams signed into law the Act for the Relief of Sick and Disabled Seamen. A year later, Congress extended the act to cover every officer and sailor in the US Navy.

1871: John Maynard Woodworth, the first supervising surgeon, adopted a military model for his medical staff as part of a system reform. He instituted examinations for applicants, put physicians in uniforms, and created a cadre of mobile, career-service physicians who could be assigned to various marine hospitals.

1878: The prevalence of major epidemic diseases such as smallpox, yellow fever, and cholera spurred Congress to enact the National Quarantine Act to prevent the introduction of contagious and infectious diseases into the United States.

1912: Name of the Public Health and Marine Hospital Service was shortened to the Public Health Service. Legislation enacted by Congress broadened its powers by authorizing investigations into human diseases (such as tuberculosis, hookworm, malaria, and leprosy) related to sanitation, water supplies, and sewage disposal.

1930 and 1944: US Public Health Service Corps officers expanded to include engineers, dentists, research scientists, nurses, and other health care specialists (e.g., dental hygienists), as well as physicians.

2006: The Commissioned Corps fulfills its mission to protect and promote the nation's public health. With more than 6,000 active-duty officers, it works both nationally and internationally to create a world free of preventable disease, sickness, and suffering.

Source: US Public Health Service. About the US Public Health Service: History. http://www.usphs.gov/aboutus/history.aspx. Accessed September 16, 2014.

Dental public health focuses on oral health care and education of a population with an emphasis on the utilization of dental hygiene sciences. Many agencies of the federal and state governments fund dental care delivery and the dental workforce needed to provide this care (see Chapter 3).

Did You Know?

Dental hygiene was initiated as a public health profession.

Many times dental public health is called **community dental health.** Both terms are correct and share similar meanings. Some consider community health to be a component of public health; others use the terms interchangeably. The major difference between the terms is that *community* focuses on a specific group of people whereas the connotation of *public* is thought to be wider reaching.

The delivery of dental services for individuals and the general population at national and local levels involves a variety of institutions, infrastructures, and activities. Dental public health functions need to be secured and implemented across all areas to ensure the same level of coverage, quality, and performance of services.

Dental public health practice follows steps similar to those taken by a dental hygienist in the private sector, but the focus is primarily on a population, including those who do not seek care, rather than just one patient who presents at the scheduled time. Table 1-2 ■ compares the two types of delivery. Assessment is the core public health function,

and the dental public health practitioner collects the necessary information to identify community problems, similar to an individual dental hygienist diagnosing a patient's condition. Just as a clinical dental hygienist develops a treatment plan after the diagnosis, the dental public health practitioner uses the information from the community assessment to develop policies and programs to address the problem(s). Ensuring dental public health is inherent to a dental hygienists' providing care: It involves the delivery of the services to the community.

Many dental hygienists choose to work in dental public health settings. All educational dental hygiene programs present dental public health education to dental hygiene students. The roles of the dental hygienist as related to dental public health are depicted in Table 1-3 ■ and Figure 1-4 ■. Because dental hygiene students are familiar with the role of the traditional clinical dental hygienists, it is an easy way to explain the similarities to dental public health to the existing knowledge of typical dental hygiene functions.

Public health, although an ADHA specificied role, is embedded in the clinician, educator, researcher, administrator, corporate and entrepeneurroles of a dental hygienist, since public health is encompassing in health care. An educator may teach in a public health program or educate parents during an Early Head Start home visit. A researcher may study the relationship between diabetes and periodontal disease, whereas an administrator may decide to work in a managerial position in a governmental agency. Many dental hygienists work in the corporate roles in the private dental supply and insurance industry, selling and educating dental providers on products, insurance systems and modalities. An entrepreneur initiates new dental enterprises and practices.

Table 1–2 A Comparison of Aspects of Private and Public Dental Health Models of Practice

	Dental Hygienist's Role in Private Practice	Dental Hygienist's Role in Public Health
Assessment	Conducts initial health assessment by reviewing health and dental history with patient	Conducts a needs assessment of target populations
	Conducts a comprehensive oral examination	Analyzes community needs
Dental hygiene diagnosis	Provides patients' dental hygiene diagnosis	Provides community dental hygiene diagnosis to basically prioritize the needs
Planning	Develops a treatment plan based on the diagnosis, patient interaction, and the priorities and method of payment; utilizes measurable assessment mechanisms	Develops a program based on the analysis of needs assessment data, priorities, and alternatives; community interaction; and resources available for which measurable assessment mechanisms are used
	Selects appropriate health care workers to provide comprehensive care	Selects appropriate labor to implement program
Implementation	Implements self-generated treatment plan effectively, changing it when necessary	Implements self-generated treatment plan effectively, changing it when necessary
Evaluation	Provides treatment via dental, gingival, and periodontal evaluations	Evaluates program via index and community evaluations
Documentation	Documents all findings and treatment notes during and after appointment	Documents all data gathered throughout all stages

Factors Affecting Dental Public Health

Numerous landmark reports suggest that the current dental care system in the United States is not effectively ensuring optimal oral health for all populations.[18–21] Multiple factors exacerbate the challenges to achieving oral health including the current structure of the dental care delivery system; poor distribution of providers; individuals accessing care regularly; restrictive regulatory statutes; geographic, educational, and cultural barriers; and cost of care.[18–22]

Access to Care

Although many issues impact dental public health and the care dental hygienists provide in the United States today, routinely accessing dental care is undoubtedly one of the most important. The reasons for this widespread problem vary, but one is that in many states, dental hygienists are restricted to providing care only under the supervision of dentists. Moreover, many individuals lack the financial resources or transportation needed to obtain dental care

Table 1–3 Professional Roles of the Dental Hygienist as Related to Dental Public Health

Role of the Dental Hygienist	Dental Public Health Responsibilities Embedded Throughout
Administrator	Develops and coordinates dental public health programs
Entrepreneur	Creates dental health initiatives for various target populations and lobbies to change laws to increase access to care for the underserved population
Clinician	Provides clinical care to the population
Educator	Educates and promotes dental health education and issues to various target populations
Researcher	Conducts research germane to the study of health and disease and utilization of the dental hygienist
Corporate	Supports public health efforts by providing funding, research and products for dental public health initiatives

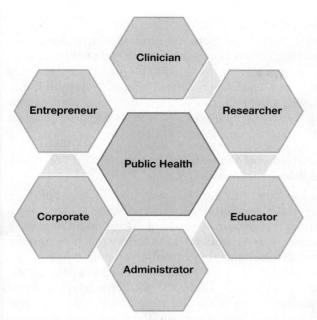

FIGURE 1–4 Roles of the Dental Hygienist

Source: Based on American Dental Hygienists' Association: Standards for Clinical Dental Hygiene Practice: June 2007. Available at http://www.adha.org/resources-docs/7261_Standards_Clinical_Practice.pdf. Accessed July 17, 2013.

services, or some simply do not value dental care until pain presents. The numerous barriers to care in the United States are discussed in more detail in Chapter 10.

Did You Know?

An increasing number of children receive preventive care during school hours from dental hygienists who work in school-based health clinics or as mobile care providers, helping to improve access to care.

Infrastructure

Exacerbating oral health disparities is the structure of the existing dental care delivery system. The practice of dentistry has remained in the private sector, providing services to those willing to access care in private offices and pay for services,

either out of pocket or by using their dental insurance coverage. The populations who need dental care the most are often without the means or desire to pay for services.

Many individuals present to the emergency rooms in local hospitals with dental caries that have progressed into major infections. Treatment of these infections costs thousands of dollars in hospital care, medicine, and operating room costs, not to mention the pain and suffering the individuals and families endure. Any level of primary, secondary, or tertiary services could prevent these problems.

Dental care is generally not as effectively positioned as comprehensive health care, nor is it practiced in a multidisciplinary fashion. Models need to be developed and implemented to address the needs of all individuals within society and to incorporate dental health care within comprehensive health care systems.

Workforce

Reports suggest the current dental care delivery system in the United States is not effectively ensuring optimal oral health for all populations. Although controversy exists regarding suggested dentists or dental hygienists provider shortages and the use of alternative providers, an updated system is needed to bring oral health care to diverse, underserved populations. Additionally, ongoing research linking oral health to general health will continue to spur demand for preventive dental services, which are often provided by dental hygienists.[23] Some suggest increasing funding for oral health services provided to those in need could be the most needed change in the system, as opposed to the possible saturation of dentists or dental hygienists or the initiation of a less educated dental provider.

The Surgeon General's *National Call to Action to Promote Oral Health Care* identifies the need to enhance the oral health workforce in the United States. Many new programs and positions have been developed to address this issue, including the Alaska Dental Health Therapist (ADHT) and the Advanced Dental Hygiene Practitioner (ADHP). The ADHT program was created in 2000 to provide workers to some Indian Health Service Dental Clinics in Alaska.[24,25] Under ADHT, the therapist provides restorative and urgent care services, including dental restorations and extractions. Although this program has not

DENTAL HYGIENIST SPOTLIGHT

Public Health Column: Dolores Malvitz, RDH, DrPH

The American Dental Hygienists' Association (ADHA) recently established the position of ADHA public health consultant. The function of this position is to consult with members who have questions regarding public health endeavors and to serve as an adviser to the Council on Public Health and ADHA staff on all

public health issues. The ADHA chose a true dental hygiene pioneer, Dolores Malvitz, as the first ADHA public health consultant.

After receiving her certificate in dental hygiene and bachelor's degree in English at the University of Michigan and Western Michigan, respectively, Dr.

Malvitz went on to earn master's and doctoral degrees in public health from the University of Michigan. She has taught dental hygiene, published numerous articles on studies she led, spoken all over the nation, been active in several professional associations, consulted with various organizations, and recently retired from the Centers for Disease Control and Prevention (CDC). Her exact title at CDC was Surveillance and Research Team Leader, Division of Oral Health, National Center for Chronic Disease Prevention and Health Promotion. She continues to be a role model and mentor to many dental hygienists, and her many accomplishments have truly motivated others in the professions.

Dr. Malvitz has received many awards. Some of the most noteworthy include:

- Special Merit Award of the American Association of Public Health Dentistry
- Distinguished Service Award from the Association of State and Territorial Dental Directors
- Outstanding Alumnus Award, University of Michigan
- Doctor of Humane Letters from the University of Detroit, Mercy (an honorary degree)
- Pfizer/ADHA Excellence in Dental Hygiene Award

She continues to be active in dental hygiene and is a true public health practitioner. Even after retirement, she is still promoting the public's health.

I asked her some questions regarding her career.

Can you provide some examples of your consulting this past year?

I attended and provided expertise at meetings of ADHA work groups—for example, Council on Public Health, ADHP Task Force. Also, I reviewed the public health portion of the ADHA Web site and suggested specific revisions. I communicated via phone and e-mail with a dental hygiene faculty member assigned to teach community health for the first time; we discussed potential content, learning strategies, and sources of information. I created and oversaw the review of content for the ADHA Web site related to the National Research Council report on fluoride. I also provided expert advice to the staff at ADHA and council members on request.

Why did you decide to go into dental hygiene?

Here is the unvarnished truth: Because I was a good student, my high school teachers were pressing me to go to college. I was not enthralled with nursing or teaching, the two careers considered appropriate for young women in that era. My boyfriend's sister-in-law taught in a suburban Detroit school system that employed a dental hygienist, and she suggested exploring this career that required only two years of college yet operated on the school calendar.

How did you get into public health? Did you need additional education?

As I began teaching in a dental hygiene program, it became clear that graduate education would be essential for success in academia. After exploring alternatives, I chose public health for my master's degree. That discipline seemed to offer a wider range of opportunities than the other logical choice, dental hygiene education. Then, my graduate school adviser encouraged me to stay for a doctorate, a decision that proved wise. Knowing more is always better than getting by with incomplete knowledge or skills—and it's critical to have the education that's expected for certain positions.

What type of advice would you give to a practicing hygienist who is thinking of doing something different?

First, the dental hygienist must decide what sorts of things she or he likes—and doesn't like—to do. What are favorite courses from the past? What aspects of the current position provide personal rewards that would be difficult to relinquish? What tasks would be a joy to never perform again?

Then, do some exploring on the Web; start moving outward via links and searches. Find some people who hold the kinds of positions that seem appealing and ask to spend some time with them. By observing carefully and asking strategic questions, the dental hygienist should be able to decide whether the new role would be satisfying, and given current obligations, whether it's possible to acquire the credentials necessary for credibility in the new role.

Do you have anything else to share or advice to provide?

I emphasize my belief that dental hygiene must ensure an ongoing cadre of well-educated and capable leaders. In education, it is important to be able to work as peers with other health professionals, who often hold master's and doctoral degrees.

Source: Christine Nathe writes the Public Health Column in *RDH* magazine published by Pennwell Publishing. For more public health spotlights please see RDH magazine online at http://www.rdhmag.com/index.html

produced a large number of providers, nor has it been replicated in other areas, the main focus of the ADHT is to alleviate infection and restore function.

In Minnesota, two models emerged to address the new workforce models. These include the dental therapist provider and the advanced dental therapist, which is a Master's level provider, who is a licensed dental hygienist before therapy training.[26] Expanding scopes of practice for dental hygienists and assistants has not translated to the maximal delegation allowed by law among network practices.[27] The effects of this new models on dental care delivery in the state will be interesting to watch.

The ADHA developed the ADHP to address the shortage of dentists and dentally underserved populations. This program provides diagnostic, preventive, restorative, and therapeutic services directly to the public.[28] Although the ADHP's main focus is preventive in nature, this provider is able to provide basic restorative care.

Dental Hygiene

From its inception, dental hygiene has had a strong foundation in managing dental care delivery. The role of the dental hygienist was created to identify and treat dental infections before they became too severe for treatment, to refer patients to the appropriate health care providers, and to prevent dental disease in all populations. Essentially, the dental hygienist is in the unique management position to provide the link to comprehensive oral health care (see Box 1-7 ■). Dr. A. C. Fones wrote in the preface to the third edition (1927) of *Mouth Hygiene,* the first textbook on dental hygiene:

> In many states the dentists have chosen to cooperate in an educational movement for mouth hygiene and they have accepted a coworker, the dental hygienist, as the logical means by which dentistry as a profession can discharge her responsibility for improving the mouth health of the masses. It is no longer a theory that the service of the dental hygienist will better the mouth health and general health of all whom she is permitted to serve. . . . The actual results secured by dental hygienists in private and public service, particularly in public schools, affords incontrovertible proof of the value of this type of preventive dentistry. Those who may still be skeptical are finding it difficult indeed to suggest any other means by which similar good results can be accomplished for large groups of people.[29]

Did You Know?

The Fones School of Dental Hygiene at the University of Bridgeport in Bridgeport, Connecticut, showcases many of Dr. Fones's original writings, instruments, and equipment.

Box 1–7 Historical Dental Standards in Connecticut

In 1921, Bridgeport's board of education voted to require a definite physical standard for every school child and after conferences with the Connecticut Department of Health, adopted resolutions that included dental standards. The Resolution stated that all schoolchildren:
  a. provide certification from the dental hygienist that there were no cavities in the permanent dentition
  b. demonstrate effectively the use of the toothbrush to remove food debris and to keep the gums in a state of health
  c. have teeth and gums in a clean and healthful condition

Source: Author developed information from: Fones, AC. *Mouth hygiene.* 3rd edition. 1927. Philadelphia: Lea & Febiger. 1927. P.315

The introduction of professional dental hygiene care, fluoride, and dental sealants have, more than any other factors, influenced the reduction in oral disease rates. Many believe the practice of dental hygiene must continue to move into health care systems and models that serve all populations. This idea is becoming a reality now that dental hygiene care is becoming available to more segments of the population with the additions to dental hygienists' scope of practice and the decrease in dentists' supervisory requirements.

Oral Health Disparities

Oral Health in America: A Report of the Surgeon General states that oral health in the United States is rife with profound and consequential disparities within the population. Demographic information shows a correlation between oral health and **socioeconomic status (SES),** which is an individual's comparative social and economic standing within a community. An individual's SES affects the person's access to dental care. Specifically, the lower the individual's SES, the more frequent are untreated dental caries.

The racial and ethnic minority population is already compromised with oral health disparities, and with this projected growth, the disparities will become even greater.[30] In the United States, people who are Hispanic, elderly, and have the lowest SES suffer more periodontal diseases than other populations.[31] Furthermore, about one in three adults living in poverty has untreated dental decay.[31]

Tooth decay remains the single most common chronic disease in children. Untreated dental decay is twice as prevalent in children and adolescents living in poverty as in their peers from families with higher incomes.[31] Children from low-income households are more likely to experience tooth decay and have higher levels of untreated tooth decay compared with children from more economically advantaged households.

Dental Care Needs of the Aging Population

One indication the increased number of dental hygienists has resulted in dental disease prevention is evident in the aging population. Because of dental hygiene and fluoride treatments, the number of people with teeth lasting a lifetime has increased. Older adults have more preventive and restorative dental care now than ever before and are also much more likely to see dental health as part of their own total health. Also, medical advances have caused longer life expectancies, resulting in the need for dental care for those who are living longer.

Dental hygienists assume a more integral role than ever in the lives of the elderly population. Older people have an increased occurrence of periodontal and other oral disease; consequently, the need for dental hygiene care increases with age.

A number of significant changes occur during aging. Fortunately, most of these normal changes do not cause oral diseases.[32,33] However, oral diseases can be exacerbated by systemic conditions such as xerostomia, caused by medicine taken frequently by older adults. Xerostomia can lead to an increase in root caries, which is frequently seen in the geriatric population. Dental hygiene science has evolved in treating these patients with often debilitating diseases.

Malpractice

Although malpractice may not seem to directly affect the public's health, it has because malpractice has had a direct impact on dental care delivery and quality. **Malpractice** is a dental hygiene professional's negligence by act or omission when the care provided is not within the accepted standards of practice and negatively affects the patient's well-being. The first medical malpractice suit, which was won in 1976, ushered in the advent of patients' rights, allowing patients to sue if the provider does not adequately diagnose and treat periodontal diseases.[34] Malpractice has improved dental care by increasing the likelihood that quality assurance mechanisms are in place to aid in validating competent care. Providers are more aware of the way they document office procedures and case notes because of the possibility of malpractice claims.

Although they are employed and supervised by dentists in most states, dental hygienists are liable for all treatment they render or fail to render and consequently should carry malpractice insurance. Upon graduation and dental hygiene licensure, it is necessary for the dental hygienists to apply for malpractice coverage.

Dental Insurance

Another factor that may not seem directly related to public health is dental insurance. However, the introduction of dental insurance has increased the number of patients seeking preventive care in private dental offices, which has undoubtedly affected the public's health. Dental insurance has probably influenced many in the population to access routine preventive care and maybe even increased the value of oral health in some individuals. Dental insurance provides comprehensive coverage of dental hygiene services and lends credence to the fact dental hygiene treatment is cost effective.

Before the advent of dental insurance in the mid 1900s, all individuals paid or bartered for dental services. When dental hygiene began, patients would pay out of pocket for dental prophylaxes. In some ways, dental insurance coverage may decrease the value many place on *paying* for dental care. In many situations, if an individual or family loses dental insurance coverage, that individual or family will choose to forgo appointments if payment is necessary.

Did You Know?

In many states, the dental insurance industry has been collaborating with dental hygienists to provide funding for public health programs that promote preventive dental care to underserved populations.

In many situations, dental insurance has had a positive effect on the quality and quantity of services provided. Because patients routinely seek preventive care when it is covered by dental insurance, early restorative care is obtained—which is less costly and less invasive—and less extensive care is needed. Not having dental insurance increases the likelihood an individual will not obtain dental care.[35]

Cultural Influences

Cultural background affects health values, knowledge, and practice. An adult patient who has never been to a dental hygienist would undoubtedly have a different value on preventive dental health care than an adult who received regular, routine preventive dental care since before kindergarten. Another phenomenon that is being witnessed is the number of people accessing dental care in hospitals. It is important to remember, if an individual comes from a culture in which dental services are routinely available in a health care system, such as a hospital, it makes sense that that individual would try to access dental services in a similar facility. Cultural influences will be discussed in Chapter 11.

Summary

Dental hygiene is historically a public health profession. It is vitally important to the public that dental hygienists be educated in the dental public health sciences. The purpose of public health is to promote overall health and prevent diseases and injuries. Public health frequently involves achieving a balance between individual versus population approaches to controlling disease.

Dental public health programs should use organized, interdisciplinary efforts to address the oral health concerns of communities and populations. The activities of dental public health programs can be classified into one of the core functions of public health organizations: assessment, policy development, assurance, and serving all functions. These activities occur at all levels of society.

Factors affecting dental health include access to care, the current infrastructure of dental care delivery including the dental workforce and the practice of dental hygiene, the aging population, malpractice, and the dental insurance industry. The fact that most dental diseases seem to be untreated in specific populations signals the presence of oral health disparities in the United States. Dental hygienists must continue to address factors and strive to promote dental public health.

Self-Study Test Items

1. What is an example of primary public health prevention?
   a. Disease prevention
   b. Periodontal debridement
   c. Fluoride treatments
   d. Restorative materials

2. Public health is credited with the dramatic increase in the average life span because of which of the following?
   a. Vaccinations
   b. Safety policies
   c. Family planning
   d. All of the above

3. What is an example of secondary public health prevention?
   a. Prevention of disease
   b. Fluoride treatments
   c. Restorations
   d. Patient education

4. What is the main health care research institution in the United States?
   a. Centers for Disease Control and Prevention
   b. Food and Drug Administration
   c. National Institutes of Health
   d. Johns Hopkins University

5. How has malpractice directly impacted dental care delivery and quality?
   a. Enabled patients to sue
   b. Decreased the number of dental providers because of the fear of malpractice suits
   c. Decreased quality of care
   d. Increased the number of suits against dental providers

References

1. World Health Organization Public Health Services. Retrieved from http://www.euro.who.int/publichealth/20070319_4 on May 8, 2008.
2. Tomar S. Public health programs. In: Harris NO, Garcia-Godoy F, Nathe C, eds. *Primary Preventive Dentistry*. 7th ed. Upper Saddle River, NJ: Pearson; 2008.
3. World Health Organization. Preamble to the Constitution. Official Records of the World Health Organization. 1946;(2):100. The Constitution was adopted by the International Health Conference in New York, June 19–July 19, 1946, and was signed July 22, 1946, by the representatives of 61 countries. It became effective April 7, 1948. The definition has not been amended since 1948. Retrieved from http://www.who.int/about/definition/en/print.html on July 17, 2013.
4. Members of the Public Health Functions Steering Committee (July 1995): American Public Health Association, Association of Schools of Public Health, Association of State and Territorial Health Officials, Environmental Council of the States, National Association of County and City Health Officials, National Association of State Alcohol and Drug Abuse Directors, National Association of State Mental Health Program Directors, Public Health Foundation, and US Public Health Service.
5. Knutson JW. What is public health? In: Pelton WJ, Wison JM, eds. *Dentistry in Public Health*. 2nd ed. Philadelphia, PA: W. B. Saunders; 1955.
6. Institute of Medicine. *The Future of the Public's Health in the 21st Century*. Washington, DC: National Academy Press; 2003.
7. IOM (Institute of Medicine). 2012. *For the Public's Health: Investing in a Healthier Future. Washington DC*: The National Academies Press.
8. American Public Health Association. What is Public Health? Fact Sheet. Washington DC, 2013. Retrieve from https://www.apha.org/what-is-public-health on July 29, 2015.
9. Pickett G, Hanlon J J. Historical Perspectives. In: *Public Health and Administration*. St. Louis: Times Mirror/Mosby College Publications; 1990:21–46.
10. South Carolina Office of Solid Waste Reduction and Recycling. A Brief History of Environmental Law. OR-0593 12/11. Office of Solid Waste, Reduction and Recycling: Columbia, SC. Retrieved from http://www.scdhec.gov/environment/lwm/recycle/pubs/environmental_law.pdf on July 18, 2013.
11. American Academy of Family Practitioners. *Practice-Based Research in Family Medicine*. Kansas City. MO: American Academy of Family Practitioners; 1986.
12. US Dept of Health and Human Services. *Historical Highlights and Timelines in Public Health*. Retrieved from http://www.hhs.gov/about/historical-highlights/index.html on July 29, 2015.
13. Vinten-Johansen P. *Cholera, Chloroform, and the Science of Medicine: A Life of John Snow*. New York, NY: Oxford University Press; 2003.
14. Baker S Josephine. *Fighting for Life*. New York, NY: Arno Press; 1974.
15. Tooth care: So easy a caveman could do it? *USA Today*. September 12, 2007:5D.
16. Institute of Medicine. For the Public's Health: Investing in a Healthier Future Report Brief. Institute of Medicine: Washington DC, 2012. Retrieved from http://www.iom.edu/~/media/Files/Report%20Files/2012/For-the-Publics-Health/phfunding_rb.pdf on July 18, 2013.

17. American Board of Dental Public Health. *Informational Brochure.* Springfield, IL: American Association of Public Health Dentistry; 2008.

18. US Public Health Service. *Healthy People 2020.* Conf ed. Washington, DC: US Dept of Health and Human Services; 2010.

19. US Dept of Health and Human Services. *Oral Health in America: A Report of the Surgeon General.* Rockville, MD: US Dept of Health and Human Services, National Institute of Dental and Craniofacial Research, National Institutes of Health; 2000.

20. US Dept of Health and Human Services. *A National Call to Action to Promote Oral Health.* Rockville, MD: US Dept of Health and Human Services, Public Health Service, Centers for Disease Control and Prevention, National Institutes of Health, National Institute of Dental and Craniofacial Research; 2003. NIH Publication No. 03-5303.

21. US Dept of Health and Human Services, Health Resources and Services Demonstration, Bureau of Health Professions. *The Professional Practice Environment of Dental Hygienists in the Fifty States and the District of Columbia;* 2001. Contract No. HRSA 230-00-0099. Retrieved from http://bhpr .hrsa.gov/healthworkforce/supplydemand/dentistry/ dentalhygieneenvironment.pdf on July 29, 2015.

22. Weaver, RG, Vachovic, RW, Hanlon, LL, Mintz, JS, Chmar, JE. Unleashing the potential; 2006. Retrieved from http:// www.adea.org on July 29, 2015.

23. Bureau of Labor Statistics, US Dept of Labor. *Occupational Outlook Handbook.* 2008-09 ed. Retrieved from http://www .bls.gov/ooh/healthcare/dental-hygienists.htm. on July 29, 2015.

24. McKinnon M, Luke G, Bresch J, Moss M, Valachovic RW. Emerging allied dental workforce models: Considerations for academic dental institutions. *J Dent Educ.* 2007;71(11): 1476–1491.

25. Nash DA, Nagel RJ. A brief history and current status of a dental therapy initiative in the United States. *J Dent Educ.* 2005:69(8):857–859.

26. American Dental Hygienists' Association.The History of Introducing a New Provider in Minnesota: A Chronicle of Legislative Efforts 2008-2009. Chicago: American Dental Hygienists' Association, 2014. Retrieved from http://www .adha.org/resources-docs/75113_Minnesota_Story.pdf on July 18, 2013.

27. Blue, CM, Funkhouse, DR, Riggs, S, Rindal, DB, Worley, D, Pihlstrom, DJ, Benjamin, P, Gilbert, GH. Utilization of non-dentist providers and attitudes toward new provider models: Findings from the National Dental Practice-Based Research Network. *J Public Health Dent.* 2013 May 14.

28. Competencies for the Advanced Dental Hygiene Practitioner. Chicago, IL: American Dental Hygienists' Association; 2008.

29. Fones AC. *Mouth Hygiene.* 3rd ed. Philadelphia, PA: Lea & Febiger; 1927:5.

30. US Census Bureau. 2010 Census Shows America's Diversity. Retrieved from https://www.census.gov/newsroom/ releases/archives/2010_census/cb11-cn125.html on July 29, 2015.

31. Beltran-Aguilar ED, Barker LK, Canto MT, Dye BA, Gooch BF, Griffin, SO. Surveillance for dental caries, dental sealants, tooth retention, edentulism and enamel fluorosis—US, 1988–1994 and 1999–2002. *MMWR Morb Mortal Wkly Rpt.* 2005;54(SS-3).

32. Baum BJ, Ship JA. Oral disorders. In: Beck J, ed. *Geriatrics Review Syllabus—A Core Curriculum in Geriatric Medicine.* New York, NY: American Geriatrics Society; 1991:332–336.

33. Beck JD. Epidemiology of dental diseases in the elderly. *Gerodontology.* 1984;3:5–15.

34. Boyce JS. Risk management: An introduction for the dental practice. *Dent Hyg.* 1987;181:504–507.

35. Dental visits among dentate adults with diabetes—United States, 1999 and 2004. *MMWR Morb Mortal Wkly Rpt.* 2005; 54(46):1181–1183.

Visit www.pearsonhighered.com/healthprofessionsresources to access the student resources that accompany this book. Simply select Dental Hygiene from the choice of disciplines. Find this book and you will find the complimentary study tools created for this specific title.

2

The Prevention Movement

OBJECTIVES

After studying this chapter, the dental hygiene student should be able to:

- Describe the history of dental hygiene in relation to dental public health
- Define the historical development and mission of the American Dental Hygienists' Association
- List and describe the current public health preventive modalities practiced today
- Defend the need for preventive modalities in dental public health practice

COMPETENCIES

After studying this chapter and participating in accompanying course activities, the dental hygiene student should be competent to do the following:

- Promote positive values of oral and general health and wellness to the public and organizations within and outside the profession
- Promote the profession through service activities and affiliations with professional organizations
- Facilitate patient access to oral health services by influencing individuals or organizations for the provision of oral health care
- Pursue career options within the health care industry, education research and other roles as they evolve for the dental hygienist.
- Access professional and social networks to pursue professional goals

KEY TERMS

Alternative restorative treatment 27
Athletic mouth guard 29
Community water fluoridation 23
Dental hygiene treatment 22
Dental sealants 26
Grass roots 21
Outreach workers 18
Tobacco cessation programs 29
Xylitol 27

The proliferation of dental hygienists in dental offices and other health care facilities is evidence of the value placed on dental hygiene in the United States. The Bureau of Labor Statistics estimates that the number of employed dental hygienists is expected to increase 33 percent from 2012 to 2022, a much higher rate than for the average for other occupations. Due to ongoing research linking oral health to general health, a demand for preventive dental services, which are provided by dental hygienists, is projected to continue.[1] The insurance industry's comprehensive coverage of dental hygiene services is further proof that the practice of prevention is necessary and logical in health care delivery.

The dental hygiene profession is at the forefront of the prevention and wellness movement that continues to grow. Dental hygiene is the only health care profession based exclusively on *preventive* care. Historically, dental hygiene services have been available in public health forums focused on preventing and controlling disease within the population.[2–6] Thus, the practice of dental hygiene complements the dental public health sciences both from a scientific and practical perspective.

Historical Development

Although dental hygiene practice dates further back than its cited inception in 1913, the preventive focus of this new profession was emphasized when Dr. Alfred Civilion Fones coined the term *dental hygienist* in the early 1900s.[6] This change in title from dental nurse to dental hygienist focused on the *preventive* dental sciences. After research results on the preventive benefits of dental hygiene were published, the college discipline of dental hygiene was created.[7]

Even though prevention was being discussed and practiced in some offices, it was Fones who actually brought dental hygiene into existence. He saw it as a distinct profession and thought it should be positioned within dental public health as opposed to being offered exclusively in private dental practices. In fact, Fones believed that the dental hygienist should provide education and treatment outside the dental office with particular focus on mass pediatric prevention. He emphasized the use of dental hygienists as **outreach workers** "outside" the dental practice to bring patients in need of restorative dental care to dental offices while providing preventive services outside the dental practice, such as in a school setting.[2–6] (See Table 2-1 ■ for more of Fones's thoughts on the dental hygiene profession.)

Did You Know?

For many years the following encrypted statement was eloquently placed on the American Dental Hygienists' Association (ADHA) stationary: *For the health of the community, especially the children.* This clearly emphasized the initial focus on pediatric prevention.

Fones educated the first dental hygienist, Irene Newman, for one year before he permitted her to treat patients in his practice. In 1913, he started the Fones School of Dental Hygiene, which continues to educate dental hygienists today within the University of Bridgeport in Connecticut. (See Figures 2-1 ■ and 2-2 ■.) Before he opened his school and began working within the Bridgeport public school system, Fones initiated the dental hygienists' role in dental public health by developing curricula for dental hygienists, but his proposal was rejected. At that time, not all dentists were aware of this new preventive concept and practice. In fact, a dentist on the board of education voted against the plan. Deciding that this action was a blessing in disguise, Fones postponed the opening of his school for a year, during which time he found instructors, wrote the first dental hygiene textbook, *Mouth Hygiene*, and chose qualified students.[8]

Did You Know?

Fones secured experienced professors and experts of medicine, basic sciences, public health, and dentistry from Yale University, Harvard University, Columbia University, and the University of Pennsylvania to begin the new college discipline of dental hygiene.[7]

Fones envisioned dental hygienists working collaboratively with other health and social service workers in providing preventive health care to the public. He stated, "Dental hygiene . . . opens up paths of usefulness, activity and inspiration hitherto undreamed of, allying her with the workers of the world who are helping humanity in masses."[1] After war was declared in 1917, dental hygienists in Bridgeport provided care and education to the military. Additionally, dental hygienists worked to create positions in hospitals and numerous factories in Connecticut.

Fones traveled the country to explain the new profession of dental hygiene to state dental associations, but some dentists were opposed to it.[7,9] Preventive dental science was a new concept, and many dentists had no experience working with a dental hygienist. Consequently, many laws were enacted that prohibited dental hygienists from working in any setting other than a private dental practice with a dentist supervising all treatment.

Possibly, if Fones had introduced the new profession to schoolteachers, school administrators, hospital administrators, and other professional health care organizations instead of state dental associations, dental hygienists most likely would have been permitted to work in a variety of settings. Dental hygiene was finally accepted in all states with a reduced educational standard for practice developed in Alabama.[10] Chapter 6 discusses the access to care issues that resulted from these restrictive practice acts.

Table 2–1 Comparison of the Writings of Dr. Alfred Fones, Founder of Dental Hygiene, with Recommendations from the US Surgeon General's Report on Oral Health 2000

US Surgeon General's Report	Fones's Mouth Hygiene, textbook of dental hygiene, 1–4 eds., 1916–1934
Perceptions regarding oral heath and ideas should be changed so that oral health becomes an accepted component of general health.	Since the days of Hippocrates, it has been known that infections of dental origin may be accompanied by serious systemic symptoms. The work of the dental hygienist is most important in the prevention of the systemic infection through the avenue of the mouth.
Accelerate the building of science and advance evidence base and apply science effectively to improve oral health.	It is no longer a theory that the service of the dental hygienist will better the mouth health and general health of all whom she is permitted to serve. The research field in preventive dentistry is gradually widening into a study of constitutional causes that are believed to have an influence on the general health, and consequently on dental health.
An effective health infrastructure that meets the oral health needs of all Americans should be built and integrate oral health effectively into general health.	Hundreds of millions of dollars in public and private funds are expended to restore the sick to health, but only a relatively small portion of this amount is spent to maintain the health of well people, even though it is definitely known that the most common physical defects and illnesses are preventable. It is not the intention to in any way belittle the efforts being made to aid the sick and needy, nor should such efforts be decreased. The vital point is that we have not commenced to cover the possibilities of true prevention.
Known barriers between people and oral health services should be removed.	The dental hygienist was created from the realization that mouth hygiene was a necessity and that the average dental practitioner could not give sufficient time to it and that the toothbrush alone would never produce it. The present need of the dental profession in solving the public health problem of mouth hygiene is an immense corps of women workers, educated and trained as dental hygienists, and therefore competent to enter public schools, dental offices, infirmaries, public clinics, sanitariums, factories, and other private corporations, to care for the mouths of the millions who need this educational service.
Public–private partnerships should be used to improve the oral health of those who still suffer disproportionately from oral disease.	The actual results secured by dental hygienists in private and public services, particularly in public schools, affords incontrovertible proof of the value of the dental hygienists. Those who may still be skeptical are finding it difficult indeed to suggest other means by which similar good results can be accomplished for large groups of people. The future of the dental hygienist in public schools work must be determined on a basis of cooperation between the dental profession and the educational authorities. The Fones's hygienists who were completing their course in 1917 when war was declared had the unique experience of completing exams and cleanings and supplying each soldier a toothbrush and individual instruction in the care of the mouth.

Source: Nathe C. Dental hygiene's historical roots in modern-day issues. *Contemp Oral Hyg.* 2003;3:24–25.

Today, dental practice laws are changing, and at least thirty-seven states now permit the practice of dental hygiene without the physical presence of a dentist, allowing dental hygienists to work more effectively in the public health arena.[11] See Figure 2-3 ■.

In fact, some states allow dental hygienists to provide direct services to patients in all settings. Dental hygienists increasingly are bringing dental hygiene services to schoolchildren, people who are elderly, and other underserved populations.

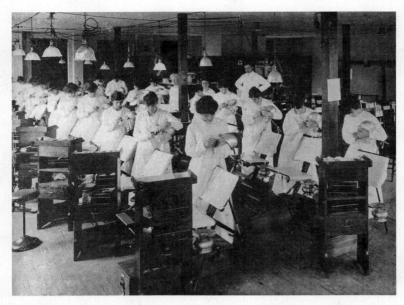

FIGURE 2–1 Fones School of Dental Hygiene, Bridgeport, Connecticut, Circa Early 1900s

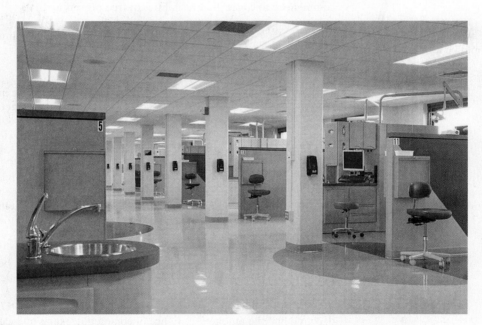

FIGURE 2–2 Fones School of Dental Hygiene, Bridgeport, Connecticut, 2008

Evolution of Organized Dental Hygiene

The Connecticut Dental Hygienists' Association was formed with nineteen members on graduation day of the first dental hygiene class in Bridgeport, Connecticut, June 5, 1914. The objective of this newly formed association was "to educate the public in, and to advance the cause of Mouth Hygiene for the mutual improvement of its members, and to assist as far as lie within its power in the prevention of disease."[12] The national association, ADHA, was formed in 1923 in Cleveland, Ohio.

Did You Know?

The first president of the ADHA was, fittingly, Irene Newman, the world's first dental hygienist.

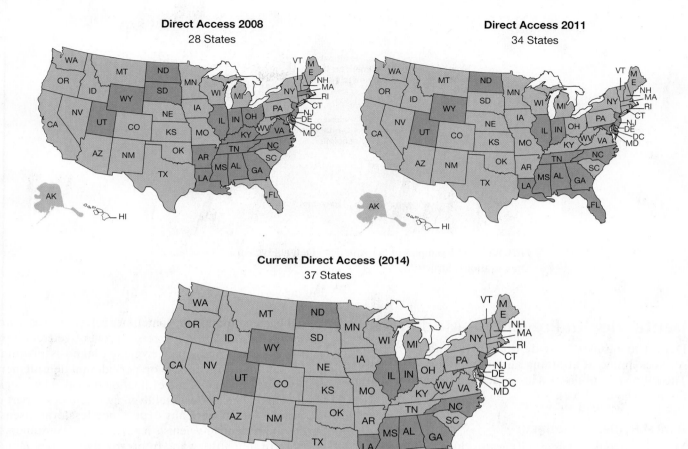

FIGURE 2–3 ADHA Direct Access Map 2014

Source: American Dental Hygienists' Association: http://www.adha.org/resources-docs/7524_Direct_Access_Map.pdf

The ADHA's mission has evolved since its inception. Its present mission is:

> to improve the public's total health by working to advance the art and science of dental hygiene by ensuring access to quality oral health care, increasing awareness of the cost-effective benefits of prevention, promoting the highest standards of dental hygiene education, licensure, practice and research and representing and promoting the interests of dental hygienists.[13]

Presently, the ADHA represents more than 185,000 registered dental hygienists and works actively in professional development and governmental affairs (Figure 2-4 ■).

Each of the fifty state dental hygiene associations is a constituent member. All 375 local dental hygiene associations are known as *component organizations.* Constituent organizations serve the components in their jurisdictions by informing them of national policies and programs and actively working on legislative issues. The components form the first line of involvement, the **grass roots,** or local, efforts to effect change and help guide policy-making decisions. Grass roots members are local dental hygienists who strive for social change to improve their communities' oral health. The components implement community services programs and educational sessions and offer ideas and information about state and national policies. The ADHA has a student membership category and provides student scholarships, networking, mentorship, employment assistance, and continuing education.

Did You Know?

The International Federation of Dental Hygienists is the professional organization that represents dental hygienists from twenty-five countries. It was informally started in 1970 and officially recognized in 1986. The IFDH will be discussed in greater detail in Chapter 4.

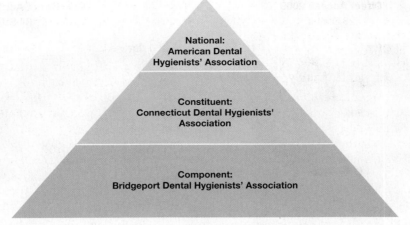

FIGURE 2–4 Examples of the American Dental Hygienists' Association Organizational Structure

Dental Health Preventive Modalities

Dental hygienists provide diagnostic and therapeutic services aimed at attaining and maintaining oral health. The following modalities are practiced to prevent dental diseases (Figure 2-5 ■).

Dental Hygiene Treatment

Many believe that community water fluoridation and the introduction of dental sealants have had the biggest impact on public dental health. However, since 1913, dental hygienists have made a tremendous impact through prevention.

Dental hygiene treatment, sometimes referred to as *dental cleanings* and *oral prophylaxes,* is preventive treatment, including assessment, dental hygiene diagnosis, planning, implementation with a focus on periodontal debridement, oral hygiene instruction, and evaluation provided by a registered dental hygienist. Dental hygiene treatment is part of the reason that Americans experience less oral disease. Furthermore, dental hygienists have educated consumers to be more oral health aware. Interestingly, *Healthy People 2020, Oral Health in America: A Report of the Surgeon General* and *A National Call to Action to Promote Oral Health* do not even address the impact dental hygiene has

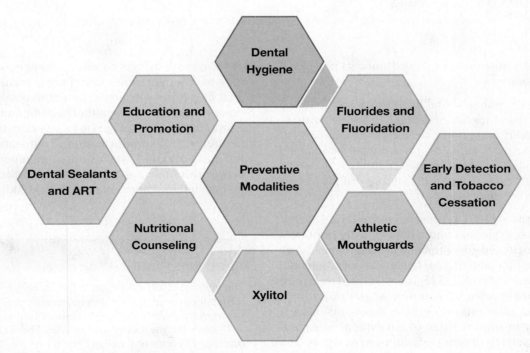

FIGURE 2–5 Modalities Practiced to Prevent Dental Diseases

had on preventive dental care in the United States.[14–16] However, this sentiment seems to be changing, and in recent years reports have focused on the utilization of dental hygienists to address oral health disease in society.[17–19]

Since the 1970s, dental hygienists have been employed in clinical positions in the United States, providing preventive, educational, and therapeutic services. However, some private dental offices and many public dental health settings still do not utilize or underutilize dental hygienists. A recent survey conducted by the American Dental Association found that only 68 percent of dentists employ a part-time or full-time dental hygienist.[20] Nevertheless, the American public indeed places great value on a healthy, beautiful smile, and the United States is often portrayed as a dentally healthy culture with an emphasis on straight, white teeth.

Countries without the benefit of dental hygiene have a higher incidence of dental caries, periodontal diseases, and cancrum oris (noma)—often of a severe nature—than the United States does. In fact, the World Health Organization (WHO) focuses much attention on the treatment of cancrum oris, a serious disease of the mouth and face.[21] Cancrum oris begins with severe gingivitis and is followed by rapidly extending ulceration within the mouth. The infection then spreads through the buccal mucosa, which becomes edematous and necrotic. If septicemia and death do not quickly supervene, a foul-smelling purulent discharge precedes massive tissue loss and secondary healing by wound contracture. This often leads to facial disfigurement with limited jaw motion. In the United States, cancrum oris is rarely seen; however, in many developing countries without dental hygienists, it is much too common.

Did You Know?

Dental hygiene was the forerunner to the prevention movement now seen in the United States.

Dental hygiene has not been studied per se as a preventive treatment modality, so no data can be cited regarding its benefits to society. The ADHA has prioritized research focusing on the cost-effectiveness of dental hygiene, focusing on the use of dental hygienists to treat the underserved.[22] The *role* of the dental hygienist in the oral health care system has been studied, however, and one recent study indicated that dental hygienists were being utilized more in 2000 than they were a decade earlier. The report suggested that dental hygienists have demonstrated their clinical ability to contribute both to quality patient care and improved access to care. Over the past decade, virtually every state has expanded the legal scope of practice of dental hygienists. When taken in conjunction with the findings of expansion initiatives in California and Colorado, which focused on direct care provided by dental hygienists without dentist's supervision, this report suggests that expanding the professional practice environment of dental

hygienists improves access to oral health services, use of oral health services, and oral health outcomes.[23]

Community Water Fluoridation

Community water fluoridation is the addition of fluoride to community water supplies. Although fluoride is present naturally in variable amounts in all soils and existing water supplies, it is also present in animal and plant food consumed by people. Community water fluoridation is an excellent method to provide benefits to most people because everyone drinks and cooks with water. Moreover, fluoridated water is used in the processing and bottling of many foods and beverages. Therefore, it is a successful, cost-effective way to decrease dental caries in a population.[24–26] The cost per person is significantly less than the cost of restoring demineralized tooth structure, and fluoride's ability to remineralize demineralized tooth surfaces is of even more value.

Dr. Frederick McKay, a graduate of a Philadelphia dental school who started practicing dentistry in Colorado Springs, Colorado, is partially credited for discovering the effects of fluoridation. He found it accidentally when he was trying to determine why long-term residents of the area had brown enamel opacities and mottling, commonly referred to as *Colorado brown stain*. Dr. McKay knew from his experience in other parts of the country that this was not a normal occurrence. In 1908, with funding from the Colorado Springs Dental Society, he began an investigation that ultimately found that an excess of naturally occurring fluoride in the water supply was causing *dental fluorosis* or chronic fluoride toxicity.[27] However, the same patients exhibited far fewer carious lesions than his other patients, thus revealing the preventive benefit of fluoridated water.[28]

As beneficial as fluoride is to prevention of dental caries, too much of it can be harmful, as McKay found. If systemic fluoride concentration is high enough for a long enough period of time, severe skeletal fluorosis (or chronic fluoride toxicity) can occur as is seen in some parts of the world. Acute fluoride toxicity that can occur after excessive ingestion of fluoride produces nausea and vomiting, which can damage the stomach wall. The condition can be severe enough to be fatal. Emergency treatment includes induced vomiting, protection of the stomach by binding fluoride with orally administered calcium or aluminum preparations (milk), and maintenance of blood calcium levels with intravenous calcium.

Dr. H. Trendley Dean, a US Public Health Service dental officer, and his staff studied fluoride in drinking water and by the late 1930s discovered that fluoride levels of up to 1.0 ppm (parts per million) in drinking water did not cause enamel fluorosis in most people and only mild enamel fluorosis in a small percentage of people.[28]

In the United States, 74.6 percent of those served by public water systems received fluoridated water in 2012.[29] A *Healthy People 2020* goal calls for 79.6 percent of the population on piped-water supplies to be serviced with optimally fluoridated water.[14] Figure 2-6 ■ graphically displays the levels of fluoridation by state.

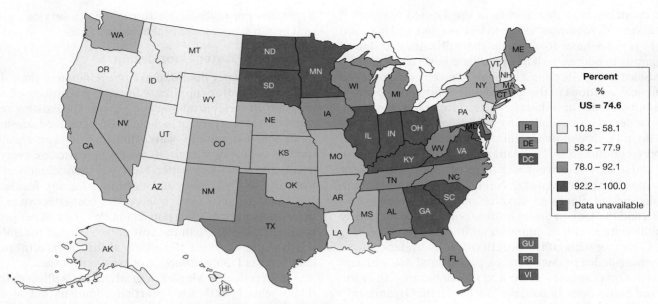

FIGURE 2–6 Public Water Supply Population Using Fluoridated Water

Source: http://apps.nccd.cdc.gov/nohss/IndicatorV.asp?Indicator=1

In areas where it is impossible to fluoridate the water, either because the residents have well water or the overwhelming opposition to fluoride, schools can fluoridate the water.

Did You Know?

Well water is needed in areas without access to a public water supply. A household well is dug as part of the house construction, and water treatment processes are needed to permit safe drinking water development. Well water can be taken to most pediatricians for fluoride level identification.

School water fluoridation is recommended only when the school has its own source of water and is not connected to a community water system. Each state is responsible for determining whether school water fluoridation is desirable and developing a written agreement between the state and appropriate school officials. Such a program must not be started unless resources are available at the state level to undertake operational and maintenance responsibilities.[30]

Fluoridated water has proved to be an effective means of preventing caries in children with an 8–37 percent reduction. Although children benefit from the systemic and topical benefits of fluoride, adults benefit only from topical (on the tooth structure) effects. Reviewed studies show that the topical effect of drinking fluoridated water reduced caries in adults from 20–40 percent.[25]

Community water fluoridation is especially beneficial for communities of low socioeconomic status.[31] These communities have a disproportionate burden of dental caries and less access to dental care services and other sources of fluoride than higher income communities do. So, community water fluoridation benefits *all* populations who drink from a public water supply, without influencing the creation of oral health disparities.

See Table 2-2 ■ for the previous recommended levels of fluoride, depending on climate. In a warmer climate, less fluoride is needed because people drink more water.

Table 2–2 Fluoride Levels Recommended by US Public Health Service for Cool and Warm Climates

Annual Average of Maximum Daily Air Temperatures (°F)	Recommended Control Limits of F Concentrations (ppm)		
	Lower	Optimum	Upper
50.0–53.7	1.1	1.2	1.7
53.8–58.3	1.0	1.1	1.6
58.4–63.8	0.9	1.0	1.5
63.9–70.6	0.8	0.9	1.4
70.7–79.2	0.7	0.8	1.3
79.3–90.5	0.6	0.7	1.2

Source: Centers for Disease Control and Prevention. Engineering and administrative recommendations for water fluoridation. *MMWR Morb Mortal Wkly Rpt.* 2001;44(RR-13):1–40.

Table 2–3 US Food and Drug Administration (FDA) Fluoride Requirements for Water Bottled in the United States

Annual Average of Maximum Daily Air Temperature (°F) of Retail Establishment Selling Bottled Water	Maximum Fluoride Concentration (mg/L) Allowed in Bottled Water	
	No Fluoride Added to Bottled Water	Fluoride Added to Bottled Water
53.7	2.4	1.7
53.8–58.3	2.2	1.5
58.4–63.8	2.0	1.3
63.9–70.6	1.8	1.2
70.7–79.2	1.6	1.0
79.3–90.5	1.4	0.8

Note: FDA regulations require that fluoride be listed on the label only if the bottler adds it during processing, but the bottler is not required to list the fluoride concentration, which might or might not be optimal. The FDA does not allow imported bottled water with no added fluoride to contain >1.4 mg fluoride/L or with added fluoride to contain >0.8 mg fluoride/L.

Source: US Dept of Health and Human Services, Food and Drug Administration. Bottled water. 21 Code of Federal Regulations CFR). 1995;60:57124–57130.

Because of the increased use of air conditioning in houses and automobiles, however, this theory may be changing.

In 2011, the US Department of Health and Human Services (HHS), proposed a new guidance to update and replace the 1962 US Public Health Service Drinking Water Standards related to recommendations for fluoride concentrations in drinking water. The US Public Health Service recommendations for optimal fluoride concentrations (were) based on ambient air temperature of geographic areas and ranged from 0.7–1.2 mg/L. HHS proposed that community water systems adjust the amount of fluoride to 0.7 mg/L to achieve an optimal fluoride level. For the purpose of this guidance, the optimal concentration of fluoride in drinking water is that concentration that provides the best balance of protection from dental caries while limiting the risk of dental fluorosis.[32] Parts per million (ppm) and milligrams/liter (mg/L) are essentially equivalent, and the terms are used interchangeably. Some documents refer to concentrations used in water fluoridation as parts per million; others use milligrams per liter. In this chapter, parts per million will be used.

Dental hygienists should be aware that bottled water often contains no fluoride or fails to identify its fluoride content on the label. See Table 2-3 ■ for bottled water requirements developed in 1995 and still in effect. The FDA has also given permission for bottled water to include enough fluoride to advertise the fluoride claim of reducing dental decay.

The only valid argument against community water fluoridation is that the addition of fluoride to water prevents personal choice. Refer to Box 2-1 ■ for some reasons people oppose public water fluoridation.

Did You Know?

Although opponents to community water fluoridation may believe that it causes diseases, including cancer and multiple sclerosis, no credible evidence supports such an association.

The US Centers for Disease Control and Prevention (CDC) recognizes the fluoridation of drinking water as one of ten great public health achievements of the twentieth century. In 2004, the Surgeon General issued a statement promoting the use of community water fluoridation

Box 2–1 Some Reasons Cited for Opposition to Water Fluoridation

- Violation of personal freedom
- Cause of disease(s) and/or medical conditions: cancer, AIDS, fatigue, etc.
- Forced medication
- Communist plot
- Abuse of police power

as a cost-effective preventive measure that benefits all individuals without creating oral health disparities.

Defluoridation is the process of removing excess fluoride naturally present in a water supply to prevent dental fluorosis. South Carolina requested the defluoridation of naturally occurring 2.0 ppm fluoride, which would have cost an estimated $12 million. The state found that few of the small communities affected were interested in defluoridating because the degree of fluorosis did not concern them. They did not suffer ill effects, but they had a lower rate of caries.[33]

Fluoride Preventive Modalities

Community water fluoridation works both systemically and topically.[24] Fluoride's systemic effects occur as the fluoride becomes incorporated into the structure of the teeth. On the other hand, fluoridated toothpastes, mouth rinses, professional gels, fluoride varnish, and water fluoridation work topically. Laboratory and epidemiological research suggests that fluoride prevents dental caries predominately after eruption of the tooth into the mouth by inhibiting demineralization, enhancing remineralization, and inhibiting bacterial activity in dental plaque.[24]

In addition to community water fluoridation, other systemic fluoride modalities include the use of fluoride supplements. Dietary fluoride supplements are available in the form of tablets, lozenges, or liquids (including fluoride-vitamin preparations) and have been used throughout the world since the 1940s. Most supplements contain sodium fluoride as the active ingredient. Tablets and lozenges are manufactured with 1.0, 0.5, or 0.25 mg fluoride. To maximize its topical effect, tablets and lozenges are intended to be chewed or sucked for one to two minutes before being swallowed. Supplements for infants are available as a liquid and used with a dropper.[24] Although the primary teeth of children aged one to six years would benefit from fluoride's posteruptive action and possibly from the preeruptive benefit to developing permanent teeth, fluoride supplements also could increase the risk for enamel fluorosis at this age.[24]

The benefits of topically applied fluoride are well documented. Fluoride gels and foams professionally applied twice a year reportedly caused an average decrease of 26 percent in caries in the permanent teeth of children residing in nonfluoridated areas.[24] Fluoride-containing prophy paste is routinely used during dental hygiene treatment and contains 4000–20,000 ppm fluoride, which might restore the concentration of fluoride in the surface layer of enamel removed by polishing, but this amount is not an adequate substitute for fluoride gel or varnish in treating persons at high risk for dental caries.

Fluoridated toothpastes are thought to decrease the prevalence of dental decay by 25 percent.[34] Over-the-counter fluoride mouth rinses decrease the prevalence of dental decay by 26 percent.[35] Patients with xerostomia, high caries rates, orthodontic therapy, or undergoing radiation treatment for cancer can decrease decay by up to 80 percent when utilizing a fluoride gel in a custom-made tray.[36] Fluoride varnishes applied by the dental hygienist are increasingly being used, although the FDA has approved them only for use as a desensitizing agent.[37] See Table 2-4 ■ for more information on fluoride modalities.

Dental Sealants

Dental sealants are plastic resins placed on tooth surfaces to prevent dental decay. Their placement is an effective means of preventing caries in pits and fissures, the areas least affected by fluoride.[38] Dental sealants (sometimes called *pit and fissure sealants*) should be placed as soon as possible after the tooth erupts and can be isolated to prevent moisture contamination. Indications for dental sealants also include a history of caries, xerostomia, orthodontics, poor oral hygiene, and incipient caries. Some contraindications for sealants include patient behavior that does not permit a dry field and the presence of open occlusal carious lesions.

Sealants are a cost-effective means to prevent occlusal, buccal pit, and lingual groove decay. On average, the cost of one surface restoration is more than the cost of a sealant placement.[39] Figure 2-7 ■ indicates sealant usage of a specific population in the United States.

Pits and fissures that remain completely sealed are well protected from caries, according to several investigations.[40] Moreover, studies have confirmed that complete retention rates after one year are 85 percent or better and after five years are at least 50 percent.[41] Sealants are effective in reducing the occlusal caries incidence in permanent first molars of children with reduction of 76.3 percent at four years when sealants were reapplied as needed. Caries reduction was 65 percent at nine years from initial treatment when sealants were not reapplied as needed.[42] Sealing the occlusal surfaces of permanent molars in children and adolescents reduces caries up to forty-eight months when compared to no sealant; after longer follow-up the quantity and quality of the evidence is reduced.[43] One review of previous studies suggested that sealants should be placed as part of an overall prevention strategy based on assessment of caries risk.[44]

Sealants are most effective when administered by a dental hygienist utilizing a dental assistant, a combination that has proved to be an effective force in public health settings. In fact, many communities have dental hygienists who travel to schools placing dental sealants. In some states, dentists are required to supervise their placement by dental hygienists, increasing the cost and subsequently decreasing cost-effectiveness. Moreover, in some states, a dentist must approve tooth surfaces before a dental hygienist places a sealant, a practice that further increases the time spent and decreases cost-effectiveness.

Table 2–4 Quality of Evidence, Strength of Recommendation, and Target Population of Recommendation for Each Fluoride Modality to Prevent and Control Dental Caries

Modality[a]	Quality of Evidence (Grade)[d]	Strength of Recommendation (Code)[d]	Target Population[ab]
Community water fluoridation	II-1	A	All areas
School water fluoridation	II-3	C	Rural, nonfluoridated areas
Fluoride toothpaste	I	A	All persons
Fluoride mouthrinse	I	A	High risk[c]
Fluoride supplements			
Pregnant women	I	E	None
Children aged <6 years	II-3	C	High risk
Children aged 6–16 years	I	A	High risk
Persons aged >16 years		C	High risk
Fluoride gel	I	A	High risk
Fluoride varnish	I	A	High risk

[a]Modalities are assumed to be used as directed in terms of dosage and age of user.

[b]Quality of evidence for targeting some modalities to persons at high risk is grade III (ie, representing the opinion of respected authorities) and is based on considerations of cost-effectiveness that were not included in the studies establishing efficacy or effectiveness.

[c]Populations believed to be at increased risk for dental caries are those with low socioeconomic status or low levels of parental education, those who do not seek regular dental care, and those without dental insurance or access to dental services. Individual factors that possibly increase risk include active dental caries; a history of high caries experience in older siblings or caregivers; root surfaces exposed by gingival recession; high levels of infection with cariogenic bacteria; impaired ability to maintain oral hygiene; malformed enamel or dentin; reduced salivary flow because of medications, radiation treatment, or disease; low salivary buffering capacity (ie, decreased ability of saliva to neutralize acids); and the wearing of space maintainers, orthodontic appliances, or dental prostheses. Risk can increase if any of these factors is combined with dietary practices conducive to dental caries (ie, frequent consumption of refined carbohydrates). Risk decreases with adequate exposure to fluoride.

[d]See US Preventive Services Task Force grading and coding systems.

No published studies confirm the effectiveness of fluoride supplements in controlling dental caries among persons aged >16 years.

Source: CDC Recommendations for using fluoride to prevent and control dental caries in the United States. *MMWR Morb Mortal Wkly Rpt.* 2001;50(RR14):1–42.

Alternative Restorative Treatment (ART)

When no restorative option is available to a patient, a provider can use a method called **alternative restorative treatment** (ART), formerly known as *atraumatic restorative treatment*. The provider removes carious lesions using hand instruments and restores the resultant cavity and adjoining fissures using a dental sealant, usually glass ionomer material.[45,46] This technique may be modified by the use of rotary instruments.[46]

ART is widely used in developing countries and in rural areas in developed countries. However, application by a dental hygienist may not be legal in some states. The WHO and the International Association for Dental Research have endorsed ART as a means of restoring and preventing dental caries.[46]

Xylitol

Xylitol is a sugar substitute that has shown promising results in reducing dental decay and ear infections. It is found in berries, fruit, vegetables, mushrooms, and birch wood. Xylitol can be delivered in teeth via mints, gums, and lozenges to help reduce dental decay.

Did You Know?

Xylitol is present in many of the frequently purchased chewing gums in the United States.

Advocates of xylitol use theorize that after chewing it, bacteria do not adsorb well on the surface of the teeth, and

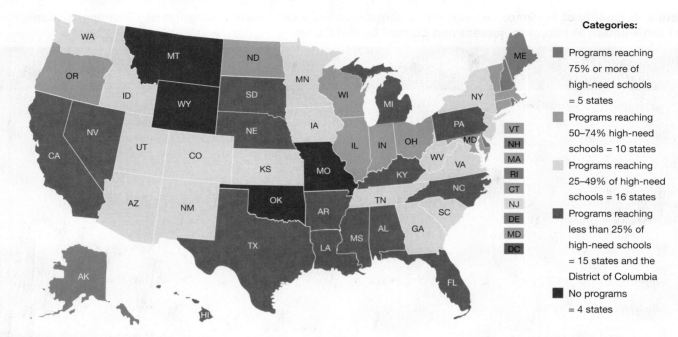

Categories:

■ Programs reaching 75% or more of high-need schools = 5 states

■ Programs reaching 50–74% high-need schools = 10 states

□ Programs reaching 25–49% of high-need schools = 16 states

■ Programs reaching less than 25% of high-need schools = 15 states and the District of Columbia

■ No programs = 4 states

FIGURE 2–7 Dental Sealant Utilization

Source: CDC and the Association of State and Territorial Dental Directors. National Oral Health Surveillance System, 2006. Data from states vary by year of reporting. Available at http://www.cdc.gov/nohss.

as a consequence, the amount of plaque decreases. However, some studies do not support the anticaries benefits.[47,48] More research is warranted.

Nutritional Counseling

In *Mouth Hygiene,* the first textbook for dental hygienists (published in 1916), the author states that normal nutrition and mouth cleanliness are the two most important factors for preventing dental pathology.[2–5] This concept is still relevant. With this in mind, the dental hygienist must remember to incorporate nutritional counseling into all regimens related to oral health care. In fact, awareness of oral health is a major contributor to good nutrition. The oral cavity is the pathway to the body, and disturbances in the mouth can profoundly affect diet and ultimately nutritional status. Conversely, good nutrition provides the foundation for optimum oral health. Diet plays a major role in the etiology and prevention of dental caries and is an important supporting factor in other oral infections.

The ADHA recommends that dental hygienists maintain a current knowledge of nutrition recommendations and effectively educate and counsel their patients about proper nutrition and oral health.[49] Furthermore, the American Dietetic Association states that collaboration between dietetics and dental professionals is necessary for oral health promotion, disease prevention, intervention, and research.[50] It is important for dental hygienists to work with dietitians in community and patient endeavors to educate and promote the importance of a healthy diet in oral health and, consequently, total health. The dental hygienist should also manage nutritional issues by making referrals to appropriate health care workers.

Early Detection and Tobacco Cessation

Tobacco use in any form is dangerous to an individual's health. Tobacco is related to tooth staining, periodontal diseases, and oral and pharyngeal cancer. Each year, oral and pharyngeal cancers, which are mainly squamous cell carcinomas, are diagnosed in approximately 45,000 US residents, and well over 8,000 persons die of these diseases.[51] Another obstacle to early discovery, and resulting better outcomes, is the advent of a virus, HPV16, contributing more to the incidence rate of oral cancers, particularly in the posterior part of the mouth (the oropharynx, the tonsils, and the base of tongue areas), which many times does not produce visible lesions or discolorations that have historically been the early warning signs of the disease process.[52] Overall, 60 percent of people with oral cancer survive for five years; however, this percentage is significantly lower for black men and women. Studies do show that diagnosing oral cancer at an early stage significantly increases five-year survival rates. Interestingly, oral cancer survival rates have steadily improved since 1975.[53]

Prevention of oral cancer is critically important and can be accomplished in four ways, by (1) understanding cause-and-effect and modifying associated risks, (2) recognizing and controlling precancerous lesions, (3) establishing the earliest possible diagnosis and administering timely and appropriate therapy, and (4) effectively managing the complications of treatment.[51] Dental professionals should

conduct oral cancer exams annually and provide educational strategies designed to increase public awareness of these diseases.

Dental hygienists in many states have the opportunity to provide OralCDx®, a brush test method combined with advanced computer analysis to be used when abnormal tissue presents.[54] Another technology available for oral cancer screening is Vizilite®, which exposes oral tissues to a light source with a specific wavelength, causing normal healthy tissue and precancerous or cancerous tissues to fluoresce differently. The change in appearance occurs because their cellular composition causes them to reflect light at different rates. Using this handheld device, dental hygienists can visually assess oral tissues for abnormalities.[55] Both of these assessment modalities need more research to determine their overall effectiveness in early diagnosis of oral cancers. The referral to an oral surgeon for any tissue abnormality is paramount.

Dentists and dental hygienists can provide counseling to patients to stop tobacco use and limit alcohol use, both of which are associated with oral and pharyngeal cancer. In fact, one study suggested that approximately 90 percent of dentists and dental hygienists ask their patients if they smoke.[56] Unfortunately, many dental professionals stop after they ask the initial question. Programs to help smokers and tobacco chewers quit the habit are plentiful, and many campaigns exist to aid tobacco users. Many dental public health and private dental settings implement **tobacco cessation programs.** These programs encourage patients to quit using tobacco by employing ADHA's Ask, Advise, and Refer program. To learn more on this program, go to the ADHA web site.[57]

Athletic Mouth Guards

An **athletic mouth guard** is a removable oral appliance that protects the hard and soft tissues of the oral cavity and brain during contact sports. Sometimes referred to as *mouth protectors*, mouth guards protect by absorbing energy during an impact, thus decreasing the likelihood of trauma to the oral cavity and brain.[58,59]

Many orofacial injuries can be prevented by wearing athletic mouth guards, yet some individuals participating in athletic activities still do not wear them. The dental hygienist must promote their use by implementing mouth guard programs in school sports and private athletic organizations as well as educating the public on the value of mouth protection during contact sports, and fabricating mouth guards for athletes.

Did You Know?

Young athletes particularly are prone to sports-related orofacial trauma because they are less experienced than professional athletes. This makes the use of athletic mouth guards vitally important to this population.

The three types of mouth guards are the store-bought, boil-n-bite, and the custom-made mouth guards fabricated in the dental office. Dental providers (including dental hygienists in most states) can fabricate them simply by taking an alginate impression of the maxillary dentition, pouring a study model, and melting a thermoplastic material using a vacuum-forming machine. Custom-made mouth guards fit better and are recommended.

Mass Education and Promotion

One of the most important functions of the dental hygienist is to provide dental health education and promote dental health to the public. For these reasons, it is important for the dental hygienist to be well versed as an educator and public speaker. Chapter 8 includes an in-depth look into dental health education and promotion.

Many dental supply companies have developed educational materials for targeted populations. These materials are helpful to the dental hygienist and can be utilized by teachers and other health care workers. Moreover, many popular children's books and videos about dental health issues are also available.

Consumers also receive dental education and promotion through advertising, both in written form and through television. Many times television sitcoms discuss dental issues and even the role of dental hygienists. Sometimes this information is correct; however, these mass messages often give the population inaccurate information. Therefore, it is important for the dental hygienist to provide accurate and evidenced-based information to the population.

DENTAL HYGIENIST SPOTLIGHT

Public Health Column: Commander Cathy Hollister, RDH, PhD

The mission of the Public Health Service (PHS) Commissioned Corps is to protect, promote, and advance the health and safety of our Nation. Commander Cathy Hollister is a dental hygienist who works as a commissioned officer with the United States Public Health Service. She has been honored with more than ten awards in the Public Health Service and recently received the Navajo Area Director's Award for Health Promotion.

Commander Hollister has published articles on health behavior models and oral health in a variety

of periodicals and has presented talks on oral health all over the nation. She has presided as chair of the American Dental Hygienists' Association Council on Public Health and contributed to the ADHA Focus on Advancing the Profession paper. She has been instrumental in enhancing the role of dental hygiene in dental public health in a variety of venues and organizations and is constantly driven to build coalitions to effectively improve oral health status and the methods used to deliver care.

Commander Hollister has many professional accomplishments. She constantly promotes the skills of dental hygienists by effectively practicing dental hygiene in a variety of roles, subsequently providing quality care to the public.

I asked her several questions regarding her career.

Why did you decide to go into dental hygiene?

I knew I wanted to be in a health-related field. After high school, I volunteered in my dentist's office. I had a chance to observe many dental procedures, and I knew I wanted to work in dental care.

After practicing dental hygiene for a few years, I considered going back to dental school. I thought about it for a long time and decided I really wanted to stay in dental hygiene. I enjoyed the preventive side of dentistry and wanted to help people stay healthy rather than treat disease after it occurred.

How did you get into dental public health? Did you need additional education?

After working in private practices for eight years, I went to work in a community health center. That was my introduction to public health. I conducted a fluoride mouthrinse program in the schools and offered classroom education in many schools. Many of the students in the schools rarely saw a dentist, and the education they received at school was their only opportunity to learn about dental health and take control of their own oral health. I saw this as a real opportunity to improve the oral health of a large group of people, many of whom could not or did not have regular dental visits.

I knew I wanted to work in public health. I also knew I needed more education. At the time, I had an associate's degree in dental hygiene. I entered a certificate completion program to finish my bachelor's degree. Immediately following, I began to work on my master's degree in public health (MSPH). I had some public health education in my dental hygiene programs, but my MSPH gave me an excellent foundation for my present position.

I work in the US Public Health Service and after seven years in PHS, I entered a program to earn a doctorate in health services. I thought this education would help me improve the delivery of oral health services. I did my doctorate at a distance education university that allowed me great flexibility. I was able to study issues in oral health that affected utilization of health services, health education, and health care systems.

What is your current position?

Currently, I am the dental prevention officer with the Indian Health Services Gallup Service Unit, in Gallup, New Mexico. Additionally, I am the director of a dental hygiene clinic I developed and chair of the Medical Ethics Committee at Gallup Indian Medical Center. I also am an adjunct faculty member at the University of New Mexico, Division of Dental Hygiene in Albuquerque.

Please discuss any particularly interesting experiences you have had in your dental public health positions.

I have found it quite interesting to learn about the political side of health care. When I first began working in schools, I found that teachers may want to offer health education or services but could not because of so many demands on classroom time.

Nursing home aides wanted to do oral hygiene for the residents but often did not because of lack of time or because many residents needed dental services and none were available to them.

Public health has caused me to think about more than "How many patients do I have to see in a day?" It also has caused me to look past individual clinical care and look for community partners. I have had the opportunity to work with Head Start; Women, Infants and Children (WIC); diabetes programs; nursing homes; and schools. The most interesting and challenging aspect of working in public health has been finding common ground with nondental groups to increase oral health education, empower individuals to take charge of their own oral health, and increase access to dental services.

What type of advice would you give to a practicing hygienist who is thinking of doing something different?

First, enter a field you have a passion for. Second, make sure it is the right time in your life to make a change. Third, get adequate education or training. On-the-job training may be adequate if the change is very closely related to your current position, but if it is a major change, consider a degree program.

Source: Christine Nathe writes the Public Health Column in *RDH* magazine published by Pennwell Publishing. For more public health spotlights please see RDH magazine online at http://www.rdhmag.com/index.html.

Summary

Dental hygiene was the forerunner of the prevention movement now prevalent in public health care. Educating dental hygienists about preventive treatment modalities is vitally important to the public. Those involved in dental hygiene must continue to strive to meet the needs of the public by educating dental hygienists to provide effective preventive public-based care. Since the profession's inception, dental hygienists have worked to increase access to dental hygiene care provided by educated providers throughout the world, decrease barriers to the optimum level of dental hygiene care, and continue to provide care based on the evidence derived from dental hygiene research and practice.

Self-Study Test Items

1. What is referred to as a constituent member in the ADHA organization?
   a. National organizations
   b. State organizations
   c. Local organizations
   d. Student organizations

2. When is school fluoridation recommended?
   a. When an independent water source is available
   b. For children who have caries
   c. For children who have brown discolored areas on enamel
   d. None of the above

3. Demineralization, enhancement of remineralization, and inhibition of bacterial activity are examples of what?
   a. Water fluoridation
   b. Topical fluoridation
   c. Systemic fluoridation
   d. Fluoride supplements

4. Which type of fluoride increases children's risk of developing dental fluorosis?
   a. Supplements
   b. Systemic
   c. Topical
   d. Both a and b

5. When are sealants most effective?
   a. When applied without etchant
   b. When an assistant is utilized
   c. In the presence of saliva
   d. When material is cured for one minute

References

1. Bureau of Labor Statistics, US Department of Labor, *Occupational Outlook Handbook, 2014-15 Edition*, Dental Hygienists. Retrieved from http://www.bls.gov/ooh/healthcare/dental-hygienists.htm on September 17, 2015.

2. Fones AC. *Mouth Hygiene*. Philadelphia, PA: Lea & Febiger; 1916:59–504.

3. Fones AC. *Mouth Hygiene*. 2nd ed. Philadelphia, PA: Lea & Febiger; 1927:307–335.

4. Fones AC. *Mouth Hygiene*. 3rd ed. Philadelphia, PA: Lea & Febiger; 1927:307–335.

5. Fones AC. *Mouth Hygiene*. 4th ed. Philadelphia, PA: Lea & Febiger; 1934:329–359.

6. Fones AC. Origin and history. *J Am Dent Hyg Assoc.* 1929;(3):9–10.

7. Motley WE. *History of the American Dental Hygienists' Association 1923–1982*. Chicago, IL: American Dental Hygienists' Association; 1983.

8. Ottolengui R. The inauguration of a serious effort to establish a system of education for the dental hygienist. *Dent Items of Int.* 1914;36(1):6.

9. Personal Notes. Alfred C. Fones, DDS. Bridgeport, CT. Circa 1900s.

10. Code of Alabama/Alabama Dental Practice Act Alabama State Code & Rules of the Board of Dental Examiners of Alabama Published by Board of Dental Examiners of Alabama updated August 2013. Retrieved from http://www.dentalboard.org/pdf/Code-Rules%20for%20Web%20complete%20Aug%202013.pdf on September 22, 2014.

11. *Direct Access States*. Chicago, IL: American Dental Hygienists' Association; 2014. Retrieved from http://www.adha.org/resources-docs/7513_Direct_Access_to_Care_from_DH.pdf on July 30, 2015.

12. History of the Connecticut Dental Hygienists' Association. *J Am Dent Hyg Assoc.* 1931;5:26.

13. American Dental Hygienists' Association. Bylaws Code of Ethics. Chicago, IL: American Dental Hygienists' Association; Adopted June 23, 2014. Retrieved from https://www.adha.org/resources-docs/7611_Bylaws_and_Code_of_Ethics.pdf on July 30, 2015

14. US Public Health Service. *Healthy People 2020*. Washington, DC: US Dept of Health and Human Services; 2010.

15. Tooth care: So easy a caveman could do it? *USA Today*. September 12, 2007:5D.

16. US Dept of Health and Human Services. *A National Call to Action to Promote Oral Health*. Rockville, MD: US Dept of Health and Human Services, Public Health Service, Centers for Disease Control and Prevention, National Institutes of Health, National Institute of Dental and Craniofacial Research; 2003. NIH Publication No. 03-5303.

17. The Role of Dental Hygienists in Providing Access to Oral Health Care. January 2014. National Governor's Association: Washington DC. Retrieved from http://www.nga.org/cms/home/nga-center-for-best-practices/center-publications/page-health-publications/col2-content/main-content-list/the-role-of-dental-hygienists-in.html on July 30, 2015.

18. *Improving Access to Oral Health Care for Vulnerable and Underserved Populations*. Washington, DC: The National Academies Press. Retrieved from http://iom.nationalacademies.org/Reports/2011/Improving-Access-to-Oral-Health-Care-for-Vulnerable-and-Underserved-Populations.aspx on July 30, 2015.

19. PEW Charitable Trust. Children's Dental Policy: Most States Lack on Dental Sealants. Washington DC: PEW. 2014. Retrieved from http://www.pewtrusts.org/en/multimedia/data-visualizations/2013/most-states-lag-on-dental-sealants on July 30, 2015.

20. American Dental Association. *2010 Survey of Dental Practices.* Chicago: American Dental Association Store.

21. Peterson PE. World Health Organization global policy for improvement of oral health – World Health Assembly 2007. *International Dental Journal* (2008) 58, 115–121. Retrieved from http://www.who.int/oral_health/publications/IDJ_June_08.pdf

22. American Dental Hygienists' Association. *National Dental Hygiene Research Agenda.* Chicago, IL: American Dental Hygienists' Association; 2007.

23. The Professional Practice Environment of Dental Hygienists in the Fifty States and the District of Columbia, 2001. National Center for Health Workforce Analysis, Bureau of Health Professions, Health Resources and Services Administration; 2004. Contract No. HRSA 230-00-0099; Newbrun E. *Fluorides and Dental Caries.* Springfield, IL: Charles C. Thomas; 1986; National Research Council. *Health Effects of Ingested Fluoride.* Washington, DC: National Academy Press; 1993.

24. Recommendations for using fluoride to prevent and control dental caries in the United States. *MMWR Morb Mortal Wkly Rpt.* 2001;50(RR14):1–42.

25. Newbrun E. Effectiveness of water fluoridation. *J Public Health Dent.* 1989;49:279–289.

26. Kamel MS, Thomson WM, Drummond BK. Fluoridation and dental caries severity in young children treated under general anaesthesia: an analysis of treatment records in a 10-year case series. *Community Dent Health.* 2013 Mar;30(1):15–18

27. The relation of mottled enamel to caries. *JADA.* 1928;15:429–437.

28. The Story of Water Fluoridation. Bethesda, MD: National Institute of Dental and Craniofacial Research; 2008. Retrieved from http://www.nidcr.nih.gov/oralhealth/topics/fluoride/thestoryoffluoridation.htm on July, 22, 2013.

29. Centers for Disease Control and Prevention. 2012 Water Fluoridation Reporting System (WFRS). Retrieved from http://www.cdc.gov/fluoridation/statistics/2012stats.htm on September 17, 2015.

30. Engineering and administrative recommendations for water fluoridation, 1995. *MMWR Morb Mortal Wkly Rpt.* 1995;44(RR-13):1–40.

31. Riley JC, Lennon MA, Ellwood RP. The effect of water fluoridation and social inequalities on dental caries in 5-year-old children. *Int J Epidemiol.* 1999;28:300–305.

32. Federal Register/Vol. 76, No. 9/Thursday, January 13, 2011/Notices. Page 2384.

33. Newbrun E. *Fluorides and Dental Caries.* Springfield, IL: Charles C. Thomas; 1986; National Research Council. *Health Effects of Ingested Fluoride.* Washington, DC: National Academy Press; 1993.

34. Topping G, Assaf A. Strong evidence that daily use of fluoride toothpaste prevents caries. *Acta Odonto Scand.* 2003;61(6):347–355.

35. Marinho VCC, Higgins JPT, Logan S, Sheiham A. Fluoride mouthrinses for preventing dental caries in children and adolescents. *Cochrane Database of Systematic Reviews.* 2003;3(CD002284.DOI:10.1002/14651858.CD002284).

36. Englander HR, Keyes, PH, Gestwicki M. Clinical anticaries effect of repeated topical sodium fluoride applications by mouthpieces. *JADA.* 1967;75:638.

37. Marinho VCC, Higgins JPT, Logan S, Sheiham A. Fluoride varnishes for preventing dental caries in children and adolescents. *Cochrane Database of Systematic Reviews.* 2002;3(CD002279. DOI: 10.1002/14651858.CD002279).

38. Dental sealants in the prevention of tooth decay. *NIH Consens Dev Conf Consens Statement 1983.* 1983;4(11): 1–18.

39. Simonsen RJ. Retention and effectiveness of a single application of white sealant after 10 years. *JADA.* 1987;115:31–36.

40. Griffin SO, Oong E, Kohn B, et al. The effectiveness of sealants in managing caries lesions. *Dent Res.* 2008;87: 169–174.

41. Beltrán-Aguilar ED, Barker LK, Canto MT, et al. Surveillance for dental caries, dental sealants, tooth retention, edentulism, and enamel fluorosis—United States, 1988–1994 and 1999–2002. *MMWR Morb Mortal Wkly Rpt.* 2005;54(3):1–44.

42. Bravo M, Montero J, Bravo JJ, Baca P, Llodra JC. Sealant and fluoride varnish in caries: a randomized trial. *J Dent Res.* 2005;84(12):1138–1143.

43. Ahovuo-Saloranta A, Forss H, Walsh T, et al. Sealants for preventing dental decay in the permanent teeth. *Cochrane Database Syst Rev.* 2013 Mar 28;3:CD001830. doi: 10.1002/14651858.CD001830.pub4.

44. Azarpazhooh A, Main PA. Pit and fissure sealants in the prevention of dental caries in children and adolescents: a systematic review. *J Can Dent Assoc.* 2008 Mar;74(2):171–177.

45. Frencken JE, Leal SC, Navarro MF. Twenty-five-year atraumatic restorative treatment (ART) approach: a comprehensive overview. *Clin Oral Investig.* 2012 Oct;16(5):1337–1346. doi: 10.1007/s00784-012-0783-4. Epub 2012 Jul 24.

46. American Academy of Pediatrics Dentistry Policy on alternative restorative treatment (ART). *Reference Manual.* 2008;29(7). Retrieved from http://www.aapd.org/media/Policies_Guidelines/P_ART.pdf on July 18, 2013.

47. Stecksén-Blicks C, Holgerson PL, Twetman S. Effect of xylitol and xylitol-fluoride lozenges on approximal caries development in high-caries-risk children. *Int J Paediatri Dent.* 2008;18(3):170–177.

48. Bader JD, Vollmer WM, Shugars DA, et al. Results from the Xylitol for Adult Caries Trial (X-ACT). *J Am Dent Assoc.* 2013 Jan;144(1):21–30.

49. *American Dental Hygienists' Association: Bylaws.* Chicago, IL: American Dental Hygienists' Association; 2013.

50. Position of the American Dietetic Association: Oral health and nutrition. *J Am Diet Assoc.* 2007;107(8):1418–1428.

51. Oral Cancer Facts. Retrieved from http://www.oralcancer-foundation.org/facts on September 8, 2015.

52. Rautava J, Syrjänen S. Human papillomavirus infections in the oral mucosa. *J Am Dent Assoc.* 2011 Aug;142(8):905–914.

53. Oral Cancer 5-Year Survival Rates by Race, Gender, and Stage of Diagnosis. Retrieved from http://www.nidcr.nih.gov/datastatistics/finddatabytopic/oralcancer/oralcancer5yearsurvivalrates.htm on July 19, 2013.

54. OralCDx BrushTest. Retrieved from http://www.sopreventable.com/brushtest.htm. On April 23, 2008.

55. Ebihara A, Krasieva TB, Liaw LL, et al. Detection and diagnosis of oral cancer by light-induced fluorescence. *Lasers in Surg and Med.* 2003;32:17–24.

56. Tobacco control activities in US dental practices. *JADA.* 1997;18:172.

57. Ask, Advise, Refer Tobacco Cessation Program. American Dental Hygienists' Association. Retrieved from http://jdh.adha.org/content/78/3/5.full.pdf. onJuly 30, 2015.

58. Nathe CN. Athletic mouthguards. In: Harris, NO, Garcia-Godoy, F, Nathe, CN, eds. *Primary Preventive Dentistry*. 7th ed. Upper Saddle River, NJ: Pearson; 2008:388.

59. American Dental Association. Using mouthguards to reduce the incidence and severity of sports-related oral injuries. *J Am Dent Assoc.* 2006;37:1712–1720.

Visit www.pearsonhighered.com/healthprofessionsresources to access the student resources that accompany this book. Simply select Dental Hygiene from the choice of disciplines. Find this book and you will find the complimentary study tools created for this specific title.

Dental Care Delivery in the United States

OBJECTIVES

After studying this chapter, the dental hygiene student should be able to:

- Describe the state of dental health in the United States
- Identify the government agencies related to dental hygiene
- Compare the functions of federal, state, and local government in dental care delivery
- Describe dental workforce issues
- Define *need, supply, demand*, and *utilization*

COMPETENCIES

After studying this chapter and participating in accompanying course activities, the dental hygiene student should be competent to do the following:

- Assess the oral health needs and services of the community to determine action plans and the availability of resources to meet health care needs
- Facilitate patient access to oral health services by influencing individuals or organizations regarding the provision of oral health care
- Pursue career options within health care, industry, education research and other roles as they evolve for the dental hygienist.
- Access professional and social networks to pursue professional goals

KEY TERMS

Demand *41*
Dental care delivery *35*
Medicaid *39*
Need *41*
Supply *41*
Utilization *41*
Workforce *38*

Science photo/Shutterstock

Dental care delivery refers to the way dental care is provided to the public. In the United States, dental care delivery involves a number of different private and government entities. Although most dental hygienists are employed by private practice dentists, many dental hygiene positions are available with government- or community-based organizations that may be funded by government or private sources. This chapter describes the infrastructure including the federal and state entities that play a role in dental care as well as concepts germane to the utilization of dental care services and dental workforce models.

Landmark reports suggest that all populations within the United States do not access oral health care in an equitable fashion.[1,2,3,4] Although dental diseases are preventable, many disparities in preventive dental care exist. Untreated dental disease is more prevalent in individuals from lower-income households and ethnic minorities.[1–4]

Oral health is an integral part of total health. Research has associated periodontal diseases to heart, lung, and a number of other systemic diseases, diabetes, pneumonia, and premature, low-birth-weight babies. Prevention and early intervention are strategies long recognized across health disciplines as being effective in terms of dollars spent on health care and minimizing or eliminating human pain and suffering. Dental hygiene science, which emphasizes disease prevention and treatment of oral infection, fits perfectly into an interdisciplinary model to provide comprehensive health care to all populations.

Delivery of Dental Care in the United States

Private dental practices for the most part provide dental care delivery in the United States. Figure 3-1 ■ depicts the agents involved in the delivery of dental care: dentists, dental hygienists, dental assistants, denturists (in some states), dental therapists or advanced dental therapists (in some states), expanded function dental providers, and dental laboratory technicians. Historically, many Americans obtained their care from private dental and dental hygiene providers with employer-offered dental insurance or out-of-pocket as the reimbursement mechanism. The trend may be changing as more Americans depend on publicly funded sources to pay for dental care

services. The government plays a role in funding and regulating dental care delivery.

Did You Know?

Denturists are dental providers who construct and deliver removable oral prostheses (dentures and partial dentures) directly to the patient.

Many federal and state governmental entities impact dental care delivery. Additionally, states impose practice acts and rules and regulations to govern the practice of dental hygiene, which is discussed in Chapter 6.

Federal Structure of Dental Public Health

The executive branch of the federal government has a direct impact on dental care delivery. The Department of Health and Human Services (HHS) is responsible for many entities providing dental care.

Department of Health and Human Services

The HHS is the government's principal agency for protecting the health of all Americans and providing essential human services, especially for those who are least able to help themselves. The HHS includes more than 300 programs, covering a wide spectrum of activities. (See Box 3-1 ■.) The HHS administers more grant dollars than all other federal agencies combined, and the Medicare and Medicaid programs provide health care insurance for one in three Americans. The HHS works closely with state and local governments, and many HHS-funded services are provided at the local level by state or county agencies or private sector grantees. See Figure 3-2 ■ for the HHS organizational chart. The secretary of the department, who directs the HHS, is appointed by the president of the United States.

US Public Health Service Commissioned Corps

The US Public Health Service (PHS) works to improve and advance the health of our nation's people. It includes

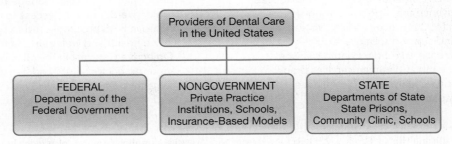

FIGURE 3–1 Dental Care Delivery in the United States

several separate entities. The PHS Commissioned Corps, which is directed by the US Surgeon General, was established by Congress in 1889. Congress organized the PHS along military lines with titles and pay corresponding to army and navy grades. Officers are currently commissioned in twelve professional categories representing the breadth of health care professionals. Dental hygienists, with a bachelor's degree are eligible to be commissioned as a US PHS Health Services Officer.

National Institutes of Health

The National Institutes of Health (NIH), headquartered in Bethesda, Maryland, is the government's medical research organization, supporting some 38,000 research projects nationwide in diseases such as cancer, Alzheimer's disease, diabetes, arthritis, cardiovascular diseases, and AIDS. The NIH has twenty-seven separate health institutes, including the National Institute of Dental and Craniofacial Research (NIDCR), which focuses on research in the oral health sciences. Dental hygienists with advanced degrees may have opportunities in this research organization.

Food and Drug Administration

The Food and Drug Administration (FDA), which was established in 1906 and headquartered in Rockville, Maryland, ensures the safety of foods and cosmetics as well as the safety and efficacy of pharmaceuticals, biological products, and medical devices. It is responsible for regulating dental materials, dental equipment, and over-the-counter dental care products.

Did You Know?

Products regulated by the FDA represent almost 20 cents out of every dollar in consumer spending in the United States.

Centers for Disease Control and Prevention

The Centers for Disease Control and Prevention (CDC) provides a system of health surveillance to prevent the outbreak of diseases and monitor any that do occur. It also

Box 3–1 Strategic Plan of the US Department of Health and Human Services

- Strategic Goal 1: Strengthen Health Care
  - **Objective A:** Make coverage more secure for those who have insurance, and extend affordable coverage to the uninsured
  - **Objective B:** Improve health care quality and patient safety
  - **Objective C:** Emphasize primary and preventive care, linked with community prevention services
  - **Objective D:** Reduce the growth of health care costs while promoting high-value, effective care
  - **Objective E:** Ensure access to quality, culturally competent care, including long-term services and supports, for vulnerable populations
  - **Objective F:** Improve health care and population health through meaningful use of health information technology
- Strategic Goal 2: Advance Scientific Knowledge and Innovation
  - **Objective A:** Accelerate the process of scientific discovery to improve health
  - **Objective B:** Foster and apply innovative solutions to health, public health, and human services challenges
  - **Objective C:** Advance the regulatory sciences to enhance food safety, improve medical product development, and support tobacco regulation
  - **Objective D:** Increase our understanding of what works in public health and human services practice
  - **Objective E:** Improve laboratory, surveillance, and epidemiology capacity

- Strategic Goal 3: Advance the Health, Safety, and Well-Being of the American People
  - **Objective A:** Promote the safety, well-being, resilience, and healthy development of children and youth
  - **Objective B:** Promote economic and social well-being for individuals, families, and communities
  - **Objective C:** Improve the accessibility and quality of supportive services for people with disabilities and older adults
  - **Objective D:** Promote prevention and wellness across the life span
  - **Objective E:** Reduce the occurrence of infectious diseases
  - **Objective F:** Protect Americans' health and safety during emergencies, and foster resilience to withstand and respond to emergencies
- Strategic Goal 4: Ensure Efficiency, Transparency, Accountability, and Effectiveness of HHS Programs
  - **Objective A:** Strengthen program integrity and responsible stewardship by reducing improper payments, fighting fraud, and integrating financial, performance, and risk management
  - **Objective B:** Enhance access to and use of data to improve HHS programs and to support improvements in the health and well-being of the American people
  - **Objective C:** Invest in the HHS workforce to help meet America's health and human services needs
  - **Objective D:** Improve HHS environmental, energy, and economic performance to promote sustainability

Source: Department of Health and Human Services. 2014. Retrieved from http://www.hhs.gov/about/strategic-plan/index.htmlon July 31, 2015.

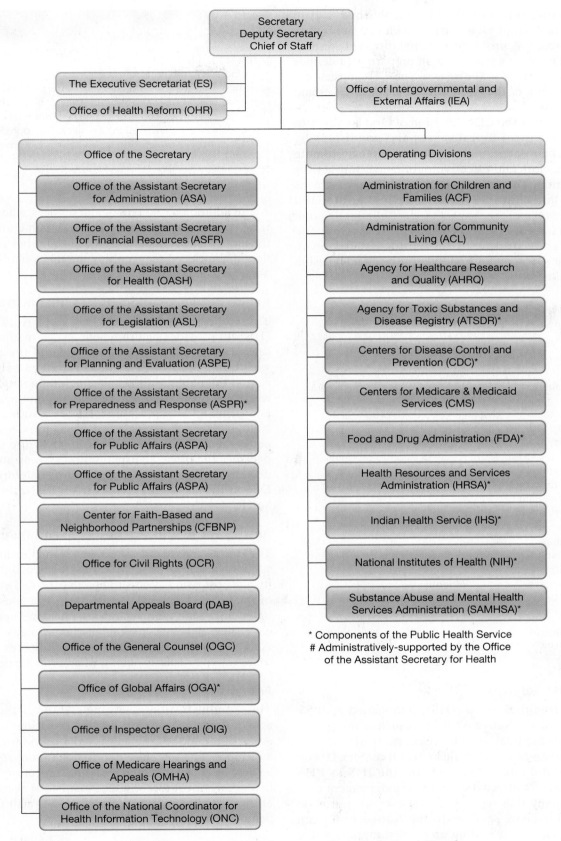

FIGURE 3–2 US Department of Health and Human Services: Organizational Chart

Source: http://www.hhs.gov/about/orgchart.html. Accessed September 2, 2008.

maintains national health statistics. Established in 1946 and located in Atlanta, Georgia, it provides immunization services to guard against international disease transmission. The CDC plays a major role in preparing guidelines for the prevention of oral diseases. The CDC director is also administrator of the Agency for Toxic Substances and Disease Registry.

The mission of the CDC Division of Oral Health is to prevent and control oral diseases and conditions by building the knowledge, tools, and networks that promote healthy behaviors and effective public health practices and programs. They have identified goals such as preventing and controlling dental caries, periodontal disease, and oral and pharyngeal cancers; eliminating oral health disparities; promoting dental prevention; and increasing state oral health program effectiveness. Box 3-2 ■ lists the specific strategies of the CDC Division of Oral Health.

Box 3–2 CDC Division of Oral Health

The CDC's Division of Oral Health (DOH) works to improve the oral health of the nation and reduce inequalities in oral health by—

- Helping states improve their oral health programs
- Extending the use of proven strategies to prevent oral disease by—
  - Encouraging the effective use of fluoride products and community water fluoridation
  - Promoting greater use of school-based and -linked dental sealant programs
- Enhancing efforts to monitor oral diseases, such as dental caries (tooth decay) and periodontal infections (gum disease)
- Contributing to the scientific knowledge base regarding oral health and disease
- Guiding infection control in dentistry
- Helping states improve their oral health programs

Source: CDC Work 2014. Retrieved from http://www.cdc.gov/oralhealth/about/index.htm on November 5, 2014.

Indian Health Services

The Indian Health Service (IHS), established in 1955, provides 1.8 million Native Americans, including Alaskan Natives, with medical and dental care. It also assists thirty-four urban Native American health centers. Dental hygienists and dentists can work for the IHS as PHS commissioned officers, civil servants, or independent contractors. In many IHS settings, dental assistants provide some dental hygiene services to the Native American population, including scaling and polishing and some restorative services. In fact, because of the shortage of dentists in rural Alaska, dental therapists provide restorative services.

Did You Know?

The federal government first offered health services for Indians in the early nineteenth century when US army physicians took steps to curb smallpox and other contagious diseases among tribes living in the vicinity of military posts. By 1880, the first federal hospital was built in Oklahoma making health care available to Indians. By 1913, dentists were visiting reservations and schools to provide dental services.[5]

In addition to the IHS dental services, many individual tribes offer dental services and maintain clinics. Each of the more than 560 federally recognized tribes govern tribal dental clinics and may employ dental hygienists, dentists, and dental assistants.

Health Resources and Services Administration

The Health Resources and Services Administration (HRSA) provides health resources for medically underserved populations and works to build the health care **workforce,** the workers whose members deliver health care to the public. This agency operates a nationwide network of community health centers, migrant health centers, and primary care programs. HRSA also maintains the National Health Service Corps, which provides services to people with AIDS through the Ryan White CARE Act, oversees the organ transplantation system, and works to decrease infant mortality and improve children's health. Dental hygienists may serve with the National Health Service Corps.

Agency for Healthcare Research and Quality

The Agency for Healthcare Research and Quality (AHRQ) supports research on health care systems, health care quality and cost issues, access to health care, and effectiveness of medical treatments. AHRQ also provides evidence-based information on health care outcomes and quality of care. These data include oral health information. Using the AHRQ reports on dental use, expenditures, and payer source are particularly helpful when studying dental issues.

Administration on Aging

The Administration on Aging (AOA) is the principal agency designated to carry out the provisions of the Older Americans Act of 1965 and is responsible for enhancing and supporting the older population's independence. The agency has been involved in dental education in geriatric dental care. Most recently, the AoA has worked to identify and promote community-based programs that provide dental services to older adults.

Administration for Children and Families

The Administration for Children and Families (ACF) is responsible for federal programs that promote the

economic and social well-being of families, children, individuals, and communities and is responsible for the Early Head Start and Head Start programs, which provide educational, social, medical, dental, nutritional, and mental health services to pregnant mothers and children up to five years old from low-income families.

Did You Know?

In many states, dental hygienists provide education and preventive treatment to children enrolled in Head Start programs. The title Head Start describes giving children in need a "head start" to their future.

Centers for Medicare & Medicaid Services

The Centers for Medicare & Medicaid Services (CMS), formerly known as the Health Care Financing Administration (HCFA), is the federal agency responsible for administering the Medicare, Medicaid, Children's Health Insurance Program (CHIP), Health Insurance Portability and Accountability Act (HIPAA), Clinical Laboratory Improvement Amendments (CLIA), and several other health-related programs. CMS also oversees the federal portion of the Medicaid program and has full responsibility for the Medicare program. Medicare funds cover medical care for people who are elderly and/or disabled. In specific cases, Medicare may provide reimbursement for dental procedures carried out in the hospital on elderly or disabled individuals, but it generally does not fund dental care.

Medicaid is the program that traditionally funds dental care to the indigent population and is administered by states. Medicaid insurance can be paid to dentists and, in some states, dental hygienists in private practice or community clinical settings.

Medicare and Medicaid are the two largest federal health care programs and account for about 80 percent of annual federal health care expenditures. The CMS also runs CHIP, the largest effort by Congress since Medicaid was enacted thirty-two years ago to provide health insurance to vulnerable children throughout the United States. Enacted as part of the Balanced Budget Act of 1997, it addresses the health care needs of 10 million medically uninsured children. CHIP is distinct from Medicaid in that it entitles states, but not individual children, to allotments of federal funds to purchase child health assistance; it pays a 30 percent higher share of program costs than Medicaid, and it gives states more latitude in program design, including eligibility, benefits, cost sharing, and administration. Chapter 5 discusses in detail the financial aspects of Medicaid and CHIP.

Other Federal Dental Health Programs

Many other federal departments impact dental health, including the Departments of Agriculture, Defense, Education, Justice, Labor, State, Treasury, and Veterans Affairs. Dental hygienists have opportunities to work in various federal government positions and settings. (See Table 3-1 ■.) To qualify for a civil service dental hygiene position, a candidate must be a US citizen and undergo a thorough background investigation to receive a security clearance. In many instances, a bachelor's degree may be required.

Table 3–1 Federal Dental Hygiene Settings and Positions

Department/Agency	Settings/Positions
Agriculture	Women, Infant, Children (WIC) preventive educator
Defense	Military base dental clinician
Justice	Federal prison dental clinician
Health and Human Services	Public Health Service commissioned officer
	Early Head Start and Head Start dental educator/provider
	CDC/HRSA/NIDCR researcher/administrator
Peace Corps (Agency)	Developing country dental clinician/educator
State	Civil service position with military, VA hospital, or other governmental agency
Veterans Affairs	VA hospital dental clinician

Food, nutrition counseling, and access to health and dental services are provided to low-income women, infants, and children under the Special Supplemental Nutrition Program for Women, Infants, and Children (WIC). Specifically, its programs collaborate with dental hygiene programs and community dental clinics to offer dental screenings and dental health education. The Food and Nutrition Services of the Department of Agriculture administers WIC at the federal level, providing federal grants to states for their WIC programs. Most state WIC programs provide vouchers that participants use at authorized food stores.

The Department of Defense oversees the dental care of military dental personnel and their dependents often provided by dentists in the military and enlisted dental technicians. One interesting facet of dental care delivery in the military is that in some military branch dental settings, enlisted dental technicians provide supragingival scalings and coronal polishing, which are termed prophylaxis without having graduated from an accredited dental hygiene program or taking the national and regional dental hygiene board examinations. This practice, however, is becoming less common. Dental hygienists may work as civil servants or independent contractors for the Department of Defense, and dental hygienists with Bachelor of Science degrees may be commissioned as military officers. Dependents of military personnel generally receive care through the dental providers participating in the dental insurance program available to them through military benefits.

Did You Know?

Dental hygienists are being hired more frequently to provide dental hygiene care and education in military bases around the United States.

In the United States, inmates have a constitutional right to health care. The Department of Justice is responsible for the Federal Bureau of Prisons and therefore the dental care provided to prisoners. Dentists and dental hygienists may work as US PHS officers, civil servants, or independent contractors. Settings can vary from prison camps for minor offenders to maximum-security prisons. Providing dental hygiene to this population decreases cost by decreasing the need for restorative services.

Many dental hygienists practice in facilities under the Department of Veterans Affairs (VA), treating veterans with service-connected dental disabilities. Dentists, dental hygienists, assistants, and technicians are usually employed as civil servants. Occasionally, VA dental services treat members who have left military service but did not complete their dental care as well as veterans who reside in long-term care facilities at the individual VA medical centers. With the increase in the number of veterans during the past decade, dental hygienists in this setting are able to provide a variety of services, including educating patients and nurses and offering clinical treatment within the dental clinic and at the bedside.

The Bureau of Labor Statistics (BLS), which is organizationally housed within the Department of Labor, is the principal fact-finding agency for the federal government in the broad field of labor, economics, and statistics. BLS collects, processes, analyzes, and disseminates essential statistical data to the American public, the Congress and federal agencies, state and local governments, business, and labor. The BLS forecasts dental and dental hygiene workforce need and demand for future years. Box 3-3 ■ depicts some of the information BLS updates annually regarding dental hygiene.

Box 3–3 Bureau of Labor Statistics Information on Dental Hygienists

Quick Facts: Dental Hygienists	
2012 Median Pay	$70,210 per year $33.75 per hour
Entry-Level Education	Associate's degree
Work Experience in a Related Occupation	None
On-the-job Training	None
Number of Jobs, 2012	192,800
Job Outlook, 2012–22	33% (Much faster than average)
Employment Change, 2012–22	64,200

Source: Bureau of Labor Statistics, US Department of Labor, *Occupational Outlook Handbook, 2014–2015 Edition.* On the Internet at http://www.bls.gov/ooh/healthcare/dental-hygienists.htm (visited November 05, 2014).

The Department of Treasury is responsible for the manufacturing and labeling of alcohol and tobacco products. This work is important in promoting health-related problems that are often acquired by use of these products. Box 3-4 ■ depicts the warnings of which one must appear on smokeless tobacco products.

The Department of Education's (DOE) mission is to ensure equal access to education and to promote educational excellence for all Americans. The DOE provides federal financial aid policies to many dental hygiene students.

The Peace Corps, an independent agency within the executive branch of the federal government, was formally initiated in 1961. The president of the United States appoints the Peace Corps director and deputy director who must be confirmed by the Senate. The Senate Foreign Relations Committee and the House Committee on International Relations have general oversight of Peace Corps activities and programs.

Box 3–4 Warning Label Statements on Smokeless Tobacco Products

WARNING: This product can cause mouth cancer

WARNING: This product can cause gum disease and tooth loss

WARNING: This product is not a safe alternative to cigarettes

WARNING: Smokeless tobacco is addictive

Source: Section 3 of the Comprehensive Smokeless Tobacco Health Education Act of 1986 (15 U.S.C. 4402). Retrieved from http://www.fda.gov/syn/html/ucm261997.htm on November 5, 2014.

Did You Know?

Dental hygienists can provide dental hygiene treatment and education as Peace Corps volunteers.

Structure of State Dental Public Health

All states, Washington, DC, and US territories have departments that provide health and human services to those in need. The departments may have different names, but all share a similar mission that includes preventing disease and promoting health, ensuring access to health care, and managing public health resources.

State health departments include dental divisions whose directors work as dental consultants within the state. Dental hygienists may be employed as state dental directors in many states. Many of these departments work to implement water fluoridation within communities, school-based prevention programs, school sealant programs, and fluoride mouth rinse programs. Some state health departments are in charge of the CHIP program as well. The human services division of the state health department usually operates Medicaid programs, which are often operated by a third party, generally an insurance company.

Did You Know?

The American Association of State and Territorial Dental Directors (AASTDD) provides leadership to advocate a governmental oral health presence in each state and territory and to assist in the development of initiatives for prevention and control of oral diseases.

Many states operate community clinics to provide dental care, and some states own and operate community clinics, many of which employ dental hygienists to provide services. Some of these clinics are private, and many are nonprofit but sometimes receive sliding scale reimbursements and Medicaid payments. State dental clinics can be federally qualified heath centers (FQHCs), meaning that they qualify for enhanced reimbursement from Medicaid and other benefits. FQHCs must provide services for an underserved area or population, offer a sliding fee scale, provide comprehensive services, have an ongoing quality assurance program, and have a governing board of directors.

Did You Know?

Some clinics actually are designated as FQHC's Look-Alikes and operate much like a FQHC.

Although some of these clinics are in an urban or metropolitan setting, many operate in rural or small town settings. Populations can be underserved whether they live in a rural setting or metropolitan setting depending on factors discussed in Chapter 10.

State or private organizations operate state prison systems that are separate from the Federal Bureau of Prisons. Sometimes dental hygienists are hired directly by a state prison system, but many times they are hired by a private health care organization to provide care in a state prison setting.

States may also have tribal dental clinics that usually follow guidelines established within the tribe. In some instances, the IHS provides assistances. Dental hygienists are often employed in these clinics and may provide care in migrant clinics as well.

Many states provide dental care to the elderly and those populations with disabilities in residential dental clinic settings. Care to these groups is difficult to obtain in private dental practices because of the difficulty in transportation, low reimbursement rates, treatment specialization needed, and financial instability.

Dental Health Care Workforce

In the United States, *pluralism* refers to the way of organizing and providing health care services because of the diversity of values, populations, and entities involved.[6] The dental care delivery system is a mixture of organizations, practitioners, financing mechanisms, and innovative approaches to health care.

Those concerned with planning to meet health labor force requirements attach a specific meaning to the concepts of need, demand, utilization, and supply. **Need** can be defined as a normative, professional judgment as to the amount and kind of health care services required to attain or maintain health. The particular or desired frequency of dental care utilized by a population is **demand,** and the amount of dental care services available can be termed **supply. Utilization** is the number of dental care services actually consumed, not just desired, which can be important when speculating on the available supply of personnel to meet the demand and/or need. One example of the difference between need and demand is demonstrated with children's athletic teams. Players on these teams have high

rates of oral-facial injuries and concussions, and professional recommendations mandate the use of mouth guards, preferably custom-made; however, many young athletes across the country do not wear them. In this case, the need is present—oral health professionals have determined that using mouth guards will maintain health—but the demand by consumers is not because they are not using them as desired. Now, assume that consumers' demand is great, but their communities lack the dental providers to fabricate the mouth guards. This scenario would change the equation by not having the supply to meet the demand and the need.

Another example could include a constituent (state) dental hygienists' association conducting a study of the number of unfilled dental hygiene appointments per week as reported by dental hygienists (demand). In that very same state, the state dental division conducted a study on the prevalence of periodontal diseases in the state among adults (need). If results suggested that there were many dental hygiene appointment left unfilled and there were also a majority of adults with periodontal disease, that would imply that the need is greater than the demand. Adults are not accessing dental care (demand), but they should be because of the prevalence of periodontal disease (need).

The federal guidelines forecast the number of dentists needed for a population but do not include the number of dental hygienists necessary. Adequate dental capacity as suggested by the National Health Professional Shortage Area (HPSA) is designated as one dentist per 5000 population.[7,8] Furthermore, the appropriate dentist-to-population ratio for a special consideration population, such as a state facility or reservation, has been estimated at one dentist per 4000 population.

Dental Workforce Issues

The landmark 2000 Oral Health in America report concluded that the public health workforce was not sufficient to meet the dental needs of the underserved.[1] The reasons for this include barriers to oral health care access, lack of insurance or payment options, tremendous growth of the aging population, limited means of transportation, and insufficient availability of dental providers.[1-4] These issues have resulted in the development of innovative models of delivery and proposed additions to the dental team.

MODELS OF CARE   Although the provision of dental hygiene originated in schools, in most states it has not been practiced there. However, schoolchildren in an increasing number of states are receiving preventive dental care. In some states, schools also provide restorative care. Sometimes this is accomplished with mobile dental programs,

but recently school-based health clinics have begun to hire dental hygienists. Preventive dental care also is being brought into Early Head Start and Head Start programs, WIC programs, and nursing facilities.

Another opportunity to bring prevention to the people is to place dental hygienists in pediatric offices, primary care clinics, and hospitals. Positioning dental hygienists within health care systems allows them to provide the missing link between total health and oral health. This also provides an effective referral mechanism with local dentists. Bringing care *to* populations in need is one solution to the oral health disparities witnessed today.

DENTIST WORKFORCE   Although the American Dental Association (ADA) projects an increase in the aggregate number of dentists over the next two decades, the increase will not keep pace with the projected population growth.[9] Additionally, the BLS projects that the number of dentists is expected to grow by 16 percent from 2012 to 2022, faster than the average for all occupations. Dentists will continue to see an increase in public demand for their services as studies continue to link oral health to overall health.[10]

A large number of aging dentists are projected to retire from practice during the next ten to fifteen years.[11] During the next decade, two dentists will retire for every new graduate.[12] In addition, geographic distribution of dentists remains unbalanced. In large metropolitan areas, the dentist-to-population ratio was 61 per 100,000 as compared to 29 dentists per 100,000 in rural areas.[13]

In many instances, individuals from rural or frontier areas of the country have more difficulties accessing dental care than their counterparts in urban or metropolitan areas, because where there are fewer people living, there are also fewer dentists residing. Many times individuals living in remote locations need to travel long distances to access dental care. (See Figure 3-3 ■.)

Although these data suggest a possible issue with the dental workforce, more dental schools have been opening, existing dental schools have increased enrollment, and there may be a trend in decreasing dental visits by Americans due in part to the economic downturn in the past several years. With this in mind, it is difficult to state that there is a shortage or surplus of dentists in the United States.

DEMAND FOR DENTAL HYGIENISTS   Dental hygiene continues to grow as a profession, and the market continues to dictate the need for dental hygiene providers. Dental hygienists held about 192,800 jobs in 2012, and employment of dental hygienists is expected to grow by 33 percent from 2012 to 2022, much faster than the average for all occupations.

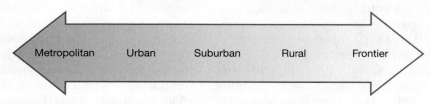

Metropolitan   Urban   Suburban   Rural   Frontier

FIGURE 3–3 Geography and Population Terms

Ongoing research linking oral health and general health will continue to spur the demand for preventive dental services, which are often provided by dental hygienists.[14]

To meet the increasing demand for dental hygiene, facilities that provide dental care, particularly dentists' offices, will increasingly employ dental hygienists, and more per office, to perform services that dentists have performed in the past. Older dentists who have been less likely to employ dental hygienists are leaving the profession and will be replaced by recent graduates, who are more likely to employ dental hygienists. In addition, as dentists' workloads increase, they are expected to hire more hygienists to perform preventive dental care, such as cleaning, so that they may devote their own time to more complex procedures.[14]

DENTURISTS *Denturists* are trained to provide complete oral examinations and evaluation of patients and to directly provide them removable dentures and fit them properly.[15] They are legally allowed to practice in only a few states. Although fairly new to the United States, denturists have the potential to provide care to many older adults.

DENTAL THERAPISTS Beginning in 2000, Alaska Native tribal health organizations developed the Alaska Dental Health Therapist Initiative, within the US PHS, a new solution to address rural Alaska's dental needs.[16] This included the Alaska dental health aide therapist (DHAT) concept that is an accepted primary model of care in more than fifty countries. The Alaska DHAT student completes a two-year program and focuses on providing restorative care in patients in remote areas under the supervision of a dentist who is responsible for writing standing orders and being the point of contact for the therapists through telehealth.[11] Telehealth is the delivery of health services using telecommunications, such as a non-dentist providing care in an unsupervised setting and communicating any questions to the dentist via the telephone or computer.

At present, DHATs may practice only in the state of Alaska, within specific tribal clinics. Minnesota recently began programs at the bachelor's degree level for dental therapists and at the master's degree level designed for practicing dental hygienists to become advanced dental therapists. The graduates of these programs have now begun practicing in Minnesota.

PROPOSED PROVIDERS The *National Call to Action to Promote Oral Health* identified the need to enhance oral health workforce capacity in the United States. The DHAT program was a response to that call as were the following proposed dental care providers.

Advanced Dental Hygiene Practitioner The American Dental Hygienists' Association developed the position of *advanced dental hygiene practitioner* (ADHP) to improve the underserved public's health. Specifically, the ADHP as a mid-level provider will provide diagnostic, preventive, therapeutic, and restorative services as well as referrals to dentists and other health care providers in a variety of settings. The focus of care for this provider will still be prevention, but the ADHP will also have the ability to stop infection by restoring demineralized tooth surfaces and prescribing medicine. ADHPs will be educated in master's degree programs.[13]

The concept of a mid-level provider is well accepted in the medical field and integrated into the health care arena. For example, the nursing profession has developed the nurse practitioner position in response to unmet public health needs. Applied to the dental health field, the mid-level practitioner model will allow greater access to care. At present, many states are proposing legislation to approve this provider model.

Community Dental Health Coordinator The American Dental Association has proposed the addition of the community dental health coordinator (CDHC) in response to the *National Call to Action*.[17] The CDHC would perform many duties, such as oral hygiene instruction and coronal polishing, that dental assistants and dental hygienists do today but must be supervised by a dentist at all times.[11] Table 3-2 ▪ compares these proposed new models of dental providers.

Table 3–2 Comparison of New Models of Dental Health Providers

	Advanced Dental Hygiene Practitioner (ADHP)	Alaska Dental Therapist (DHAT)	Community Dental Health Coordinator (CDHC)
Proposed or currently available	Proposed	Currently practiced in Alaska Indian Health Service Clinics	Proposed
Developing organization	American Dental Hygienists' Association	United States Public Health Service	American Dental Association
Degree	Master's degree	No degree required	No degree required
Physical presence of dentists required for clinical care	No	No	Yes
Clinical focus	Prevention and primary restorative	Restorative	Prevention
State license required	Yes	No	No

DENTAL HYGIENIST SPOTLIGHT ·····························

Public Health Column: Beth McKinney, RDH, MS

Beth McKinney is a dental hygienist and case manager with the Montgomery County, Maryland, Public Health Department. She graduated with honors from both the University of Maryland with a Bachelor of Science degree in Dental Hygiene and from Old Dominion University with a Master's of Science degree in Dental Hygiene.

Ms. McKinney previously worked as a patient care coordinator with the National Institutes of Health in Bethesda, Maryland. She treated medically compromised and acutely ill patients and provided oral health education for health care providers. She also coordinated hospital care for patients in several research studies and participated in research studies. Ms. McKinney has taught as an adjunct faculty member with dental hygiene programs in the area as well. She has also worked for the US Department of the Navy as a dental hygienist and in the dental insurance industry as a quality assurance coordinator.

Ms. McKinney is a member of Sigma Phi Alpha, the national dental hygiene honor society, and was bestowed the Outstanding Performance Award, Naval Dental Clinic; the Employee Service Award at the National Institutes of Health (NIH); and recently was honored as the recipient of the Sunstar Butler/ RDH magazine Award of Distinction, which is presented to dental hygienists of distinction (September 2005, RDH).

Clearly, Ms. McKinney's career in dental public health has been multifaceted. A dental hygienist who has the skills to practice in public health and by advancing his or her education will find opportunities more easily.

I asked Ms. McKinney a few questions.

Why did you decide to go into dental hygiene?

I'm not sure it was a conscious decision. I was a dental assistant for a while out of high school. I wanted to work in the health care profession, but all of my relatives were nurses, and they always complained about their jobs. So I thought dental hygiene might be the way to go.

How did you get into dental public health? Did you need additional education?

Surprisingly, I have to say that I found all of my jobs in public health through ads in the paper. Traditionally, this is not reputed to be the best way to network and make career moves. I got into this right out of school

when I took a job doing quality assurance for a dental insurance company. The only days I have ever spent in private practice as a hygienist have been as a temp. I quickly found that I loved the variety and autonomy that come with working in public health.

In order to be successful in public health, I really think a bachelor's degree is necessary. An advanced degree certainly helped me be very competitive for jobs. Familiarity with statistics, research, budgets, and program management are all essential skills for working in the public health sector. Most of that kind of education you get in an advanced program. Having that knowledge made it very easy to adapt to the roles I've been called upon to fill.

What are your current positions?

I currently work for a county health department. I'm responsible for the program that treats children and pregnant women. I deliver care, manage cases, and do statistical reporting. I'm also responsible for clinic management and the supply budgets for three clinics. I teach students on rotation from a nearby dental hygiene program. I'm responsible for OSHA compliance, infection control, and quality assurance audits conducted on all dental programs the county offers. I do some group education, too, when I can fit the requests into my schedule.

Can you discuss any particularly interesting experiences you have had in your dental public health positions?

I have a ton of stories. Once when I was working at NIH, I treated a patient who was there for a bone marrow transplant. He required ten packs of platelets prior to the scaling visit. When I was cleaning up, I picked up the instrument cassette where an explorer was poking out from underneath and punctured my finger. Up at occupational medicine, when responding to the questions about the source, I had to tell them there were eleven sources and they'd have to contact the blood bank. Even so, I still had to get in line behind the guy who had been bitten by a monkey. At NIH, I worked with an oral medicine resident who was researching oral manifestations of McCune-Albright syndrome. One of my jobs while helping him turned out to be spinning urines to look for vitamin D excretion levels. That brought a new meaning to how we're always telling people the mouth is connected to the body.

When I worked for the navy, the clinic had a mobile dental van. It was always fun to get the opportunity to go out to the submarines and see patients. When I worked for the dental insurance company, I used to travel all over the country inspecting dental offices. I saw some interesting things back in the late 1980s. There was the dentist who sterilized his instruments in a toaster oven. There was another who sterilized his instruments in a GE kitchen oven he kept in an operatory.

What type of advice would you give to a practicing hygienist who is thinking of doing something different?

Do it. You won't regret it, and you'll never "burn out." You may need to expand your skills or get additional education. Expect to make less money at first. But also expect a better benefit package. And remember, benefits add about 30 percent to your salary. All in all, public health is much less stressful and much more fun than private practice.

Source: Christine Nathe writes the Public Health Column in *RDH* magazine published by Pennwell Publishing. For more public health spotlights please see RDH magazine online at http://www.rdhmag.com/index.html.

Summary

Many barriers to dental care delivery exist in the United States. In fact, the current system has proven ineffective in providing care to all segments of the population. Creating dental hygienist positions in existing interdisciplinary public health settings can help alleviate this problem. The governmental structure in relation to dental hygiene care is intricate and offers numerous opportunities for dental hygiene employment. New solutions and innovative approaches to dental care delivery will most definitely occur in the next decade as organizations respond to the current issues.

Note

Much of the information on the federal government was taken directly from the Web sites http://www.hhs.gov, http://www.ed.gov, http://www.va.gov, http://fns1.usda.gov, and http://www.dol.gov.

Self-Study Test Items

1. What has been recognized as a major unmet need in the United States?
   a. Geriatric awareness
   b. Oral health
   c. Access to health care
   d. All of the above

2. What branch of the federal government has a direct impact on dental care delivery?
   a. Legislative
   b. Executive
   c. Judicial
   d. All of the above

3. Who or what directs the US Public Health Service?
   a. US Surgeon General
   b. Centers for Disease Control and Prevention
   c. Johns Hopkins University
   d. Dental Public Health Committee

4. Which organization provides a system of health surveillance to monitor and prevent outbreaks of disease and maintain national health statistics?
   a. National Institutes of Health
   b. Centers for Disease Control and Prevention
   c. Food and Drug Administration
   d. Indian Health Service

5. Which organization is responsible for the Head Start program?
   a. Administration on Aging
   b. Centers for Medicare and Medicaid Services
   c. Administration for Children and Families
   d. Indian Health Services

References

1. US Department of Health and Human Services. *Oral health in America: A Report of the Surgeon General.* Rockville, MD: Department of Health and Human Services, National Institute of Dental and Craniofacial Research, National Institutes of Health; 2000.
2. US Department of Health and Human Services. *Healthy People 2020: Understanding and Improving Health.* 2nd ed. Washington, DC: US Government Printing Office; 2020.
3. US Department of Health and Human Services. *A National Call to Action to Promote Oral Health.* Rockville, MD: US Department of Health and Human Services, Public Health Service, Centers for Disease Control and Prevention, National Institutes of Health, National Institute of Dental and Craniofacial Research; 2003. NIH Publication No. 03-5303.
4. National Research Council. *Advancing Oral Health in America.* Washington, DC: The National Academies Press; 2011.
5. Murphy, CG. Dental hygiene in the Indian Health Service with information from Ann Witherspoon. Paper presented at: DEHY 442: Dental Public Health Course, University of New Mexico, October 1, 2008.
6. DeFriese G, Barker B. *Assessing Dental Manpower Requirements.* Cambridge, MA: Ballinger Publishing; 1982.
7. Dental HPSA Designation Overview. Bethesda, MD: US Department of Health and Human Services; 2013. Retrieved

from http://bhpr.hrsa.gov/shortage/hpsas/designationcriteria/dentalhpsaoverview.html on July 31, 2015

8. Shortage Designation Branch, Bureau of Health Professions, Health Resources and Services Administration. Retrieved from http://www.hrsa.gov/shortage/ on September 17, 2015.

9. Weaver RG, Valachovic RW, Hanlon LL, Mintz JS, Chmar JE. *Unleashing the Potential.* Washington, DC: American Dental Education Association; 2006. Retrieved from http: www.adea.org. on July 31, 2015.

10. Dentists. *Occupational Outlook Handbook.* 2014–2015 ed. Retrieved from http://www.bls.gov/ooh/healthcare/dentists.htm on September 17, 2015.

11. McKinnon M, Luke G, Bresch J, Moss M, Valochovic RW. Association Report: Emerging Allied Dental Workforce Models: Consideration for Academic Dental Institutions. *J Dent Ed.* 2007;71(11):1476–1491.

12. Beazoglou T, Bailit H, Jackson-Brown L. Selling your practice at retirement: Are there problems ahead? *J Am Dent Assoc.* 2000;31(12):1693–1698.

13. Competencies for the Advanced Dental Hygiene Practitioner. Chicago: American Dental Hygienists' Association; 2008.

14. Dental Hygienists. *Occupational Outlook Handbook.* 2014–2015 ed. Retrieved from http://www.bls.gov/ooh/healthcare/dental-hygienists.htm on September 17, 2015.

15. National Denturists Association. What denturists do. http://www.nationaldenturist.com/about%20us.html. Accessed on September 17, 2015.

16. Alaska Native Tribal Health Consortium. Dental Health Therapist. http://www.anthc.org/cs/chs/dhs/index.cfm. Accessed on September 17, 2015.

17. Fox K. ADA House creates new options for dental team. American Dental Association; 2015. Retrieved from http://www.ada.org/en/public-programs/action-for-dental-health/community-dental-health-coordinators. on July 31, 2015.

4

Dental Hygiene Care Delivery in the Global Community

OBJECTIVES

After studying this chapter, the dental hygiene student should be able to:

- Describe the evolution of dental hygiene in countries other than the United States
- Identify global oral health challenges and the positioning of dental hygiene care
- Describe the global workforce distribution and access to dental hygiene care
- Explain global dental hygiene education and work roles
- Explain professional regulation models
- Describe portability of licensure and other professions providing care
- List and define the international professional organizations involving dental hygiene

COMPETENCIES

After studying this chapter and participating in accompanying course activities, the dental hygiene student should be competent to do the following:

- Promote the values of the dental hygiene profession through service-based activities, positive community affiliations and active involvement with local organizations
- Promote positive values of oral and general health and wellness to the public and organizations within and outside the profession
- Access professional and social networks to pursue professional goals

KEY TERMS

Dental nurses 57
Dental therapists 57
Fédération Dentaire
  Internationale (FDI) 48
International Federation of
  Dental Hygienists (IFDH) 49
World Health Organization
  (WHO) 48

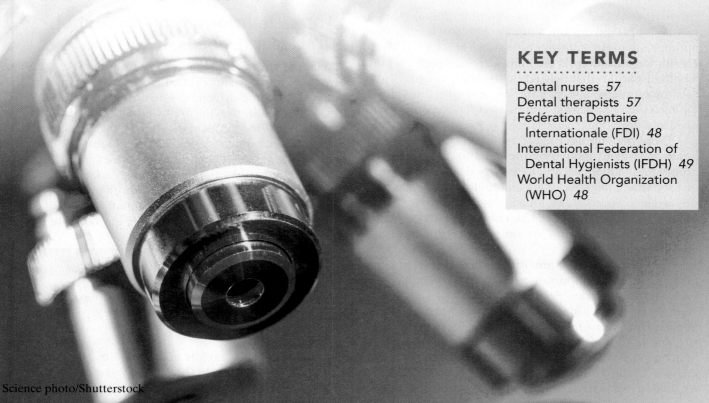

Science photo/Shutterstock

The methods in which dental care is provided on a global basis differ widely. Variations between industrialized nations and developing nations exist. Specifically, delivery systems are affected by political, cultural, and socioeconomic factors and can change frequently. Some countries have no set oral health policy, and in others more structured policies are practiced.

Dental hygienists place oral health as a priority issue, but for the majority of countries oral health is low on the list. Government health policies too often exclude oral health or it is hidden in the text among nutrition or general health policies. Even in these enlightened times, oral health promotion is often not prioritized within health care.

Over the past decades, in many industrialized regions effective preventive strategies have contributed to a decreased incidence of dental disease. These strategies included the addition of fluoride to toothpastes, community water systems, milk products, and table salt; community efforts to educate the public about oral health risk factors; the application of dental sealants; the use of non-cariogenic sweeteners; and the introduction of the dental hygiene profession as a discipline of prevention. Life expectancy is increasing, and teeth are more likely to be retained.

However, oral health disparities exist in many nations with dental hygienists. According to the *Global Goals for Oral Health 2020* report, one of the goals actually states that emphasis should be placed on reducing disparities in oral health between different socioeconomic groups and inequalities in oral health across countries.[1] This report was a truly global initiative; thus, the importance of addressing oral health disparities is paramount. Although common dental diseases are preventable, not all community members are informed of or are able to benefit from appropriate oral health-promoting measures.[2] The **World Health Organization (WHO)** has identified profound oral health disparities that may relate to socioeconomic status, race or ethnicity, age, gender, or general health status. Underserved population groups are found in both developed and developing countries.[2]

These findings have led to the development of public health strategies guided by the need to identify at-risk groups and individuals and to modify risk behaviors with an established negative effect on oral health, such as poor oral hygiene, sugar intake, tobacco use, and excessive alcohol consumption. However, risk reduction can be possible when oral health systems are oriented to primary health care and prevention.

Thus, to plan for the provision of oral health care for a given society, it is important to gather reliable evidence-based information on treatment needs, oral health care systems, costs, workforce numbers, and education for the dental team.[2] In some regions of the world, dental hygienists, due to their primary preventive orientation, play an important role in providing access to oral health care. The majority of the world's dental hygienists practice in societies that have a high demand for prevention, esthetics, and

wellness, as well as the recognition that oral health is an integral part of general health and quality of life.[3] Because of this, most dental hygienists provide care on an individual basis in dental or dental hygiene offices and serve the increasing number of persons who have maintained a functional dentition as a consequence of preventive or restorative dental work, and implants.[4]

Dental hygiene varies greatly among countries. For instance, in Norway, dental hygienists already act as primary oral health care providers in the public health system. In lower-income populations with a lack of basic dental care, as in the Dominican Republic and Nepal, some dental hygienists have been involved in public health initiatives and other grassroots projects promoting oral health.[5-6] Even in developed nations, however, the need is ever increasing for dental hygienists to facilitate oral health equity for underserved populations and to respond to the current and future demographic changes of an aging population with natural teeth, some of whom require services while residing in permanent care facilities.

This chapter examines the global distribution of dental hygienists and national and regional community oral health care needs and demands. Additionally, the chapter explores workforce roles and extended professional positions that would enable dental hygienists to make a greater contribution to global public oral health care provision in response to specific regional needs. Finally, the chapter presents examples of the role dental hygienists play in public health to stimulate other projects of global and local impact.

Access to Information on Global Oral Health Needs

Action plans for promoting the prevention of oral disease frequently rely on surveys that monitor disease patterns. To ensure outcome-driven oral health programs, the WHO maintains statistics on the prevalence of dental diseases from more than 170 countries in its Global Oral Health Database. Data on both dental caries and periodontal diseases are accessible.[7-9] WHO methodology has stimulated the gathering of epidemiological data in a large number of countries. These data are combined with information from the WHO Country Profiles Project and are available to administrators for planning and evaluating oral care services.

Did You Know?

Dental caries and periodontal diseases are the most widespread of all human diseases.

Another data bank is maintained by the **Fédération Dentaire Internationale (FDI),** the organization that represents the international community of dentists.[10] In

addition to some epidemiological data on nearly 130 countries, the FDI Web site provides detailed information about dentistry and the dental team in participating member countries including demographics and numbers concerning the dental workforce, institutions for dental and dental hygiene education, type of oral health care system, fluoridation levels, existence of a public health policy, and information on free dental coverage for children. However, figures pertaining to the dental hygienist workforce must be viewed with caution, especially for countries in which the profession has not been officially introduced or schools are reported but are not accredited.

The Council of European Chief Dental Officers (CECDO) maintains another databank.[11] Key data relate to the oral health workforce, dental education, costs, and oral health indicators including epidemiological data on decayed, missing, and filled teeth (DMFT). CECDO data also include information on the numbers of registered and active dental hygienists in Europe.

The Council of European Dentists (CED) maintains a databank on 30 European countries containing detailed descriptions of national oral health systems, workforce, and public health care demographics.[12] The association was established in 1961 and is composed of 32 national dental associations from 30 European countries.

Since 1987, Johnson has monitored patterns and changes pertaining to the dental hygiene profession in membership countries of the **International Federation of Dental Hygienists (IFDH),** the organization representing the international community of dental hygienists.[13] Her international longitudinal study, which began with thirteen countries, had been extended to twenty-two by 2001 and to twenty-six by 2007. Her latest survey may be accessed through the IFDH Web site (Visit www.ifdh.org).[13–15]

Meaningful international comparisons concerning the equity and quality of oral health care must be based on a precise epidemiological assessment of treatment needs, demands, and information on how these are being met.[3] For strategic planning, it is imperative that data be evidence based, consistent, reproducible, and comparable. Unfortunately, finding reliable data is still a major challenge in global dental public health.[3]

Epidemiology of Dental Caries

The prevalence of caries tends to be most commonly measured with the DMFT index. Key ages for data collection are twelve years, thirty-five to forty-four years, and sixty-five years and older. A mean DMFT between 0.0 and 1.1 is considered low; one of 6.6 or more is high. Although some populations report that the WHO goals for the year 2000 were achieved or even exceeded, they remain a remote hope for a significant part of the world's population.[1] (See Table 4-1 ▪.)

Some question the reliability of these data. Eaton conducted an extensive analysis concerning the validity and comparability of data accessible through international data banks.[3] Even though most countries still provide

Table 4–1 WHO Goals for "Health for All" by the Year 2000

By the age of	Goal
5–6 years	50% should be caries free
12 years	Fewer than 3 decayed, missing, and filled teeth
18 years	85% should have retained all their teeth
34–44 years	50% reduction in the number of persons with no teeth
65 + years	25% reduction in the number of persons with fewer than 20 teeth

Source: www.who.int/oral_health/action/information/surveillance/en/index.html.

epidemiological evidence in DMFT scores, results showed that existing epidemiological data are inadequate and the studies performed to gather the data are not comparable. No universally accepted criteria appear to be used for the diagnosis of caries, and most international surveys lack interexaminer calibration to ensure consistency.[16] In addition, sampling facilities tend to lack dental chairs, lights, and a supply of compressed air. These factors lead to lower estimates of caries experience.

Did You Know?

Interexaminer calibration means that all examiners have a degree of consistency among themselves when evaluating outcomes during a research study whereas *intraexaminer calibration* means that all examiners have a degree of consistency within themselves.

The International Caries Detection and Assessment System (ICDAS) is a collaborative initiative with the goal of finding closer agreement between the outcomes of caries epidemiology and caries clinical trials.[17] The system provides consistent criteria based on evidence-based dentistry designed to generate more meaningful and comparable data. ICDAS has been used in pilot studies in a number of countries such as the United States, United Kingdom, Denmark, Colombia, Mexico, and Iceland and has been shown to be valid and practical.

The Significant Caries Index has been proposed to replace the ICDAS because DMFT scores do not account for the skewed distribution of caries prevalence within a given population.[18] This proposed index would bring attention to individuals with the highest caries in each population.

As a consequence, public health programs could be targeted to benefit these groups.

Epidemiology of Periodontal Diseases

Data collection on periodontal disease appears to pose an even greater challenge for the scientific community. Over the years, significant differences pertaining to severity and incidence of periodontal diseases have been reported, again due to nonstandardized methods of sampling. To improve methodology, the WHO introduced the Community Periodontal Index of Treatment Needs (CPITN, sometimes to referred to as CPI) to evaluate periodontal disease in population surveys.[19] (See Box 4-1 ■.)

After the inception of the CPI, a wealth of global data was generated, but no uniform criteria for the assessment of periodontal diseases have yet been established globally. Furthermore, it has been shown that broad indices such as the CPI produce such severe inconsistencies in the methodologies employed in epidemiological studies that it is unclear whether this group of diseases represents a growing, stable, or declining problem.[3] Consequently, it has been concluded that no reliable epidemiological method currently exists for assessing periodontal disease and that data used to assess treatment needs have been of questionable value and are not comparable. The underestimation of periodontitis may not only adversely affect treatment recommendations and public health strategies but also service cost studies, service demand estimation, or workforce planning.[20,21]

Currently available information on oral health care systems, costs, and workforce numbers also appears inadequate for planning the provision of oral health care on a scientific basis.[22] Problems persist in the collection of information with which to calculate the supply of dental hygienists and their ratio to dentists and the population for the same year.[14]

International Dental Hygiene

Theoretically, the ratio of dental hygienists and dentists to the population would suffice to meet preventive and restorative oral health care needs. However, most countries still report a lack of access to dental hygiene services. Reasons include insufficient funding for preventive service and educational facilities, limitations inherent in the legal restraints on the profession, and a social and cultural lack of awareness of the benefits of preventive care.[14]

Historical Perspective

Dental hygiene is a comparatively young profession. The profession has steadily progressed, and many schools of dental hygiene around the world have based their curriculum on the American method of education. Certainly, it can be said that training programs in other countries evolved based on the American educational model and career structure. Other than the United States, England recorded one of the earliest histories of establishing the profession of dental hygiene. The beginnings came in the form of training of dental hygienists in 1942 to ensure that pilots in the Royal Air Force (RAF), flying fighter planes during World War II, had good dental health and were not troubled by dental pain, which can occur when flying at high altitudes, particularly in unpressurized aircraft.

At that time, the RAF had dentists who had an interest in oral hygiene and had trained further in periodontics in the United States, having heard about the training programs involving dental hygienists. These pioneering, enthusiastic dentists were instrumental in urging the British government's Department of Health to start training "civilian" hygienists at the Eastman Dental Institute, London, in 1949, after the war had ended. A number of schools around the world were influenced by the British example such as those in Australia, New Zealand, and Nigeria (once, all members of the British Commonwealth). The School in Nigeria, in fact, was set up by one of the first civilian hygienists, Vera Creaton, who originally trained in the RAF and then taught at the Eastman Dental Institute. For many years the school, which was a school for training dental therapists, ran parallel with the British courses and was regulated by the General Dental Council (GDC) of the United Kingdom. However, since then the Nigerian course has devised its own method of training dental hygienists and is run independent of the GDC. (See Table 4-2 ■.)

Box 4–1 Community Periodontal Index (CPI) of Treatment Needs

A specially designed periodontal probe is used for the examination using specifically designated index teeth. The highest score for each sextant is used for treatment recommendations.

- **0:** Healthy: No signs of periodontal disease: Promote self-assessment of oral health, (Oral Hygiene Instruction)
- **1:** Gingival bleeding after gentle probing: OHI
- **2:** Presence of supra- or subgingival calculus: OHI, supra- and subgingival scaling
- **3:** Presence of periodontal pockets of 4–5 mm: OHI, supra- and subgingival scaling
- **4:** Presence periodontal pockets ≥ 6 mm: Need for more complex periodontal therapy

Source: WHO Oral Health Country/Area Profile Programme. Community Periodontal Index (CPI). Periodontal country profiles. http://www.who.int/oral_health/databases/niigata/en/ Retrieved on November 6, 2014.

Did You Know?

Dental hygiene is still a relatively young profession around the world.

Table 4–2 **Chronology of Dental Hygiene Education and Legal Recognition by Country**

Country	1st Education	Legal Regulation
Norway	1924, 1971	1979
Great Britain	1948	1954
Japan	1948	1948
Canada	1951	1947, 1952
Nigeria	1958, 1961	1993
R. South Korea	1965	1973
The Netherlands	1968	1974
Sweden	1968	1991
South Africa	1972	1969
Denmark	1972	1986
Switzerland	1973	1975*, 1991*
Australia	1975	1972
Finland	1976	1972
Italy	1978	1988
Israel	1979	1978
Iceland	pending 2008	1978
Hong Kong	1977	1970
Jordan	1980s	missing
Poland	1973	1973
Portugal	1984	1988
Saudi Arabia	1985	missing
Spain	1989	1986
Hungary	1994	1995
Latvia	1996	1996
Lithuania	1996	missing
Czech Republic	1996	1996
New Zealand	1993	1988
Austria	No DH education	DHs work in legal "grey zone"
Belgium	No DH education	Not legally recognized**
France	No DH education	Not legally recognized**
Germany	CE model***	DHs work in legal "grey zone"
Greece	No DH education	Not legally recognized**

aPractice could have begun earlier; this is when dental hygiene practice was legally defined.

bApplies to different cantons.

cA few internationally educated dental hygienists work there.

NA = No information available.

Source: Luciak-Donsberger, C. Dental Hygiene Care Delivery in the Global Community in Nathe, CN. *Dental Public Health and Research*. 3rd Edition. Upper Saddle River, NJ: Pearson, 2011.

Global Workforce Distribution and Access to Dental Hygiene Care

Although the ratio of dental hygienists and dentists to the population indicates that they cannot presently meet preventive and restorative oral health care needs, most countries still lack dental hygiene services.

A global analysis indicates that dental hygiene has been introduced in more than thirty countries. However, a closer look at the demographics reveals that access to care mainly exists in economically developed countries that have an increased life expectancy. These countries exhibit an overall decline in caries prevalence, and interest in wellness and esthetics, possibly an improvement in periodontal health but no significant improvement in the incidence of oral cancer, at least in Europe. Even in these countries, access to dental hygiene varies significantly according to income levels as the Report of the US Surgeon General in 2000 stated.[23] Populations living in remote areas may also lack access to care. This applies to large countries, such as Australia and Canada, where most people are mainly residing in cities with less people living in remote rural areas.

However, for most people living in industrialized countries, going to the dentist and seeing a dental hygienist is relatively easy, although costly. Therefore, cost is a major factor in preventing people from accessing dental care. Dental treatment free to patients is usually (if at all) provided only for children. Even in countries that subsidize care for adults, not all services are covered.

A survey of the dental hygiene workforce in 1998 concluded that Canada, Japan, and the United States had more than fifteen times as many dental hygienists as the former eighteen-member states of the European Economic Area (EEA) although the combined populations and the total number of dentists working in these three countries are broadly similar to those in the EEA.[24] Because the countries with the most dental hygienists have the most educational institutions, their workforce naturally will continue to expand the fastest. According to estimates, today's European Union (EU), composed of thirty countries, has more than 30,000 dental hygienists (no information is available as to whether they are educated in accredited institutions or preceptorship trained) and 340,000 active dentists. (See Table 4-3 ■.) Japan, Canada, and the United States still have seventeen times more dental hygienists than the expanded European Union. Seven EU countries still report no or few dental hygienists. In some countries, such as Austria and Germany, clinical care is frequently provided by preceptorship-trained dental assistants at a significant loss of quality and safety to the public.[25,26] Access to qualified dental hygiene care is therefore not equitable among EU countries.

With access to dental hygienists in the EU mainly through private dental offices in industrialized countries, care tends to be preventive, cosmetic, and therapeutic, which favors a team approach to maximize access and profit.[22] Only a few countries, such as Finland, Norway, and Sweden, report the public health sector as the predominant workplace for a dental hygienist.

Table 4–3 Estimated Ratios of Dental Hygienists to Dentists and to the Population

Country	Population (millions)	Dental Hygienists (number)	Ratio Dental Hygienists: Dentists	Ratio Dental Hygienists: Population
Australia	22.00	900	1:14	1:25,500
Austria	8.00	8	1:350	1:1,000,000
Canada	33.00	18,500	1:1	1:1800
Denmark	5.50	1800	1:3	1:3100
Fiji	0.80	50	1:1	1:16,000
Germany	82.00	150	1:300	1:550,000
Hungary	10.50	900	1:5	1:10,400
Ireland	4.25	300	1:8	1:14,000
Italy	60.00	3000	1:12	1:20,000
Israel	7.20	1030	1:8	1:6700
Japan	127.00	150,000	1:1	1:846
Latvia	2.30	200	1:80	1:11,000
Netherlands	16.50	2000	1:30	1:8000
New Zealand	4.30	250	1:90	1:17,000
Norway	4.50	1200	1:50	1:3700
Portugal	11.00	340	1:15	1:32,000
Slovakia	5.50	300	1:11	1:18,000
South Africa	48.00	2000	1:2.5	1:24,000
South Korea	49.00	31,000	1:0.5	1:1500
Sweden	9.00	3200	1:20	1:2800
Switzerland	7.50	1700	1:2.5	1:4100
United Kingdom	60.00	4500	1:80	1:13,300
United States	300.00	180,000	1:0.9	1:1700

Sources: Luciak-Donsberger C. Questionnaire presented to delegates of the IFDH and representatives of CECDO, 2007–2008; FDI and WHO databanks.

Did You Know?

In most other parts of the world, the dental hygiene workforce is still nonexistent.

Oral health has experienced no change or even deterioration in many developing or underdeveloped countries. A large workforce is needed to promote oral health and educate the public about fluoride, home care, smoking cessation, and nutrition. The total population in Brazil, China, India, Indonesia, and the Russian Federation is nearly

3 billion. According to estimates cited earlier,[14,15,22] the ratio of dental hygienists and dentists per capita is too small for them to plan and implement programs, provide treatment, or educate hundreds of millions of people about the consequences of increased consumption of sugar, processed foods, and carbonated drinks as well as the positive effects of fluoride toothpaste and prophylactic care. This explains the vicious cycle of dental caries remaining largely untreated and very little knowledge about preventive measures such as the benefits of fluorides and the effects of cariogenic nutrition on oral health. India, Pakistan, and Thailand train personnel in basic oral health education and oral hygiene instruction. These providers tend to work in public dental health clinics or go out to villages where they demonstrate toothbrushing and encourage individuals to adopt a preventive attitude toward dental diseases. But even they are far too few in number to make a significant impact.

Data compiled by the FDI suggest that the highest number of dental hygienists is found in countries with the highest dentist-to-population ratios and the greatest reduction of dental diseases as in Canada, Sweden, Switzerland, and the United States. (See Table 4-3 ■.) These data suggest that there is no need to fear that dental hygienists will replace dentists but that a larger workforce is needed to treat and maintain the oral health of a growing and aging population that cares for and retains its natural teeth. Dental hygienists and dentists truly work in a collaborative manner.

Current Status of Dental Hygiene Education

Education serves to socialize and validate knowledge, and educational credentials ensure a standard of care. Currently, dental hygiene education is eclectic, which means that it varies considerably in many different areas from country to country. Studies indicate that it varies in prerequisites, duration, and institutional settings. Dental hygiene education in Europe is becoming increasingly academic.[27] Requiring specific education to gain entry into the profession is a response to the increasing complexity in dental hygienists' work roles.

In most countries, dental hygiene education seeks to qualify students in evidence-based clinical care, diagnostic assessment and intervention planning, lifestyle consulting, and risk behavior modification counseling as well as in public health promotion, teaching, research, and program administration. In some countries, dental hygienists are educated to polish amalgam restorations, administer local anesthesia and/or local antibiotic therapy, place and remove temporary restorations and/or orthodontic bands, and even prepare and treat primary caries. These applications require increased responsibility and critical thinking based on research. As the profession is becoming increasingly autonomous, dental hygiene education must transmit technical efficiency with critical evidence-based decision making coupled with the ability to recognize one's own professional limitations in order to judge when it is time to refer to a dentist.[14,25]

In most countries, entry into the dental hygiene profession is preceded by graduation from an accredited program and independent testing of clinical ability and theoretical knowledge.[14,25] Dental hygiene educational institutions range from private schools to technical colleges and universities that award diplomas as well as associate's, bachelor's, master's, and doctoral degree levels. Duration of study to enter the profession varies from two to four years with an average of three years. Globally, and even within the European Union, a variety of models of dental hygiene education exists.

Two- to three-year diploma programs still exist in many countries, but in Europe the tendency is to replace them with degree programs or, as is the case in Sweden, offer an optional third year of education to attain bachelor's degree levels at all schools. Some countries already require a bachelor's degree for entry into practice, and several more report a planned academic upgrade of the educational process.

The European Union is increasingly adapting degree program curricula to the European credit transfer system (ECTS). The European Ministers of Education introduced this system in Bologna in 1999 to make academic studies more attractive, transparent, and transferable and to promote quality assurance. Under this system, students earn sixty credits per year (forty-two weeks of study) for a total of 1680 hours of study. Bachelor's programs in Denmark, Finland, Italy, the Netherlands, Portugal, the Republic of Ireland, Sweden, and the United Kingdom either already have or are about to introduce this system. The European Dental Hygienists' Federation proposed 198 ECTS units for the study of dental hygiene, which totals 5200 hours.

Postgraduate-level programs such as those for master's or doctoral (PhD) degrees in related health fields are open to all dental hygienists with bachelor's degrees. Sweden, Italy and the United States offer master's programs in dental hygiene.[28] The United States has the highest number of master's programs in dental hygiene. More are pending in Australia, Italy, and Norway in response to the need for evidence-based research in dental hygiene care by providing scientifically oriented educational opportunities.

In some countries, students may graduate with a degree in both dental hygiene and dental therapy.[28] However, these dual degree programs have caused some concern about the disappearance of stand-alone dental hygiene education because professionals educated in

preventive and restorative care might lose their predominantly preventive orientation.

Germany has chosen so far an eclectic model of dental hygiene education. It is a continuing education model for actively working dental assistants, not comparable to the two-, three-, and four-year full-time diploma or degree courses found in accredited dental hygiene education. The only three-year full-time diploma course in Germany, which followed the Swiss model of education, closed in 2006. However, there is discussion about implementing programs at bachelor's levels at technical colleges.

Although the length of study and entry requirements to the profession vary, all students in countries in which the profession is registered complete examinations at the end of their courses to obtain a national qualification. In the larger countries, such as in the United States, Australia, and Canada, state or province examinations (sometimes called *boards*) are also required to practice in that particular region.

Did You Know?

The length of dental hygiene education tends to be extended as curricula are being expanded with an increase in academic orientation.

The movement toward extended education is associated with an increase in the scope of practice and a decrease in regulation. In the Netherlands, for instance, students acquire skills in extended functions, including the restoration of primary caries. This change occurred in response to an aging population coupled with a significant decline in the dentist workforce due to retirement.

Professional Regulation

Regulation of health occupations under public statute ensures quality and safety of patient care. Although the dental profession still exercises control over the dental hygiene profession, requirements for becoming a dental hygienist in many countries include legislative changes and self-regulation.[29] (See Table 4-4 ■)

Interestingly, the dates of the onset of dental hygiene education rarely coincide with the profession's legal recognition. This means that, in several countries, dental hygienists were providing patient care, usually under the supervision of dentists, long before their services were legally regulated. In some cases, the legal acceptance of the profession, which organized dentistry often opposed, required years of lobbying by supporters, most of them also dentists. Foreign-educated dental hygienists working in Austria, Belgium, Germany, and France still face this situation; these countries continue to resist developing the profession or employing dental hygienists, especially because preceptorship- (on-the-job) trained dental assistants work

Table 4–4 Regulation of the Dental Hygiene Profession by Country

Country	Regulating Authority
Australia	Dental board
Canada	Self-regulation in 6 provinces (representing 90% of DHs); dental board/council in 4 provinces
Denmark	Board of Health
Finland	Social and Health Ministry
Hungary	Ministries of Health and Education and Culture
	Institute for Basic and Continuing Education of Health Workers
Ireland	Dental Council
Italy	Ministry of Health
Israel	Division of Dental Health of Ministry of Health
Netherlands	Ministry of Health
New Zealand	New Zealand Dental Council
Norway	Health Personnel Act
Portugal	Ministry of Health
South Africa	Health Professions Council of South Africa
South Korea	Ministry of Health and Welfare
Sweden	Board of Social Welfare
Switzerland	Swiss Red Cross
United Kingdom	General dental council
United States	Individual state boards

for less than educated and licensed dental hygienists, even though the fees charged to the public are often roughly the same.[30]

National differences in legislative practices affecting dental hygiene tend to reflect the impact of the dental profession's organized lobby to retain control of dental hygiene care. Some countries still legally prohibit anyone other than dentists to provide patient care. In those countries, dental hygiene may not be implemented at all. Barriers to change may include the fear that this will financially affect too many dentists who might provide dental

hygiene care themselves and that they will lose control and status. Frequently, such fears can result from a lack of understanding of exactly what dental hygienists can do. Dental schools that favor a team approach by integrating dental and dental hygiene education may foster mutual understanding and recognition of task-related boundaries.

However, data show that regulations imposed to tie dental hygiene care to work settings controlled by dentists are gradually beginning to disappear. Increasingly, dental hygienists may practice autonomously, free of any supervision of dentists. In such settings, they may be consulted as primary oral health care providers.

Movement Toward Autonomy

International dental hygienist regulation is decreasing, resulting in increased autonomy. However, the definition of independent practice in one country is not necessarily the same in another. Some countries allow dental hygienists to operate their own practices and provide treatment without the referral of a dentist. Other countries may not allow them to operate their own practices but allow them to work in the public sector without supervision.

Models of Supervision

The shift toward an increase in professional autonomy is reflected in the definition of a dental hygienist found in the Dutch curriculum for dental hygiene education. The dental hygienist is an independent preventive professional within the dental healthcare sector, with his/her own responsibility and specific expertise.[4] Discussion of the models of supervision (or lack thereof) is summarized in Table 4-6 ■ below.

DIRECT SUPERVISION   In countries employing direct supervision, legal requirements state that dentists not only decide and authorize dental hygiene treatment but must be physically on-site during the delivery and, in some cases, may have to be in the room or examine the patient after treatment. Once the predominant model of care, this supervisory method has essentially disappeared or is applied to selected treatments such as the administration of local anesthesia.[5]

GENERAL SUPERVISION   Countries such as the Czech Republic and Israel legally stipulate that dentists prescribe and authorize dental hygiene care but need not be physically on-site while treatment is rendered. Generally, care is provided at a facility owned or managed by dentists or at public health clinics managed by them.

INDEPENDENT REFERRED PRACTICE   Legislation in some countries permits dental hygienists to practice in their own facilities or in institutions that provide preventive services only if the patient is referred by a dentist. Treatment decisions are thus made in collaboration with dentists. This practice is found in some Canadian provinces, Germany (one practice in Munich), the United Kingdom, and Latvia.

UNSUPERVISED, AUTONOMOUS, OR INDEPENDENT PRACTICE   Some countries have enacted legislation that permits dental hygienists to practice without the supervision of a dentist. Dental hygienists autonomously decide treatment plans and render care in their own facilities or in the public sector without the referral of a dentist and refer patients to dental care when they diagnose a problem that is beyond their scope of practice or are uncertain about a diagnostic decision. This practice has been introduced in the United States and in some Canadian provinces, Denmark, Finland, Italy, the Netherlands, Norway, and Sweden and in all but one of the Swiss cantons. In these cases, the public may choose dental hygienists as primary oral health care providers. South Africa and Fiji so far permit this practice only in the public sector.

Trends reflect a strong movement toward independent dental hygiene practice. Standardization of autonomy would facilitate dental hygiene services in remote areas, public health care settings, permanent care facilities, and mobile dental units, which are underserved by dentists in all countries surveyed. For instance, dental hygienists in South Africa may not own their own practice (change may be pending) but may perform their full scope of services in all public health settings independently of a dentist. They provide care in much needed fissure-sealant and brushing programs, HIV and home-based care projects, correctional services programs, and rural programs. Dental hygiene education increasingly prepares students for independent decision making and the ability to recognize when to refer patients to dentists.

Professional self-regulation and autonomy in providing care may be the key to a gradual change in the profession's image.[14] Independent practice is empowering—not only to operators but also to patients who may freely choose care providers. One-third of all dental hygienists in the Netherlands have their own practice, probably the highest percentage worldwide. Globally, relatively few dental hygienists work in this manner. Financial considerations of investing in an office and the responsibilities of office maintenance and administration may be deterrents. As role models increase, however, more and more dental hygienists may recognize the rewards of being in charge of their own business, job sharing, flexible work and vacation times, and choice of how and where to practice. The need for a cooperative arrangement between independent dental hygienists and general dentists and dental specialists is not in question.

In summary, in the Scandinavian countries, dental hygienists increasingly work as independent professionals, academics, and public health experts with significant decision-making responsibilities and may be chosen as primary oral health care providers by the public. In Eastern Europe, Asia, and in the Middle East, dental hygienists frequently work as rigidly controlled and supervised auxiliaries who perform dental assisting functions and are underutilized in clinical care.[31,32]

DENTAL HYGIENIST SPOTLIGHT ···

Public Health Column: Ron Knevel, RDH

Ron Knevel is a graduate of the University of Amsterdam's School of Dental Hygiene. He has worked full-time as a dental hygienist at the department of periodontology at the Academic Centre for Dentistry (ACTA) and in a general practice. After earning his teacher's degree at the Free University, he became a teacher at the Dental Hygiene Program in Amsterdam. He has become more and more involved in dental hygiene curriculum development and is now planning to begin work on a doctoral degree.

I asked him some questions concerning his work and the status of dental hygiene in the Netherlands.

What is your current position?

When the European Union began funding projects for exchange within it, and Amsterdam Dental Hygiene School started to develop partnerships with others for student exchange, I became an international coordinator and therefore came into contact with many colleagues in other countries. I introduced the concept of the international week, and at international conferences, I discussed the benefits of internationalizing dental hygiene. I believe that student and teacher mobility can lead to more respect and understanding for different cultures and treatment options.

I started a project in Nepal to promote oral health based on sustainability and equity. It focuses on oral health promotion based on the culture of Nepal, not on Western approaches. I am also involved in the curriculum development of the dental hygiene school in Kathmandu. This project also involves conducting research to determine the impact of the oral health promotion activities on the oral health of children and oral-related aspects of quality of life. I will probably start a similar project in Sri Lanka.

How does the department of periodontology charge for its services?

Patients pay a small nominal fee for the complete treatment, which almost all patients can afford and whose quality is important. The prevalence of caries is decreasing, but the incidence of periodontal diseases is growing. General oral health promotion focuses on identifying and targeting groups at risk for oral health problems.

Have economic and social changes in the Netherlands influenced the way the university operates?

Yes, in the Netherlands, it is important for departments to generate their own financial resources.

How have the same factors influenced the national health insurance?

Although the demand for dental care is high and there is a shortage of dentists and dental hygienists, the national health insurance and basic dental insurance began covering fewer treatments for economic reasons. Dental care is covered by national insurance for children and young adults up to eighteen years (depending on the parents' financial situation; otherwise, the parents need extra insurance to cover the children). People older than eighteen are required to have extra dental insurance, which can be rather expensive and not affordable for many. This situation eventually led people to avoid dental checkups.

How has the country's approach to dental care changed?

A special advisory group of the government concluded that to improve the availability of dental care, a new team approach was needed. The team includes dentists, dental specialists, dental hygienists, dental assistants, and dental technicians who work closely together to offer patients integrated dental care. This approach has led to a different type of dental hygiene education. The program (which had been changed from two to three years not long before) was changed to a four-year course of study. Now dental hygienists in the Netherlands must have a bachelor of health degree, and their duties have been extended to include the preparation and restoration of simple (primary) cavities with composite.

The prolonged education was necessary because additional preparation was required. To provide this training, the dental faculty offered some teachers the opportunity to become skilled in restorative techniques and be trained in evidence-based practice.

Source: Christine Nathe writes the Public Health Column in *RDH* magazine published by Pennwell Publishing. For more public health spotlights please see RDH magazine online at http://www.rdhmag.com/index.html.

Effects of Gender Politics on Dental Hygienists

It is worth noting, that worldwide, approximately 98 percent of all dental hygienists are women. This raises the question of whether this female-dominated profession, perceived as auxiliary to the historically male-dominated profession of dentistry, has been affected by gender politics.[26] A 2003 report commissioned by the Austrian Federal Ministry of Science, Education, and Culture explored whether a correlation exists between national differences found in the dental hygiene profession and gender-related disparities found in other work-related areas. Results showed that, while the scope of practice tends to be similar around the world, the gender bias in the dental hygiene profession has impaired equal access to education and equal occupational opportunities for dental hygienists within the European Union and beyond.

In northern Europe, higher educational attainment in the field of dental hygiene increased professional responsibility, and opportunities for self-employment in autonomous practice tend to correlate with increased equality in the workforce at large. In Eastern Europe, lower educational and professional opportunities in dental hygiene correlate with gender disparities found in other work-related areas. In some western European countries, the profession may not be implemented because of the political impact of male-dominated organized dentistry.

Portability of Licensure

Many hygienists would like to be able to travel and work in countries other than their own. Large countries such as Australia, Canada, and the United States require state or provincial and national qualifications. Within the European Union, an equivalency ruling exists, permitting the regulatory body to assess whether training in one EU country is equivalent to another. If the finding is positive, the dental hygienist is permitted to work. Of course, hygienists are permitted to work only in those European countries that recognize them. One disadvantage could be the inability to speak the language of the country in which one wishes to work.

The European Union regulates a profession when it is legally registered in at least two-thirds of the member countries. This goal is almost reached and actively pursued by the European Federation of Dental Hygienists. Such a regulation would lead to free movement of the dental hygiene workforce within the European Union.

Other Dental Professions Providing Care

Dental therapists provide restorative care under the general supervision of dentists. They are mostly found in the United Kingdom and in former countries of the British Commonwealth, such as Australia, Canada, and Nigeria. Until recently, their services were restricted to public health facilities and school dental services where they would examine and treat children under the prescription of dentists. Therefore, in New Zealand, they are also referred to as school **dental nurses.** Generally, their services include dental hygiene care, but their main focus is on children's restorative needs. Dental nurses may restore both the primary and permanent dentition of children and extract primary teeth. While they initially worked only at community dental services, dental therapists now may provide services for children and adults in private practice settings.

Orthodontic assistants are trained in Canada and Australia and will soon be in the United Kingdom. They tend to be qualified dental assistants who attend a postgraduate course in orthodontics. They assist orthodontists in technical tasks by making and fitting bands, taking impressions, and fitting arch wires. They also ensure that the patient undergoing treatment maintains a high level of daily oral hygiene practices.

Developing countries have programs for oral health educators who dispense information in a culturally sensitive manner to raise oral health awareness of large poor populations who frequently live in remote areas. Little can be gained by training a highly skilled professional to undertake costly and complex clinical tasks when the population requires simple oral hygiene education and oral health promotion programs.

Some countries require *dental assistants* to graduate from training programs that have high standards, meet specified qualifications, and be registered before being considered a professional member of the dental team. In other countries, however, their skills may not be rated so highly and not be recognized by regulatory authorities. Many receive only preceptorship training with no formal theoretical education to support evidence-based practice. Clearly, the standard of training is inconsistent.

A formally trained and registered professional is more likely to receive public confidence. No regulation or deregulation allows more opportunity for substandard care by individuals with no recourse to an authority should the need arise. For instance, assistants in Austria operating in a legal "grey zone" perform prophylactic treatments and nonsurgical periodontal therapy, sometimes without any coursework at all, which has been shown to have a detrimental effect on treatment efficacy and patient safety.[25] Countries endeavoring to standardize education are slowly recognizing this risk. Society has the right to expect that educated and qualified professionals will provide its oral health care. In this context, the International Federation of Dental Hygienists, representing the views of its members, objects to calling these grey-zone assistants "dental hygienists." The title is protected in a number of countries and has an international definition, which is, in most cases, tied to the advanced educational requirements described in this chapter.

Challenges to the Profession

The WHO Oral Health Report 2003 shows that for some societies, dental diseases (especially caries) have declined while certain at-risk groups carry the bulk of the burden of

oral diseases around the globe.[33] It is estimated that in developing countries, nearly 90 percent of the population is unable to receive standardized caries treatment.[34] There is a dire need to promote oral health on a large-scale basis.

The Role of the WHO in Promoting Global Oral Health Equity

The World Health Organization (WHO) in conjunction with the Fédération Dentaire Internationale (FDI) established the first global oral health goals in 1981 to combat rising levels in dental caries due to an increase in sugar consumption. These goals were formulated to be achieved by some industrialized countries by 2000.[35] (See Table 4-1 ■.) In 2003, the FDI, the WHO, and the International Association for Dental Research (IADR), jointly presented new global oral health goals for 2020. (See Box 4-2 ■.) This document presents two goals, ten objectives, and sixteen targets at which community public health programs may be directed.[36] Objectives are population based and guided by the principles of disease prevention and health promotion. The new goals emphasize an evidence-based approach to practice and a stronger public health orientation with a focus on modifiable oral risk behaviors. The targets are formulated in more general terms without absolute values and are intended to serve as a useful framework for health planners at regional, national, and local levels, taking into account global variations in the epidemiology of oral diseases and socioeconomic realities. One specific target is the decrease periodontal disease.[37]

In 2007, WHO issued the document "Oral Health: Action Plan for Promotion and Integrated Disease Prevention," which includes step-by-step suggestions for framing policies and strategies for oral health.[38] It is hoped that this initiative will unite public health providers in effective strategies to reduce barriers to oral health care.

Box 4–2 Global Goals for Oral Health 2020

- To promote oral health and to minimise the impact of diseases of oral and craniofacial origin on general health and psychosocial development, giving emphasis to promoting oral health in populations with the greatest burden of such conditions and diseases
- To minimise the impact of oral and craniofacial manifestations of general diseases on individuals and society, and to use these manifestations for early diagnosis, prevention and effective management of systemic diseases.

Note: Adopted by the FDI General Assembly September 18, 2003.

Source: FDI policy. http://www.who.int/oral_health/media/en/orh_goals_2020.pdf. Accessed June 8, 2009.

Impact of Global Dental Hygiene on Oral Health Equity

Generally, it appears that public dental health is not perceived as a priority service in many countries. Dental hygienists can play a major role in influencing health services to place more importance on their dental public health programs. In addition to improving the quality of life and general health, preventing oral diseases translates into long-term cost savings.

Many countries have community and school dental services within the public health sector in which dental hygienists provide a significant part of services. Some hygienists are actively involved in clinical work; others work solely in oral health promotion.

Did You Know?

In Norway, the majority of hygienists work in community dental services.

Dental hygienists worldwide have been involved in oral health promotion for children and in giving oral hygiene instruction to disadvantaged groups in the community. Under the stewardship of the WHO, community programs and health care settings provide opportunities to expand oral disease prevention and health promotion knowledge and practices among the public. To implement global oral health strategies and community programs, the WHO promotes partnerships with national and international nongovernmental organizations through its Collaborating Centres on Oral Health.[39] Dental hygienists, in their traditional role as oral health prevention specialists, are ideally qualified to become proactive in this collaboration.[40] Dental hygienists have also been effective in achieving another WHO objective, that of promoting healthy lifestyles by incorporating tobacco cessation programs and nutritional counseling into their practices.[2] In a study with periodontal patients, success rates in smoking cessation (up to one year later) following the advice of dental hygienists trained in smoking cessation counseling were better than national quit rates achieved in specialist smoking cessation clinics.[41]

An increased collaboration of the WHO with dental hygienists would not only save financial resources but might relax many barriers and legislative restrictions that currently interfere with the full use of dental hygienists in the delivery of public oral health promotion and care.[40, 42]

Autonomous dental hygiene care has the potential to significantly impact the quality of mobile dental care, a service model in which oral health care facilities are transported to a nonmobile population. With the aging of society, mobile dentistry is gaining importance not only in less developed countries but also in industrialized nations.[42] Extended function dental hygienists (such as in the Netherlands) could meet many challenges presented by

the care for this population through their minimal interventive approach. This includes the assessment of the risk of disease with a focus on early detection and prevention, techniques for remineralization, and the treatment of primary coronary or root caries, erosion, abrasion, demineralization, compensation for salivary dysfunction, and management of high plaque levels.[43]

Many countries have structures in place, but the dental hygiene workforce is too scarce and the scope of practice too restricted to have a significant impact on access to care. (See Table 4-5 ∎.)

National Oral Health Policies

Few countries have formal national published oral health policies or strategies provided by the government, but Japan, South Korea, and the United Kingdom do provide them. Denmark, France, Germany, Kenya, New Zealand, Nigeria, Norway, Portugal, Slovenia, and Sweden also have policies in place.[10] They range from statements about entitlement to dental treatment to strategies explaining in detail what the government is striving to achieve. In the past, the Council of European Chief Dental Officers proposed an oral health strategy for Europe.[11]

Mass fluoridation programs were popular at one time. However, research has shown that they have decreased in number. This may be due in part to the success that fluoride toothpaste has had on reducing caries, community leaders trying to reduce short-term costs, or societal resistance to what some may feel is forced governmental medicine. Examples of community water fluoridation are found, for instance, in the United States and the Republic of Ireland. However, in the poorest nations, even access to community water resources is generally scarce.

Public Health Initiatives and Campaigns

Most countries have some public dental health services administered by states or provinces within the country. In some countries, such as Germany and the United Kingdom, specifically trained oral health promoters offer the programs. In the United Kingdom, a dental professional (dental hygienist, dental therapist, or dental assistant) often provides the service. Many governments are, however, reducing their financial support for national oral health promotion programs in part because of the absence of evidence-based research providing a rationale for the continuation of such government spending.

Many countries increasingly are having significant dental public health campaigns and health promotion days, weeks, or months. Some of the major campaigns are Japan's 8020 campaign, which focuses on retaining twenty teeth by eighty years of age; South Korea's 10 Principles of Dental Health poster campaign; the Netherlands' extensively documented Bottle It Up, Take a Cup campaign to reduce the incidence of nursing caries; and the United Kingdom's Early Years campaign that reflects principles similar to those of the Netherlands. Refer to Table 4-6 ∎ for examples of groups lobbying for oral health.

Successful Public Health Initiatives Involving Dental Hygienists

"SONRISAS," AN ORAL HEALTH CARE PROJECT FOR THE UNDERPRIVILEDGED IN THE DOMINICAN REPUBLIC In 1986, while on vacation in the Dominican Republic, Elina Katsman, a Canadian dental hygienist, noticed the poor oral health condition of the local youth and initiated a project to provide free dental treatment and oral health education to underprivileged children. She started giving lectures with two local nurses whom she trained in the principles of oral hygiene and related primary health care. Through relentless lobbying, she was able to gain support and funding for dental clinics to provide much-needed care. Today, the Sonrisas project runs eight dental clinics and five mobile units that serve remote areas and have benefited more than 1.7 million people. This project was honored with the 2007 Sunstar World Dental hygienists' award.[6]

ORAL HEALTH CARE ON THE PHELOPHEPA TRAIN IN SOUTH AFRICA The Phelophepa (meaning "good clean health") Train is a project to provide health care to rural South Africans. It began in 1903 as an eye clinic with three coaches. Today, the train has thirteen coaches traveling through rural areas to deliver comprehensive, affordable, accessible health care to remote rural areas in which people have limited access to care. The train reaches more than 130,000 people each year. The dental coach has six dental chairs for providing hygiene care, restorations, and extractions and a special x-ray unit. Prescreenings are performed outside the coach.[44]

DYSPHAGIA MANAGEMENT FOR THE ELDERLY IN JAPAN A three-year dental hygiene curriculum in Japan introduced a dysphagia management course in a residential care facility for elderly people.[45] Dental hygiene care was performed on a patient who was bedridden after suffering from a stroke. Oral health personnel had difficulty providing daily oral hygiene routines because the patient suffered from severe muscle tension around the oral cavity. After monthly treatments for five months, results showed a relaxation of oral muscles and a decrease in plaque accumulation and gingival inflammation. Through the positive results of this intervention, students gained first-hand knowledge of the importance of professional oral care to organic and functional oral health improvements for elderly people.

NATIONAL PERIODONTAL SCREENING IN AUSTRIA When the Austrian national health insurance updated its periodic health examination in 2005, a US-educated dental hygienist was approached to design a periodontal screening program to be administered by general physicians as part of this

Table 4–5 Requirements for Supervision of Dental Hygiene Practice per Country

Country	Independ. Practice	Indep. Ref. Practice	Off Site Supervision	On-site Supervision	Expected Changes
Australia	✓[a]	✓[b]	✓		More autonomy
Canada	✓[b]	✓			More autonomy; direct insurance. reimbursement
Czech Republic			✓		Move toward independent practice
Denmark	✓				Expanded functions
Fiji	✓[a]				Missing
Finland	✓				Missing
Germany		✓[c]	✓[d]		Missing
Hungary				✓	—
Iceland		✓			Missing
Israel			✓[e]		More autonomy
Italy	✓				More independent practices
Japan			✓		Missing
Latvia		✓	✓		Missing
Lithuania			✓		Missing
Netherlands	✓				More independent practices
New Zealand			✓[e]		More autonomy
Norway	✓				More independent practices
Portugal			✓		Expanded functions
R. Ireland			✓[e]		Independent practice
R. S. Korea		✓[a]		✓	Missing
R. Slovakia			✓		Independent practice
South Africa	✓[a]				Autonomous practice in private settings
Spain			✓		Greater autonomy
Sweden	✓				More independent practices
Switzerland	✓[e]				More independent practices
UK		✓			Removal of referral

[a]Only in public sector.

[b]One autonomous practice in Munich run by US-educated and Swiss-licensed DH.

[c]Eclectic dental hygienist (DH) education; DH not licensed.

[d]DH treatment plan decided with dentist

[e]Direct supervision during administration of local anaesthesia

Source: Luciak-Donsberger C. Questionnaire presented to delegates of the IFDH and representatives of CECDO, 2007–2008.

Table 4–6 Oral Health Lobbying Groups by Country

Country	Lobbying Groups
Germany	Toothfriendly Germany (Aktion Zahn-freundlich e.v.) for sugar-free confectionery and drinks
New Zealand	New Zealand Dental Health Foundation
Switzerland	Toothfriendly Switzerland (Aktion Zahn-freundlich) for sugar-free confectionery and drinks
United Kingdom	Action and Information on Sugars (watchdog on misinformation on sugars through poor labeling and advertising)
	Food Commission (watchdog on food industry including sugar issues)
	Chuck Sweets Off the Checkout
	Toothfriendly UK for sugar-free confectionery and drinks

examination. Austria, where the dental hygiene profession has not been introduced, has a high incidence of untreated periodontitis because prevention and treatment are excluded from national social insurance coverage. Goals of this periodontal screening are to raise public awareness of prevention and treatment, refer persons at risk to periodontal care, include treatment coverage in the national insurance coverage, and make evident the need for qualified care provided by dental hygienists. This project may be viewed as an initiative to integrate oral health into primary health functions, a step the WHO recommends.[46]

Future of Dental Hygiene Worldwide

Dental hygiene is an expanding profession. Changes in demographics, epidemiology of oral diseases, and longevity call for cost-effective, flexible health care that is best provided by a team approach. In health care, knowledge utilization commonly manifests through evidence-based decision making in practice as well as in public health initiatives.[47] Many examples have shown that autonomous dental hygienists with expanded functions and higher educational attainment are better able to provide quality, cost-effective clinical care and to initiate and manage scientifically based public oral health initiatives. Such dental hygienists may contribute to a wider practical application of scientific knowledge, which has been shown to improve oral health and general health.

The change toward an increasingly academic orientation in dental hygiene education enables a growing number of graduates to engage in research, interpret research results, and apply new scientific achievements to benefit the public.

Researchers in dental hygiene are needed to gather evidence-based data about the effectiveness of clinical dental hygiene care, behavior modification strategies, and public initiatives. They are needed to collaborate in epidemiological research with relevant organizations in the collection of reliable data. In their traditional role as oral health prevention specialists, dental hygienists may also play a more significant role in workforce partnerships with other health practitioners and academics in conducting evaluations of national and community oral health programs. However, a 2007 survey of all members of the House of Delegates of the IFDH revealed that dental hygienists so far have not participated in such initiatives in any significant way.

In addition to their clinical skills, dental hygienists have an established role as oral health promoters and educators. The new WHO goals emphasize an evidence-based approach to practice and a stronger public health orientation with a focus on modifiable oral risk behaviors. A policy statement of the Proceedings of the 2003 European Workshop on Oral Care and General Health acknowledges that as *clinicians, dental hygienists have the advantage of meeting patients on a regular basis*. This allows dental hygienists to play a key role in changing behavior patterns, thus improving both oral health and quality of life for the patient.[48] Dental hygienists may apply their excellent motivational skills to modify risk behaviors by providing smoking and alcohol cessation counseling and promoting healthy nutrition.

With expanded skills, the dental hygiene workforce may be utilized in a more flexible and accessible way—from private practice to mobile oral health care. The aging population in industrialized regions presents new challenges. Many in this population have heavily restored dentitions and implants that require extensive flexible maintenance care for the rest of their lives.[45] In some countries, dental hygienists are beginning to respond to the need to work in such facilities. Barriers preventing educated members of the dental team to provide autonomous cost-effective preventive and minimal interventive restorative care must be removed.[42]

In addition, in some countries, in an effort to detect oral cancer, dental hygienists have been allowed to administer minimally invasive brush biopsies combined with an advanced computer analysis of nuclear DNA contents, taken from suspicious oral lesions. This process may lead to early referral and to a better prognosis for a cure.

Did You Know?

Dental hygienists have been effective in lobbying for oral health campaigns and programs and are acting as local and national policy advisers in health promotion.

In developing countries, autonomous dental hygienists with extended functions may not only initiate preventive oral health programs but also begin to tend to the primary,

minimal interventive restorative needs of millions of untreated children and adults.

Concerns have been voiced about dental hygienists being replaced by preceptorship-trained assistants. However, a closer look at the information presented in this chapter reveals a steady growth of the dental hygiene workforce, a tendency toward higher academic educational attainment, and extended functions as well as increased autonomy and self-regulation. Evidence supports the increased employment and extended roles for dental hygienists after appropriate training. When viewing this development in the context of an increased need for care due to demographic changes coupled with a decline in the dentist workforce, the future of the dental hygiene profession appears to be secure.

Key International Organizations

In addition to the World Health Organization, a number of other organizations seek to promote dental health worldwide.

Fédération Dentaire Internationale (FDI)

One of the oldest international health organizations, the FDI was founded in 1900 in Paris. It has member associations in about 120 countries and has established standing commissions and programs on a number of dental-related issues including oral health. FDI began official relations with the World Health Organization (WHO) in 1948 and collaborates with the WHO on the planning and development of global goals for oral health.

International Association for Dental Research (IADR)

The mission of the International Association for Dental Research (IADR) is to advance research and increase knowledge for the improvement of oral health worldwide. It consists of divisions and sections that establish and support programs to promote oral health research and IADR activities. IADR collaborates with other international dental associations, industries, health agencies, and scientific and educational professional organizations.

Council of European Chief Dental Officers (CECDO)

The Council of European Chief Dental Officers (CECDO) promotes dental public health and ethics and exchanges views on dental matters throughout EU and European Economic Area member countries with the goal to harmonize dental professions and access to care within Europe.[10]

Council of European Dentists (CED)

The Council of European Dentists (CED) represents the interests of more than thirty dental associations across Europe. It maintains a databank on thirty European countries with detailed descriptions of national oral health systems, workforce, and public health care demographics.[11]

European Federation of Periodontology (EFP)

The main goal of the European Federation of Periodontology (EFP), which first met officially in 1994, is "the promotion of periodontal health in Europe."[49] The EFP strongly believes that some minimum standards in all fields of dental education should be provided and enforced and has published recommendations concerning undergraduate and specialist education in periodontology.

International Federation of Dental Hygienists (IFDH)

The International Federation of Dental Hygienists (IFDH) was officially formed in 1986 in Oslo, Norway. It is an international nonprofit organization uniting dental hygiene associations from around the world in their common cause of promoting access to quality preventive oral services and to raise public awareness about the prevention of dental disease.[50] The IFDH is a growing organization with twenty-eight countries current members.

IFDH has forged strong links with international organizations that have similar outlooks on oral health promotion such as the FDI, EFP, and WHO (Oral Health Unit). Resources on its Web site include information about work requirements for each member country.

Did You Know?

IFDH publishes the quarterly periodical *International Journal of Dental Hygiene* that contains peer-reviewed scientific articles and international issues involving dental hygiene.

European Dental Hygienists' Federation (EDHF)

The European Dental Hygienists' Federation (EDHF) was founded in 1999 by Spain, Italy, Portugal, Austria, Germany, the Netherlands, and Switzerland and has since expanded.[51] The focus is on the recognition of the dental hygiene profession and the harmonization of dental hygiene education within Europe. The work of this organization is essential in light of directives from the European Union pertaining to free movement of EU workers and the right of its citizens to equitable access to health care, education, and work opportunities.

Summary

This chapter has provided an overview of the ways in which dental hygienists are involved in dental public health on a global basis. Many countries lack basic facilities for sophisticated oral health promotion programs and are not able to utilize a dental hygienist in the traditional role developed in the United States. Therefore, dental hygienists should remain flexible in their approach to delivering oral hygiene.

Oral health issues are not recognized as health problems in many countries; consequently, periodontal diseases and oral hygiene are neglected and programs addressing them do not exist or are underfunded.

Oral health should embrace other health issues in order to make a case for priority funding in national health programs such as tobacco cessation, nutrition, and diet in efforts to prevent disease.

This is an exciting time for dental hygienists, and the profession will continue to grow in importance and status within the dental team. It is possible to significantly reduce oral disease on a global basis if dental public health systems include dental hygienists.

Self-Study Test Items

1. Which European country has a history of establishing the dental hygiene profession?
   a. England
   b. Italy
   c. Germany
   d. Portugal

2. Which of the following is a reason for the lack of access to dental hygiene services worldwide?
   a. Insufficient funding
   b. Lack of social and cultural awareness
   c. Legal restraints
   d. All of the above

3. Delivery systems are affected by which of the following?
   a. politics
   b. culture
   c. socioeconomic factors
   d. All of the above

4. In industrialized nations, where do dental hygienists mainly practice?
   a. Public health clinics
   b. Educational institutions
   c. Government positions
   d. Private dental clinics

5. What organization is a nonprofit group that unites dental hygiene associations from around the world in their common cause of promoting access to quality preventative oral services and to raise public awareness of the prevention of dental disease?
   a. American Dental Hygiene Association
   b. European Dental Hygienists' Federation
   c. International Federation of Dental Hygienists
   d. European Federation of Periodontology

Note

The author wishes to thank Sue Lloyd, contributor of this chapter in the first and second editions; Claudia Luciak-Donsberger, for her contributions during the third edition and her research on international dental hygiene; and Patricia M. Johnson for her continuing contributions to research on dental hygiene worldwide.

References

1. Hobdell M, Petersen PE, Clarkson J, Johnson N. Global goals for oral health 2020. *Int Dent J.* 2003;53:285–288.

2. World Health Organization. Strategies and Approaches in Oral Disease Prevention and Health Promotion. http://www.who.int/oral_health/strategies/cont/en/index.html. Accessed November 12, 2007.

3. Eaton, KA. Factors affecting community oral health care needs and provisions. (Dissertation). London, UK. University of London, 2002. Retrieved from http://discovery.ucl.ac.uk/952008 on November 6, 2014.

4. Pine CM, Pitts NB, Steele JG, Nunn JN, Treasure E. Dental restorations in adults in the UK in 1998 and implications for the future. *Br Dent J.* 2001;190(1):4–8.

5. Katsman E. Report on the activities carried out by "Sonrisas" to promote oral health: The experience of a Canadian dental hygienist in the Dominican Republic. *Int J Dent Hyg.* 2007;5(3):139–144.

6. Knevel RJM, Neupane S, Shressta B, de Mey L. Buddhi Bangara Project—a 3–5 year collaborative program combining support, education, and research. *Int J Dent Hyg.* 2008 Nov;6(4):337–46.

7. World Health Organization. Global Oral Health Database. Retrieved from http://www.who.int/oral_health/database/global//en/index.html on November 6, 2014.

8. World Health Organization. Periodontal Country Profiles. Retrieved from http://www.dent.niigata-u.ac.jp/prevent/perio/contents.html on November 6, 2014.

9. Federation Dentaire International. Data Hub for Global Health. Retrieved from http://www.fdiworldental.org/data-hub/atlas.aspx on September 18, 2015.

10. Federation Dentaire International. Dental Schools. Retrieved from http://www.fdiworldental.org/media/78385/72_map_oral_health_2.pdf on September 29, 2015.

11. Council of European Chief Dental Officers. CECDO database. Retrieved from http://www.cecdo.org/pages/database%20intro.html on August 4, 2015 on November 6, 2014.

12. Council of European Dentists. About the CED. Retrieved from http://www.eudental.eu. on August 4, 2015.

13. Johnson PM. Dental hygiene practice: international profile and future directions. *Int Dent J.* 1992;42:451–459.

14. Johnson PM. International profiles of dental hygiene 1987 to 2001: a 19-nation comparative study. *Int Dent J.* 2003;53:299–313.

15. Johnson PM. International profiles of dental hygiene from 1987–2006: a 21 nation comparative study. *Int Dent J* 2009;59;63–77.

16. Bader JD, Shugars D. Need for change in standards of caries diagnosis—epidemiology and health services research perspective. *J Dent Educ.* 1993;57:415–421.

17. Ismail AI, Sohn W, Tellez M, et al. The International Caries Detection and Assessment System (ICDAS): an integrated system for measuring dental caries. *Community Dent Oral Epidemiol.* 2007;35(3):170–178.

18. Bratthall D. Introducing the Significant Caries Index together with a proposal for a new global oral health goal for 12 year-olds. *Int Dent J.* 2000;50:378–384.

19. Ainamo J, Barmes DE, Beagrie BG, Cutress TW, Martin J, Sardo Infirri J. Development of the World Health Organization (WHO) Community Periodontal Index of Treatment Needs (CPITN). *Int Dent J.* 1982;32:281–291.

20. Bassani DG, da Silva CM, Oppermann RV. Validity of the "Community Periodontal Index of Treatment Needs" (CPITN) for population periodontitis screening. *Cad Saude Publica.* 2006;22(2):277–283.

21. Baelum V, Papapanou PN. CPITN and the epidemiology of periodontal disease. 1996: commentary. *Community Dent and Oral Epidemiol.* 24;6:367–368.
22. Chaudhry Z, Scully C. Dental manpower: many questions, weak data and inadequate answers. *Br Dent J.* 1998;184: 432–436.
23. US Department of Health and Human Services. *Oral Health in America: A Report of the Surgeon General.* Rockville, MD: US Department of Health and Human Services, National Institute of Dental and Craniofacial Research, National Institutes of Health; 2000.
24. Eaton KA, Newman HN, Widsröm E. A survey of dental hygienists numbers in Canada, the European Economic Area, Japan and the United States of America in 1998. *Br Dentl J.* 2003;195:595–598.
25. Luciak-Donsberger C. Origins and benefits of dental hygiene practice in Europe. *Int J Dent Hyg.* 2003;1:29–42.
26. Luciak-Donsberger C. The effects of gender disparities on dental hygiene education and practice in Europe. *Int J Dent Hyg.* 2003;1(4):195–212.
27. Luciak-Donsberger C. *The Study of Dental Hygiene in Europe: Education and Legal Regulation in Eight Additional Countries. Current Developments in Six Countries.* Vienna, Austria: Federal Ministry of Education, Science and Culture; 2003.
28. Luciak-Donsberger, C and Eaton, KA. Dental hygienists in Europe: trends towards harmonization of education and practice since 2003. *Int Jour Dental Hygiene* 7, 2009;273–284.
29. McKeown L, Sunell S, Wickstrom P. The discourse of dental hygiene practice in Canada. *Int J Dent Hyg.* 2003;1:43–48.
30. Luciak-Donsberger C. *The Study of Dental Hygiene in Europe: Education and Legal Regulation in Eight Additional Countries. Current Developments in Six Countries.* Vienna, Austria: Federal Ministry of Education, Science and Culture; 2003.
31. Cheng YA, Huang ST, Hsieh ST. A predictive study on the role and function of the dental hygienist in Taiwan. *Int J Dent Hyg.* 2007;5(2):103–108.
32. Luciak-Donsberger C, Chan C. Dental hygiene in Hong Kong: A global perspective. *Int J Dent Hyg.* 2003;1(2):84–88.
33. Petersen PE, Kwan S. Evaluation of community-based oral health promotion and oral disease prevention—WHO recommendations for improved evidence in public health practice. *Community Dent Health.* 2004;21(suppl 4):319–329.
34. Robert Y, Sheiham A. The burden of restorative dental treatment for children in Third World countries. *Int Dent J.* 2002;52(1):1–9.
35. Global goals for oral health in the year 2000: FDI. *Int Dent J.* 1982;32:74–77.
36. World Health Organization Sixtieth World Health Assembly, A60/16 Provisional Agenda Item 12.9 22. http://apps.who.int/gb/ebwha/pdf_files/WHA60/A60_16-en.pdf. Accessed March, 22 2007.
37. World Health Organization. Global goals for oral health 2020 Retrieved from http://www.who.int/oral_health/publications/goals2020/en/ on September 29, 2015.
38. World Health Organization. **Oral health: action plan for promotion and integrated** disease prevention. Retrieved from http://apps.who.int/gb/ebwha/pdf_files/EB120/b120_r5-en.pdf on September 29, 2015
39. World Health Organization. WHO collab centres. Retrieved from www.who.int/whocc. on August 4, 2015.
40. Monajem S. Integration of oral health into primary health care: the role of dental hygienists and the WHO stewardship. *Int J Dent Hyg.* 2006;4(1):47–51.
41. Nasry HA, Preshaw PM, Stacey F, Heasman L, Swan M, Heasman PA. Smoking cessation advice for patients with chronic periodontitis. *Br Dent J.* 2006;200(5):272–275.
42. Correa da Fonseca, A. *An Analysis of Mobile Dentistry in Austria in Comparison to International Scenarios* [master's thesis]. Krems, Austria: Danube University; 2007.
43. Chalmers JM. Minimal intervention dentistry: Part 2. Strategies for addressing restorative challenges in older patients. *J Can Dent Assoc.* 2006;72(5):435–440.
44. Phelophepa Train. Retrieved from http://www.mhc.org.za. on November 12, 2007.
45. Nishimura T, Takahashi C, Takahashi E. Dental hygiene residential care in a 3-year dental hygiene education programme in Japan: towards dysphagia management based on the dental hygiene process of care. *Int J Dent Hyg.* 2007;5(3):145–150.
46. Luciak-Donsberger C, Piribauer F. Evidence-based rationale supports a national periodontal disease screening program. *J Evid Based Dent Pract.* 2007;7(2):51–59.
47. Cobban SJ. Evidence-based practice and the professionalization of dental hygiene. *Int J Dent Hyg.* 2004;2(4):152–160.
48. Policy Statement—Proceedings of the European Workshop on Oral Care and General Health. Opportunities for the Dental Hygienists in Health Education in the New Century. *Oral Health and Prev Dent.* 2003;1(suppl 1):340.
49. European Federation of Periodontology. Vision. www.efp.net. Accessed November 12, 2007.
50. International Federation of Dental Hygienists. Retrieved from http::www.ifdh.org on September 18, 2015.
51. European Dental Hygienists' Federation. About us. Retrieved from http://www.edhf.eu/ on August 4, 2015.

Visit www.pearsonhighered.com/healthprofessionsresources to access the student resources that accompany this book. Simply select Dental Hygiene from the choice of disciplines. Find this book and you will find the complimentary study tools created for this specific title.

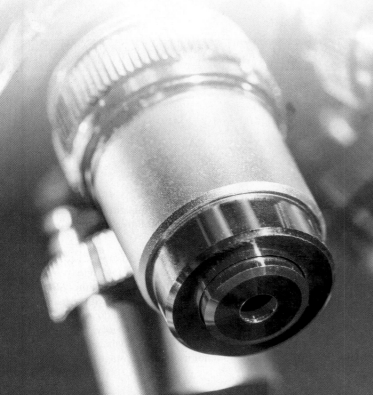

5

Financing of Dental Care

OBJECTIVES

After studying this chapter, the dental hygiene student should be able to:

- Describe current methods of payment for dental care
- Define and apply terminology associated with financing dental care
- Identify the different insurance plans available for dental care
- Describe the role of the government in financing dental care

COMPETENCIES

After studying this chapter and participating in accompanying course activities, the dental hygiene student should be competent to do the following:

- Assess the oral health needs and services of the community to determine action plans and availability of resources to meet the health care needs.
- Provide screening, referral, and educational services that allow patients to access the resources of the health care system.
- Evaluate reimbursement mechanisms and their impact on the patient's access to oral health care

KEY TERMS

Barter system *71*
Benefit *80*
Capitation plan *70*
Copayment *80*
Deductible *80*
Dental claim *80*
Dental necessity *80*
Encounter fee plan *71*
Explanation of benefits *80*
Fee-for-service plan *70*
Health maintenance organization (HMO) *71*
Medicaid (Title XIX) *80*
Medicare (Title XVIII) *80*
Preexisting condition *80*
Preferred provider organizations (PPOs) *71*
Premium *80*
Usual, customary, reasonable (UCR) fee *70*

Science photo/Shutterstock

Historically, the financing of dental care was the responsibility of the patient in need of treatment and the dental practitioner involved in managing the dental practice. However, in today's economy, the financing of dental care in the United States involves numerous entities in both the private and public sectors.

Although health insurance began in the early 1900s, dental insurance did not become commonplace until the 1970s. The first model for dental insurance actually began in 1954, when dentists formed dental service organizations in California, Oregon, and Washington to provide dental benefits with employee benefits programs for organized labor unions. By 1966, this movement became part of what is now called Delta Dental Plans Association.[1]

Public funding for dental care was not created until 1965 by the addition of Title XIX to the Social Security Act. Basically, Medicaid was created as a program to help states provide medical coverage for low-income families and other individuals who meet eligibility requirements such as those who are blind, aged, disabled, or pregnant. States are required to offer Medicaid dental coverage to children from low-income families, and some states choose to offer dental coverage to adults in need as well. So, many dental hygienists who practiced before the 1970s were not accustomed to the role private insurance or public funding had in dental hygiene care.

Of the total health care expenditures in the United States in 2010, only 2.9 percent was spent on dental services.[2] Nearly 91 percent was paid for by private funds whether by the patient (47.5 percent) or by private insurance (43.1 percent), and approximately 5.8 percent was funded by Medicaid.[1] (See Table 5-1 ■.)

Approximately 60 percent of the population had private dental coverage during 2007. In 2007, a higher percentage of adults ages 21–44 had public dental coverage only than in 1997.[3] The differences in dental coverage status between 1997 and 2007 did not vary significantly by race/ethnicity.[3] (See Figures 5-1 ■, 5-2 ■, and 5-4 ■.)

Use of dental services—the percentage of individuals who had at least one dental visit—also remained relatively unchanged at around 40 percent from 1996 to 2010.(4) Dental coverage through Medicaid or the State Children's Health Insurance Program (CHIP), which was established in 1997, rose from 9 to 13 percent. The increase was due primarily to an increase in the number of children covered by these federal-state health programs with mandated pediatric dental coverage.[4] Medicaid and CHIP beneficiaries, children in particular, showed increases in the use of dental services, but still visited the dentist less often than privately insured children.[4]

FIGURE 5–1 Dental Visits per Coverage Status

	1996	2004	2010
Private	56.4	57.3	56.9
Medicaid	27.7	31.6	33.6
Unknown[a]	33.5	34.8	31.8
None	25.8	21.7	18.0

Notes: Data are from the Medical Expenditure Panel Survey (MEPS). This table includes only the noninstitutionalized population with a dental visit. For 2004 and 2010, Medicaid includes children enrolled in the State Children's Health Insurance Program.

[a]Individuals in the unknown category indicated that they had other types of public medical coverage, including state or federal programs such as Medicare or veteran's benefits. These programs might not have included dental coverage, or might have provided limited dental coverage to certain individuals. For these programs, the MEPS survey methodology did not allow us to identify which beneficiaries actually had dental coverage. Beneficiaries in these programs with a dental claim paid by insurance during the period were counted as having private coverage. For example, Medicare Advantage enrollees who had a claim paid by private insurance were counted in the private insurance category. Medicare beneficiaries who did not have a claim paid by insurance were included in the unknown category because they might have had dental coverage such as under a Medicare Advantage plan, but did not use their coverage during the survey period.

Source: http://www.gao.gov/assets/660/657454.pdf on page 15.

Table 5–1 **Dental Service Expenses in the United States, 2012**

Population Characteristic	Population (in thousands)	Percent with Expense	Per Person with an Expense		Total Expenses (in millions)	Percent Distribution of total Expenses by Source of Payment				
			Median	Mean		Out of Pocket	Private Insurance[a]	Medicare	Medicaid	Other[b]
Total	313,490	40.4	243	670	84,818	48.5	42.1	0.9	5.5	3.0
Age in years										
Under 65	268,219	39.9	230	634	67,856	42.9	47.1	0.2*	6.7	3.1
Under 5	19,946	19.2	129	233	892	20.9	45.8	0.0*	30.5	2.8*
5–17	53,967	56.3	200	706	21,434	41.8	44.9	0.0*	11.3	2.0
18–44	111,957	33.3	232	586	21,872	40.7	50.0	0.1*	5.1	4.1
45–64	82,349	43.2	270	666	23,658	46.8	46.4	0.4*	3.1*	3.2
65 and over	45,271	43.1	330	870	16,962	70.7	22.0	4.0	1.0	2.3
Sex										
Male	153,191	37.4	236	637	36,517	47.9	43.1	0.8	4.8	3.5
Female	160,299	43.2	248	698	48,301	49.0	41.3	1.0	6.0	2.6
Race/ethnicity										
Hispanic	53,517	29.0	174	532	8,243	40.7	38.2	1.8	14.3	5.0
White, Non-Hispanic	197,943	46.1	260	700	63,880	51.5	41.4	0.7	3.8	2.5
Black, Non-Hispanic	37,888	29.0	183	543	5,962	34.7	45.5	1.6	13.4	4.8
Amer. Indian/ AK Native/ Multi. Races, non-Hisp.	6,945	39.4	262	722	1,975	35.1	51.7	1.7*	7.8*	3.8*
Asian/ Hawaiian/ Pacific Islander, non-Hispanic	17,197	34.8	271	794	4,756	43.9	49.5	1.0*	2.9	2.6*
Health insurance status[c]										
<65, Any private	178,072	47.5	248	674	57,085	42.5	56.0	0.0*	0.7	0.8
<65, Public only	50,545	31.8	133	421	6,772	30.4	0.0*	1.6*	60.9	7.1
<65, Uninsured	39,603	15.9	249	633	3,999	70.4	0.0*	0.0*	0.0*	29.6
65+, Medicare only	16,439	37.7	330	805	4,983	83.5	0.0*	11.0	0.0*	5.5
65+, Medicare and private	23,387	52.7	330	910	11,219	65.3	32.4	0.9*	0.5*	0.9*
65+, Medicare and other public	4,749	16.5	200	817	640	74.8	0.0*	4.6*	17.0*	3.5*
65+, No Medicare	—	—	—	—	—	—	—	—	—	—
Poverty status[d]										
Negative or Poor	46,993	26.5	163	516	6,419	38.2	15.7	0.4*	34.4	11.3

(*continued*)

Table 5–1 Dental Service Expenses in the United States, 2012 (*continued*)

Dental Services-Median and Mean Expenses per Person With Expense and Distribution of Expenses by Source of Payment: United States, 2012 All Dental Visits

Population Characteristic	Population (in thousands)	Percent with Expense	Per Person with an Expense		Total Expenses (in millions)	Percent Distribution of total Expenses by Source of Payment				
			Median	Mean		Out of Pocket	Private Insurance[a]	Medicare	Medicaid	Other[b]
Near-poor	15,846	24.7	186	456	1,783	46.2	18.1	2.6*	24.6	8.5
Low income	44,609	29.1	200	595	7,725	51.1	26.0	2.2	13.5	7.2
Middle income	94,168	39.0	241	665	24,427	49.1	44.0	1.1*	3.5	2.3
High income	111,875	54.1	272	735	44,464	49.3	48.6	0.6	0.3*	1.2
Metropolitan statistical area (MSA)										
MSA	268,925	40.9	247	691	76,046	48.6	42.9	1.0	4.6	2.9
Non-MSA	44,565	37.0	215	531	8,772	47.2	35.2	0.2*	13.8	3.6*
Census Region										
Northeast	55,698	42.5	240	653	15,436	48.7	40.4	1.2*	7.4	2.4*
Midwest	66,851	46.3	244	661	20,457	46.7	44.5	0.9	5.8	2.2
South	117,018	35.4	230	642	26,570	50.8	40.1	0.9	4.8	3.5
West	73,923	41.3	272	732	22,354	47.3	43.4	0.9	4.9	3.4
Perceived Health Status										
Excellent	99,661	44.4	224	612	27,061	45.6	46.9	0.4	4.7	2.3
Very Good	100,372	42.9	247	668	28,763	49.2	43.3	0.7	4.2	2.6
Good	78,157	37.3	250	741	21,622	50.5	37.8	1.2	7.7	2.8
Fair	25,490	29.7	279	738	5,590	49.2	33.5	3.5	6.6	7.1*
Poor	9,244	26.5	300	728	1,781	54.5	27.0	0.8*	10.1	7.6*
Missing	–	–	–	–	–	–	–	–	–	–

[a] Private insurance includes Tricare (Armed-Forces-related coverage).

[b] Other includes other public programs such as Department of Veterans Affairs (except Tricare); other Federal sources (Indian Health Service, military treatment facilities, and other care provided by the Federal Government); other State and local sources (community and neighborhood clinics, State and local health departments, and State programs other than Medicaid); and other public (Medicaid payments reported for persons who were not enrolled in the Medicaid program at any time during the year). Other also includes Worker's Compensation; other unclassified sources (e.g., automobile, homeowner's, liability, and other miscellaneous or unknown sources); and other private insurance (any type of private insurance payments reported for persons without private health insurance coverage during the year, as defined in MEPS).

[c] Uninsured refers to persons uninsured during the entire year. Public and private health insurance categories refer to individuals with public or private insurance at any time during the period; individuals with both public and private insurance and those with Tricare (Armed-Forces-related coverage) are classified as having private insurance; 65+, No Medicare refers to persons age 65+ without Medicare but with private, or Medicaid, or uninsured.

[d] Poor refers to incomes below the Federal poverty line; near poor, over the poverty line through 125 percent of the poverty line; low income, over 125 percent through 200 percent of the poverty line; middle income, over 200 percent to 400 percent of the poverty line; and high income, over 400 percent of the poverty line.

[†] Standard error approximately zero because of poststratification to Census Bureau population control tables.

[–] Less than 100 sample cases.

[*] Relative standard error equal to or greater than 30%.

Sources: Agency for Healthcare Research and Quality. Dental Services-Mean and Median Expenses per Person With Expense and Distribution of Expenses by Source of Payment: United States, 2012. Medical Expenditure Panel Survey Household Component Data. Generated interactively. (January 13, 2015)

FIGURE 5–2 Dental Visit per Coverage

	1996	2004	2010
Dental visit	42.9	43.6	41.3
No dental visit	57.1	56.4	58.7
Total	**100.0**	**100.0**	**100.0**

Source: GAO analysis of HHS data.

Notes: Data are from the Medical Expenditure Panel Survey (MEPS). This table includes only the noninstitutionalized population.

Source: http://www.gao.gov/assets/660/657454.pdf on page 15

FIGURE 5–3 Dental Coverage Status, 1996, 2004, and 2010

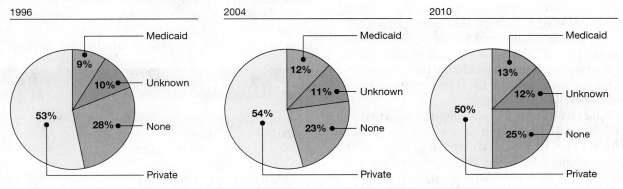

Notes: Data are from the Medical Expenditure Panel Survey (MEPS). This figure includes only the noninstitutionalized population. For 2004 and 2010, Medicaid includes children enrolled in the State Children's Health Insurance Program. Individuals in the unknown category indicated that they had other types of public coverage, including state or federal programs such as Medicare or veteran's benefits. These programs might not have included dental coverage, or might have provided limited dental coverage to certain individuals. For these programs, the MEPS survey methodology did not allow us to identify which beneficiaries actually had dental coverage. Beneficiaries in these programs with a dental claim paid by private insurance during the period were counted as having private coverage. For example, Medicare Advantage enrollees who had a claim paid by private insurance were counted in the private insurance category. Medicare beneficiaries who did not have a claim paid by private insurance were included in the unknown category because they might have had dental coverage, such as under a Medicare Advantage plan, but did not use their coverage during the survey period.

Source: Data are from the Medical Expenditure Panel Survey

FIGURE 5–4 National Expenditures for Dental Services, Adjusted for Inflation, 1996–2011

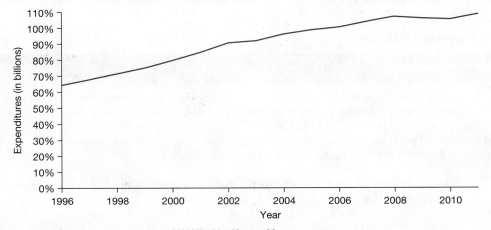

Source: http://www.gao.gov/assets/660/657454.pdf page 32.

Payment Methods

Generally, there are four types of payment methods in dental care delivery. These include the fee-for-service arrangements, capitation plans, encounter fee plans, and the barter system. (See Table 5-2 ■.) Although these reimbursement mechanisms can be unique to different parts of the country, they have similarities.

The **fee-for-service plan** is based on a fee scale for all covered services, and bills the patient for the services rendered by a dental hygienist, dentist, or denturist. It is the most commonly used payment method in the United States. The patient and/or an insurance company may pay the fee. These set fees are referred to as **usual, customary, and reasonable (UCR) fees,** which are the average dentist fee per service in the immediate local region. *Usual* implies that the fee is what is most often charged by dental providers for a given dental or dental hygiene service. *Customary* refers to a schedule of maximum fees charged by dental providers with similar training and service within a specific and limited geographic area as determined by the administrator of a dental plan based on submitted fees. *Reasonable* indicates that the fee meets the usual and customary definitions and is therefore justifiable.

Some clinics have instituted a sliding-fee scale to make services more affordable for patients with a low income. The fees for services may be decreased depending on the patient's income and family size. This type of reduced-fee program is available through federal grants.

Indemnity plans are traditional fee-for-service insurance plans that operate by a submission and reimbursement method. The dental practitioner provides a service and either bills the patient, who pays the fee and submits the bill to an insurance company for reimbursement, or bills the insurance company, which makes direct payment to the practice. Usually, patients with an indemnity plan may choose any dentist but may be required to obtain preauthorization (prior authorization) for certain procedures. Preauthorizations involve sending information to the insurance company for approval of reimbursement for the prescribed procedure. So, this involves a waiting period for patients, and in some cases, a prior approval may be required for periodontal scaling and root planning per quadrant treatment.

The term waiting period is used to define a time period in which the dental insurance company may not pay or reimburse a patient for certain procedures, which are usually not preventive procedures. The dental insurance company may define a waiting period to decrease the likelihood of a patient buying insurance only when there is significant dental work to be done or to decrease a patient needing periodontal scaling annually. Not all dental insurance companies have waiting periods.

Most indemnity plans require an annual deductible payment, and after the patient has paid that amount, the plan typically pays a percentage of UCR rates for covered services. For example, the insurance company may pay 80 percent of the UCR and the patient may be required to cover the remaining 20 percent. Most plans require the patient to make a copayment for a visit, which is deducted from the 20 percent the patient, not the plan, covers.

Did You Know?

Copayments are often used to discourage the overuse of services.

Many fee-for-service payment methods offer a discounted fee for a target population. For example, a dental office may lower fees by 10 percent for senior citizens or participants in a prepaid group.

Most dental practices accept fee-for-service plans that provide an incentive for dental practitioners to provide all necessary treatments. Generally, these plans increase the production of an office because it is paid based on the number of services produced. The clinic or provider creates the fee scale, usually similar to the UCR.

With the **capitation plan,** a dental provider contracts with a third party to provide all or most of the services to a specified group of people in return for a fixed monthly

Table 5–2 Types of Payment Methods

Payment Method	Definition
Fee for service	Fee scale is developed for all services provided by the dental provider, and a payment is then developed for the service(s) rendered. This is the most common payment method used in the United States.
Capitation	Dental provider contracts with a program to provide all or most dental services to the program's subscribers in return for payment on a per capita basis.
Barter system	Dental provider and patient negotiate payment by exchanging goods or services without utilizing money.
Encounter	Payment is based on an office visit and is always the same regardless of the service(s) rendered.

payment, which is determined according to the number of individuals or families in the group. The dental provider receives the payment whether the patients use the care or not. The patients are sometimes charged a copayment for specified treatments. The philosophy behind capitation plans is that it is more cost effective to keep people healthy than it is to treat their disease. The incentive is to keep people well and out of the health care provider's practice. Costs are kept low so the patient benefits and patient demand are also kept low, which benefits the practice.

Dental managed care organizations typically provide capitation plans. Managed care organizations were created in 1973 by the Health Maintenance Organization Act. Participating physicians of a **health maintenance organization (HMO)** provide comprehensive health care to enrolled individuals and families in a specified region and receive fixed periodic payments. Some suggest that because of their primarily preventive care, HMOs actually reduce costs for participants by reducing hospitalization and the use of costly services. Some dental providers do not support dental managed care plans because of the reduction in reimbursement and the decrease in control of treatment that they can recommend. Most HMOs provide medical coverage but do not cover routine dental care.

In some instances, capitation plans may not benefit the patient. For example, a dental practice that receives a set payment each month from a plan has little incentive to provide preventive treatment to the plan-covered patients. In other words, a practice that is paid whether it provides treatment or not may choose not to prioritize scheduling (and/or provide treatment) to capitation plan members but instead to schedule as many fee-for-service patients as possible. In this way, the office could collect the monthly stipend from the capitation plan and still collect fees for services provided to fee-for-service patients.

The **encounter fee plan** basically pays for each care encounter regardless of the service provider. For example, if a patient visits a provider on one day for an exam and prophylaxis, on the next day for two amalgam restorations, and the third day for a class-V glass ionomer restoration, each encounter generates the same reimbursement fee.

The encounter fee plan may tend to decrease productivity overall because some dental clinics offer only one service per visit to capitalize on the number of encounters and thus fees paid. This would obviously inconvenience the patient and may subsequently decrease the likelihood of the patient's receiving comprehensive care. Some clinics go so far as to have a new patient appointment take at least three visits by scheduling one visit for radiographs, one for an exam, and another for the dental prophylaxis.

The **barter system,** used only in the private sector, involves exchanging goods and services without using money. The dental provider and the patient negotiate the exchange. For instance, the dental practitioner may provide dental care in return for the patient's carpentry services. Although not common, this payment method is still in place in many private dental offices.

Insurance Plans

Dental service corporations are legally constituted nonprofit organizations incorporated in a state and sponsored by a dental society to negotiate and administer programs. These programs are contractual agreements with dentists to provide care to eligible beneficiaries using UCR fees. Generally, dental providers accept payment at 90 percent of fees as payment in full. Their patient charts are regularly audited for fees and inspected. Currently, the largest dental benefits carrier in the United States is Delta Dental Plans Association[1] operated on a state-by-state basis. See Figure 5-5 ■ for a Delta Dental of New Mexico summary of covered dental services.

Health service corporations offer limited dental coverage as part of their hospital-surgical-medical policies. A common health service corporation is Blue Cross/Blue Shield.[5]

Many dental practices in the United States participate in **preferred provider organizations (PPOs).** The practitioners contract with a PPO to provide dental care services for lower than average fees in order to attract patient subscribers who are seeking lower costs. This gives the dental practitioners a competitive edge over nonparticipating practitioners.

Individual practice associations (IPAs) are legal entities organized for individual participating dental practitioners to enter into contracts collectively to provide prepaid dental services to enrolled patients. They may contract directly with a group or an insurance carrier. This is usually referred to as *managed care* and uses the capitation method of reimbursement.

Concordia Plus Dental Program is an example of a prepaid dental plan that focuses on preventive care and the early diagnosis of dental problems.[6] Under Concordia Plus, members select a primary dental office (PDO) from a contracted and credentialed network of providers. The PDO handles the member's dental care needs, including referrals to specialists when necessary. Members select their own PDO from the Concordia Plus network of participating dentists.

See Table 5-3 ■ for a comparison of the various types of insurance plans.

Dental Provider Billing

Dental providers generally bill insurance companies for dental procedures utilizing a *dental claim form.* (See Figures 5-6 ■ and 5-7 ■ for an example of a fee slip and a claim form, respectively.) These forms generally require the

FIGURE 5–5 Summary of Delta Dental of New Mexico Covered Dental Services

Summary of Dental Plan Benefits

Benefit Period: January 1 through December 31

Deductible: $50 deductible per person total per Benefit Year limited to a maximum deductible of $150 per family per Benefit Year

Maximum Benefit Amount: $1,000 per person total per Benefit Year

Orthodontic Lifetime Maximum: $1,000 per person total per Lifetime

Covered Services:	Delta Dental PPO℠ Dentist	Delta Dental Premier® or Non-Participating Dentist*
	You Pay	**You Pay***
Diagnostic and Preventive Services		
Diagnostic and Preventive Services – exams, cleanings, topical fluoride, and space maintainers	No Charge	No Charge
Emergency Palliative Treatment – to temporarily relieve pain	No Charge	No Charge
Sealants – to prevent decay of permanent teeth	No Charge	No Charge
Brush Biopsy – to detect oral cancer	No Charge	No Charge
Radiographs – images	No Charge	No Charge
Periodontal Maintenance – cleanings following periodontal therapy	No Charge	No Charge
Basic Services		
Minor Restorative Services – fillings	20%	20%
Endodontic Services – root canals	20%	20%
Periodontic Services – to treat gum disease	20%	20%
Oral Surgery Services – extractions and dental surgery	20%	20%
Other Basic Services – misc. services	20%	20%
Major Services		
Crown Repair – to individual crowns	50%	50%
Major Restorative Services – crowns	50%	50%
Relines and Repairs – to bridges, dentures, and implants	50%	50%
Prosthodontic Services – bridges, dentures, and implants	50%	50%
TMD Treatment – medically necessary treatment of the disorder of the temporomandibular joint, including diagnostic imaging	50%	50%
Orthodontic Services		
Orthodontic Services – braces	50%	50%
Orthodontic Age Limit	to the end of the month of age 19	to the end of the month of age 19

*Selecting a non-participating dentist may result in higher out-of-pocket expenses. Non-participating dentists do not accept Delta Dental's Maximum Approved Fees.

Source: © Pearson Education, Inc.

Table 5–3 Types of Insurance Plans

Insurance Plan	Definition	Example
Dental service corporations	Not-for-profit organizations that negotiate fees for providing dental care; incorporated on a state-by-state basis and sponsored by a constituent dental society to negotiate and administer programs	Delta Dental Plans Association
Health service corporations	Organizations that offer limited dental coverage as part of their hospital-surgical-medical policies	Blue Cross/Blue Shield
Preferred provider organizations (PPO)	Providers of dental benefits and third-party contractors with employer to offer services to employer's employees at reduced prices	Aetna U.S. Healthcare Dental PPO
Individual practice associations (IPA)	Legal entities organized for dental providers to enter into contracts collectively to provide prepaid dental services to enrolled groups	MD Individual Practice Associates, Inc.

(continued)

Table 5–3 Types of Insurance Plans (*continued*)

Insurance Plan	Definition	Example
Commercial insurance plans	Operate for profit and designed as an indemnity plan	Unicare 200
Prepaid group practice	Large group practice that contracts with groups of subscribers	Golden West Dental and Vision
Health maintenance organization (HMO)	Developed in 1973 by the HMO act, organization provides comprehensive health care to enrolled individuals and families in a specified region by participating providers, financed by fixed periodic payments; initially designed to decrease health care costs	Presbyterian Health Plan
Capitation plan	Offers per capita payment for a defined population provided by specific dental providers; payment made to provider regardless of use	Concordia Plus

	I. DIAGNOSTIC SERVICES		
00120	Periodic Oral Evaluation		
00140	Limited Oral Evaluation (Emergency)		
00150	Initial Comprehensive Oral Evaluation		
	RADIOGRAPHS	TOOTH	ARCH
00210	Intraoral Comp Series-Inc. BW		
00220	Intraoral Periapical-1st Film		
00230	Intraoral P.A.-Ea. Addl. Film		
00240	Intraoral Occlusal Film		
00270	Bitewing-Single Film		
00272	Bitewing-Two Films		
00274	Bitewings-Four Films		
00330	Panoramic Film		
	II. PREVENTIVE SERVICES	TOOTH	
01110	Prophylaxis - Adult		
01120	Prophylaxis - Child		
01203	Topical Floride - Child (without Prophy)		
* 01204	Topical Floride - Adult (without Prophy)		
01351	Sealant - Per Tooth (multiple teeth)		
01510	Space Maint-Fixed-Unilateral		
01515	Space Maint-Fixed-Bilateral		
01550	Re-cement Space Maintainer		
	III. RESTORATIVE SERVICES	TOOTH	SURFACE
02140	Amalgam-1 Surface, Prim. or Perm.		
02150	Amalgam-2 Surfaces, Prim. or Perm.		
02160	Amalgam-3 Surfaces, Prim. or Perm.		
02161	Amalgam-4+ Surfaces, Prim. or Perm.		
02330	Resin-based comp.-1 Surface, Anterior		
02331	Resin-based comp.-2 Surfaces, Anterior		
02332	Resin-based comp.-3 Surfaces, Anterior		
02335	Resin-based comp-4+ Surfaces or Incisal, Ant.		
02390	Resin-based composite crown, Anterior		
02391	Resin-based composite-1 Surface, Posterior		
02392	Resin-based composite-2 Surfaces, Posterior		
02393	Resin-based composite-3 Surfaces, Posterior		
02394	Resin-based composite-4+ Surfaces, Posterior		
	CROWNS	TOOTH	SURFACE
* 02710	Crown Resin (Indirect/Laboratory)		
02740	Crown-Porc/Ceramic Substrate		
02750	Crown-Porc. High Noble Metal		
* 02751	Crown-Porcelain to Base Metal		
* 02752	Crown-Porcelain to Nobel Metal		
02790	Crown-Full Cast. High Noble Metal		
* 02791	Crown-Full Cast. Base Metal		
* 02792	Crown-Full Cast. Nobel Metal		
02910	Recement Inlay		
02920	Re-cement Crown		
02930	Stainless Steel Crown-Primary		
02931	Stainless Steel Crown-Permanent		
02932	Prefabricated Resin Crown		
02940	Sedative Filling		
02950	Crown Buildup, including any pins		
02951	Pin Retention, per tooth, in addt'n to estoration		
02952	Cast Post & Core, in addt'n to crown		
02954	Prefab Post & Core, in addt'n to crown		
* 02960	Crown Repair by report		
06930	Recement Fixed Partial Denture (Bridge)		
	IV. ENDODONTIC SERVICES	TOOTH	
03220	Therapeutic Pulpotomy		
* 03310	Anterior RCT (Exel. Rest.)		
* 03320	Biscuspid RCT (Excl. Rest.)		
* 03330	Molar RCT (Excl. Rest.)		
03410	Apicoectomy-Anterior		
03421	Apicoectomy/Periadicular Bicuspid		
03425	Apicoectomy/Periadicular Molar		

* Services allowed by Medicaid, but must be pre-authorized

	Con't. ENDODONTIC SERVICES	TOOTH	
03426	Apicoectomy/Periadicular ea. Addt'l root		
03430	Retrograde Filling, Per Root		
03450	Root Amputation, Per Root		
	V. PERIDONTAL SERVICES	TOOTH	QUAD
* 04210	Gingivectomy Or Gingivoplasty (Per Quad)		
04320	Provisional Splinting, Intracoronal		
04321	Provisional Splinting, Extracoronal		
* 04341	Scaling & Root Planing, 4+ teeth, Per Quad		
* 04342	Scaling & Root Planing, 1-3 teeth, Per Quad		
* 04910	Periodontal Maintenance		
	VI. REMOVABLE PROSTHODONTIC SERVICES		
* 05110	Complete Denture-Maxillary		
* 05120	Complete Denture-Mandibular		
* 05130	Immediate Denture-Maxillary		
* 05140	Immediate Denture-mandibular		
* 05211	Maxillary Partial-Resin Base		
* 05212	Mandibular Partial-Resin Base		
* 05213	Maxillary Partial-Cast Metal Framework		
* 05214	Mandibular Partial-Cast Metal Framework		
05410	Adjust Complete Denture-Maxillary		
05411	Adjust Complete Denture-Mandibular		
05421	Adjust Partial-Maxillary		
05422	Adjust Partial-Mandibular		
	X. ORAL SURGERY SERVICES	TOOTH	QUAD
07111	Coronal Remnants-Deciduous Tooth		
07140	Extraction, Erupted Tooth or Exposed Root		
07210	Extraction, Surgical Removal-Erupted Tooth		
07220	Extraction-Impacted Tooth-Soft Tissue		
07230	Extraction-Impacted Tooth-Partial Bony		
07240	Extraction-Impacted Tooth-Full Bony		
07241	Extraction-Unusual Tooth-Full Bony w/ compl.		
07250	Extraction-Residual Root-Surgical		
07270	Tooth Reimplantation-Accident (Avulsed)		
07281	Surgical Exposure to Aid Eruption		
07285	Biopsy of Oral Tissue-Hard		
07286	Biopsy of Oral Tissue-Soft		
07320	Alveoloplasty-No Extractions-Per Quad		
07510	I & D Intraoral Abscess		
07520	I & D Extraoral Abscess		
07960	Frenulectomy		
	XII. ADJUNCTIVE GENERAL SERVICES	TOOTH	
09110	Palliative (Emerg) Treatment-Minor Procedure		
09410	House Call (nursing home visits)		
09420	Hospital Call		
09630	Other Drugs and Medicaments, by report		
0359Y	DD Dental Special Needs		
	OTHER SERVICES RENDERED (NOT LISTED ABOVE)		

Location: ____________ Tax ID#: 00-0000001

Provider: ____________

Date of Service: ____ / ____ / ____

PATIENT IDENTIFICATION

Last First I.

FIGURE 5–6 Fee Slip Hard Copy, University of New Mexico Division of Dental Hygiene

Source: Fee Slip. Albuquerque, NM: University of New Mexico, Division of Dental Hygiene, 2009.

DENTAL CLAIM FORM

1. ☐ Dentist's pre-treatment estimate ☒ Dentist's statement of actual services Provider ID #	2. ☐ Medicaid Claim ☐ EPSDT Prior Authorization # Patient ID #	3. Carrier Name and Address **Fones Dental of New Mexico** **2500 Newman Blvd.** **Bridgeport, CT 06601**

PATIENT COVERAGE INFORMATION

4. Patient Name **Mary Jones**	5. Relationship to employee ☐ Self ☐ Child **Child** ☐ Spouse ☐ Other	6. Sex M F **F**	7. Patient birthdate MM DD YY **07/02/1995**	8. If full time student school city

9. Employee/subscriber name and address **John Jones** **1234 Main St.** **Albuquerque NM 87120**	10. Employee/subscriber dental plan I.D. number **123-45-6789**	11. Employee/subscriber birthdate MM DD YY **02/05/1966**	12. Employer (company)	13. Group number

14. Is patient covered by another dental plan **No** Is patient covered by a medical plan? yes no	15-a. Name and address of carrier(s)	15-b. Group no.(s)	16. Name and address of other employer

17-a. Employee/subscriber name (if different than patient's)	17-b. Employee/subscriber dental plan I.D. number	17-c. Employee subscriber birthdate MM DD YY	18. Relationship to patient ☐ Self ☐ Parent ☐ Spouse ☐ Other

19. I have reviewed the following treatment plan and fees. I agree to be responsible for all charges for dental services and materials not paid by my dental benefit plan, unless the treating dentist or dental practice has a contractual agreement with my plan prohibiting all or a portion of such charges. To the extent permitted under applicable law, I authorize release of any information relating to this claim. > **SIGNATURE ON FILE** **09/04/2009** Signed (Patient or parent if minor) Date	20. I hereby authorize payment of the dental benefits otherwise payable to me directly to the below named dental entity. > **SIGNATURE ON FILE** **09/04/2009** Signed (Employee/subscriber) Date

BILLING DENTIST

21. Name of Billing Dentist or Dental Entity **Dental Hygiene DH0000** **University of New Mexico Dental Hygiene**	30. Is treatment result of occupational illness or injury?	No	Yes	If yes, enter brief description and dates.
22. Address where payment should be remitted **2320 Tucker NE, Novitski Hall**	31. Is treatment result of auto accident?	**N**		
23. City, State, Zip **Albuquerque, NM 87131-1391**	32. Other accident?	**N**		
24. Dentist SSN or T.I.N. **00-0000000** 25. Dentist License no. **DH-1230** 26. Dentist phone no. **(505)555-4106**	33. If prosthesis, is this initial placement? **N**	(if no, reason for replacement)	34. Date prior placement

27. First visit date current series	28. Place of treatment Office Hosp. ECF Other **X**	29. Radiographs or models enclosed? No Yes How **N** many? **0**	35. Is treatment for orthodontics? **N**	If services already commenced enter:	Date appliances placed	Mos. treat. remaining **0**

36. Identify missing teeth with 'X' Facial (tooth chart diagram) Right Left Lingual Facial	37. Examination and treatment plan - List in order from tooth no. 1 through tooth no. 32 - Using charting system shown.						For administrative use only
	Tooth # or letter	Surface	Description of service (including x-rays, prophylaxis, materials used, etc.)	Date of service performed Mo. Day Year	Procedure number	Fee	
			Periodic Oral Evaluation	10/26/2001	00120	30.00	
			Prophylaxis, Child	10/26/2001	01120	50.00	
			Topical Fluor.(not proph)Child	10/26/2001	01203	20.00	

38. Remarks for unusual services

39. I hereby certify that the procedures as indicated by date have been completed and that the fees submitted are the actual fees I have charged and intend to collect for those procedures. > **Christine Nathe, R.D.H** **DH-1230** **05/04/2010** Signed (Treating Dentist) License no. Date	41. Total Fee Charged **100.00**
	42. Payment by other plan
40. Address where treatment was performed **2320 Tucker NE, Novitski Hall**	**Albuquerque, NM 87131-1391** City, State, Zip
	Max Allowable
	Deductible
© American Dental Association, 2008 Claim # 5781	Carrier %
	Carrier Pays
	Patient Pays

FIGURE 5–7 Dental Claim Form Hard Copy

Source: American Dental Association. CDT-4. 2002. Chicago: American Dental Association. http://www.ada.org/en/publications/ada-catalog/cdt-products cdt-4

use of five-character, alphanumeric codes to identify and define certain procedures (e.g. D2110). See Figure 5-8 ■ for examples of CDT codes and their meanings. The maintenance of these codes is the responsibility of the Council on Dental Benefit Programs with consultation from the Health Insurance Association of America, Blue Cross/Blue Shield, the Health Care Financing Association, National Electronic Information Corporation, and the ADA recognized dental specialty organizations. The *Code on Dental Procedures and Nomenclature* of the American Dental Association (ADA) provides current dental terminology (CDT).[7] The ADA updates the CDT approximately every five years.

Did You Know?

The "6 month" prophy appointment that is generally covered by dental insurance plans may have come from an ad for Pepsodent Tooth Power in the early 1900s.

Source: Amos 'n' Andy Continuity Script, 1 April 1932, Box 13, Folder 1, NBC Records.

A patient who is on a self-pay program generally pays for the dental procedures immediately at the end of the appointment. Many dental offices offer payment plans to patients to make their treatments more affordable, and some use dental credit cards as a financial payment plan for patients.

FIGURE 5–8 CDT 2015 Definitions of Billable Oral Exams

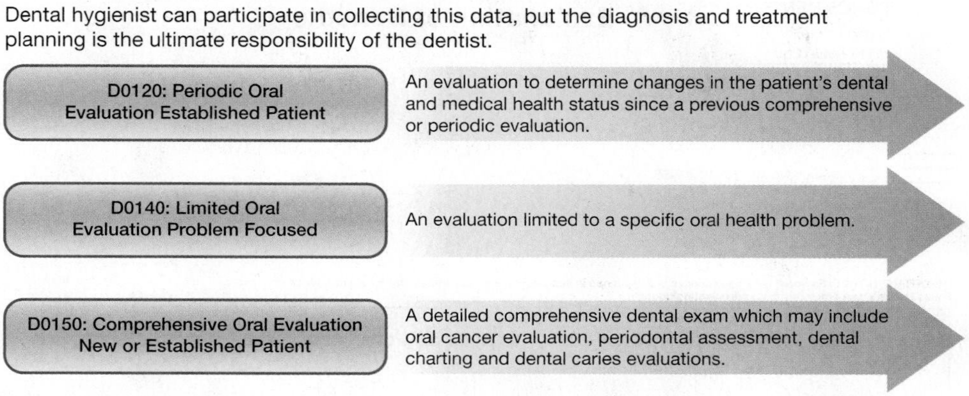

Dental hygienist can participate in collecting this data, but the diagnosis and treatment planning is the ultimate responsibility of the dentist.

D0120: Periodic Oral Evaluation Established Patient	An evaluation to determine changes in the patient's dental and medical health status since a previous comprehensive or periodic evaluation.
D0140: Limited Oral Evaluation Problem Focused	An evaluation limited to a specific oral health problem.
D0150: Comprehensive Oral Evaluation New or Established Patient	A detailed comprehensive dental exam which may include oral cancer evaluation, periodontal assessment, dental charting and dental caries evaluations.

Source: Adapted from American Dental Association. CDT-4. 2002. Chicago: American Dental Association. http://www.ada.org/en/publications/ada-catalog/cdt-products cdt-4.

If a patient is covered by insurance and the office files the claim, it sends the form to the insurance company either electronically or in hard copy. The insurance company decides on payment and sends an *explanation of benefits* (EOB) to the patient and the provider with an accompanying payment to the provider for the allowed amount if the company covers the procedure. (See Figure 5-9 ■.)

Some dental practices prefer to bill patients who pay them for procedures rendered, and then the patients submit the charges to their insurance company for possible reimbursement. Many times these practices are referred to as *cash-only* or *no-insurance practices.*

Did You Know?

Dental hygienists are responsible for choosing which code(s) to report and are legally responsible for that choice.

Insurance fraud is committed with the intent to falsely obtain payment from an insurer. Entering a date other than the actual date of treatment and entering a code for a procedure that was not provided are forms of insurance fraud. Even choosing codes incorrectly is considered a form of insurance fraud, so it is important that dental hygienists enter the proper coding and maintain the necessary documentation for all services rendered.

Governmental Roles in Funding Dental Care

In the United States, the total federal, state, and local governments' share of expenses for dental care is approximately 4 percent.[8] Basically, the federal government funds dental care delivery through a variety of programs for the express purpose of improving the nation's capacity to provide improved oral health care (Table 5-4 ■).

The government funds programs that provide research, disease prevention, and control (e.g., water fluoridation, fluoride mouth rinse programs—"swish and spit"—and dental sealants in schools); the planning and development of dental programs; regulation by means of quality assurance programs and assessment; and education of dental professionals (via scholarship, loan forgiveness programs, and financial aid). Chapter 21 provides more information on current government incentives for dental hygiene students.

Did You Know?

The recently enacted Affordable Care Act (ACA) does not seem to generate any additional funding for oral health care. However, although there are no additional revenues geared toward oral health, there may be more patients who are eligible to receive Medicaid benefits due to the ACA, which could increase demand.

The federal government provides funding to programs concerned with providing dental care services, such as the US Public Health Service and the National Health Service Corps. It also funds dental services for federal prisoners, military personnel, veterans with dental service-connected disabilities, Native Americans via the Indian Health Service, and children enrolled in Head Start and Early Head Start programs.

Did You Know?

Dental hygienists may be eligible for loan repayment programs when practicing in settings defined to provide care for the underserved.

Federal block grants also cover some dental services, especially for children. A *block grant* is an unrestricted

FIGURE 5–9 Explanation of Benefits Form

FONES DENTAL

Fones Dental
2500 Newman Blvd.
Bridgeport, CT 06601
555-3161 or 1-555-375-3320

Explanation of Benefits
(THIS IS NOT A BILL)

Check No.:	NO CHECK
Issue Date:	08-25-2010
Receipt Date:	08-20-2010

Patient Name: MARY JONES
Relationship Code: 03
Subscriber Name: JOHN JONES
Dentist: Alfred Fones, DDS

Document No.: 0123
Document Type: 1

Pay To: S=Subscriber
P=Provider

IMPORTANT NOTICE: Payment for these services is determined in accordance with the specific terms of your dental plan and/or Fones Dental's agreements with its participating dentists.

Tooth Code	Date of Service	Procedure Code	Procedure Description	Submitted Amount	Approved Amount	Allowed Amount	Deductible	% Co-Pay	Patient Payment	Plan Payment	Pay To
GROUP NO:	000123		NAME: Dental Hygiene Corp.								
SUBGROUP NO:	0001		NAME: Dental Hygiene Corp.								
	08/05/09	D1120	CLEANING	60.00	60.00	.00	.00		.00	60.00	P
POLICY CODE:	966										
	08/05/09	D1203	FLUORIDE	24.00	24.00	.00	.00		.00	24.00	P
POLICY CODE:	966										
			TOTAL	84.00	84.00	.00	.00		.00	84.00	

THE FOLLOWING POLICIES ARE APPLIED TO EXPLAIN BENEFITS PAYABLE AND ARE NOT INTENDED TO ALTER
THE TREATMENT PLAN DETERMINED BY THE DENTIST AND PATIENT:
966. THE PATIENT'S DENTAL COVERAGE WAS NOT IN EFFECT WHEN THIS SERVICE WAS
PERFORMED OR SUBMITTED FOR PREDETERMINATION. PLEASE VERIFY THE CLAIM
WAS SUBMITTED TO THE PROPER CARRIER BASED ON THE DATE OF SERVICE AND
THE CORRECT SOCIAL SECURITY NUMBER WAS PROVIDED.

Payment for these services is determined in accordance with the specific terms of your dental plan and/or Fones Dental's agreements with its participating dentists. For inquiries regarding participating dentists, please call the number above. Fones Dental's payment decisions do not qualify as dental or medical advice. You must make all decisions about the desirability or necessity of dental procedures and services with your dentist.
If your claim was denied in whole or in part so that you must pay some amount of the claim, upon a written request and free of charge, we will provide you with a copy of any internal rule, guideline or protocol or, if applicable, an explanation of the scientific or clinical judgment relied upon in deciding your claim. If you think Fones Dental incorrectly denied all or part of your claim, you may ask to have the claim reviewed. Your written request for a formal review must be sent within 180 days of your receipt of this EOB to the address on the upper-left hand corner. You may submit any additional materials you believe support your claim. A decision will be made no later than 30 days from the date we receive your request. Refer to your Dental Benefit Handbook for a complete description of Fones Dental's Claims Appeal process. You are not required to file a formal appeal to Fones Dental prior to arbitration or taking civil action.

Insurance fraud significantly increases the cost of health care. If you are aware of any false information submitted to Fones Dental, you can help us lower these costs by calling our toll-free hotline. You do not need to identify yourself. Only ANTI-FRAUD calls can be accepted on this line.

ANTI-FRAUD TOLL-FREE HOTLINE
1-800-000-0000

IlldladadldlddIhhldhudhulhadldhndldlddl
#BWNCYPW
#S0041334569NM6#
JOHN JONES
1234 MAIN ST
ALBUQUERQUE NM 87120-6066

PAGE 1 OF 1

federal grant given to a state or local government that does not specify how it is to be spent. The Maternal and Children's Health Services (MCHS) Block Grant Title V and Preventive Health and Human Services are usually used to provide preventive services and may cover dental services for children.

Many dental clinics utilize federal and state grants to help cover their operational costs. Dental treatment for children with craniofacial deformities, cleft lip and palate, and certain other conditions is funded by state and federal governments. In some states, dental hygiene services are offered to individuals participating in the Women, Infants and Children (WIC) program.

State governments generally fund dental services for inmates of state prisons and detention centers. A state often contracts with a private agency to deliver the services. State dental departments also may provide consulting services for developing and managing dental health programs. Some state dental clinics offer services to a target population, which usually includes children, patients with special needs, older adults, and indigent (impoverished) patients.

Local governments may provide dental care in school or community clinics. In many instances, the funding for these clinics is from federal, state, private, and local entities. Funding for community water fluoridation usually falls under the auspices of local government.

Federal and state governments jointly finance the Children's Health Insurance Program (CHIP) initiated in 1997 and is administered by the states. Within broad federal guidelines, each state designs its program and determines the eligibile groups, benefit packages, payment levels for coverage, and administrative and operating procedures. In many instances, CHIP finances dental coverage for children whose parents work but have low incomes and do not have health insurance coverage.[9]

Medicaid Dental Coverage

The federal government also funds dental services under the auspices of Medicaid and provides limited funding for medically necessary dental services, such as oral/maxillofacial needs related to a medical condition, through Medicare. As discussed in Chapter 3, Medicaid is the federal

Table 5–4 Description of Dental Coverage with Certain Federal Health Programs

Descriptions of Dental Coverage within Certain Federal Health Programs	Description of Dental Coverage
Medicaid[a] and State Children's Health Insurance Program (CHIP)	For children in Medicaid, under the Early and Periodic Screening, Diagnostic, and Treatment benefit, state Medicaid programs must provide dental services, including diagnostic, preventive, and related treatment services, for all eligible Medicaid beneficiaries under age 21. For adults in Medicaid, dental coverage varies, as states have flexibility to determine whether to provide dental benefits for adults and if so, what services to include. For example, while many states cover some dental services for adults, such as preventive exams, other states do not, limiting this benefit to trauma care or emergency treatment for pain relief and infection. States may also require that certain services have prior approval, or place limits on the total amount of services an enrollee can receive each year. When CHIP was established in 1997, coverage of dental services was not a required benefit.[b] The Children's Health Insurance Program Reauthorization Act of 2009 expanded federal requirements for CHIP programs to cover dental services.[c] Specifically, the act required states to cover dental services in their CHIP programs beginning in October 2009. It also gave states authority to use benchmark plans to define the benefit package or to supplement children's private health insurance with a dental coverage plan financed through CHIP. States that provide CHIP coverage to children through a Medicaid expansion program are required to provide the Early and Periodic Screening, Diagnostic, and Treatment benefit. States with a separate CHIP program may choose from two options for providing dental coverage: a package of dental benefits that meets the CHIP requirements, or a benchmark dental benefit package that is substantially equal to the (1) most popular federal employee dental plan for dependents, (2) most popular plan selected for dependents in the state's employee dental plan, or (3) dental coverage offered through the most popular commercial insurer in the state.
Medicare	Generally, Medicare does not cover routine preventive or restorative dental services. Medicare fee-for-service offers dental coverage under limited circumstances, for example, providing dental services that are an integral part of a covered procedure (e.g., reconstruction of the jaw following accidental injury). Medicare Advantage plans have the flexibility to offer coverage of routine preventive and restorative dental services. Medicare dental coverage varies by type of Medicare Advantage plan selected by beneficiaries.[d]
Department of Veterans Affairs (VA)	VA coverage of dental services requires enrollment, and exact coverage of dental services varies by an individual veteran's status—for example, whether the veteran has a service-connected disability. In some instances, VA may provide comprehensive dental care, while in other cases covered dental services may be limited. For example, some veterans with service-connected disabilities are eligible for any necessary dental care. Other veterans are only eligible for dental care if their dental problems may complicate existing medical conditions.
Department of Defense TRICARE	TRICARE—the Department of Defense's regionally structured health care system—offers dental benefits as a separate program that for many beneficiaries requires separate enrollment. The TRICARE Dental Program and TRICARE Retiree Dental Program are voluntary and require enrollment. The TRICARE Active Duty Dental Program supplements services provided at military dental treatment facilities for active duty service members. Benefits vary by program and eligibility—for example, families may have to purchase a supplemental dental policy outside of their medical coverage to obtain dental coverage.

Source: GAO Report: Dental Services Information on Coverage, Payments, and Fee Variation published September 2013 by the Government Accountability Office Washington DC. http://www.gao.gov/assets/660/657454.pdf on February 19, 2014.

DENTAL HYGIENIST SPOTLIGHT ·····························

Public Health Column: Marcia Brand, RDH, PhD

This month I have the pleasure of spotlighting a dental hygienist, who has worked in various entities in public health. Marcia Brand has accomplished so much during her career. If you remember from the *ADHA Focus on Advancing the Profession* report published several years ago, she is an excellent example of a dental hygienist working within governmental infrastructure. The report mentioned that dental hygienists should serve at all levels of government to administer programs that provide access to care for the public, impact and interpret the laws that regulate the profession, and improve the oral health of the nation. Here is the interview.

Why did you decide to go into dental hygiene?

I did not grow up thinking I would become a dental hygienist. Most of the women in my family whom I admired were schoolteachers, but that did not seem like the right career for me. I wanted to be different. I considered several careers in the health professions, such as nursing and medical technology. Then, during a weekend trip to West Virginia University to visit my older sister Jane, I met a friend of hers who was studying to be a dental hygienist. I knew nothing about the profession, and frankly I do not think I had ever had my teeth cleaned properly, but this was a new field, it was a challenging program to get into, and I did not know anyone who was a hygienist. I guess it is fair to say that not many people go into dental hygiene to be rebellious, but I think that was my intent. Or maybe I just wanted to be different from my six sisters.

How did you get into public health? Did you need additional education?

While my interest in government and public policy first attracted me to public health, I also pursued this path after thinking carefully about my work style. During my dental hygiene education at Old Dominion University (ODU) in Norfolk, VA, I realized that I was not very good at sitting still. Since that would be required of me as a dental hygienist, I started to think about ways to use my training and interests into my career. I observed the faculty moving between students and their patients in the clinic, sometimes teaching in the classroom, or engaging in research. The faculty members seemed to have the best of both worlds—variety and an interesting profession. So, I decided to get my Master's Degree in Dental Hygiene and become a faculty member. I really enjoyed teaching at ODU

and then at Thomas Jefferson University in Philadelphia. However, I knew that to become a tenured professor, and to achieve my ultimate goal of becoming the dean of a school of allied health, I needed a terminal degree. So, while in Philadelphia, I pursued a doctoral degree in higher education with a focus on administration. What happened next was a bit of a course correction. As a member of the Association of Schools of Allied Health Professionals, I was selected to travel to Washington, DC, for a fellowship program that placed me in a Congressional office. I went to work for Senator Robert Byrd from my home state of WV, and at the end of the internship, Senator Byrd offered me a full-time position. I was the legislative aide for health, education, agriculture and veterans affairs! I really enjoyed working in the Senate and I spent two years there, but when a position came open at the Health Resources and Services Administration (HRSA) that focused on allied health education and policy, I knew that was the right fit for my skills and experience. I really enjoy working in government.

What is your current position?

I am currently the Deputy Administrator of the Health Resources and Services Administration (HRSA). HRSA is one of twelve agencies that compose the US Department of Health and Human Services (eg, FDA, CDC, NIH). HRSA seeks to provide access to care for the nation's most vulnerable and underserved populations. It has an $8 billion dollar annual budget. People often know it better by its programs that by its acronym—community health centers, maternal and child health, Ryan White HIV/AIDS care, health professions training programs, organ transplantation. All targeted to improve the nation's health. Through these programs and policies, I work every day to help improve the public's health. As Deputy Administrator, I provide leadership for the Agency's grant programs, health policy, and operational efforts. I am "second in command," and I represent the Agency at meetings attended by HHS staff and external stakeholders. I help with strategic planning, budget oversight, and evaluation. We have a great staff at HRSA—about 1800 people—and I work with our team to make sure that they have the resources and training they need to get their work done, and as a result, accomplish our mission.

I did not get to this position right away. I actually have had several positions at HRSA. I have worked as a grants Project Officer and Policy Analyst, and

on a variety of issues, including health professions education and rural health policy. Each position was challenging and required learning about new grant programs and health policy concerns. As Director of the Office of Rural Health Policy, we worked on all issues related to health care delivery—health care financing, access to primary and specialty care, oral and behavioral health. It was good to be from West Virginia—it gave me credibility with my stakeholders!

Can you discuss any particularly interesting experiences that you have had in your public health positions?

I have testified before Congressional committees—it certainly was an "interesting" experience. It has been very interesting to engage with HRSA's many external stakeholders and learn their views about how government programs and policies can help them achieve their mission. Sometimes they give you a "wake-up call." I was meeting with representatives from the National Association of State and County Health officials about rural health concerns. They described challenges in accessing primary care and behavioral health in their communities. At the end of the meeting, I asked them if access to oral health care was a problem in the communities they serve. One fellow said "it's the area of greatest unmet need." I asked him why he didn't raise it with us, and his response was that "there's just nothing to be done." As one of eight children, a college professor, and an aide to Senator Byrd, I am the wrong person to tell there's just nothing to be done.

I was very proud when in 2011, HRSA funded the Institute of Medicine to support two studies, "Advancing Oral Health In America" and "Improving Access to Oral Health Care for Vulnerable and Underserved Populations." It had been ten years since the Surgeon General had released a landmark report on oral health and it was time to reexamine the importance of oral health to overall health and look at oral health financing, education, sites of care and workforce. The recommendations in these reports can serve others in public health policy and prove that indeed, there is something that can be done.

What type of advice would you give to a practicing hygienist who is thinking of doing something different?

I would encourage a practicing hygienist who is interested in working in public health and government to be engaged in professional organizations, such as the state oral health coalitions. Through these types of organizations and coalitions, you can learn about oral health issues and opportunities to address them. You'll meet people who are engaged in this kind of work who can help you think through opportunities that might be available to you at the county, state, or national level. You may need an advanced degree for some of these positions, but there are many opportunities to do graduate work in a way that fits into your schedule. And by the way—it took me six years to get my doctoral degree. Most folks think of dental hygienists as clinicians, and of course we are, but we also know about community health, epidemiology, research, practice management, and health literacy. You may have to make those connections. Finally, you have to be flexible and maybe just a little brave. It would be great to go into health policy meetings and find fellow dental hygienists seated at the table.

Dr. Marcia Brand is an excellent role model for dental hygienists wishing to pursue other roles in dental hygiene. And as evidenced in her response to experiences she has had, having a dental hygienist in a governmental position, has been a positive influence for the promotion of oral health in America. Thank you Dr. Brand!

Source: Christine Nathe writes the Public Health Column in *RDH* magazine published by Pennwell Publishing. For more public health spotlights please see RDH magazine online at http://www.rdhmag.com/index.html.

program enacted in 1965 that distributes funds to states for providing health care services to the indigent. Dental care is an option that requires additional funding from the state.[10] Each state decides whether to offer Medicaid dental coverage as a traditional fee-for-service plan or a capitation agreement. In many states, private insurance agencies operate Medicaid coverage.

Because of the states' freedom to apply the federal money in various ways, Medicaid dental coverage differs from state to state. Some states cover cleanings twice per year for adults, while some may cover cleanings only once per year. Basically, services covered are different in all states. Some states provide coverage only to children

under the age of twenty-one; others choose to insure all low-income individuals regardless of age. A state that limits coverage to children has more money to spend on each child, and the state is able to pay providers UCR rates. This option theoretically motivates more providers to see children covered by Medicaid. However, when only children are covered, many other individuals are left with no dental coverage.

Although many states fund dental care to the indigent population through Medicaid, historically, that population may have had difficulty accessing it. Many dental practitioners choose not to enroll as Medicaid providers so that they do not have to accept indigent patients. In recent

Box 5–1 Terminology of Dental Care Financing

Benefit: Amount that the insurance entity will pay for covered dental services described in its policy

Children Health Insurance Program (CHIP): Federal program created to cover medical care for children whose families have incomes too high to qualify for state medical assistance but cannot obtain private insurance; all states participate, but some do not cover dental care

Claims processing: Entering procedures rendered and determining whether payment will be approved or denied

Commercial insurance plan: Plan that operates for a profit

Contract: Legal agreement between an insurance entity and a group or individual

Copayment: Portion of the cost of each service a patient pays

Deductible: Amount an individual enrolled in an insurance plan must pay for covered services before the insurance entity begins paying

Dental claim: Patient's formal request for insurance payment for a dental procedure that was rendered

Dental claim form: Standard dental document used to file a claim or request authorization for a procedure

Dental necessity: Service provided by a dental provider that has been determined as a generally acceptable dental practice for a specific diagnosis and treatment

Early and periodic screening, diagnosis and treatment (EPSDT): Service for persons under twenty-one years of age for medical, dental, and vision care paid for by Medicaid

Exclusive provider arrangement (EPA): Contract between dental care providers and an employer (which eliminates the third party) stating the negotiated fees for services offered to the employer's employees

Explanation of benefits: Form sent to the patient and provider explaining the approval or denial of payment for procedures rendered

Fee slip: Form a dental practice uses to detail the services rendered a patient

Managed care: Integration of health care delivery and financing

Medicaid (Title XIX): Federal program that distributes funds to states for health care services provided to certain groups including aged, blind, and disabled people; those with low incomes; and certain members of families with dependent children

Medicare (Title XVIII): Federal insurance program supported by a trust fund; provides limited funding for medically necessary dental services, such as oral/maxillofacial needs related to a medical condition for all people sixty-five years of age and older

Preexisting condition: Medical condition that exists prior to the person's coverage by an insurance entity.

Premium: Amount a group or an individual pays to the insurance entity for coverage

Prepaid group practice: Large group of dental providers contracted to provide services to groups of patients

Procedure number: Identification given to a specific procedure as designated in the *Codes on Dental Procedures and Nomenclature* published by the ADA

Provider: Legally licensed dental hygienist or dentist operating within a scope of practice

Single procedure: Specific procedure designated by a specific code

Sound natural teeth: Either primary or permanent teeth that have adequate hard and soft tissue support

Three-party system: Program in which a dental provider renders the service for which the patient's sponsor (insurance company or employer) pays

TRICARE: Health care program serving active-duty service members, National Guard and Reserve members, retirees, their families, survivors, and certain former spouses worldwide; formerly known as Civilian Health and Medical Program of the Uniformed Services (CHAMPUS)

Two-party system: Program in which a dental provider renders the service for which the patient pays

---

years, many dental companies began treating primarily the Medicaid population, so this previous trend is changing. This means that patients with Medicaid may have more options for providers to access care.

See Box 5-1 ■ for a list of terms used in financing dental care.

Summary

Most dental care in the United States remains in the private sector, but federal, state, and local governments fund dental care to certain populations. The federal government also funds dental research and education of dental providers. Dental insurance plans have made preventive dental care

affordable to many individuals and have focused on prevention as a means to decrease restorative dentistry costs. To become a consumer advocate, dental hygienists must understand dental funding in both private and public organizations.

Self-Study Test Items

1. Which of the following does financing of dental treatment involve?
   a. Private sector
   b. Dental practitioner
   c. Public sector
   d. Both a and c

2. What payment is based on an office visit and is always the same regardless of the services rendered?
   a. Encounter
   b. Fee-for-service plan
   c. Capitation
   d. Barter system

3. What term refers to a portion of the cost of each service that the patient pays—in other words, the part of the payment not covered by the third party?
   a. Insurance payment
   b. Copayment
   c. Deductible
   d. Exchange

4. What is defined as the number given to a specific procedure as designated in the *Codes on Dental Procedures and Nomenclature* published by ADA?
   a. Premium number
   b. Procedure number
   c. Contract number
   d. Benefit number

5. What form is sent to the patient and provider explaining the payment or denial for procedures rendered?
   a. Explanation of benefits
   b. Managed care
   c. Exclusive provider arrangement
   d. Dental claim

References

1. Delta Dental Plans Association History of Dental Benefits Expertise. Retrieved From https://www.deltadental.com/public/company/mission.jsp on August 4, 2015.
2. Rohde F. Dental Expenditures in the 10 Largest States, 2010. Rockville, MD: Agency for Healthcare Research and Quality; 2010. Statistical Brief 415. Retrieved from http://meps.ahrq.gov/mepsweb/data_stats/Pub_ProdResults_Details.jsp?pt=Statistical Brief&opt=2&id=1113 on July 29, 2013.
3. Manski, R.J. and Brown, E. *Dental Coverage of Adults Ages 21–64, United States, 1997 and 2007*. Statistical Brief #295. October 2010. Agency for Healthcare Research and Quality, Rockville, MD. Retrieved from http://www.meps.ahrq.gov/mepsweb/data_files/publications/st295/stat295.shtml on August 4, 2015.
4. Dental Services: Information on Coverage, Payments, and Fee Variation GAO-13-754: Published: Sep 6, 2013. Publicly Released: Sep 12, 2013. Retrieved from http://www.gao.gov/products/GAO-13-754 on August 4, 2015.
5. BlueCross BlueShield of Illinois. Retrieved from http://www.bcbsil.com/insurance-basics on August 4, 2015.
6. Concordia Plus. Retrieved from https://www.unitedconcordia.com/dental-insurance/. on August 4, 2015.
7. *Current Dental Terminology*. Chicago: American Dental Association; 2015.
8. U.S. Healthcare Costs: Background Brief. KaiserEDU.org. See also Trends in Health Care Costs and Spending, March 2009 - Fact Sheet. Kaiser Permanente.
9. State Children's Health Insurance Plan. Retrieved from http://www.medicaid.gov/chip/chip-program-information.html. on August 4, 2015.
10. Medicaid overview. Retrieved from http://www.medicaid.gov/medicaid-chip-program-information/program-information/medicaid-and-chip-program-information.html. on August 4, 2015.

Visit www.pearsonhighered.com/healthprofessionsresources to access the student resources that accompany this book. Simply select Dental Hygiene from the choice of disciplines. Find this book and you will find the complimentary study tools created for this specific title.

6

Federal and State Legislation Affecting Dental Hygiene Practice

OBJECTIVES

After studying this chapter, the dental hygiene student should be able to:

- Explain the legislative process in the United States
- Identify the major bodies of law in the United States
- Describe the entity responsible for regulation of the dental hygienist
- Advocate for the utilization of a dental hygienist without restrictive barriers
- Describe the legislative initiatives affecting dental hygienists in the United States

COMPETENCIES

After studying this chapter and participating in accompanying course activities, the dental hygiene student should be competent to do the following:

- Adhere to state and federal laws, recommendations, and regulations in the provision of oral health care
- Promote positive values of oral and general health and wellness to the public and organizations within and outside of the profession
- Facilitate patient access to oral health services by influencing individuals and/or organizations for the provision of oral health care

KEY TERMS

Administrative law 86
Bodies of law 86
Branches of government 86
Common law 86
Constitutional law 86
Executive 86
Judicial 86
Legislative 86
Legislature 86
Regulation 87
Statute 86
Statutory law 86

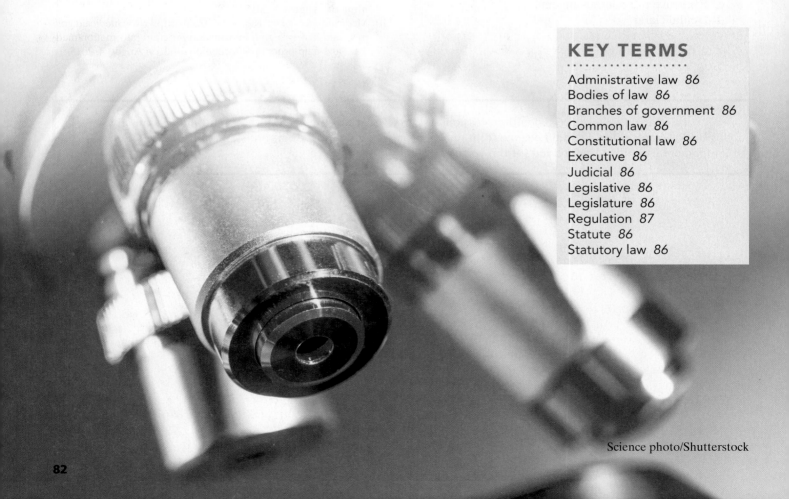

Science photo/Shutterstock

Many legislative initiatives affect the practice of dental hygiene. Legal changes to practice scope or supervision can impact the public's access to dental hygienists. Most states make changes to dental hygiene rules and regulations annually. These changes can be accessed at any time at www.adha.org, which updates the changes throughout the year.

Public health and the law have always been interdependent. Public health law focuses on issues in public health practice and how they affect practice. Generally, three major areas of public health law are police power, disease and injury prevention, and populations. *Police power* includes laws enforced by governmental agencies, such as dental boards or emergency health operations. *Disease and injury prevention* includes legal activities such as prevention initiatives and Occupational Safety and Health Agency (OSHA) regulations. *Population law* uses epidemiology to analyze health issues, such as the environment and community water fluoridation.

Historical Perspective of Practice Issues

The first statutes pertaining to dental hygiene were written in Connecticut based on the legislative initiative of Dr. Alfred Fones.[1] Since then, all states have added statutes that define dental hygiene practice. Historically, many state dental hygiene associations have worked to expand the settings and the scope of dental hygiene practice. Additionally, dental hygiene organizations have worked to allow the regulation of dental hygienists by dental hygienists.[2] In contrast, many state dental organizations had worked to permit the practice of on-the-job-trained personnel (preceptorship).[3,4] Resolutions passed by the American Dental Association (ADA) support this alternative education model of preceptorship.[5]

Did You Know?

In 1915, an amendment was added to Connecticut state dental law to regulate dental hygienists and dental hygiene practice.

Within the past decade, many states have passed statutes giving dental hygienists the ability to provide dental hygiene in any setting without the supervision of dentists.[6] One of the first states to make this change was New Mexico. The state's health policy commission, not the dental hygiene association, brought about the impetus for the change. The reason for the change, which is termed *collaborative practice,* was to increase access to care for underserved populations. This initiative created a precedent, and most states have made similar changes to their practice acts so that dental hygienists can treat patients without the physical presence of dentists.[7] (See Figure 6-1 ■.) Instituting laws or regulations that permit dental hygienists to treat

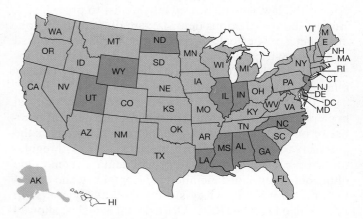

FIGURE 6–1 Direct Access Map

Source: http://www.adha.org/resources-docs/7524_Current_Direct_Access_Map.pdf

patients without the dentist's presence or supervision does not change the scope of services or the way that dental hygiene is practiced, it merely makes it easier for a dental hygienist to work when a dentist is not present.

Changes in policy and even terminology can impact the legal aspects of dental hygiene practice. Within the past decade, the *Current Dental Terminology (CDT)* published by the ADA redefined oral prophylaxis as a dental prophylaxis performed on transitional or permanent dentition that includes scaling and/or polishing procedures to remove coronal plaque, calculus, and stains. In other words, a dental assistant could provide a polishing, which would be legal in many states, and then bill it as a cleaning. Fortunately, the ADA unanimously rescinded this decision after the American Dental Hygienists' Association (ADHA) explained the significance of this wording change.[8] The dental insurance industry would not want to fund preventive services such as prophylaxis when a polishing was done without the necessary scaling to remove plaque and calculus.

Did You Know?

Although legislative action is not required for changing billing definitions, it can directly affect the provision of patient care. Policies, rules, and regulations are other initiatives that affect practice.

Regulations by state boards concerning the delivery of dental hygiene services are not always in accord with the law. In 2003, the South Carolina Board of Dentistry passed an emergency regulation that restricted dental hygienists from providing preventive dental services—including cleanings, sealants, and fluoride treatments—to children who had not previously been examined by a dentist in state schools. The Federal Trade Commission (FTC) issued

a complaint, stating that the regulation violated federal laws, and in 2007, the FTC issued a consent order that upheld the law, which allowed a hygienist to provide services without a previous dentist exam of the child if conducted in a public health setting. It also required the board of dentistry to publicly announce its support of the law and to notify the FTC if it considered altering any policies related to preventive dental care services in the future.[9]

In 2009 in California, new legislation gave a dental hygiene committee of four consumers, one general practice or public health dentist, and four dental hygienists the authority to regulate the licensure, education, and regulatory enforcement of the profession of dental hygiene. One of the dental hygienist members is a dental hygiene educator and another is a Registered Dental Hygienist in Alternative Practice (RDHAP), a dental hygienist allowed to practice independently in California. The legislation in California marks the first time a state dental hygiene committee has been granted the full authority to make rules and regulations that apply to the profession.[10]

Most recently, Minnesota has expanded the scope of practice to include additional assessment and restorative services that can be provided by a dental hygienist who completes a Master's Degree Program in Dental Therapy.[11] This may be a trend that will continue to meet the dental needs of Americans.

In fact, the US Surgeon General's 2003 *Call to Action* requested an increase in the diversity, capacity, and flexibility of the oral health workforce.[12] The ADHA House of Delegates, recognizing the need to increase the organization's efforts to address the public's unmet oral health needs, approved the development of the advanced dental hygiene practitioner (ADHP), a mid-level provider. As a result, the ADHP will extend primary oral health care to all while improving the health of underserved groups by providing access to early interventions, quality preventive oral health care, and referrals to dentists and other health care providers.[13] This new position will move the profession one step closer to meeting the changes the Surgeon General's report requested.

DENTAL HYGIENIST SPOTLIGHT ·····································

Public Health Column: Kathy Kane, RDHAP, BS

The dental hygienist spotlight this month focuses on a California RDHAP who has her own practice serving those in need. She is a very educated dental hygienist as well. Kathy Kane, RDHAP graduated from Riverside Community College with 1998 with an Associate of Science Degree in Dental Hygiene, in 1992 from Loma Linda University with a Bachelor of Science Degree in Dental Hygiene and she earned her RDHAP certification from the University of the Pacific.

She established *On the Go* Dental Hygiene Practice in 2005 to provide underserved populations access to preventive dental hygiene services. Kathy is an active member of national, state and local dental hygienists' associations. Since 1998, she has worked in private practice and she has spent 6 years as an Infection Control and OSHA consultant, providing staff training and seminars to dental professionals. She created the manual "Exposure Control Program for the Mobile Dental Hygienist." Kathy is currently the dental provider for the WIC Dental Days Program of Sonoma County. She is part founder and clinical consultant for Community Dental Health Consultants, a branch of Sonoma County Community Action Partnership, where she focuses on educating healthcare professionals about oral health, and providing training and program implementation for oral health care access programs. Quite an amazing dental hygiene

career as you can see. Recently I found out even more about this entrepreneurial dental hygienist.

Were you involved in the creation of the RDHAP in California and, if so, do you have any comments about the development process?

I was not involved in the creation of the RDHAP, but I was in the first class of the UOP program and feel that many of us in that first class have continued to spearhead changes in the RDHAP profession through our membership and involvement in component and state activities. A group of us started meeting shortly after we became RDHAPs and started to address issues that the RDHAP profession was experiencing.

1. How did you get into public health and/or RDHAP?

I have always felt the need to give back to our community so volunteering has always been a part of my professional development. I volunteered with community clinics health fairs, Give Kids a Smile events and gave oral health classes to different professional groups and to my children's elementary classes when they were young. Even after the kids were grown, the teachers continued to have me come in every year to present. When the RDHAP profession became a reality I knew this was a path that I wanted to follow.

Once I became an RDHAP it was these early connections and the people that I met through volunteering that have led to the opportunities that I have today.

What is your education level?

I have a Bachelor's Degree in Dental Hygiene from Loma Linda University, a certificate and state licensure for the RDHAP and am currently entertaining the idea of starting my Masters in Public Health.

What are your current positions?

I continue to work two days a month in private practice and have been there for years so many of my patients feel like my family and friends. Plus my dentist, Dr. Robert Leach, is a great boss and has supported my growth along the way even as it has slowly taken me out of his practice. I work in my own RDHAP business two days a week. I have a variety of patients ranging in age from 0-103. I work in Skilled Nursing Facilities, Developmentally Disabled Group Homes and am the primary provider for the Dental Days at WIC program in Sonoma County. I also work part-time at Community Action Partnership (CAP) of Sonoma County in their Health Services Department. I help develop and implement oral health programs for at-risk populations in the county. Our department runs such programs as the annual Give Kids a Smile event, School Smile program and I recently just finished screening over 1700 children in our county·as part of our countywide Smile Survey. We have also taken the WIC model and developed it into a medical-dental integration model for our county FQHC clinics. We placed an RDHAP directly into the medical clinics to provide care to the patients of the medical clinic. It has created collaboration within the medical and dental staff and the patients benefit from increased access to preventive dental care. Along with Dr. Susan Cooper, who is the Health Services Director at CAP, we also developed a consulting branch of our department as a result of getting many requests from other agencies and persons around the state asking us how to implement our programs in their areas. Also part of our goal was to create a larger RDHAP workforce and opportunities for them so I also began helping new RDHAPs with business start up. Business start up is often the most daunting part of becoming and RDHAP. We were taught hygiene, not business,

so if I am able to help an RDHAP with all the start-up licensing, business and provider applications, marketing materials and business focus, then they are able to get out there and start working sooner.

What type of advice would you give to a practicing hygienist that is thinking of doing something different?

Go for it! Take a risk. The opportunities are out there and sometimes you have to make your own opportunities. Find like-minded people in your community. Find a mentor. Mentorship can lead to several successful collaborations and gathering a larger countywide network of support your programs. Work with other hygienists. When I first became an RDHAP there were only a few in our county. I wanted to be able to work together so I started hosting a quarterly networking meeting that we could just share ideas, ask questions and help other RDHAPs with their businesses and job opportunities. We continue to invite new RDHAPs in the county and any RDH who is interested in the RDHAP profession. At our first meeting we had 6 attendees, two of who went on to become RDHAPs. Our numbers continue to grow. Get involved in what's going on in your local, state and national levels. We would not even have the RDHAP profession if it was not for our state association. They continue to fight for changes within our profession and it is important to show support through your membership dollars and your voice. Attend meetings and meet new people. Attending meetings allows me the opportunity to talk with other RDHAP's across the state, visit with friends and expand my network.

Kathy Kane embodies the entrepreneurial spirit that seems to be common skill of public health dental hygienists that I spotlight. Another common thread is the additional education level that most of these dental hygienists obtain. Networking with other dental hygienists and oral health stakeholders is paramount in increasing access to care for those in need and Katherine Kane is a perfect example of this!

I believe the RDHAP profession is on the doorstep to so many new paths for growth in preventive dental health. There is so much focus now on "placed based services" and the RDHAP has the ability to be directly involved in this.

Source: Christine Nathe writes the Public Health Column in *RDH* magazine published by Pennwell Publishing. For more public health spotlights please see RDH magazine online at http://www.rdhmag.com/index.html.

State Government Overview

Although the federal laws discussed in Chapter 15 affect dental hygiene *science*, the laws that affect dental hygiene *practice* are enacted and enforced by individual states. The federal government does not play a major role in governing the dental hygiene practice, but it is the model after which each state's system of government is fashioned. See Table 6-1 ■ for a comparison of the branches of federal and state governments.

Table 6–1 Comparison of State and Federal Governments

Branch	Federal Government	State Government
Legislative	Congress	State legislature
Executive	President	Governor
Judicial	Federal courts	State courts

Did You Know?

The federal government has no responsibility or authority for the regulation of dental hygiene in states.

The governments of the United States and its individual states have three sections, or **branches of government:** legislative, executive, and judicial. Each branch has a specific function and limited areas of authority, which is exclusive to that branch. (See Table 6-2 ■.) The **legislature,** or **legislative** branch, of each state makes its laws, including the licensure and practice of the dental hygienist. The **executive** branch executes, or carries out, the laws passed by the legislature. The **judicial** branch, composed of courts, interprets the laws the legislature passes, but it does not make them.

A **body of law** refers to the rules of conduct or action prescribed or formally recognized as binding or enforced by a controlling authority. In the United States, the major bodies of law are common, statutory, constitutional, and administrative. (See Table 6-3 ■.) Courts create **common law** through judicial decisions that in many cases other courts can change. It contains notions of common sense and precedent. **Statutory law** is the legislature-enacted, written law, which serves to promote justice. Only the legislature can change statutory law. **Constitutional law** deals with the interpretation and implementation of a government's codified constitution. The people, through their legislators, created it, and the people, also through their legislators, have the power to change it. It takes precedence over both common and statutory law. The fourth body of law is **administrative law,** which refers to the body of rules, regulations, orders, and decisions created by a government's administrative agencies.

Table 6–2 Function of State Government Branches

Branch of Government	Function
Legislative	Create laws
Executive	Enforce laws
Judicial	Interpret laws

Table 6–3 Major Bodies of Law

Body	Definition
Common	Created and changed only by courts
Statutory	Created and changed by legislature
Constitutional	Created and changed by people through their legislators
Administrative	Delegated legislative power to an administrative agency

Agencies such as state dental boards fall within this law. The legislature has the authority to say whether and when administrative agencies can develop rules and regulations.

Generally, a state legislature includes two legislative bodies, the Senate and the House of Representatives, sometimes referred to as the Assembly or House of Delegates. In most states, the legislature meets each year for up to six months.

State Laws and Their Passage

To become a state law, a concept (or bill) must be reviewed by specific committees within each house of the legislature, which may amend, or change, it. If the committees accept it, both houses must vote to approve it. (See Figure 6-2 ■.) Although a bill often "dies" in committee, its most vital provisions may be incorporated in a totally different bill. If either house fails to pass the bill, it will not become a law. If both houses pass it, the governor must sign it. If the governor vetoes the bill, both houses may override the veto by a two-thirds majority vote.

Laws pertaining to dental hygiene are generally found in the state dental hygiene law(s) regarding scope of practice, many times referred to as the dental hygiene practice act. However, policies enacted at the federal level pertaining to dental insurance and Medicaid may impact state dental hygiene practice. For instance, if federal Medicaid law allows dental hygienists to be reimbursed for performing oral examinations, oral prophylaxis, and other procedures, states must ensure that their laws and rules do not conflict with it in order to receive Medicaid funding. These funds can support dental hygiene care delivered in schools or practice settings other than private dental offices and to the underserved. In this case, the state may even push for the passage of a **statute**—a law enacted by a government's legislature—to allow dental hygienists to be reimbursed for providing such care.

Dental hygienists lobby for the support of bills that could impact dental hygiene care delivery. *Lobbying* is the act of educating legislators and promoting specific bills that would benefit the lobbyists; for dental lobbyists, this could involve supporting legislation to enhance dental care or opposing bills that are detrimental to dental care delivery.

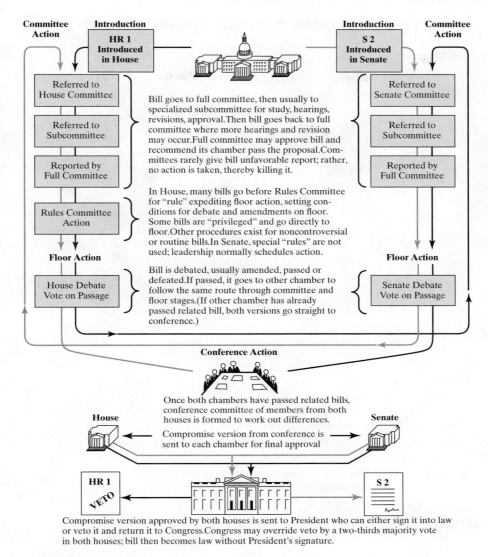

FIGURE 6–2 How a Bill Becomes a Law

State Dental Boards

A state's laws pertaining to dental hygiene practice describe its allowable scope, supervision, and licensure requirements, and procedures for suspension and revocation of license. Aiding in the interpretation of practice laws are regulations and rules. **Regulations** are orders imposed by an executive authority or government agency governing practice, which in this case could be a state dental board.

Rules implement and interpret the law or define the practice and procedure requirements of a state government's agency; an example is a state dental board's interpreting and implementing a law concerning educational requirements. Thus, a mandatory rule establishes a requirement, fee, or fee rate; sets a standard; provides a set procedure; pronounces how a law will be implemented; gives guidance for compliance with a law; describes the structure of an organization; or instructs members of the public how they must deal with any agency. The rule-making process is

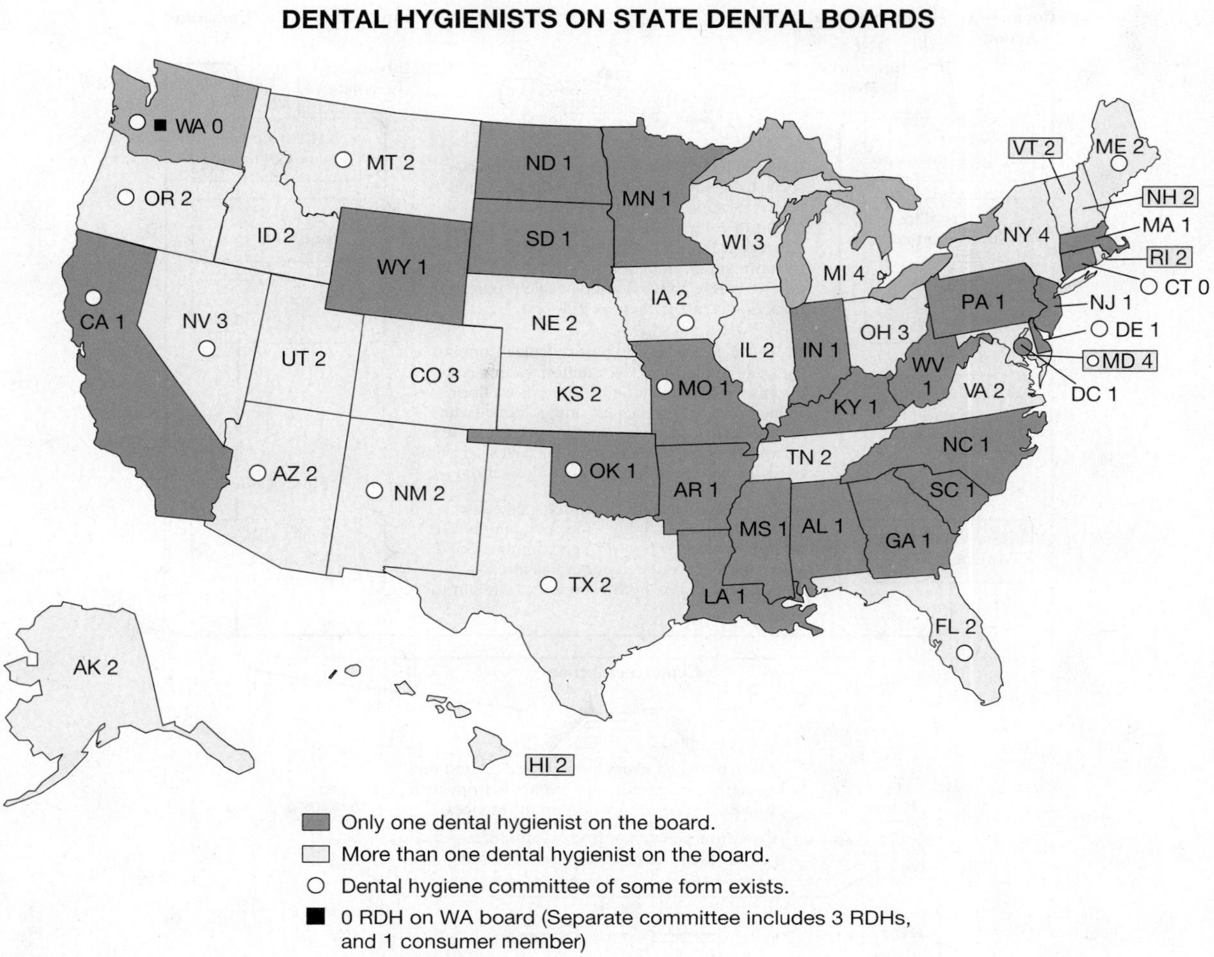

DENTAL HYGIENISTS ON STATE DENTAL BOARDS

FIGURE 6–3 State Dental Board Representation

Source: American Dental Hygienists' Association

ongoing. State dental boards may promulgate rules at any time provided they follow state law and, by applying the rule-making process, can change a rule it believes should be changed or in response to a petition.

The state dental board is responsible for regulating dentistry and dental hygiene, usually by interpreting or further defining the law as well as granting and suspending or revoking licenses. Some states have dental hygiene committees or advisory boards that have a role in governing but do not have full authority to regulate practice. Most state dental boards are composed primarily of dentists, one or two dental hygienists, and one or two public members. This representation on the board means that dental hygienists in the state are basically governed by dentists. The dentists, usually the majority board members, can interpret the law to limit the practice of dental hygiene while increasing the functions of on-the-job trained dental personnel. Unfortunately, in many instances, the profession of dental hygiene has not had power to affect its own practice. With recent legislation allowing self-regulation by its dental hygiene committee, California became the exception to this. (See Figures 6-3 and 6-4 ■.)

Supervision of Dental Hygienists

Many states have requirements dictating the situations in which dentists are to supervise dental hygienists. In more than thirty states, dental hygienists may provide services in certain settings under various forms of unsupervised practice. Moreover, in sixteen states, dental hygienists may enroll as Medicaid providers, billing and collecting for services rendered.[14] Supervision is a major problem because it usually restricts the practice of dental hygiene to dental offices and decreases the effectiveness of public health efforts.[6] Both direct and indirect supervision generally require the physical presence of a dentist during dental hygiene treatment. This practice can decrease the availability of dental hygiene care and possibly increase the cost effectiveness of such care. See Table 6-4 ■ for the definitions of different forms of supervision of dental hygienists. Each and every state practice act defines supervision or direction for their specific state, so these definitions are a synthesis of the most common found in practice acts.

FIGURE 6–4 State Dental Hygiene Committees

The following states have dental hygiene advisory committees or varying degrees of self regulation for dental hygienists.

1. **Arizona** The Arizona Dental Hygiene Committee consists of one dentist and one dental hygienist from the board, plus four additional dental hygienists and one public member. The committee serves as a forum for discussion of dental hygiene issues and advises the board on rules and proposed statute changes concerning dental hygiene education, regulation and practice. In addition,the committee evaluates CE classes for expanded functions and monitors dental hygienists' compliance with CE requirements. R4-11-605

2. **California** The Dental Hygiene Committee of California is a self-regulating dental hygiene committee in conjunction with the Department of Consumer Affairs. The committee consists of four dental hygienists, four public members, and one dentist appointed by the governor. The responsibilities of DHCC include issuing, reviewing, and revoking licenses as well as developing and administering examinations. Additional functions include adopting regulations, determining fees and continuing education requirements for all hygiene licensure categories.

3. **Connecticut** Connecticut is unique because dental hygiene is directly under the Department of Public Health. Although there is no standing dental hygiene committee, the department director has the ability to appoint an ad hoc committee of dental hygienists, if there is a need to address rules or disciplinary matters.

4. **Delaware** Delaware's Advisory Committee is appointed by the governor and consists of three dental hygienists. The committee writes the examination for dental hygiene licensure (in conjunction with the dental board). In addition, the committee votes with the board on issues of dental hygiene licensure by credentials, disciplinary decisions, continuing education requirements for dental hygiene licensure, disciplinary action involving dental hygienists and issues involving the policy and practice of dental hygiene but not the scope of practice. Delaware Code 24

5. **Florida** Florida has both dental hygiene and dental assisting councils. The dental hygiene council is composed of four dental hygienists, one of whom sits on the board, and one dentist member of the board. The council is expected to develop all dental hygiene rules to submit to the board for its approval.

6. **Iowa** Beginning in 1999, both dental hygienists on the dental board and one of the dentists became a dental hygiene committee of the board. This committee has the power to make all rules pertaining to dental hygiene. The board is required to adopt those rules and enforce the committee rules.

7. **Maine** Maine has a Subcommittee on Dental Hygienists. The subcommittee consists of five members: one dental hygienist who is a member of the board; two dental hygienists appointed by the governor; two dentists who are members of the board and appointed by the president of the board. The duties of the subcommittee are to perform an initial review of all applications for licensure as a dental hygienist, submissions relating to continuing education of dental hygienists, and all submissions relating to public health supervision status of dental hygienists.

7. **Maryland** Maryland's committee consists of three dental hygienists, one dentist, and one public member, all of whom are full voting members of the dental board. The committee was created during a sunset review as a compromise to the creation of a separate dental hygiene regulatory board. According to statute, all matters pertaining to dental hygiene must first be brought to the committee for its review and recommendation.

8. **Michigan** This six member committee, comprised of two dental hygienists and two dentists, one dental assistant, and one public member, considers matters related to the dental hygiene profession and makes recommendations to the full board of dentistry. All members of the committee are voting members on the board. The existence of the committee is not mandated by state rules or statutes, but instead is a committee appointed by the chairperson of the board.

9. **Missouri** A five member advisory commission, composed of the dental hygienist on the dental board and four dental hygienists appointed by the governor was created by the state legislature in 2001. The commission makes recommendations to the board concerning dental hygiene practice,

FIGURE 6–4 State Dental Hygiene Committees (*continued*)

licensure, examinations, discipline, and educational requirements.

10. **Montana** In 2002, the board assigned both dental hygienist members and one dentist member to be a standing committee to consider and address dental hygiene issues in a timely fashion. The committee formulates specific recommendations to bring to the entire board for action.

11. **Nevada** Legislation in 2003 added a third dental hygienist to the board who, together with a dentist appointed by the board, constitute a dental hygiene committee that formulates recommendations on dental hygiene rules for the board.

12. **New Mexico** New Mexico has a Board of Dental Health Care comprised of five dentists, two dental hygienists and two public members. There is a dental hygiene committee comprised of five dental hygienists, two public members and two dentists. The committee selects two of its dental hygiene members to serve as the dental hygienists on the board. The board's public members and two of its dentist members are the dentist and public members of the committee. The committee adopts all the rules pertaining to dental hygiene and is also responsible for the discipline of dental hygienists. The board enforces the dental hygiene committee's rules.

13. **New Hampshire** The New Hampshire Dental Hygienists' Committee is a five member advisory committee, comprised of one dental hygienist member of the board, one dentist member of the board and three addition dental hygienist members appointed by the governor. The Dental Hygienists' Committee proposes rules concerning the practice, discipline, education, examination, and licensure of dental hygienists. The rules proposed by the committee may be accepted by the Board of Dental Examiners for adoption.

13. **Oklahoma** The Dental Hygiene Advisory Committee is comprised of the dental hygiene board members and four additional dental hygienists appointed by the board.

14. **Oregon** Under its authority to create standing committees, the Oregon dental board has appointed a dental hygiene committee to advise the board concerning dental hygiene issues.

15. **Texas** In 1995, a dental hygiene advisory committee, comprised of three dental hygienists and two public members appointed by the governor and one dentist appointed by the board, was established.

16. **Washington** The state of Washington has a uniform disciplinary code which applies to all health professions and creates the regulatory bodies to implement each practice act. Dentistry and dental hygiene have separate practice acts. Dentists are regulated by the Dental Quality Assurance Commission (an independent dental board with no dental hygiene members). Dental hygienists are regulated by the Department of Health, but the statute requires that the department develop rules and definitions to implement the dental hygienist act in consultation with the Dental Hygiene Examining Committee. The committee is comprised of three dental hygienists and one public member appointed by the department.

Source: American Dental Hygienists' Association New http://www.adha.org/resources-docs/75111_Self_Regulation_by_State.pdf

Table 6–4 Types of Supervision of Dental Hygienists

Supervision Type	Generally Accepted Definition
Unsupervised, independent, collaborative practice	Dental hygiene practice without any supervision required from a dentist. Dental referral is necessary. In many states, a dental hygienist may practice only in certain public health settings.
General supervision	Dental hygiene practice without a dentist's "physically present" supervision. The patient must be a patient of record of a dentist in some states. Many states have additional stipulations, such as the patient must have had an exam within 30 days prior to or 30 days after dental hygiene treatment.
Indirect supervision	The dentist must be in the facility during dental hygiene treatment.
Direct supervision	The dentist must be in the treatment operatory during dental hygiene treatment.

Summary

Dental hygienists must understand the function of governmental entities in order to make legal changes benefiting the public and the profession. Dental hygiene organizations continually strive to increase access to dental hygiene care. The profession supports the concept that to effectively prevent dental diseases, dental hygienists must become empowered in the political process and act as the voice for underserved populations who currently face barriers to care.

Self-Study Test Items

1. State agencies such as dental boards fall within which type of law?
   a. Common
   b. Statutory
   c. Constitutional
   d. Administrative

2. Which branch of government makes laws for the state?
   a. Legislative
   b. Executive
   c. Administrative
   d. Judicial

3. Laws that explain what services dental hygienists can provide are found in
   a. Medicaid rules
   b. State law
   c. Federal law
   d. Health care regulations

4. Judges do not make laws, but they interpret them.
   a. The first statement is true, but the second statement is false.
   b. The first statement is false, but the second statement is true.
   c. Both statements are true.
   d. Both statements are false.

5. Because federal laws regulate dental hygiene practice, federal senators are involved with state regulation.
   a. The first statement is true, but the second statement is false.
   b. The first statement is false, but the second statement is true.
   c. Both statements are true.
   d. Both statements are false

References

1. Motley WE. *History of the American Dental Hygienists' Association 1923–1982*. Chicago, IL: American Dental Hygienists' Association; 1983:39.
2. American Dental Hygienists' Association. Policy Manual. Chicago, IL: American Dental Hygienists' Association; 2014. Retrieved from http://www.adha.org/resources-docs/7614_Policy_Manual.pdf on January 13, 2015.
3. Alabama Dental Hygiene Program. Hoover, AL: Board of Dental Examiners of Alabama; 2015. Retrieved from http://www.dentalboard.org/adhp2b.htm on January 13, 2015.
4. American Dental Hygienists' Association. *What is ADHA doing to fight Preceptorship?* Chicago, IL: American Dental Hygienists' Association. Retrieved from https://www.adha.org/resources-docs/7524_Preceptorship_What_ADHA_is_Doing.pdf. on January 13, 2015.
5. American Dental Association Current Policies 1954-2013.Chicago: American Dental Association. Retrieved from http://www.ada.org/~/media/ADA/Member%20Center/FIles/2013%20Current%20Policies%20Final.aspx on January 13, 2015.
6. American Dental Hygienists' Association. Direct Access Chart 2015. Chicago: American Dental Hygienists' Association. Retrieved from http://www.adha.org/resources-docs/7513_Direct_Access_to_Care_from_DH.pdf on January 13, 2015.
7. American Dental Hygienists' Association. *Direct Access to Care by a Dental Hygienist*. Chicago, IL: American Dental Hygienists' Association; 2008.
8. American Dental Hygienists' Association. Prophylaxis Definition Restored in CDT-4 [presss release]. Chicago: American Dental Hygienists' Association. http://www.adha.org/profissues/cdt.htm. Accessed December 9, 2008.
9. Federal Trade Commission. South Carolina Board of Dentistry settles charges that it restrained competition in the provision of preventive care by dental hygienists: FTC complaint alleged conduct limited needy children's access to care. Retrieved from http://www.ftc.gov/enforcement/cases-proceedings/0210128/south-carolina-state-board-dentistry-matter on January 13, 2015.
10. California Self Regulation Signed into Law. http://www.cdha.org/downloads/FINALSB853-6-13-08.pdf. Accessed August 27, 2008;(11)
11. Minnesota Board of Dentistry. Advanced Dental Therapist Scope of Practice. Retrieved from http://www.dentalboard.state.mn.us/Portals/3/Licensing/Dental%20Therapist/ADT-SCOPE.pdf on September 18, 2015.
12. US Department of Health and Human Services. National Call to Action to Promote Oral Health. Rockville, MD: US Department of Health and Human Services. Public Health Service, National Institutes of Health, National Institutes of Dental and Craniofacial Research. NIH Publication No. 03-5303, Spring 2003.
13. *Competencies for the Advanced Dental Hygiene Practitioner (ADHP)*. Chicago, IL: American Dental Hygienists' Association; 2008:1–32.
14. Medicaid direct reimbursement of dental hygienists. Retrieved from http://www.adha.org/reimbursement. on August 4, 2015.

Visit www.pearsonhighered.com/healthprofessionsresources to access the student resources that accompany this book. Simply select Dental Hygiene from the choice of disciplines. Find this book and you will find the complimentary study tools created for this specific title.

7

Advocacy for Dental Care

Shari Peterson, RDH, MEd

OBJECTIVES

After studying this chapter, the dental hygiene student will be able to:

- Identify four roles that the dental hygienist can assume as an agent of change
- Describe the various levels of change agent performance
- Utilize tools and resource models to implement change
- Identify the role of the change agent in policy making
- Promote partnership and coalition development
- Describe inter- and intraprofessional collaborations
- Identify components of grant writing

COMPETENCIES

After studying this chapter and participating in accompanying course activities, the dental hygiene student should be competent to do the following:

- Promote the profession through service-based activities, positive community affiliations, and active involvement with local organizations
- Promote positive values of oral and general health and wellness to the public and organizations within and outside the profession
- Assess the community's oral health needs and the quality and availability of resources and services
- Facilitate patient access to oral health services in a variety of settings
- Advocate for effective oral health care for underserved populations
- Access professional and social networks to pursue professional goals

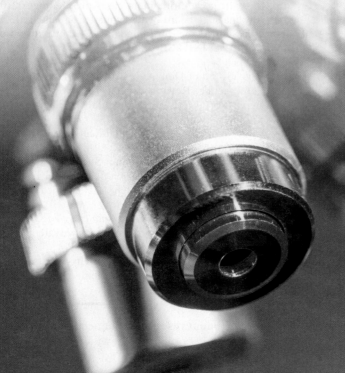

KEY TERMS

Advocate 93
Change agent 93
Coalition 102
Collaboration 101
Empower 93
Ethics 99
Facilitator 103
Grantsmanship 104
Interprofessional 103
Intraprofessional 103
Lobbying 100
Networking 101
Partnerships 101
Policy 99
Request for proposals (RFP) 104
Stakeholder 102

Science photo/Shutterstock

The majority of policies and programs within the dental profession would not have come to fruition without advocacy. Alfred C. Fones advocated for a new preventive health care professional within dentistry that eventually led to the development of the registered dental hygienist. The United States government advocated for a new division within its structure to enact policies and treat infectious and communicable diseases occurring in the coastal port towns that gave rise to the National Institutes for Health and Public Health Service. Citizens within the state of Minnesota advocated for a new dental hygiene professional to address disparities in access to dental care that resulted in the advanced dental hygiene practitioner. All of these changes and many more were the result of advocacy and change.

Advocacy involves an individual or individuals with an issue and a plan for remedy. Usually advocacy is needed to make some change for the betterment of society. An **advocate** is an individual or group of individuals with a common concern who join efforts to educate, promote or lobby others who can assist with establishing policy, programs, or funding. The advocates are usually individuals closely related to the issues and work or serve with the populations or policies of concern. Within the realm of dental care, advocacy is commenced on the behalf of underserved or uninsured populations. The ultimate product of advocacy is change within society.

The concept of *social advocacy* spans many disciplines but is predominantly associated with the business and legal worlds. A social advocate is frequently referred to as a **change agent,** an individual who intentionally or unintentionally causes social, cultural, or behavioral change. A change agent proactively bases action not only on a vision but also on well-defined goals and measurable objectives.

A change agent is not as effective without the collaboration of others motivated by both external and internal factors to pursue change. Rarely is a sole person entirely responsible for a total evolution, and rarely does a true change agent take credit as the sole individual responsible for change. Often a person is considered a change agent because of specific abilities to coordinate change or **empower** others to take action or make a change.

An important part of the art of being a change agent is to know what resources are available and the position that those who oppose changes take. *Change* is a process of evolution and is better facilitated when the change agent follows a pathway that allows for professional growth and increased ability to perform.

This chapter explains the process of change and how dental hygienists can recognize and effect change in dental public health. To help dental hygienists develop as agents of change, the chapter discusses the roles and responsibilities of change agents, the significant actions that change agents must perform, and ways to apply these skills. As dental hygienists develop an understanding of these components and abilities, they can become competent social advocates and be more effective in the community and in public health programs.

Understanding Change and its Agents

Advocates for dental public health are needed to implement change in regard to delivering dental care and ensuring program sustainability for various populations. In fact, dental public health would not be readily available if it were not for individuals empowered to change the existing systems and provide alternative concepts and pathways.

A basic understanding of the link between change and dental public health is critical to the dental hygiene profession. The number of dental hygienists entering the field of dental public health and involved with policy making and networking with other health care providers continues to increase. Changing dental public health should be a primary concern and interest of dental hygienists. They must advocate for patients' health by effecting changes in their behavior, in dental office protocols, in products used in practice, and in dental hygiene practice through the legislative and regulatory systems.

Did You Know?

The dental hygiene profession originated in a public health setting and then was removed from public health in most states because of legal restrictions. This resulted in limiting dental hygiene positions to private dental offices. In the past decade, however, the presence of dental hygienists and dental hygiene advocates in the public health sector has increased, and a movement by the profession to return to its roots has occurred.

Change is recognized as an evolution or transformation from one state to another state. It can be abrupt or happen slowly over time. It can be only one person's decision impacting that person or large numbers of people uniting for a particular cause with decisions that affect many or all of them. For an idea to evolve into an action, many things must occur, but interaction is first. For change to take place, the individual must engage others through interaction. To understand how individuals behave in certain situations is sound preparation for managing barriers to change and achieving success. The key to successful change is to understand others and resolve to work with them regardless of whether they share the change agent's goals or interests.

Understanding programs or policies that need change and identifying the people responsible for bringing about change is necessary. A person acting on behalf of a particular group has a responsibility to represent its best interests regardless of personal opinion. This can create a conflict if the change agent does not have a vested interest in the desired change or if the change agent is not completely sold on doing things differently.

To create policy change, it is necessary to create change in individuals who govern that policy. A policy is the outward manifestation of a collective opinion. Because

people create policies, advocates of change must devote a significant amount of time convincing the policies' creators of the need for change. The receptiveness of the target individual(s) must be determined.

Roles and Responsibilities

Four roles have been identified for the dental hygiene change agent: catalyst, solution giver, resource linker, and process helper.[1]

A *catalyst* is defined as an agent that provokes or speeds significant change or action; to be one, a person must understand what needs to change and motivate others to transform their opinions and actions. Positive dental hygienists motivate patients to invest in themselves as a priority. The change agent can facilitate change by brainstorming of ideas, projecting excitement in the process of change, maintaining a positive disposition, and encouraging others to be positive during oral health education.

The *solution giver* is a problem solver who is vital to establishing or maintaining rapport among a group of individuals such as a dental office. A solution giver is often a person or a group who can "think outside the box," offer creative problem solving, and break a problem into individual components that can then be examined and addressed. A community dental hygienist, for example, may assemble a group of stakeholders to develop solutions to the oral health disparities seen in specific populations.

The *resource linker* is a facilitator. For example, dental hygienists can bring together individuals who share interests, abilities, monetary support, and common goals. There is strength in numbers, and change agents recognize the abilities of others and link together people who are suited to similar tasks or have similar abilities. Linking people with different perspectives on a problem is often crucial to the success of an endeavor, but balancing groups is also important. A dental hygienist may act as a resource linker by scheduling social services for prospective patients to help them find dental funding for specific needs. Individuals who have been involved in the organization or cause for a significant time period can mentor, and inexperienced individuals can draw wisdom from veterans.

The *process helper* understands all aspects of the change process and provides help where it is needed, focusing on goals rather than stumbling blocks or obstacles. The process helper often jumps into roles that have been abandoned or neglected or convinces others to assume those roles.

Actions

Change as a verb implies action. The actions of modifying, altering, and transforming imply a movement from one state or condition to another. To *modify* something means to make basic or fundamental changes without losing essential components. A modification is usually a more acceptable form of change as a starting point. Within the dental hygiene profession, most states allow for administration of local anesthesia. The acts of administration of local anesthesia is very broad and nonspecific within dentistry, but when allowed as a duty within dental hygiene, the act is modified to become more specific. With state autonomy, some states list only that a dental hygienist can perform local anesthesia if they have been formally educated. Some states specify the education setting, clinical hours, and procedures. Some states require a clinical demonstration of competency in local anesthesia after formal education. These modifications to the act of local anesthesia still allow for the practice without losing the essential components necessary to have patients comfortable during invasive procedures that cause discomfort.

To *alter* is to deviate from what is normal or expected or to make different without changing into something else. In some cases, an alteration may prevent returning to the original status or method. Alterations should be carefully weighed and considered before they are made. Within the dental hygiene profession, the rules and regulations that govern how a dental hygienist can perform duties are determined by the actions of a Dental Board. An example of alteration would be to change the dental hygienists' scope of practice from indirect supervision to general supervision. This change still allows the dental hygienist to perform the same duties within the dental office; however, indirect supervision (the dentist must be present in the office) is changed to general supervision (the dentist does not need to be present in the office given specific parameters). The supervisory requirement is altered and expands the scope of practice. It is unlikely that the scope of practice would be returned back to the original rule. Expansion allows for a movement forward in the profession as well as greater access to care. To *transform* is to change something from one state to a completely different one. For example, it results in abandoning one concept or procedure for a completely different one. This is a substantial change that cannot be taken lightly. Change agents must foresee the impact of a transformation and make plans to address problems that result from it. This process usually occurs over a period of time to allow for responsible changes. In 2006, the California legislature transformed how the practice of dental hygiene is regulated by passing a law that allowed for the separation of dental hygiene regulation from the California Board of Dental Examiners. This allowed the newly created Board of Dental Hygiene to not only enact self-regulation but also act autonomously for the profession. Although self-regulation in some form exists for a few states, no other state has a specific Board of Dental Hygiene at the time of this printing. This transformation was the result of years of advocacy and will take many years post-implementation to refine the impact to both dentistry and dental hygiene. Many modifications and alterations to current policy may be needed in the future (Figure 7-1 ■).

FIGURE 7–1 Actions of Change

Actions of Change			
Issue	**Action**	**Advocacy**	**Change**
General act of local anesthesia	Modification of rule to specify requirements of education and clinical experience for dental hygienists	1. Formal education within an ADA accredited program or State Board approved course post-graduation 2. Number of clinical experiences with specific block injections	Comparable education and clinical experience that can be compared to other states for reciprocity in licensure
Supervision requirements for the practice of dental hygiene	Alteration of supervision requirements in the dental practice act to allow a dental hygienist to work when the doctor is not present	1. Allow a dental hygienist to work under general supervision if the patient is a patient of record and has had an examination and treatment plan within the last 18 months	Increased scope of practice for the dental hygienist and increased access to care for patients
Self-regulation of the dental hygiene profession	Transformation of the current regulatory structure to allow for the regulation of the dental hygiene profession by dental hygienists	1. Establish a Board of Dental Hygiene with representation of six appointed dental hygienists and a consumer member 2. Power to create rules and regulations pertaining to the profession of dental hygiene	Establishment of self-regulation in a formal Board structure and the ability of dental hygienists to regulate the requirements of education, licensure, and discipline

Procedures and Applications

The process of change becomes tangible when it is incorporated into specific procedures. Planned changes can be integrated into the dental hygiene process. (See Box 7-1 ■). The familiarity and versatility of the model described in Box 7-1 makes it easy for dental hygienists to see how to become involved in the process of change. The concepts of assessment, diagnosis, planning, implementation, evaluation, and documentation are identified with procedures to incorporate into an action plan. Action plans become "recipes" for carrying out procedures.

The cyclic nature of the dental hygiene process of care allows for continual change. During the various stages of the process, regular meetings between all involved should be held to allow for immediate changes in procedures. Additionally, a final evaluation of outcomes helps to establish a need for future change. In dental public health settings, dental hygienists can easily adapt a model similar to that just discussed to their communities or create their own model within the parameters of their state laws and regulations; doing so is essential for clarifying how a dental hygienist practices. As scopes of practice change, models will need to be adapted.

Having teams of change agents at various levels of experience increases the likelihood that a dental hygienist will manage change effectively. In participating in the change process, the dental hygienist gains self-confidence and accepts additional roles and responsibilities, thus increasing competence. Competence is the achievement of a predetermined level of special skill derived from education, experience, and task completion.[2] Competency is directly related to understanding and experience. It is inherent in the dental hygienist to strive to attain competency in all abilities. The key competencies for dental change agents identified in Box 7-2 ■ can be used as a dental hygienist's personal standard.

Did You Know?

The competent change agent has refined abilities of vision, collaboration, communication, and negotiation.

The most important contributions of a competent change agent are those that sustain an organization's

Box 7–1 Components of a Planned Change

Assessment

- Recognize when a change is needed.
- Collect data to verify the problem to be solved through change and identify the desired situation that will result from the change

Diagnosis

- Identify the problem that has created a need for change.

Planning

- Plan solutions/approaches and alternatives to the problem for which change is needed. Analyze the alternative approaches in terms of advantages, disadvantages, consequences of each, resources needed, cost, and level of support. Decide on a course of action from the alternatives analyzed.
- Design a plan for change: state objectives, outline methods, develop a timetable, involve people, assign responsibilities, assign resources, and monitor stability.

Implementation

- Implement the plan for change.
- Monitor for unforeseen problems.

Evaluation

- Determine whether the desired outcome and stated objectives have been achieved as a result of the implemented change.
- If necessary, reassess the situation and modify the plan for change.
- Stabilize the change by directing human and material resources to make the change permanent. Rewards and incentives should meet the human needs of the people involved.

Documentation

- Throughout process
- Record all data, evaluation, policies and agreements

Modified from: Darby M, Walsh M. 2010. *Dental hygiene theory and practice.* 3rd edition. Canada: Saunders.

Box 7–2 Key Competencies of Dental Change Agents

Vision

- Sensitivity to changes in dental care delivery, professional perceptions, technology, and in the way in which each impacts the health of the public
- Ability to develop clearly defined, realistic goals for a project of change
- Generalized perspective of priorities

Collaboration

- Ability to bring together key stakeholders and establish effective partnerships
- Networking skills to establish and maintain appropriate contacts within and outside the organization
- Management skills to establish working groups and to define and delegate respective responsibilities clearly

Communication

- Effective interpersonal skills, predominantly listening to and recognizing the concerns of others
- Ability to express enthusiasm in partnership ideas and stimulate motivation and commitment in others
- Ability to convey effectively the need for adaptation to colleagues and partners

Negotiation

- Skills to influence others to commit to plans and ideas by creating a desirable and challenging vision of the future
- Tolerance of uncertainty about the causes and effects of change
- Fosters cohesiveness
- Political awareness in identifying potential hazards and balancing conflicting goals and perceptions

current performance and ensure its future performance. Competency enables people to work effectively as they plan, implement, and experience change; it also increases their ability to manage future change.

Barriers to Change

The process of change frequently must overcome impediments for various reasons. Typical barriers are unexpected changes in external conditions, lack of commitment to implementation, resistance of the people involved, and lack of resources.

Unfortunately, the implications of failed change go well beyond the unmet objectives. Because of the many problems and risks associated with change projects, the change agent affects not only the success or failure of the project but also the extent of negative outcomes, which can result in a lack of motivation among those involved. As a result, some may never again be willing to commit to

DENTAL HYGIENIST SPOTLIGHT ·······································

Public Health Column: Shari Peterson, RDH, MEd

Professor Shari Peterson, RDH, MEd, is a dental hygiene educator who epitomizes the word *mentor* for dental hygienists interested in the public health path. She has great enthusiasm for community health and has educated hundreds of students about public health. Professor Peterson serves on numerous state and national committees that focus on community oral health endeavors and continually strives to improve the dental care delivery system in Nevada. She is the recipient of the Student American Dental Hygienists' Faculty Advisor Award from the American Dental Hygienists' Association, the Outstanding Dental Hygienists' Award from the Southern Nevada Dental Hygienists' Association, and a Letter of Commendation for Community Water Fluoridation from Dr. David Satcher, US PHS Surgeon General.

I asked her some questions regarding her career.

Why did you decide to go into dental hygiene?

I was always interested in biological sciences, but my mother is the one who convinced me to seek a career in dental hygiene. She felt it was important to pursue a career that was flexible and would allow me to work my schedule around motherhood. My mother had always taken me to dentists who did their own cleanings. When I was in high school, she worked as a dental receptionist, and I enjoyed watching the dentist work, but dentistry as a profession didn't interest me. When my mom left her job, she looked for another dentist closer to our home to take our family to for care. She decided on Dr. Robert Racine in Grass Valley, California. His wife, Rue, was his dental hygienist, and I have to credit her with inspiring me to pursue dental hygiene as a career. She let me sit by her chair for an afternoon while she worked with her patients. I loved the fact that she could provide care directly to the patients in her own operatory, and I was really impressed by how she educated her patients: She connected with them on a personal level and made the appointments pleasant for them. All of my previous cleanings had been very rough, but she was gentle.

Watching her that day, I knew that I wanted to be just like her. She gave me the phone number for ADHA; I called and requested information and a list of programs. I was accepted at Idaho State University and headed to school with only $500 to my name. The program director, Denise Bowen, was fantastic in setting me up with grants, loans, and scholarships. I would not have been able to go to school otherwise.

How did you begin to educate hygienists about public health? Did you need additional education?

Well, I was always interested in teaching. My mother had taught elementary school too. After working for ten years in private practice, I returned to college and obtained a master's degree in education from the University of Nevada–Las Vegas. I thought that maybe someday I would pursue a teaching career, but someone at the local dental hygiene school (College of Southern Nevada) found out I was working on my master's degree and asked if I would accept a part-time teaching position there. Several years later, I applied for a full-time position in the program.

I became passionate about dental public health after being invited to participate in a prophy/sealant clinic for homeless children organized by my local dental hygiene component. It was a fantastic event, but I was frustrated with the lack of organized dental public health opportunities that existed in Nevada at that time. A friend, Cathy Lytle, kept me in the loop about opportunities to serve and help with the programs we did have. We worked together on many projects over the years. Chris Wood with the Nevada State Health Division also became a mentor for me on developing programs and grant writing. She helped me understand the intricacies of government and legislation.

What are your current positions?

Currently, I am the program director for the Associate of Science and Bachelor of Science degrees in dental hygiene at the College of Southern Nevada. Prior to becoming program director I was the Community Outreach/Community Dental Health Course Director and adviser to the American Dental Hygienists' Association Student Chapter at the College of Southern Nevada. I teach many of the public health track courses in our online baccalaureate completion program.

Can you discuss any particularly interesting experiences you have had in your dental public health and/or educational positions?

Wow, there are so many! Most of my inspiring experiences have happened as a result of being a member of ADHA and advocating returning public health dental hygiene back to the scope of practice for dental hygienists in my state. With these changes, dental hygienists are allowed to practice

unsupervised in public health settings with a public health endorsement from our Board of Dental Examiners.

My most interesting and memorable experiences have occurred when working with our statewide dental sealant program. Most of the time, we see rampant decay in the second grade children; however, this last year I have seen a dramatic drop in the amount of decay our children are experiencing. I believe this can be attributed to the combination of sealant placement and community water fluoridation that was established in Clark County around 2001. It is awesome to have visible results.

What advice would you give to a practicing hygienist who is thinking of doing something different?

I would say serve your community first. There is so much to offer in your own community. The feelings you get from helping others are incredible. The reality check of working in dental public health puts into focus the true nature of prevention that dental hygienists committed to when they pledged their oath. And service is free; giving of yourself has tremendous value to others. Pursuing a career in public health also increases your leadership abilities and your capacity for changing the profession to make it more beneficial for the public.

Source: Christine Nathe writes the Public Health Column in *RDH* magazine published by Pennwell Publishing. For more public health spotlights please see RDH magazine online at http://www.rdhmag.com/index.html.

change initiatives. Some will become skeptical of any future change project and consider the process to be just another elaborate idea from leadership bringing much work and few benefits.

The change agent can become competent by acknowledging and adapting the concepts presented in various models. The multifaceted road to competence can be visualized as a road map. See Table 7-1 ■ for the roles of the change agent, concepts of change and the change model, and the significance of each in the change process. The table indicates the reciprocal relationship of change and competency.

Dental hygienists as agents of change have made substantial contributions in the field of dental public health. Although many states had expanded the scope of practice for

Table 7–1 PAUSE: A Collaborative Style for Reaching an Agreement

Prepare	
Acquire facts.	Plan an alternative to a negotiated agreement.
Identify issues and interests.	Select an appropriate time and place to meet.
Use ethical principles.	Plan opening remarks.
Develop options.	Seek counsel.
Anticipate reactions.	
Affirm Relationships	
Courteously communicate.	Seek solutions that satisfy all.
Acknowledge personal issues.	Confront in a gracious manner.
Respect leaders' authority.	Allow face-saving.
Seek to understand others' position(s).	Praise valid points.
Discuss participants' responses.	
Understand Interests	
Focus on interests rather than positions.	Determine coinciding or conflicting points.
Seek to fully understand interests.	Use caution in revealing personal interests.

(continued)

Table 7–1 PAUSE: A Collaborative Style for Reaching an Agreement (*continued*)

Search for Creative Solutions	
Invent solutions based on need.	Expand the topic with additional interests.

Evaluate Options Objectively and Reasonably	
Keep an open and fair mind.	Identify concession points for both sides.
Use rules of reason, laws, ethics, and culture.	Identify unbendable points for both sides.
Discover reasons behind objections.	Identify and focus on agreeable points.

Source: Sande K. *The Peacemaker.* Baker Books: Grand Rapids, MI; 1997.

dental hygienists to provide care in public health settings, some under collaborative practice or unsupervised practice, the sustainability of these practices was and is a constant barrier. It was realized that although you may have a willing practitioner to provide services, supplies are needed to deliver care and money is needed to purchase the supplies. Many well-planned public health dental hygiene programs or practices struggle or fail without a strong fiscal component. Most of the public health dental hygiene programs or practices were heavily dependent on grant money and donations. Grant money is competitive, and many excellent programs are not chosen for funding despite having merit. Also, grant money is usually fixed to a specific time frame, and when the term expires, the program administrators need to find continued funding resources to ensure that the programs still function. This financial barrier can limit the ability of the program to maintain consistent care.

Due to state laws that define health care providers, the dental hygienist has been excluded from the list of providers. Insurance companies or service reimbursement providers limit those who can qualify and receive reimbursement for dental services to those that are on the state recognized lists. In some states, the Medicaid administrators changed their policies to allow dental hygienists to apply for Medicaid insurance provider status. This allowed dental hygienists who were approved by state Medicaid to bill Medicaid for services provided to their insured. This policy change improved the sustainability of some programs. But barriers still exist in that states determine who can receive Medicaid benefits. Some states indicate only children, some indicate children and pregnant women, and other states include the geriatric population. Even with this policy change within the Medicaid system, barriers still exist for populations. In some states, public health dental hygiene programs are limited to populations for which the programs can be sustained through available funding.

The remaining sections of this chapter discuss factors related to making change. The scope of practice for dental hygienists varies significantly from state to state, so it is imperative that public health dental hygiene be practiced according to the specific state's governing and regulatory agencies.

Did You Know?

Dental hygienists are program managers, public health administrators, state dental board members, oral health researchers, community advocates, coalition leaders, grant managers, legislators, and elected officials. Each role brings its own set of required skills.

Becoming acquainted with policy making, collaboration and partnership, coalition building, and grant writing in the dental hygienist's state is essential. Whether directly involved with managing these processes as a change agent or as an active participant, the dental hygienist must have a clear picture of how these processes occur.

Making Governmental Policy

In the field of health care, research is conducted and technology is explored to find better ways to do things. The results of these findings are used to create **policy,** a written description of rules, regulations, and stipulations to govern individual actions and procedures. Policies can be as formal as laws or rules with accountability and consequences or as loosely structured as guides or advisory opinions with no binding legality. Policy in the form of a practice act can be open to interpretation by a body of peers recognized in their field.

In the regulatory environment that governs licensed health care providers, a set of ethics is assumed to be the standard of professionalism. **Ethics** are guiding principles for individuals or groups based on what is right and what is wrong. In policy related to health care, ethical behavior has no legal binding. However, ethical standards can be adopted or utilized to assess the degree to which policies are followed or ignored, and a breach of these standards can result in disciplinary action imposed by a regulatory body.

In the evolution of society, government—persons elected or appointed to represent society—has predominantly set policy. The scope of governments and the policies they enact affect dental care, specifically dental public health.

National Health Policy

The federal government has adopted national policies on behalf of and in the best interest of the public as a whole. It does this through federal agencies that have been delegated the authority to research and record the status of health in the country and to determine guidelines and set goals to effect change in the nation's health. In addition to policy development, the federal government allocates funds through initiatives to the states so that national policies can be implemented.

Examples of federal health initiatives that impact dental care are *Healthy People 2020* and the Surgeon General's *A Call to Action to Promote Oral Health.* Both of these issued benchmarks of achievement in dental care that are essential to public health. These benchmarks, such as the increase in the use of dental sealants and community water fluoridation, should become the goals of all entities that advocate for quality dental care.

State Health Policy

The federal government manages policies and funds; the states are the change agents that develop and implement programs supported by those funds. State health divisions bear the responsibility of carrying out federal policy as well as developing protocols for implementation. In regard to oral health, each state has a designated dental director or representative who manages the state's oral health programs, which are extremely varied in composition, functions, and goals.

Some states implement clinical programs and services directly, using state personnel; others execute programs indirectly by subcontracting nonstate agencies, such as professional associations, community advocates, private partnerships, and local governments. Subcontracting usually comes as a response to a request for proposed work.

Did You Know?

Examples of state oral health programs are statewide sealant programs, community water fluoridation enactment, and Head Start fluoride varnish programs.

Some policies at the state level may need to be changed to implement these programs effectively. State regulatory practice acts governing dentistry and dental hygiene need to be reviewed to ensure that programs comply with practice standards and to be evaluated for change opportunities.

Local Health Policy

Local health departments or city or county governments develop health policy. Professional associations with financial support from local businesses, private foundations, and educational institutions represent a growing presence in local policy establishment and enactment. The success of these partnerships has brought together experts and advocates to create an environment in which to consider and create change agents. These partnerships will be discussed in more detail in another section.

Did You Know?

Examples of local oral health programs are community clinics, professional association–sponsored oral health programs, and the activities of individual practitioners, such as a direct access dental hygienist who works in public health settings.

To change policy at the national, state, or local level, change agents must thoroughly understand the organization and be persistent. Government policy is not easily changed. When Surgeon General Richard Carmona wrote *A Call to Action to Promote Oral Health,* public forums were held in various locations for individuals to provide input for his consideration. The administration identified the workforce as the experts in their field with valued comments. Many states hold oral health summits of stakeholders to facilitate strategic planning. This active process brings together varied viewpoints to determine strategies for a state's office of oral health to pursue and extend resources. By participating as an agent of change, each individual's voice can be heard in helping to establish legislative policy. Change agents are broadly used to implement and monitor programs in addition to proposing legislation.

Lobbying for Policy Change

The act of **lobbying** is attempting to influence or sway others to take or support a desired position or action. In simple terms, it is the "art of the sell." Lobbying formally seeks to influence legislators to enact desired legislation and informally to persuade others. A lobbyist can be a representative of an association or organization, a government employee, a corporation, or a public interest group. There is no specific credential to become a lobbyist, but there is a requirement that you establish a rapport with legislators or other decision makers and provide reputable information and dedication toward an issue. Lobbyists can be paid or unpaid members of the organization they represent. Most commonly, you will find professional lobbyists at the legislature whose full-time job is to represent multiple organizations' interests. These lobbyists spend the majority of their time actively in the legislative climate. They have established relationships with legislators and can read or predict how an issue will be received not only by individual legislators but also by legislative committees or legislative houses that make up the legislature. Professional lobbyists are paid for their services on a fee-for-service or contract basis. All states require paid and unpaid lobbyists to register with the legislature and complete reports of their activity.

Professional lobbyists' most valued assets are their established relationships, which provide access to those whom the change agent wants to influence, but they do not

guarantee success in securing change. The lobbyist is a tool to provide advice on strategies, tactics, and procedures to maximize effectiveness. An organization's professional or other lobbyist should be considered the expert in understanding the dynamics and motivation for change. The "sell" ultimately comes from agents of change who have done their homework, invested themselves emotionally, and persevered.

Several ADHA state components have legislative committees that actively advocate for change in dental care and the practice of dental hygiene. Some state components may even employ or retain a professional lobbyist to watch the legislative initiatives, establish relationships with legislators, and keep the association abreast of any legislation that may affect the dental profession. Other ADHA state components assign members of their legislative committees to act as unpaid lobbyists.

An example of regulatory change within a state may be to seek a change in the dental hygiene practice act to allow the duty of placing amalgam and composite restorations. Acting as a lobbyist for your professional association initially entails information gathering. ADHA has a large database of information pertaining to scope of practice for dental hygienists in all states. This is usually the best starting point to determine what policies and strategies already exist. It is best to attend state Dental Board meetings to get to know their formal process of rule making. Each state Dental Board sets policy for acceptance of requests, formal work sessions to take public testimony on issues, and then formal meetings to vote on policy change. It is also important to understand the climate of the Dental Board in general as well as the individual members of the Board. The most important thing to consider in making a regulatory change is that the charge of the Dental Board is to protect the public. This information is then taken back to the component officers to aid in determining organization policies, strategies, or position statements. Special consideration needs to go into the drafting of the association strategic plan and request for change. How will the request for change be in the best interest of the public? How does this request affect or protect the public?

Once the professional association determines a strategy to pursue the regulatory change, the lobbyist is instrumental in drafting the request for change that needs to follow the legal language typically used in the dental practice act. In addition to the proposed language, the association will need to compile background data on the issue to inform the members of the Dental Board as well as those who will be affected by the change (i.e., other dental professionals and the public). These data are presented in the form of a "white paper" that lobbyists will use as their primary communication platform. The white paper is distributed as the position of the association and usually includes the formal request language. It is a lobbying strategy to place the data in bullet format or short paragraphs to keep the paper concise and contained within one page if possible. Decision makers might not have the time to read through pages of literature. It is also a misnomer that the white paper has to be white. In fact, a colored document is preferred because this will stand out from among the other white pages of literature that they will read when making their decisions.

Once the request has been made to the Dental Board, if accepted for consideration, public forums will be scheduled for public testimony. The lobbyist is the essential representative that needs to be in attendance and most versed on the issue. Many times, the language can be changed based on public forum or work session discussions. The lobbyist needs to be a contributor in the discussion so that changes still reflect the intent of the original request. The lobbyist also has an important role in conveying information back to the association in a timely manner. As a key figure in advocating for change, your lobbying efforts will include all elements of the competencies of dental change agent. Competency is developed over time with exposure to many opportunities. Whether paid or unpaid, policy makers and legislators rely heavily on lobbying efforts to gain information about issues that they need to make an informed vote.

Working in Collaboration and Through Partnerships

When it comes to change, there is strength in numbers. Individuals can join partnerships, collaborations, and teams to express their beliefs on a subject to effect a greater change through synergy.

Collaboration

Collaboration is the process of working with others toward a common goal.[3] It occurs when two or more individuals or organizations work together on a task of mutual interest and benefit. The sum of the collaboration is greater than the value of the individual contributions. The predominant factor is cooperation, in which organizations or individuals work in association on tasks. Collaboration can occur without a formal agreement or partnership.

Collaborative efforts are strengthened by **networking,** or sharing resources or services to cultivate productive relationships. Networking enables an individual or group to draw on multiple resources and build a consensus to accomplish desired objectives. An important networking skill is the ability to identify resources, both financial and human, available within the community and to contact them.

In the book *The Peacemaker*, Sande discusses "the collaborative style" as a tool for effecting change.[4] The method of PAUSE found in Table 7-1 stands for *prepare, affirm relationships, understand interests, search for creative solutions,* and *evaluate options objectively and reasonably.* This collaborative style helps to balance the principles and interests of all parties.

Partnerships

A **partnership,** which can be viewed as an intense form of collaboration, is the state or condition of associating or

participating with others regularly in pursuit of a joint interest. Each member brings a unique perspective to the partnership. The need for partnerships between health care professionals within geographical communities is becoming increasingly important as new health care needs, practice changes, and issues are identified.[5] The health care system and delivery of services to the public are improved when health-related disciplines share and borrow from one another. Successful partnerships recognize that each partner may contribute different ideas and that flexibility is the key to success.

Formal partnerships have legal documents outlining each member's responsibilities, contributions, and boundaries. Partnerships created specifically to render services generally require a contract; one organization signs an agreement with another to complete services for one of them, each other, or a third entity. A partnership agreement can be a measurement tool to evaluate the partnership's effectiveness.

A *partnership agreement* does not have to be a legal document. Community-Campus Partnerships for Health, a nonprofit organization that promotes health through partnerships between communities and higher educational institutions, recommends its use. The organization establishes and promotes collaboration, health through service learning, community-based participatory research, broad-based coalitions, and other partnership strategies.[6]

Did You Know?

Formal partnerships commonly use documents stating affiliation agreements or memorandums of understanding (MOUs).

A *memorandum of understanding* (MOU) is an agreement that some formal partnerships use, but because it is not a legal document, it is not enforceable in court. In most cases, the signers of an MOU indicate that they do not intend to try to enforce its terms, although the document expresses a convergence of will between the parties, indicating an intended common line of action rather than a legal commitment. Changes or amendments to the MOU often occur during formal evaluation or the end of a fiscal cycle.

Educational institutions sometimes use an affiliation agreement, a legally binding contract made between one entity such as a clinic, hotel, or hospital and an educational institution to allow students to participate in an internship or other educational experience at the entity's location. The affiliation agreement states the terms and conditions under which the educational institution and entity agree to furnish education, training, and/or clinical experience integral to the specific institution's academic degree or course objective. Most affiliation agreements are standardized documents and very rarely amendable.

Building Coalitions

A **coalition** is an alliance of distinct organizations or persons to take a joint action. It represents an array of interests and brings together organizations and individuals to build a power base that works to accomplish change in response to a mutual concern. A well-organized, broad-based coalition can increase the potential for success in creating policy change, educating the public, creating a network, and developing innovative solutions to complex problems. **Stakeholders,** individuals in organizations who have a particular vested interest in a specific topic, issue, or initiative, usually compose coalitions.

When community problems or issues are too large and complex for any one agency or organization to address, forming a coalition of representatives of numerous segments can be an effective strategy to move everyone in the same direction to reach a common goal. That goal could be as narrow as obtaining funding for a specific intervention or as broad as trying to permanently improve the overall quality of life for most people in the community.

Common goals of coalitions follow:

- **Influencing or Developing Public Policy.** Such policy usually involves a specific issue.
- **Changing Behavior.** Reducing the incidence of smoking or caries is an example of behavior that might be changed.
- **Building a Healthy Community.** This generally involves strengthening both the community's physical health (such as performing oral prevention services, community planning, curbing substance abuse) and its social and psychological health (e.g., encompassing diversity; improving education, culture, and the art; and preventing violence).

Consistency can be particularly important in addressing a community issue, especially if a number of organizations or individuals are already working on the same issue. Having significantly different approaches and/or failing to cooperate or collaborate can lead to a chaotic situation in which very little is accomplished. If, on the other hand, the organizations or individuals work together and agree on common goals and ways to reach them, they are much more likely to be successful.

It is important to be aware of and anticipate barriers to creating a coalition to be able to prevent or overcome them. (See Box 7-3 ■.)

A broad membership is advantageous for coalitions, but the involvement of these people and groups is absolutely essential: stakeholders, community opinion leaders, and policy makers. In addition, virtually any coalition can benefit from the membership of at least some concerned citizens who may have no direct connection to the issue at hand. Such people can act as barometers of community attitudes and provide information about the coalition's work. Media groups should be involved to publicize the coalition and its efforts. People from the media who are

Box 7–3 Barriers to Creating a Coalition

Turf Issues. Organizations are often very sensitive about sharing their work, their target populations, and especially their funding. Part of creating a coalition may be to convince a number of organizations that working together will in fact both benefit all of them and better address their common issues.

Negative History. Organizations, individuals, or the community as a whole may have had experiences in the past that have convinced them that working with certain others is simply not possible. A new coalition may have to contend with this history before it can actually start the work it needs to do.

Domination by "Professionals" or Some Other Elite. All too often in their rush to solve problems or to "help the disadvantaged," agency people with advanced degrees, local politicians, business leaders, and others neglect to involve the people most affected by the issue at hand and other affected community members. Creating a participatory atmosphere and reining in those who believe they have all the answers are almost always required when starting a coalition.

Poor Links to the Community. A first step may have to be the development of hitherto nonexistent relationships among agencies and the community at large.

Minimal Organizational Capacity. It might be necessary to find a coordinator or one or more individuals or organizations to seek a way to share the burden with the new group if it is to develop beyond a first meeting.

Funding. The difficulty of finding funding is an obvious obstacle. Less obvious are the dangers of available funding that pushes the coalition in the wrong direction or requires it to act too quickly to address the issue effectively. New coalitions should be alert to funding possibilities from all quarters and be vigilant about the kind of funding they apply for and accept.

Failure to Provide and Create Leadership Within the Coalition. Coalitions demand a very special kind of collaborative leadership. It may be necessary to bring in an outside facilitator and/or to train someone in collaborative leadership to salvage the situation.

Failure to Show Benefits of Perceived—or Actual—Costs of Working Together. The task may be to find ways to increase benefits and decrease costs for individuals and organizations if the coalition is to survive.

Source: The Community Tool Box. Retrieved from http://ctb.ku.edu/en on August 4, 2015.

members of the coalition, however, may be ethically limited as to the amount of coverage they can provide.

Bringing all these entities together requires the efforts of a coalition **facilitator.** This person conducts meetings, brings diverse ideas together, and helps the group work to reach goals. The most important role of the facilitator, however, is to lay the groundwork for creating trust as the coalition develops. The facilitator should be perceived as trusted and neutral by coalition participants.

Professional Collaborations in Practice

Current trends in education are the promotion of **interprofessional** education with practical experiences. The concept of interprofessional education is not new; it has just recently become more relevant. The Center for the Advancement of Interprofessional Education (CAIPE) has provided the following definition. "Interprofessional Education occurs when two or more professions learn with, from and about each other to improve collaboration and the quality of care."[7] This concept issues a challenge to dental education programs to have their learners not only learn about other health care providers but actually engage in collaborative practical ventures to experience how the professions can unify for the benefit of providing comprehensive patient care. There is also a call to action for **intraprofessional** education in which learners within the dental professions work alongside each other to learn with each other in an effort to improve collaboration and quality of care. Although logistical challenges exist to have all dental education programs participate in intraprofessional ventures, there is a strong message that dental care providers should be collaborating in comprehensive care before seeking interprofessional collaborations. Whether it be political or logistical, this change will be initiated and governed by the new health care reform trends.

At the American Dental Education Association Commission for Change and Innovation in Dental Education 2013 annual session, examples were provided on how these inter- and intraprofessional experiences can take form.[8] Collaborations need to be developed among health care professionals that access the public in various modalities: fixed facilities, mobile delivery, and telemedicine/dentistry. The primary platform for establishing these collaborations is respectful communication and a focus on ethics and professionalism. Initially, each professional needs to share what her or his skill set and scope of responsibilities entail to educate all the professionals within and outside of their respective profession. A critical component incumbent on each participant is self-reflection on what has been presented and what personal change may need to take place to be an advocate for the goal of inter- and intraprofessional collaboration. Lastly, efforts need to be made to develop action plans whereby the collaborative professionals can work side-by-side together.

Advocacy for collaborations needs to not only encompass a meeting of the minds, but it needs to move toward active practice. The concepts of intra- and interprofessional practice mirror the declaration adopted by dental professionals that health cannot exist without oral health. Likewise, complete oral health care can exist without enlisting the efforts of a complete and comprehensive health care collaboration.

Writing Grants

This brief overview of the grant-writing process is intended to identify the various processes involved and the essential functions of change agents in grant writing. **Grantsmanship** is the art of obtaining grants for funding projects. It is also a technical skill that requires hard work, a state of readiness, information, and sometimes trial and error before having a successful outcome.[9]

A *grant* is a financial resource given to an agency, organization, or individual to address a problem or need. The grant writer prepares a written document (*grant proposal*) that requests support (funding). The grant writer also researches the availability of funds and the criteria that apply to petitioners.

Did You Know?

A request for proposals (RFP) by groups or agencies is also called *request for applications, notice of funding availability,* or *program announcement.*

An organization usually notifies the public about the availability of funding through its announcement of a **request for proposals (RFP).** The deadline for proposal submission can be as little as one month after an RFP is issued. Good grammar, accurate spelling, and cohesion are critical to a well-written proposal. The grant writer can be creative in presenting substantive elements (such as identifying the need for funding for the topic or population of interest). In some cases, innovative or creative approaches can enhance a grant proposal's likelihood of success. A grant proposal should adhere to standard guidelines. (See Table 7-2 ■.)

Features of a strong proposal that enhance the likelihood of receiving funds include:

- Well-organized proposal sections
- Well-researched and documented statement of the problem
- Creative or innovative strategies for addressing the need or problem
- Statements of *feasible* goals and objectives
- Identification of *measurable* objectives
- Inclusion of a sound evaluation plan

Table 7–2 Standard Components of a Grant Proposal

Component	Description
Cover letter	Includes the project title, name of the agency submitting the grant proposal, agency address, name of the prospective funder, beginning and ending project dates, and total amount of funds requested.
	Title page and abstract, which briefly describes the major points of the proposal.
Needs statement or statement of problem	Documents present the problem to be addressed with text, statistics, graphs, and/or charts. It should also describe the causes of the problem creating the need and identify approaches or solutions that have already been attempted.
Project description	Contains three main parts: goal(s) and objective(s), methods to address the identified problem or need, and a time line for completing each component.
Evaluation plan	Shows how the organization will measure the success of the project and outcome objectives; should include details about how information will be collected, analyzed, and shared with the funder.
Budget request and budget justification	Should contain details regarding salaried individuals, direct and indirect costs of supplies and equipment, administrative costs, and any matching donations of money or supplies.
Applicant qualifications	Should convince grant reviewers of the validity of the requesting organization's project.
Future funding or sustainability plan	Shows a continued effort to ensure the program's security and longevity.
Appendices	Provides supplemental materials that do not belong in the body of the proposal but are important data that should be shared with the funder.

Summary

Change in dental care can be accomplished as the result of the efforts of an individual, collaboration, partnership, or coalition. Understanding how change occurs, using effective tools that facilitate change, and preparing for common barriers to its occurrence can greatly enhance the change agent's success. Studying the various attributes of vision, communication, collaboration, and negotiation required for being a successful and competent change agent can help that person recognize existing qualities and areas to be developed. As technology and health care evolve, so do opportunities for new ways to practice. The dental hygienist is a valued member of the dental team and can make a difference in changing the policies of a dental practice, local coalition, state strategic organization, and even a national agency. With other stakeholders, the dental hygienist can contribute to the change process by advocating for a specific agenda such as increasing Medicaid coverage, providing community water fluoridation, or obtaining state funds for oral health programs. Understanding how policy is created on a national, state, and local level can help the change agent focus on realistic expectations of change.

Self-Study Test Items

1. Which of the following is an individual or group who causes a social, cultural, or behavioral change, be it intentional or unintentional?
   a. Coalition
   b. Change agent
   c. Lobbyist
   d. Grant writer

2. Which of the following is *not* a way in which advocates initiate change in dental public health?
   a. By delivering dental care
   b. By helping to sustain dental public health programs
   c. By determining the type of dental treatment rendered
   d. By determining who receives dental care

3. What is necessary to create change?
   a. Influencing individuals who govern policy
   b. Increasing an organization's financial status
   c. Redesigning a public health facility
   d. All of the above

4. What are the roles identified for the dental hygiene change agent?
   a. Catalyst
   b. Solution giver
   c. Resource linker
   d. All of the above

5. Making basic changes without losing the essential components is termed _____ .
   a. Modification
   b. Competency
   c. Application
   d. Networking

6. All of the following are essential for the lobbyist except one. Which one is the exception?
   a. White paper
   b. Strategic plan
   c. Proposed language
   d. Background in law

7. Which terminology refers to a working collaboration of health care professionals?
   a. Interprofessional
   b. Intraprofessional
   c. Multicollaborative
   d. Telemedicine

References

1. Parker E. The dental hygienist: change agent for the future. *Dent Hyg.* 1984;58(8):362.
2. American Dental Association Commission on Dental Accreditation. *Accreditation Standards for Dental Hygiene Education Programs.* Effective January 1, 2013. Chicago.
3. *Merriam-Webster Online Dictionary.* www.m-w.com. Accessed June 8, 2009.
4. Sande K. *The Peacemaker.* Grand Rapids, MI: Baker Books; 1997.
5. Boswell C, Cannon S. New horizons for collaborative partnerships. *Online J Issues Nur.* 2005;10(1). Retrieved from http://www.nursingworld.org/MainMenuCategories/ANAMarketplace/ANAPeriodicals/OJIN/TableofContents/Volume102005/No1Jan05/tpc26_216009.aspx. on August 4, 2015.
6. Community-Campus Partnerships for Health. Retrieved from https://ccph.memberclicks.net/ on September 21, 2015
7. Centre for the Advancement of Interprofessional Education. *Defining IPE.* Retrieved from http://caipe.org.uk/about-us/defining-ipe/ on Accessed June 23, 2013
8. Buchanan JA. *Keynote Address: Interprofessional Education: Why Now?* Portland, Oregon, June 11, 2013.
9. Gitlin L, Lyons K. *Successful Grant Writing: Strategies for Health and Human Service Professionals.* New York: Springer; 1996.

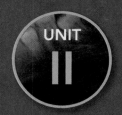

UNIT II

Dental Hygiene Public Health Programs

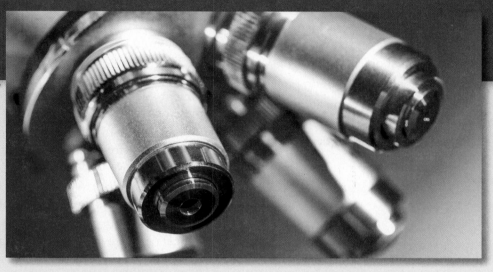

Science photo/Shutterstock

Dental hygienists practicing in public health settings strive to ensure that a given population attains oral health. As in private practice, one of the dental hygienist's most important roles is to motivate patients to change values and influence behaviors aimed at attaining oral health. When dental hygienists treat a target population, an important strategy is to provide group education.

Educating individuals in a group setting is as vital for the dental hygienist as is providing that same education to individual patients in private practice. For example, dental hygienists practicing in a prison strive to improve the oral health of the inmates they treat through education; those consulting for a Head Start program focus on helping the children attain oral health. Therefore, it is important for dental hygienists to understand the diversities of various populations and know how to effectively promote oral health for each through planning, implementing, and evaluating effective programs.

Dental Health Education and Promotion

OBJECTIVES

After studying this chapter, the dental hygiene student should be able to:

- Define dental health education and promotion
- Describe health education and promotion principles
- Describe the involvement of the population's values in behavior.
- Outline the different learning and motivation theories

COMPETENCIES

After studying this chapter and participating in accompanying course activities, the dental hygiene student should be competent to do the following:

- Evaluate factors that can be used to promote patient adherence to disease prevention or health maintenance strategies
- Promote positive values of oral and general health and wellness to the public and organizations within and outside the profession
- Provide screening, referral, and education that allow patients to access the resources of the health care
- Provide specialized treatment that includes educational, preventive, and therapeutic services designed to achieve and maintain oral health. Partner with the patient in achieving oral health goals

KEY TERMS

Behavior change *111*
Habit *111*
Health education *110*
Health literacy *109*
Health promotion *111*
Healthy behavior *110*
Values *111*

Science photo/Shutterstock

Dental hygienists frequently are asked to present information to groups regarding dental health education. Generally, these groups have underlying similarities and are referred to as *target populations*, which are discussed in Chapter 10. Although fundamental differences affect educating a group of individuals as opposed to an individual patient, many of the concepts are similar.

Communicating about health to individual patients, specific target populations, and society as a whole is paramount to dental hygienists and the profession. During the inception of the profession, one of the main constructs of the practice was the benefit derived from health communication that would help patients with their oral health and overall well-being. Oral health instruction, counseling on healthy choices and disease etiology, and demonstration of plaque removal were inherent in the first dental hygiene practices and this communication emphasis continues today.

Dental health education presented to groups can be an effective, productive, and inexpensive way to provide preventive dental care. For these reasons, all dental hygienists need to be skilled in providing such presentations to the community.

Health education historically has been paternalistic in nature. Dental hygienists typically prescribed a regimen and dictated behavior to patients. The dental hygienist was considered an expert who imparted knowledge to the patient who in turn was expected to change behaviors accordingly.[1] Now, patients are considered participants in their health care, and their social environments are important for the dental hygienist to consider when providing health education.

Did You Know?

Sometimes the paternalistic method of teaching others about health matters has been referred to as prescriptive (the provider prescribing lifestyle changes) or passive (the patient having no input into prescribed lifestyle choices).

And although patient care and education historically focused on the provider individualizing specific regimens based on his or her knowledge of disease and outcome, practice models are changing. The patient-centered model depicted in Figure 8-1 ■ focuses on health systems, institutions, and provider care revolving around the patient.[2]

Empowerment models that emphasize provider and patient working collaboratively toward treatment have become more common in recent years and are practiced routinely by dental hygienists when instructing patients on brushing and flossing. Patients become active learners during the demonstration of skills.

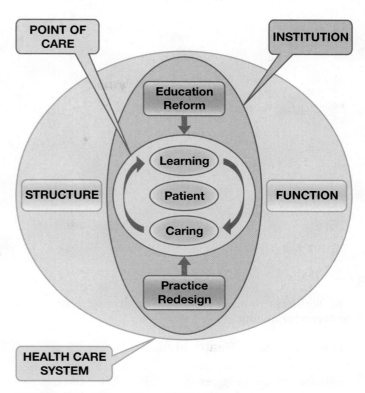

FIGURE 8–1 Patient-Centered Model

Source: Cuff PA. Interprofessional Education for Collaboration: Learning how to improve health from interprofessional models across the continuum of education to practice: Workshop Summary. Washington DC: Institute of Medicine.

Did You Know?

Patient autonomy gives a patient the right to control the course of medical treatment and participate in the treatment decision-making process, which is detailed in the ADHA Code of Ethics.

From the first use of the term *health literacy* in 1974—described as "health education meeting minimal standards for all school grade levels"—the definition of **health literacy** has evolved into a common idea that involves both the need for people to understand information that helps them maintain good health and the need for health systems to reduce their complexity.[3] Since the 1990s, health literacy has taken two different approaches: one oriented to clinical care and the other to public health.[3] Dental hygienists should focus on the empowerment of patients to become dental health literate by their education and promotion.

Principles of Health

Health has been defined as a state of physical, mental, and social well-being that involves more than just absence of disease.[4] A *wellness scale* is basically a continuum of total health to death, or a state of being from optimal health

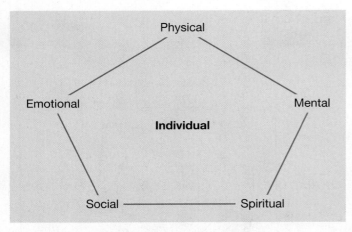

FIGURE 8–2 Five-Dimensional Health Model

Table 8–1 Five-Dimensional Health Model

Dimensions	Positive Input	Negative Input
Physical	Food, toothbrush, floss	Poor nutrition, inadequate dental care
Emotional	Trust	Mistrust, fear of dental provider
Mental	Knowledge	Ignorance
Social	Interaction with people	Withdrawal, inadequate communication skills
Spiritual	Values, morality	No value for dental health, no morality

Source: Eberst R. Defining health: A multidimensional model. *J Sch Health.* 1084;54:100.

and wellness to serious illness or disease with areas between for quality of life indicators.[5]

Five-Dimensional Health Model

Currently, the accepted view is that a person is a multidimensional being, early on this included three angles and then expanded to five dimensions: physical, mental (intellectual), social, spiritual, and emotional.[6] (See Figure 8-2 ■.) Most recently, some have added occupational and environmental dimensions. Dental hygienists should use the dimensions as need systems, each requiring specific input from the environment for an individual's complete development. (See Table 8-1 ■.) The term *input* refers to phenomena that feed each dimension in positive ways. Basically, if a dimension receives an adequate amount of input, that dimension will have the maximum potential for efficient function; conversely, if the input is lacking, the likelihood increases that a detriment to health may develop.

Maslow's Hierarchy of Needs

Keep in mind Maslow's Hierarchy of Needs (see Figure 8-3 ■) when contemplating the meaning of health. Maslow arranged

needs in lowest to highest levels. He theorized that when the needs at one level are met, those of the next higher level can be subsequently addressed in a linear, stair-step approach. In Maslow's hierarchy, the more advanced needs are not addressed until lower ones have been met. In addition, when lower needs such as hunger reappear, all higher needs momentarily vanish.[7] When adapted to dental health, this theory assumes that when individuals have not met a basic need, such as getting relief from a toothache, they cannot attain the next level, which might be flossing regularly.

Health Education and Motivation Theories

A **healthy behavior** can be defined as an action, such as daily flossing to remove plaque biofilm, that helps prevent disease and promotes health for the individual or population. **Health education** can be defined as instruction regarding health behaviors that bring an individual

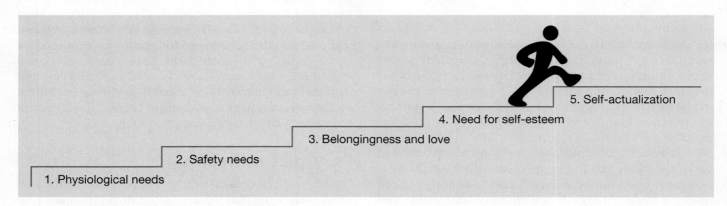

FIGURE 8–3 Maslow's Hierarchy of Needs
Source: Maslow AH. *Motivation and Personality.* 3rd ed. New York, NY: Harper and Row; 1987.

| Health Education | • DEFINED: Imparting Knowledge to Population
• EXAMPLE: Providing a group presentation to school children |
| Health Promotion | • DEFINED: Encouraging a Concept
• EXAMPLE: Providing athletic mouthguards to a youth football club |

FIGURE 8–4 Health Education and Health Promotion Comparison

to a state of health awareness, such as teaching a population the proper flossing technique. **Health promotion,** a process that informs and motivates people to adopt healthy behavior to enhance their health and prevent disease, occurs, for example, when a dental hygienist provides samples of floss at a local health fair. Health promotion is similar to health education but is geared more toward motivating people to adopt healthy behaviors. In contrast, the intention of health education is to have the learner gain accurate knowledge about healthy behaviors and lifestyles. Both promotion and education are methods to modify detrimental behaviors and promote healthy ones (see Figure 8-4).

One example of dental health promotion is the local dental hygiene association's work to ban sugary snacks and beverages from vending machines in schools in the district. The goal of this promotional activity is not to teach the effects of a sugary diet but to increase awareness of such foods' availability in the schools and to promote actions to decrease children's access to them.

The primary goal of dental health education is the prevention of disease using appropriate dental health interventions. Dental health education is a planned activity that utilizes the population's knowledge, attitudes, culture, and values to promote proper oral health practices.[8] If the local dental hygiene association held classes on dental health prevention modalities for middle school teachers who passed a test qualifying them to teach dental health to students, the dental hygiene association would have performed a dental health educational activity.

The works of several public health pioneers such as Edwin Chadwick from England and Lemuel Shattuck from the United States provide interesting examples for dental hygienists with regard to the importance of health education and health promotion. A history chapter on public health[9] compared the contributions from both. Chadwick's work to publicize the true cost of "working class" children (child labor) in England included disturbing mortality and morbidity rates. Chadwick used vivid descriptions to explain this appalling issue.[9]

Shattuck's contribution consisted of a detailed, well-research report of present and future public health needs of the nation. This report remained almost unnoticed by the community for years, and the recommendations were ignored. This was particularly interesting since the authors stated that this report, if published today, would still be ahead of its time in many respects.[9]

Chadwick's report helped get results; Shattuck's report, at the time, was not as effective. As a dental hygienist, collecting data is important, as is publishing reports, but equally important is promoting the message to many people, who may be driven to make changes for the betterment of oral health. The use of promotion is needed even when scientific evidence exists. When trying to make changes to advance the profession, make sure reports are available, but also make sure to promote the findings in such a way so that changes are adopted. Dental hygienists do have practice at changing behaviors on a patient-to-patient basis, so on a larger scale, when the need to make changes in dental care exists, they need to translate these skills to make information and ideas available to the public, to ultimately improve dental care delivery for the betterment of society.[*3]

Dental health education theory suggests that although a person may be educated on a particular health behavior, that knowledge will not impact dental health until the person positively changes the behavior, which then becomes a habit. A **behavior change** is simply changing a behavior, such as decreasing the amount of sugar in one's diet or learning how to brush properly, whereas a **habit** is a behavior that becomes automatic, such as daily brushing or routinely eating foods without added sugar. Although dental hygienists may make an effective dental health presentation that those who observe understand, they will not necessarily practice the dental health behaviors that are discussed. Therefore, a person's values regarding the behavior must be changed before the behavior is changed. **Values**—the ideas and beliefs a person possesses that influence behavior—give meaning to our lives. A person may develop values early in life from parents, grandparents, older siblings, teachers, or other influential people from whom that person seeks love and acceptance.[10] Values generally must first be changed if behavior is to change. See Figure 8-5 ■ for the steps in changing behavior. If dental hygienists could change values that the population holds toward dental health, they could dramatically decrease if not totally eliminate suffering from dental diseases. Unfortunately, changing values is a bit of a challenge.

Did You Know?

The dental hygiene student must be aware that education is the basis for any dental hygiene treatment.

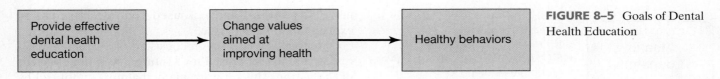

FIGURE 8–5 Goals of Dental Health Education

Theories on Methods to Change Values

Dental health education is based largely on the scientific principles of psychology and sociology that facilitate learning and behavioral change in the individual.[8] The following theories offer ideas on possible methods to use when attempting to change values.

THEORY OF THE HEALTH BELIEF MODEL The theory of the *health belief model* suggests that in order to display a readiness to take action to avoid a disease or act in a preventive manner, an individual needs to believe that he or she is susceptible or vulnerable, the disease has serious consequences, the behavior is beneficial, and the behavior is important.[11] This theory is based on the premise that when individuals have accurate information, they will make better choices including those pertaining to health. The US Public Health Service uses the health belief model for health interventions. See Table 8-2 ■ for an example of the health belief model in dental hygiene practice.

THEORY OF STAGES OF LEARNING Understanding the increments in which a person actually learns information is important. The learning ladder in Figure 8-6 ■ depicts an individual's natural progression from knowledge absorption to value adoption. This ladder has six rungs that begin with *unawareness* of the topic. *Awareness,* which occurs when education is provided, is second, followed by the *self-interest* rung characterized by the recognition of desire and involvement. The next stage, *involvement,* occurs when the person becomes involved in the learning process. *Action* is when the individual makes a change, and then a *habit* can be formed.

An example for this theory could be seen in a dental hygiene student explaining how and why flossing is important to a patient, who has never flossed and has presented to the clinic with a complaint of bleeding gums. The patient, who was unaware of the importance of flossing,

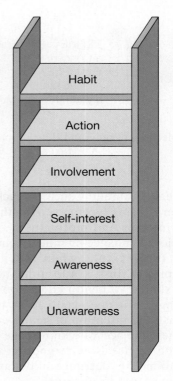

FIGURE 8–6 Learning Ladder

Source: Harris NO, Garcia-Godoy F. *Primary Preventive Dentistry.* 6th ed. Upper Saddle River, NJ: Prentice Hall; 2004.

now knows how to actually floss. The dental hygiene student has now empowered the patient by making him or her aware of flossing. The patient becomes interested in flossing, because of wanting to decrease the gum bleeding during brushing. The patient demonstrates flossing to the dental hygiene student and takes action by beginning to floss daily. When the patient arrives at the recall appointment three months later, flossing has become a habit.

Table 8–2 Example of Health Belief Model in Dental Hygiene Practice

1. Susceptibility	Individual believes he or she is susceptible to oral cancer because he or she chews tobacco
2. Serious consequences	Individual believes that oral cancer can be disfiguring and fatal
3. Benefit	Individual believes that to decrease the risk of disfigurement, illness, and possibly death, it would be beneficial to stop chewing tobacco
4. Salience	Individual makes the cessation of chewing tobacco top priority in life and stops the practice

THEORY OF THE TRANSTHEORETICAL MODEL The transtheoretical model is similar to the stages of learning and includes five stages of change through which a person travels before achieving a desired state. Each stage of readiness is characterized by certain behaviors and attitudes. These stages of change are precontemplation, contemplation, preparation, action, maintenance, and termination. A person at the precontemplation stage has no intention of taking action soon whereas someone at the contemplation stage clearly does, as evidenced by his or her contemplating an action. Upon contemplating an action, an individual prepares to take action. After changing a negative behavior or beginning a healthy behavior, the individual then needs to maintain this change. A person who never relapses from the overt behavior is said to be at the termination stage.

Assessing an individual's stage allows educators, including health care workers, to tailor the appropriate instruction[12] and is key to applying the transtheoretical model. Individuals may skip stages or lapse to previous stages, but an awareness of the individual's current stage allows the teacher, perhaps a dental hygienist, to provide appropriate assistance in meeting the stated goal. An example of this theory could be as simple as an individual contemplating daily flossing and finally taking action to floss daily.

DENTAL HYGIENIST SPOTLIGHT

Public Health Column: Mary Foley, RDH, MPH

Mary Foley is the project director for the Perinatal and Infant Oral Health Project and Oral Health Consultant for Head Start's Region I. She is the former state dental director in Massachusetts, a position she held for approximately five years. She is a graduate of the Quinsigamond Community College dental hygiene program and has a bachelor of science degree, magna cum laude, from Worcester State College. She earned a master's degree in public health from the University of Massachusetts School of Public Health and Health Policy. Ms. Foley's career epitomizes the variety of opportunities in dental public health. She has used her creative and educational skills to help further dental hygiene, which has ultimately benefited society!

I asked her several questions about her career.

Why did you decide to go into dental hygiene?

I had a good friend whose father was a dentist. One day during our sophomore year, she and I explored potential careers and colleges. In those days, men were doctors and dentists, and women were nurses and dental hygienists.

My dentist's office had no dental hygienist, so the notion of becoming a health professional in this capacity intrigued me. After investigating the courses that dental hygiene students must take, I was sold. I was strong in the sciences, and the will to help and serve others had been instilled in me from youth. The fact that it was a good-paying job—one that a woman could fall back on if something were ever to happen to her husband—made it all the more perfect a choice.

How did you get into dental public health? Did you need additional education?

When I entered the public health workforce after more than twenty years in private practice and clinical dental hygiene instruction, I went back to school to obtain a master's degree in public health (MPH). Actually, a college adviser pulled me aside the day I completed the last course of my bachelor's degree. Just when I thought I had finished, he said to me, "You have to get an MPH." He went on to say that it was a powerful degree. At the time, I didn't know what he meant, but his seriousness and intentions were so genuine that I took his wise advice. I attended the University of Massachusetts School of Public Health and Health Sciences where I earned an MPH degree in epidemiology and biostatistics with a subspecialty in cancer prevention. I loved this program. It took me nearly four years to complete on a part-time basis.

I actually entered the public health workforce as program coordinator upon graduation. I was hired to run a school-based fluoride mouth rinse program and a community water fluoridation program. On my first day of work, I was given a stack of books about eighteen inches high and was told to start reading so that I could become a fluoridation expert—so I did.

Two years later, I was appointed the state dental director, a position I never aspired to or even in my wildest dreams thought I could ever attain. I accepted it and took the position very seriously, assuming a very high level of responsibility for the broad array of constituents. I knew I had to serve the residents of the Commonwealth, my dental hygiene colleagues in Massachusetts and across the country, the dental community of Massachusetts, and a host of other groups. It was quite an opportunity as well as a distinct privilege for me to serve so many. It just goes to show one never knows what life has in store.

What are your current positions?

In late July 2007, I stepped down from my position as the Massachusetts' state dental director to move to Washington, DC, where I am currently serving as the project director for the new project Improving Perinatal and Infant Oral Health. It focuses on improving perinatal and infant oral health by providing increased access to dental care services for pregnant women and their very young children.

In addition, I am the Oral Health Consultant for Head Start's Region I (New England). In this position, I provide education and technical assistance to the eighty-four Head Start grantees/programs, the Head Start regional office staff, and others interested in improving oral health among our region's most vulnerable children.

Can you discuss any particularly interesting experiences you have had in your dental public health positions?

My dental public health experiences have been incredibly interesting and varied. I will share one that has particularly moved me. I had the wonderful opportunity of meeting *Jane* at 3 PM on the Friday of the 2001 Memorial Day weekend. I was sitting at my desk when the call came in from a woman who identified herself as "Jane." She told me that she was calling me because she had reached a dead end and had nowhere else to turn. She went on to say that she had a painful toothache and needed immediate care but was unable to access it because of a condition from which she suffers. Her physician had made calls to local dentists, but none was willing to make a home visit.

At age 60, *Jane* said that she had not left her home in more than thirty years because of the anxiety that she experienced in the outside world. She shared with me the suffering that she had encountered as a result of this condition, including the emotional pain of being unable to attend her father's funeral. Despite years of attempted therapies, hypnosis, and other medical treatments, she continued to be a prisoner in her home. Compelled by her story and the impending urgency of needed treatment, I immediately located a dentist who lived on the other side of the state to travel on the holiday weekend to care for this

woman's dental infection. The dentist, whom I consider a true saint among us, provided Betty's necessary treatment with portable dental equipment.

These qualities observed in a woman who has clearly been shortchanged on many levels have been inspirational to me and has helped me realize the many challenges that people live with. Her existence, which she may think insignificant, really reaches more people than she knows. Her way of life signifies the need for compassion by those of us who are more fortunate. Since my meeting with *Jane*, we have been able to establish routine home-care dental services for her. The dental hygienist at Tufts University's community outreach program, visits her regularly to provide routine oral assessment and preventive services.

What type of advice would you give to a practicing hygienist who is thinking of doing something different?

Dental hygiene is about promoting oral health for all Americans so that they may fully achieve their overall health and well-being. I have practiced dental hygiene for nearly thirty years. I have been fortunate to grow in the profession and experience a variety of practice roles. Every step of my journey has been critical, and I would not trade one day of it. In all aspects—private practice, education, and in public health—I have faced adversity. But each time, I have grown from it and became a better person. When we are young, adversity and challenge have a way of making us fearful, and we often back away. It is only through these tough times that we come to realize who we are, what our needs are, the needs of others, the potential we have to help others, the gifts we can offer others, and the opportunity to experience a richer and more meaningful existence.

Advancing my education was key. Some believe that advanced education is about getting a better job. I would argue it is really about personal growth. When I was in school, many people asked me what I was planning to do with my master's degree in public health. Surprisingly, I had no answer. I'm not one to plan. I just knew that I loved to learn and what I was learning was of particular interest to me. I knew that the right opportunity would present itself and that I needed to be watchful, ready, and willing when it did.

Source: Christine Nathe writes the Public Health Column in *RDH* magazine published by Pennwell Publishing. For more public health spotlights please see RDH magazine online at http://www.rdhmag.com/index.html.

THEORY OF REASONED ACTION *Reasoned action* focuses on the belief that people make rational decisions based on *behavioral intention*. A *behavior intent* is a combination of a person's *attitudes* and is therefore the most immediate and relevant predictor that the person will indeed take the intended action. Few actions that produce a healthy outcome happen without ample knowledge of and the full intention to practice the healthy behavior.[1] Two cognitive processes are at work to develop healthy behaviors: belief about what significant

others think is important, *social norms,* and personal motivation to comply with the beliefs of those significant people. Other external variables that influence attitudes, and thus behaviors, are internally processed depending on their importance to an individual.[13] Social norms formed in families, local communities, or larger societal communities and the actions or experiences of celebrities may influence social norms and, thus, behaviors such as maintaining a healthy, white smile, which may influence others to want a healthy, white smile.[1]

The following excerpt exemplifies the theory of reasoned action.

Example: Behavior/Cessation

Attitude: You know what? I think smoking is dangerous for my health.

Social Norm: I wonder if my wife would like me to quit smoking.

Behavioral Intention: I want to quit smoking right now!

Theory of Reasoned Action Outcome: As you can see, I'm not smoking anymore. Instead of taking a cigarette, when I get the cravings, I crumble paper now.[6]

SOCIAL COGNITIVE THEORY   Social cognitive theory (SCT), also known as *self-efficacy theory,* postulates that knowledge, behavior, and environment act in a reciprocal manner to continually affect each other.[14] *Self-efficacy,* the main SCT construct, is the belief that one's personal actions will have an impact on a desired outcome. Individuals with high self-efficacy practice forethought and planning, develop contingency plans, and put effort into overcoming obstacles. Self-efficacy is gained as information, behavior, and environment interact in a reciprocal manner. Lapses are a part of the learning process as the individual uses personal choices to develop behaviors consistent with individual choice and lifestyle.[14–16]

Did You Know?

The tenet of social cognitive theory behavior is conditioned by knowledge, environment, and behavior. This tenet was expanded from the social learning theory, which was a product of Skinner and other behaviorists. Bandura added the focus on personal action, which led to the social cognitive theory.

SCT reinforces the belief that social pressure is the most powerful factor in influencing social norms and emphasizes the power that social leaders have in influencing values and behaviors. An application of this model is the celebrity "Got Milk?" promotional campaign that shows celebrities with a milk mustache. In essence, SCT suggests that "social pressure" will cause people to emulate the celebrities and drink milk. See Figure 8-7 ■.

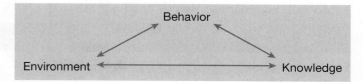

FIGURE 8–7   Social Cognitive Theory

THEORY OF THE SENSE OF COHERENCE   Antonovsky took a very different tack in health promotion and disease prevention. His central premise is that studying health is more useful than studying disease,[17] which he termed *salutogenesis,* the beginnings of health. Antonovsky's objection to the study of pathogenesis, which focuses on the origin of disease, is that it tends to classify people into either a healthy or ill state. He contends there is a continuum from "ease," or perfect health with no limitations, to *disease,* or severe disease or disability resulting in severe limitations of daily life. Most individuals exist somewhere between these two extremes.[17]

Antonovsky's sense of coherence (SOC) theory is a method of seeing the world and one's specific place in the world. Individuals who have a strong network of resistance resources will develop an overall SOC that can be used in any situation to deal with various stressors. Individuals with this type of SOC find problems manageable, comprehensible, and meaningful. If they have sufficient resources to handle the situation and the means to use those resources, these individuals can manage stressors, which are comprehensible if they are predictable or make sense and are meaningful if the individuals are willing to expend time and energy to deal with those stressors.[17]

For example, suppose that a thirty-five-year-old female patient presents with multiple carious lesions. She says her family has "soft teeth," so she thinks her decay rate is completely out of her control. Through questioning, the dental hygienist discovers the patient has very good oral hygiene skills but lacks knowledge about nutrition related to oral health. She had the habit of slowly sipping on a sugar-sweetened soft drink throughout the day. The dental hygienist identifies resources available to the patient for improved health, thereby increasing her SOC. By identifying resources, the dental hygienist has helped make oral health manageable. When the patient understands that decay is the result of personal behavior, the oral health becomes comprehensible. Through conversations with the patient, the dental hygienist learned that oral health is very important to the patient who believed that tooth loss was inevitable. She now believes that she can save her teeth; therefore, she now believes that her oral health is meaningful and is willing to expend time and effort needed to ensure good oral health.[1]

THEORIES OF MOTIVATION   *Motivation,* or the will of the individual to act, is an important factor in learning. Motivation is a drive that propels an individual to satisfy a

Table 8–3 Summary of Health Behavior Models

Theory	Major Elements
Health belief model	1. Perceived susceptibility 2. Perceived seriousness 3. Beneficial 4. Salience
Transtheoretical model	Behavior changes move through a predictable set of stages including: 1. Precontemplation 2. Contemplation 3. Preparation 4. Action 5. Maintenance 6. Termination
Theory of reasoned action	1. People make rational decisions based on behavioral intent (combination of knowledge, values, and attitudes). 2. Intentions and behavior changes are affected by attitudes and social norms.
Stages of Learning	1. Unawareness 2. Awareness 3. Self-interest 4. Involvement 5. Action 6. Habit
Social cognitive theory (SCT)	1. Extension of social learning theory that emphasizes personal actions 2. Self-efficacy is the belief that personal actions will affect outcomes. 3. Self-efficacy is gained as information, behavior, and environment interact in a reciprocal manner. As self-efficacy increases, individuals plan for contingencies and persevere through difficulties.
Theory of the sense of coherence (SOC)	1. Health lies on a continuum of ease to disease. 2. Stressors move an individual to the disease end of the continuum. 3. Individuals develop a network of general resistance resources that reduce stressors. 4. Individuals with high SOC find stressors manageable (they have the resources to cope), comprehensible (stressors make sense), and meaningful (willing to spend resources to deal with the stressor).

Source: Modified from: Hollister M. Health Education and Promotion Theories. In: Nathe C. *Primary Preventive Dentistry*. 8th ed. Upper Saddle River, NJ: Pearson; 2014. Modified from original.

need.[8] Remember that the individual must be aware of the need before he or she can be motivated.

Motivational models generally identify the considerations that must be present for values to change.(11–21)[8-18] Dental hygienists initiating a change must be aware of their own values and must recognize and understand those of the patient. Determining what motivates the patient and to understand his or her knowledge of dental care, hygienists must not thrust their own values on patients. An example of this would be a patient who is motivated to decrease bleeding "gums." When explaining the relationship between daily flossing and gingival bleeding, the dental hygienist has the perfect patient motivation to propel the action of daily flossing. A *need* must exist for changes to be considered. *Attitude* is a powerful influence on human behavior and motivation because together they determine the learner's investment in the desired outcome. *Stimulation* is an experience that makes a learner active when affect is a major influence on the learner's emotion, because of the actual experience. *Competence* occurs when an individual masters a skill.[18]

Behavior Modification Theories

Changing behavior requires more than education; behavior modification also is necessary. In fact, at one time or another, most if not all people have considered taking some type of action for change, often to improve health. Some may have started exercising or dieting at the beginning of the year or before an important event, and many may have promised themselves to get more sleep or stop smoking.

Psychologists have theorized that behavior modification is accomplished by classical conditioning, operant conditioning, or modeling. *Classical conditioning* as by Pavlov described in the late 1920s maintains that animals become conditioned to act in a specific way in response to specific stimuli. An example of classical conditioning applied to oral hygiene might be the inclination of a patient who is praised at an appointment for flossing to maintain the practice to receive the same praise at subsequent appointments.[19] *Operant conditioning*, described by Skinner, is based on the concepts of rewarding good behavior and punishing bad behavior. This theory suggests, for example, that a dental hygienist who gives a pediatric patient treats following good behavior while being treated is reinforcing positive behavior; a parent's discipline of a child exhibiting bad behavior during treatment may prevent that behavior at subsequent appointments.[20] *Modeling* behavior can facilitate learning through imitation. For example, if a child is present when an older sibling receives a treat for exhibiting good behavior, that child may imitate the good behavior.

The behavior modification model suggests that traveling through different stages is necessary in order to have

behavior changed. Important to note is that all of these theories suggest that behaviors can indeed be changed.

These health theories can help dental hygienists understand human motivation to change behaviors and work to improve health. (See Table 8-3 ■.) No single theory applies to all situations or is effective for all people. Combining pertinent elements of several theories often produces the best results.[1] Researchers have suggested that multidimensional models may prove to be the most effective, particularly for conditions with multiple risk factors, such as early childhood caries.[21]

Before deciding on a course of behavior modification for an individual, the dental hygienist must consider the patient's values and beliefs, readiness to change, perception of control, perception of the effectiveness of personal actions, behavioral and social norms, and available resources. If the dental professional is considering proposing a change of policy for a community, school, or other group of people, the primary considerations may be social norms, community resources, and level of knowledge.[1]

Summary

Dental hygienists should be able to conduct effective education to successfully transform knowledge into positive behaviors. The key word here is *successfully*. The ultimate goal of education should be to instill the value of dental health and thus change an individual's behavior.

Dental health educators must remember that education involves much more than simply relaying information. Effective dental health education should develop positive values toward dental health and cause behavior changes. Therefore, dental health educators must fully understand a specific population's knowledge level and be aware of the importance of values on health practices and decisions.

The theories discussed in this chapter involve many common themes. These main themes are similar, and the most important constructs involve understanding the difference between education and promotion and the effect individual values have on health and societal practices.

Self-Study Test Items

1. Empowerment models that focus on patient autonomy and collaborative relationships are paternalist regimens. These regimens are led by patients whose knowledge of health and disease increases the likelihood that healthy behaviors are attained.
   a. The first statement is true, but the second statement is false.
   b. The first statement is false, but the second statement is true.
   c. Both statements are true.
   d. Both statements are false.

2. Which of the following aspects is part of the multidimensional model of health?
   a. Spirituality
   b. Knowledge
   c. Behavior
   d. Values

3. The local dental hygiene association worked on policy change that banned sugary beverages from school vending machines. This is an example of
   a. Healthy behavior
   b. Health action
   c. Health education
   d. Health promotion

4. For behavioral change to occur, an individual must reach what milestone?
   a. Value the change
   b. Understand the healthy behavior
   c. Understand unhealthy behavior
   d. Understand why a behavior was chosen

5. A patient who receives praise for having healthy gums during two routine dental hygiene appointments will be more likely to maintain good home care to ensure that the praise will continue at subsequent appointments. This theory is called
   a. Classical conditioning
   b. Operant conditioning
   c. Modeling
   d. Empowerment

References

1. Hollister M. Health education and promotion theories. In: Harris NO, Garcia-Godoy F, Nathe C. *Primary Preventive Dentistry.* 8th ed. Upper Saddle River, NJ: Pearson; 2013.
2. Cuff PA. Interprofessional Education for Collaboration: learning how to improve health from interprofessional models across the continuum of education to practice. Workshop Summary. Washington, DC: Institute of Medicine.
3. IOM (Institute of Medicine). 2013. *Health literacy: Improving health, health systems, and health policy around the world: Workshop summary.* Washington, DC: The National Academies Press. Retrieved from http://www.iom.edu/Reports/2013/Health-Literacy-Improving-Health-Health-Systems-and-Health-Policy-Around-the-World.aspx on August 5, 2015.
4. *Constitution of the World Health Organization—Basic Documents.* 45th ed. (suppl); Switzerland: World Health Organization; 2006.
5. World Health Organization. WHOQOL measuring quality of life. Introducing the WHOQOL instruments [Internet site]. Retrieved from http://www.who.int/mental_health/media/68.pdf on September 24, 2015.
6. Meeks-Mitchell L, Heit P. *Health: A Wellness Approach.* Columbus, OH: Merrill Publishing; 1987:6.
7. Maslow AH. *Motivation and Personality.* 3rd ed. New York, NY: Harper & Row; 1987.
8. DeBiase CB. *Dental Health Education Theory and Practice.* Philadelphia, PA: Lea & Febiger; 1991:6.
9. Pickett G, Hanlon JJ. Historical perspectives. In: *Public Health and Administration.* St Louis, MO: Times Mirror/Mosby College Publications; 1990:21–46.
10. Seaward BL. *Managing Stress Principles and Strategies for Health and Well-Being.* Sudbury, MA: Jones and Bartlett; 1999:83–90, 181–190.
11. Becker MH. *The Health Belief Model and Personal Health Behavior.* Thorofare, NJ: Charles B. Slack; 1974.
12. Prochaska JO, Norcross JC, DiClemente CC. *Changing for Good.* New York, NY: Avon Books; 1994.
13. Ajzen I, Fishbein M. *Understanding Attitudes and Predicting Social Behavior.* Upper Saddle River, NJ: Pearson; 1980.
14. Bandura A. *Social Foundation of Thought and Action: A Social Cognitive Theory.* Englewood Cliffs, NJ: Prentice Hall; 1986.
15. Bandura A. Social cognitive theory: an angentic perspective. *Annu Rev Psychol.* 2001;52:1–26.
16. Bandura A. *Self efficacy: The Exercise of Control.* New York, NY: Freeman; 1997.
17. Antonovsky A. *Health Stress and Coping.* San Francisco, CA: Jossey-Bass; 1979.
18. Chopoorian K. How adults learn: the dental hygienist as an educator. *Dental Hygienist News.*1996;9:3–6.
19. Pavlov IP. *Conditional Reflexes.* New York, NY: Dover Publications; 1960. This edition is an unaltered republication of the 1927 translation by Oxford University Press.
20. Skinner BF. *About Behaviorism.* New York, NY: Dover Publications; 1974.
21. Freire MC, Hardy R, Sheiham A. Mothers' sense of coherence and their adolescent children's oral health status and behaviours. *Community Dent Health.* 2002;19:24–31.

9

Lesson Plan Development

OBJECTIVES

After studying this chapter, the dental hygiene student should be able to:

- Explain the dental hygiene process of care
- Describe the process of lesson plan development
- Develop goals and objectives for a lesson plan
- Describe learning levels and domains
- Identify and describe teaching methods
- Identify the characteristics of an effective teacher
- Develop a lesson plan

COMPETENCIES

After studying this chapter and participating in accompanying course activities, the dental hygiene student should be competent to do the following:

- Promote the values of the dental hygiene profession through service-based activities, positive community affiliations, and active involvement in local organizations
- Communicate effectively with diverse individuals and groups, serving all persons without discrimination by acknowledging and appreciating diversity
- Promote positive values of oral and general health and wellness to the public and organizations within and outside the profession
- Provide screening, referral, and educational services that allow patients to access the resources of the health care system

KEY TERMS

Dental hygiene process
  of care *120*
Lesson plan *123*
Teaching methods *124*

Science photo/Shutterstock

Dental hygienists are routinely asked to present dental health and preventive focused lessons in the community. Although not all dental hygienists are excited about public speaking, it is one of the founding principles of the profession. Public speaking dates back to the classroom instructions on toothbrushing in the Bridgeport Public Schools, which is depicted in an old photo entitled Toothbrushing Drills. (See Figure 9-1.)

All dental hygienists provide one-on-one patient education during routine dental hygiene appointments. Many dental hygienists provide education that is termed population-based or community focused in schools, support groups, to other health care organizations, and in numerous other venues. This chapter is devoted to preparing the dental hygiene student with providing group or population-based education, which is very similar to individualized education, in an effective manner. Dental hygienists should always prepare a lesson when providing community education to ensure effectiveness.

Dental Hygiene Process of Care

Planning an effective presentation of dental hygiene principles to a target group involves understanding the **dental hygiene process of care.** This process can be described as the assessment, dental hygiene diagnosis, planning, implementation, evaluation, and documentation of dental hygiene care of a target population. (See Figure 9-2.) Documentation has recently been added to the dental hygiene process of care. Utilizing the dental hygiene process of care enables the dental hygienist to follow logical steps in developing an effective lesson. Never underestimate the importance of planning the presentation. Although dental hygienists frequently educate individual

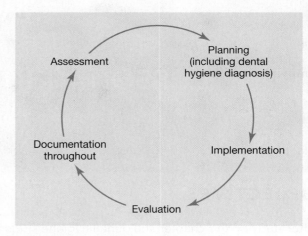

FIGURE 9–2 Dental Hygiene Process of Care

patients on the importance of oral health care, when presenting to a group, planning is crucial.

The best way to ensure that a presentation will be effective and successful is to be prepared. Preparation and strong organization decrease the initial nervousness some dental hygienists feel when asked to present to a group. Use of the steps in the dental hygiene process of care as outlined in Table 9-1 can ensure an effective lesson plan and aid in making an effective presentation.

Table 9–1 Lesson Plan Development Using Dental Hygiene Process of Care

Stage	Action
Assessment	Assess target population's needs, interests, abilities, and resources Assess dental status
Dental hygiene diagnosis	Formulate findings from assessment Prioritize goals
Planning	Select broad goal formulation Identify specific objectives Select teaching method(s)
Implementation	Prepare for various scenarios Demonstrate effective teacher characteristics
Evaluation	Use qualitative measurement Use quantitative measurement Provide follow up information to appropriate parties

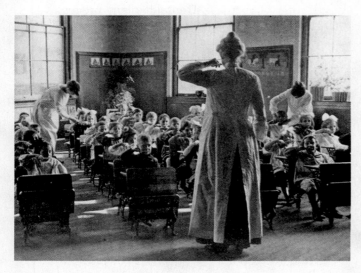

FIGURE 9–1 Toothbrushing Drills.
Source: Fones School of Dental Hygiene, Bridgeport, CT.

Assessment

Before the planning phase begins, the dental hygienist must assess the audience population. Assessment entails identifying needs, interests, and resources. Assessment is not evaluation. Assessment is done to determine the level of understanding by the learner, while evaluation is a tool to determine how well a program or educator teaching the course is conveying messages.[1] Assessment merely suggests to the presenter what the intended audience knows about dental health and how well they know the information. This stage is similar to the initial discussion a clinical dental hygienist has with the patient. It is during this time, that the dental hygienist determines what the patient knows and how well he or she understands it. When providing a presentation to a group, the dental hygienist must take the time to adequately assess the group, just as is done in the previous example from clinical practice. If this stage is skipped, the presentation may not be pertinent to the target audience.

It is important never to assume things about a target population. Consider this example. A long-term care facility asks a dental hygienist to present dental health information to its nurse's aides. Without assessing this population, the dental hygienist decides to discuss periodontal diseases based on the assumption that nurse's aides would find that information valuable because older adults generally have periodontal diseases. However, the most pressing issue in this facility is difficulties with dentures: The residents keep losing them and have trouble keeping them clean. Consequently, the nurse's aides are hoping to learn more about denture identification and care. The nurse's aides—the target population—leave the presentation feeling disappointed that only during the last three minutes, when they were able to ask questions, were their specific needs addressed. To avoid this situation, the dental hygienist could have talked with the head nurse regarding the group's particular needs, interests, and abilities *before* planning the presentation. Doing so would have better prepared the dental hygienist to present on a desired topic and answer questions.

Assessment also includes defining the target population's level of dental knowledge. Many groups have similar levels of dental health knowledge, but some do not. Although dental knowledge can be assessed at the beginning of a presentation, researching before the presentation is a better way to plan for the group's knowledge level. Discussing the topics the specific population is interested in with a contact person is one assessment method; providing a brief survey to the group prior to planning the presentation is an excellent one. The presenter can use the survey to question the group about topics that interest them.

Another important assessment goal is to learn what resources are available at the site. The dental hygienist should ask about the availability of a screen or a projector before planning a PowerPoint feature. Not having the expected resources can sabotage the presenter's confidence and effectiveness.

Dental Hygiene Diagnosis

After a thorough assessment of the target population has been conducted, the diagnosis phase of the process of care plan can begin. When diagnosing a group, the dental hygienist does not need to talk with each member but can identify the topic after speaking to one or two contacts about the group's particular needs, interests, and capabilities. Specifically, dental hygiene diagnosis requires analyzing and identifying dental needs that can be fulfilled through dental hygiene education.

Did You Know?

The diagnosis phase is included because it is part of the process of care plan. It is not necessary to refer to it as a diagnosis, but basically the dental hygienist is coming up with a diagnosis of a group per se.

An example of a dental hygiene case presentation with corresponding diagnosis follows. Before giving a presentation to a support group for patients with diabetes, the dental hygienist contacted the group leader and staff nurse regarding this group's needs, interests, and capabilities. The dental hygienist learned that many members complained of bleeding and sore gums and wanted to learn more about gum disease associated with diabetes. The dental hygiene diagnosis for this group was periodontal disease associated with diabetes. Basically, the diagnosis is the step that describes the primary need found during the assessment phase.

Planning

After assessing and developing a dental hygiene diagnosis for a group, the dental hygienist begins the planning phase by determining a goal for the presentation and identifying several objectives, which is similar to planning individualized instruction. This activity helps the hygienist plan the specific information to present to the group and how to present it effectively. Carefully preparing the lesson organizes the teacher's thinking process and builds confidence in presenting the material. The process includes gathering and organizing the information and developing the presentation of this information. Effective planning should include rehearsing the presentation that has been developed and timing it to make sure it fits within the given time limitations. In addition, consider and prepare for the questions the

DENTAL HYGIENIST SPOTLIGHT ·····················

Public Health Column: Christine Murphy, RDH, BS

Christine Murphy graduated with a bachelor of science degree in dental hygiene in 1997. She received numerous awards in college and has been inducted as a member of Sigma Phi Alpha, the National Dental Hygiene Honor Society. Since graduation, she has been busy! She has held various positions as an officer in the local dental hygienists' association, worked in private practice, and taught part-time at the University of New Mexico.

Ms. Murphy is currently the dental director at Pueblo of Isleta Dental Clinic. She started at Isleta as a staff dental hygienist shortly after graduation. Within a year, she had taken the managerial role of dental director. The clinic has grown with many more staff. Her efforts have allowed the clinic to treat more patients and enhance dental care for the Pueblo. In addition, she wrote the proposal to allow the Pueblo of Isleta to run the program separately from the Indian Health Service, thereby dramatically increasing the budget.

I asked her some questions about her career.

Why did you decide to go into dental hygiene?

I had four small children and my husband's back went out. He suggested I go back to school to become a dental hygienist because he knew I could not support our family as a dental assistant. It was a difficult decision because I had been out of high school for fifteen years at that time. I wasn't a great student in high school, but age does wonders. I graduated from dental hygiene school with a 3.98 GPA summa cum laude and have realized that I love dental hygiene!

How did you get into dental public health? Did you need additional education?

I didn't need additional education because I graduated from University of New Mexico with a bachelor's degree in dental hygiene. I got into public health slowly but surely.

When I graduated from UNM, I wasn't sure exactly what I wanted to do. I worked in private practice one day a week, taught at UNM two days a week, and worked for a temp service one day a week. I answered an advertisement for a full-time hygiene position at the Isleta Dental Clinic but informed the dentist that I was available only part-time because of

my teaching commitment. I started out at the clinic two days a week. Within six months, I had quit temping and private practice and was working three days a week with the tribe. Eventually, the tribe offered me the position of dental director, and I currently work four days per week.

What is your current position?

I am the dental director for the Pueblo of Isleta, and I see patients in the clinic two days per week. Additionally, I serve as an adjunct faculty member for the University of New Mexico dental hygiene students who rotate through my clinic.

Can you discuss any particularly interesting experiences you have had in your dental public health career?

Not long after starting here, I began trying to learn some of the Pueblo language. It is beautiful but not written, so each person must learn from another. I quickly learned that you should be very careful whom you ask to teach you the language. I asked one patient how to say a particular phrase, but when I repeated it, the meaning was definitely not what I intended. It could have been quite embarrassing, but the person I repeated the phrase to was very understanding.

What advice would you give to a practicing hygienist who is thinking of doing something different?

Try anything and everything. In school I never even considered public health as an option. I had been a dental assistant in private practice for years, so I just assumed that's where I would practice dental hygiene. When I got into public health, I realized how much I loved being able to practice hygiene to the best of my ability without any other factors involved. I don't have to worry about whether or not the patient can afford scaling and root planing or anyone making me sell dentistry.

Working in public health has been such a great experience. I have met the most fantastic people—not just the patients I see but also the providers whom I work with . . . and not just in my clinic but across the nation.

Source: Christine Nathe writes the Public Health Column in *RDH* magazine published by Pennwell Publishing. For more public health spotlights please see RDH magazine online at http://www.rdhmag.com/index.html.

audience is likely to ask; having the opportunity to pose questions will increase audience participation.

First, it is necessary to prioritize the group's particular needs. Consider, for example, the situation in which a parent teacher association (PTA) has asked the dental hygienist to come to its meeting to discuss dental care for fifteen minutes. After questioning contacts, the dental hygienist learns that the PTA group's primary interests in this presentation were access to dental care for families with Medicaid insurance, motivating their children to brush, and helping parents find quick and easy nutritional food choices. In addition, some parents were interested in learning more about periodontal surgery, implants, and bleaching. The dental hygienist realized that comprehensive dental health education on all of these topics could not be delivered in only fifteen minutes and therefore prioritized the most beneficial and important topics for inclusion in the presentation. The next step is to prepare a **lesson plan,** which is a written document used in planning a presentation.

Lesson Plan Preparation

GOALS   The first step in writing a lesson plan is to identify the presentation's goal, which is a broad statement of the final outcome that the instructor expects from the target group upon completing the presentation.[2–5] It is important to write only one or two broad goals you expect the group to accomplish. After setting the overall goal, the instructor identifies the specific outcomes that are intended to result.

OBJECTIVES   An objective includes a specific, observable action or behavior that a learner will perform or exhibit.[6] Many times, objectives include a target group, a condition, and measurement. The *audience* is the target group. The *condition* entails relevant factors affecting the actual performance, such as time or environment, and the *measurement* is the way to evaluate the level of achievement the audience is to attain or the acceptable performance. For example, consider the objective "following the presentation, the physician's assistants will be able to describe the dental caries process according to the presented information." The audience is physician's assistants; the condition is that, following the presentation, they can describe the dental caries process. The measurement could be how many audience members can describe it according to the presented information.

Did You Know?

Writing objectives allows the dental hygienist to plan in detail the information that will be presented and discussed.

When writing an objective, it is important to be aware of three learning domains.[7] (See Table 9-2 ■.) The

Table 9–2 Domains of Learning

Domain of Learning	Example
Psychomotor	To describe actions
Cognitive	To describe behavior
Affective	To describe feelings
Levels of Learning	
Knowledge	To know
Application	To apply
Problem solving	To problem solve

psychomotor domain describes actions. The behaviors in this domain are the easiest to identify with precise verbs. An example of an objective written for the psychomotor domain would be "Following the dental health presentation, the nurse's aides will clean dentures effectively." This behavior is concrete and observable, and the verbs that refer to them denote a neurophysical activity. See Box 9-1 ■ for a list of verbs commonly used in the psychomotor domain.

The *cognitive domain* represents intellectual skills. The verbs used to describe behavior in this domain (presented in Box 9-2 ■) are slightly more abstract than those in the psychomotor domain. An example of an objective in this domain is "Following the presentation, the first-grade students will identify three healthy snacks from the chart."

Finally, the domain that includes feelings, attitudes, values, and interests is referred to as the *affective domain*. See Box 9-3 ■ for verbs used in this domain. Although it can be measured by qualitative assessment, the affective domain is not directly observable and not as easily measured as the behaviors in the other two domains. For those in the dental hygiene profession, however, the affective domain is extremely important. An objective for this domain is "Following completion of the current issues course, the dental hygienist will be able to defend, in writing, the dental hygienist's role in consumer advocacy with a passing grade."

See Box 9-4 ■ for a list of verbs whose meanings are open to interpretation and should be avoided when writing objectives.

The levels of learning should also be considered when identifying objectives. The three levels are *knowledge, application,* and *problem solving.* (Refer to Table 9-2.) The knowledge level is the lowest and simply requires that knowledge be gained. The application level requires applying the new knowledge. Being able to solve a problem implies that the learner has mastered the problem-solving level.

Box 9–1 Verbs Used in the Psychomotor Domain

- Brush
- Clean
- Demonstrate
- Detect
- Disinfect
- Eat
- Exercise
- Experiment
- Floss
- Identify
- Irrigate
- Measure
- Probe
- Screen
- Sterilize

Box 9–2 Verbs Used in the Cognitive Domain

- Classify
- Collect
- Compare
- Contrast
- Describe
- Design
- Diagnose
- Explain
- Indicate
- Label
- List
- Recognize
- Record
- Show
- Solve

Box 9–3 Verbs Used in the Affective Domain

- Advocate
- Assess
- Believe
- Challenge
- Debate
- Deduct
- Defend
- Discuss
- Evaluate
- Judge
- Lead
- Live out
- Persuade
- Suggest
- Value

Box 9–4 Verbs Whose Meaning as Objectives Can Be Unclear

- Appreciate
- Comprehend
- Empathize
- Familiarize
- Grasp
- Have Faith
- Interpret
- Know
- Like
- Realize
- Think
- Understand

Teaching Methods

Another important aspect of planning is deciding which teaching strategies or methods to use. A **teaching method** is the approach or method used in instruction. The instructor must decide which method(s) to use to obtain the desired outcome. Furthermore, the method(s) should be appropriate for the activities involved and resources available. Most important, the method should be interesting and motivate the audience.

Lecture is probably the most well-known and traditional method of teaching. It is effective if a formal presentation of information is needed and the information is appropriate for the audience's knowledge level. Lecturing is also effective when the intention is to create awareness of various ideas, issues, and beliefs. The lecture method is best used in conjunction with other methods.

Did You Know?

The drawback to using the lecture method is that it does not involve the audience, which may decrease motivation and learning.

The *discussion* method involves interaction between the students and the instructor and more easily arouses interest, which helps students to develop reasoning abilities. *Presentation* is defined as employing the lecture and discussion methods together. *Demonstration* can be used with lecture, discussion, or presentation methods when the desired outcome is learning a behavior, such as the proper way to brush.

The *inquiry* method, more commonly referred to as *problem-based* learning, uses case studies in which the teacher acts as a facilitator and the student is responsible for gaining the correct information.[4] Group or individualized games and activities usually increase motivation and learning. Examples are DVD– or Internet-based interactive activities such as playing a version of dental health Jeopardy as a group. Role-play and simulation activities can also be utilized as a group.

Understanding the domains and levels of learning will enable the dental hygienist to adequately define and plan the lesson. After planning the lesson, the next step is to determine how the material will be presented or taught.

Visual Aids

The use of visual aids can add a great deal to a presentation by engaging the learners and contributing an organizing aspect to the lesson. They include PowerPoint slides, DVDs, and flip charts. If used improperly, however, visual aids can be a distraction. For instance, instructors often pass a tooth model around the class during a presentation, but this can be disruptive to the learning process because the students must listen to the instructor and inspect the tooth. By planning the presentation well, effective integration of a tooth model can be useful. See Table 9-3 ■ for more information on using visual aids effectively.

Refer to Box 9-5 ■ for an example of a lesson plan prepared to teach eighth-grade students about dental hygiene careers during a career month at school when they were preparing to register for high school classes. More than

Table 9–3 Using Visual Aids

Visual Clarity
Each visual needs to be clear and understandable on its own.

- limit each slide to only one topic
- state sources where appropriate
- know the audience: avoid abbreviations and jargon unfamiliar to them
- use meaningful graphics when they reinforce the written message
- highlight key information on figures to help focus the audience's attention
- make points concise yet meaningful—avoid being cryptic

Organizational Consistency
Balance and consistency are important when creating a presentation package.

- keep type sizes and fonts consistent
- format headings consistently
- use no more than two fonts per slide (one for headings and one for main text) or choose different sizes of the same font for headings and main text
- spread the information out so that it fills the screen
- choose contrasting colors (e.g., dark background with light lettering)
- use color consistently but avoid overuse—two to four colors per slide
- be aware of the connotations behind colors (e.g., red on a financial statement comes with the negative connotation of having a cash deficit)
- use parallel grammar for points (e.g., begin each point with the same part of speech)

Readability
Visuals are only effective if the audience can physically see them.

- use 24–28 point font for main text and 32–40 point font for headings
- if writing by hand on overhead slides, make the letters at least 1/2" (1.0 cm) high
- avoid distracting, unnecessary graphics and excessively complex backgrounds
- use clear, standard fonts such as Times New Roman, Arial, or Helvetica
- consider using boldface lettering to make text thicker
- avoid putting much text in italics or all upper-case letters—this slows down reading
- ensure diagrams are not too intricate to be visible from the back of the room
- limit each point to one line whenever possible to limit reading time

Emphasize Important Information
Effective visuals should aid the audience, not the presenter.

- write only main points on visuals, not the details that support them
- avoid giving the audience the entire presentation to read
- put the key words on the visuals (repetition is acceptable in presentations, since it helps audience retention)
- make points discrete: do not simply break up paragraphs
- assume the audience will copy down everything presented on a visual—keep information clear, simple, and minimal

Source: http://cte.uwaterloo.ca/teaching_resources/teaching_tips/tips_activities/using_visual_aids.pdf. Accessed June 9, 2009

Box 9–5 Sample Lesson Plan

Dental Hygiene Presentation

Audience
24 eighth-grade students

Time
15 minutes

Goal
To promote the career of dental hygienist

Objectives
Following this presentation, the students will be able to:

1. Describe the functions of a dental hygienist
2. Describe the settings in which dental hygienists work
3. Identify careers available in the dental field

Teaching Methods
Lecture
Discussion
Role-playing
Audiovisual Aids
Dental Hygiene Career DVD (5 minutes)
PowerPoint slide series
Dental hygiene career pamphlets

Introduction
Today we will be discussing the career of dental hygienists, their functions in dental care delivery, and other careers available in the dental field.

Rationale
It is important for you as eighth graders to be aware of career opportunities available so that next year when you begin taking classes in high school, you can identify courses that will help prepare you for college course work pertaining to the career that interests you.

Dental Hygienist Defined
A dental hygienist is a health care provider who practices the art and science of preventive oral health. (Give examples.)

Educational Preparation
The University of New Mexico in Albuquerque offers a dental hygiene program. All neighboring states offer dental hygiene programs in university and community college settings. Dental hygienists can receive associate's, bachelor's, and master's degrees in dental hygiene.

When preparing for a dental hygiene career in high school, remember that dental hygienists must have a strong background in basic health and social sciences. Recommended subjects include biology, chemistry, physics, anatomy, physiology, algebra, geometry, calculus, English, and social science courses.

Roles of the Dental Hygienists
The six roles of dental hygienists are manager, clinician, educator/health promoter, researcher, consumer advocate, and change agent. (Provide examples.)

Practice Settings
Dental hygienists work in private dental offices; public schools; nursing homes and hospitals; military, state, and federal public health programs; the dental industry; and business and research facilities. They provide oral health services through preventive, educational, diagnostic, and therapeutic sciences.

View DVD and answer questions concerning the material it presents.

Careers Available in the Dental Field
Additional roles in the dental field include dentist, dental assistant, dental technician, consultant, and dental office manager/receptionist. (Provide examples of these careers.)

Conclusion
Today we discussed the dental hygiene career, education needed to become a dental hygienist, and other careers available in the dental field.

---

fifty different individuals presented information about possible careers during the month.

Upon completion of planning the lesson, it is important to practice the actual presentation methods. Practicing by oneself initially and then upon feeling comfortable have a fellow student, friend, or family member role play as the potential audience as preparation for an upcoming presentation. Ask for feedback to help make the presentation more effective—and keep practicing. Remember being prepared is key for a successful presentation.

Implementation

The most important aspect of implementation is preparation. By completing the first three phases—assessment, dental hygiene diagnosis, and planning—the dental hygienist should be well organized and feel confident about the presentation.

Classroom Management

An instructor who feels prepared and confident can effectively manage many different situations that may occur when making a presentation. Surprisingly, managing a classroom of adults can be as challenging as managing children. Signals such as frequent talking, shuffling, or sleeping indicate that the presentation is not being well received. Staying calm and conveying your enthusiasm, knowledge, and expectations can stop these signals. Moreover, being well organized will increase instructor confidence and decrease the likelihood of losing control of the class.

Characteristics of an Effective Teacher

Effective teaching involves motivating the students to learn the information presented and apply it. To accomplish this, communication skills are vital for an educator.

Box 9–6 Characteristics of Effective Teachers

- Ability to interact with students, their families, and colleagues
- Enthusiasm
- Flexibility
- Broad knowledge
- Organizational skills
- Patience
- Pleasant personality
- Willingness to learn

Box 9–7 Self-Evaluation Example

Oral Cancer Prevention Strategies Pretest

1. Smokeless tobacco products do less harm to oral tissues than cigarettes.
   True
   False

2. Alcohol use increases the risk of oral cancer.
   True
   False

3. Regular dental hygiene examinations include oral cancer examinations.
   True
   False

Oral Cancer Prevention Strategies Posttest

1. Smokeless tobacco products do less harm to oral tissues than cigarettes.
   True
   False

2. Alcohol use increases the risk of oral cancer.
   True
   False

3. Regular dental hygiene examinations include oral cancer examinations.
   True
   False

Teachers need to be able to effectively communicate to groups of students and students on an individual basis. Being available before and after a course is important for those students who have questions or ideas. See Box 9-6 for a list of some characteristics of effective teachers.

Did You Know?

Being prepared is definitely the best way to increase the likelihood that a presentation will be effective.

Effective teachers are prepared and organized. By carefully preparing a lesson, the teacher will have an organized thinking process and should be confident in presenting the material. Other important attributes of a teacher are flexibility and fairness. Being flexible with student learning is a key to motivating students to learn. Fairness is important in all aspects of life, which of course includes learning and teaching by example.

Fear of Public Speaking

Many people, including dental hygienists, may initially be nervous when speaking to an audience. The best way to prevent this nervousness is to practice. A presenter should practice in front of an audience, even if it is only one other person, until feeling completely confident. Fear of public speaking should be improved by repeated presentations. Public speaking can actually become close to a habit if done consistently. In other words, the more a dental hygienist presents to groups, the easier it should become.

Evaluation

Evaluation is an ongoing process and should be considered in the planning phase when objectives and goals are developed. Writing effective, measurable objectives ensures that the dental hygienist can accurately evaluate the presentation's effectiveness. Learning outcomes include a detailed description of what a participant should be expected to do when they successfully complete a program.[5] The smoothness of the talk and audience interest and participation can also help in evaluation. Teachers should be well aware of the motivation level of a class. Remember that the more interested the students are and the more they participate, the more likely it is that the objectives will be met. Students who are motivated are more likely to adopt these effective dental health behaviors promoted during the presentation.

Refer to Box 9-7 for a pretest/posttest evaluation for seventh-grade students. In this example, a dental hygienist is presenting a lesson plan on the prevention of oral cancer and is planning to evaluate the lesson with the pretest/posttest evaluation. The same questions are asked before the presentation and afterward to assess the degree of learning. Other methods of evaluation can include games, activities, computer games and quizzes, or simply group questioning of the information presented.

Documentation

As is always the case, the dental hygienist should remain vigilant with documentation. During individual patient care, this is important for evaluation and legal purposes, in public health this is important for evaluation and

operation of the program. When educating an audience, documentation is important to preserve the knowledge presented for the audience after the talk and for use in subsequent presentations.

Informational material, including brochures, slide shows, posters and video links is a great source of documentation to leave with participants. This can be used to facilitate further learning and reinforce concepts presented. Attaining documented evaluations from participants can be used to improve future presentations.

Evaluating the dental hygienist's effectiveness as an information conveyor is imperative. See Boxes 9-8 ■ and 9-9 ■ for evaluation criteria for lesson plans and presentations. By following the phases of creating effective presentations, the dental hygienist increases the likelihood of meeting those criteria.

Box 9–8 Lesson Plan Evaluation Checklist

- Displays organization
- Demonstrates evidence of research of topic
- Presents effective introduction
- Presents lessons on level of target population's understanding
- Presents expected behavioral objectives
- Asks appropriate questions
- Material is covered in appropriate length of time
- Develops and utilizes appropriate visual aids
- Presents effective conclusion
- Implements self-evaluation strategies

Box 9–9 Presenter Evaluation Checklist

- Shows evidence of research of topic
- Includes instruction on level of target population's understanding
- Indicates appropriate teaching methods
- Includes the use of effective visual aids
- Timed to meet requirements
- List appropriate probing questions to ask
- Presents professional appearance
- Maintains proper eye contact
- Projects voice meaningfully
- Demonstrates a prepared, organized manner

Summary

The dental hygiene process of care involves assessment, dental hygiene diagnosis, planning, implementation, evaluation, and documentation of dental hygiene care of a

target population. The dental hygienist should thoroughly assess the target population's needs to develop an appropriate lesson and determine an appropriate dental hygiene diagnosis. Thorough planning, including developing goals and objectives with an emphasis on identifying measurable outcomes, should follow. Being prepared is the most important step in providing effective dental health education to groups.

Self-Study Test Items

1. The best way to ensure an effective presentation is to
   a. Decrease the number of participants
   b. Utilize audiovisual aids
   c. Have at least ten objectives for each presentation
   d. Be prepared

2. "Following the presentation, the audience will be able to compare ten healthy and unhealthy snack choices" is an example of a(n)
   a. Goal
   b. Lesson plan
   c. Objective
   d. Healthy behavior

3. Lecturing is always an effective way to teach dental health education. Lecture always includes the inclusion of the problem-based method of learning.
   a. The first statement is true; the second is false.
   b. The first statement is false; the second is true.
   c. Both statements are true.
   d. Both statements are false.

4. Which verb pertains to the psychomotor domain?
   a. Demonstrating
   b. Comparing
   c. Advocating
   d. Defending

5. When used in an objective, the verb *understand*
   a. Is easily measured
   b. Is open to misinterpretation
   c. Always requires skill
   d. All of the above

References

1. Cuff PA. Interprofessional education for collaboration: learning how to improve health from interprofessional models across the continuum of education to practice: workshop summary. Washington, DC: Institute of Medicine. Retrieved from http://www.nap.edu/openbook.php?record_id=13486 on January 29, 2015.
2. DeBiase CB. *Dental Health Education: Theory and Practice.* Philadelphia, PA: Lea and Febiger; 1995.
3. Dignan MB, Carr, PA. *Program Planning for Health Education and Health Promotion.* Philadelphia, PA: Lea and Febiger; 1987.

4. Smith TC. *Making Successful Presentations: A Self-Teaching Guide.* New York, NY: Wiley; 1984.
5. The Difference Between Goals and Objectives. South Dakota State University. Retrieved on http://go.sdsu.edu/dus/ctl/files/03053-Lexicon_Goals_Objectives_Outcomes_draft_Apr-14.pdf. January 29, 2015.
6. Gagliardi L. *Dental Health Education: Lesson Plan and Implementation.* 2nd ed. Upper Saddle River, NJ: Pearson; 2006.
7. Tolle L. Dental Hygiene 400/500 Oral Health Promotion Course-Pak. Anaheim, CA: Copytron; 1988.

Visit www.pearsonhighered.com/healthprofessionsresources to access the student resources that accompany this book. Simply select Dental Hygiene from the choice of disciplines. Find this book and you will find the complimentary study tools created for this specific title.

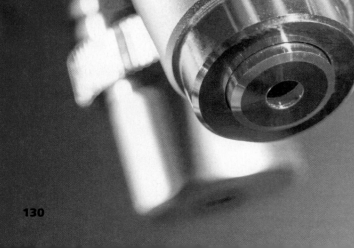

10

Target Populations

OBJECTIVES

After studying this chapter, the dental hygiene student should be able to:

- Define target populations to whom dental hygienists may provide services
- Describe faith-based initiatives
- Define target profiles
- Identify barriers to dental hygiene care
- Identify governmental resources for target populations

COMPETENCIES

After studying this chapter and participating in accompanying course activities, the dental hygiene student should be competent to do the following:

- Promote the values of the dental hygiene profession through service-based activities, positive community affiliations, and active involvement in local organizations
- Promote positive values of oral and general health and wellness to the public and organizations within and outside the profession
- Communicate effectively with diverse individuals and groups, serving all persons without discrimination by acknowledging and appreciating diversity
- Identify individual and population risk factors, and develop strategies that promote health-related quality of life
- Initiate consultations and collaborations with all relevant health care providers to facilitate optimal treatments
- Respect the goals, values, beliefs, and preferences of all patients
- Provide screening, referral, and educational services that allow patients to access the resources of the health care system
- Advocate for effective oral health care for underserved populations

KEY TERMS

Barriers to care *141*
Faith-based initiatives *141*
Target population profile *139*
Target populations *131*

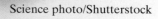
Science photo/Shutterstock

The term **target population** refers to a clearly identified segment of the population. A target population can be broad or narrow; for example, it can represent all three-year-old children, a group of youths involved in a local church group, or older adults in an assisted living community. Age can be a factor of a target population, but it usually has other common characteristics as well. For instance, the three-year-old children mentioned may be further identified by other shared characteristics, such as attending the same Head Start program, living in the same geographic area, or coming from families with similar incomes.

Target Populations

Dental hygienists provide service and education to many different groups and frequently are asked to present dental health information to these groups, which can be referred to as *target populations*. Dental hygienists should consider what type of information is appropriate to present to the target population.

Dental hygienists typically work with target populations in settings other than private dental practices. A dental hygienist may work in a school-based health center or mobile dental clinic providing care to preschool and schoolchildren or may work in a public health clinic delivering education to pregnant women in collaboration with a WIC Program. A dental hygienist may work in a nursing home, military base clinic or Veterans Affairs hospital as a clinical dental hygienist and may practice and consults as a member of an interdisciplinary team. Dental hygienists may work in a state or federal prison or work as a commissioned officer with the US Public Health Service. Basically, dental hygiene is no longer confined to only private dental practices; in fact, trends suggest the dental care delivery systems may be changing.[1]

Did You Know?

In the community setting, dental hygienists frequently treat a population rather than an individual patient, but the concept of dental hygiene treatment does not change.

Working with target populations may encompass clinical care or may focus on education and promotion. Of importance to the dental hygienist is the communication of health information, which entails the development of health literacy within the population. The dental hygienist should strive to fully understand each population and what methods are most effective at developing health-literate communities.

Dental Hygienists' Colleagues

In their professional capacities, dental hygienists serve a number of different populations. They may work with individuals as colleagues in advisory capacities, providing advice and acting as resources for dental care issues. Clinical care or population-based programs are areas in which dental hygienists may serve a variety of target populations.

FAMILY CAREGIVERS   Family caregivers provide daily care to their family members. These caregivers may be parents, grandparents, children, other relatives, or close friends. The care may be as comprehensive as dispensing medicine, both orally and intravenously, to a family member; helping the member with hygiene and sanitary functions; cooking; and feeding. These individuals usually assume some responsibility specifically pertaining to oral hygiene care. Many hospitals and health care organizations provide this group with health education and caregiving classes, which should include oral hygiene care. For instance, dental hygienists could present information to this population on how to care for the oral cavity during cancer treatments.

HEALTH CARE WORKERS   This target group provides direct patient care and/or treatment. These providers may include nurses, physicians, physician assistants, physical and occupational therapists, speech pathologists, and nurses' aides. This group has considerable knowledge about the diseases of the population they treat but may need additional information on the impact that the disease or condition has in relation to oral health. Dental hygienists should be knowledgeable about diseases and ask health care workers about their experiences treating and caring for individuals suffering from the diseases. Integrating an oral health component into health care is an excellent way to promote oral health as well as overall health.[2]

HOSPICE WORKERS   This group includes a variety of professionals who work together to make terminal illness more tolerable and comfortable for the patients and their families. Dental hygienists can alleviate oral pain by educating hospice workers, providing dental hygiene treatment, and facilitating treatment by a dentist when needed. Dental hygienists may coordinate dental care for the hospice program.

TEACHERS   Teachers can influence students a great deal and are particularly important to dental hygienists. Theorists suggest that teachers' discussion of dental health is more influential for students than is information provided by a dental hygienist once a year during dental health month. For this reason, teachers must have proper dental knowledge and be motivated to instill positive dental health behaviors in their students. Teachers should be able to recognize noticeable dental disease and know a dental hygienist within the community to contact. Dental hygienists can be effective in changing dental behavior by educating and collaborating with teachers.

SOCIAL WORKERS   A *social worker* is a professional who helps individuals, groups, and communities to enhance or restore their capacity for social functioning and to create societal conditions favorable to reaching the goals they set.[3] Social workers influence the populations they

serve, and dental hygienists can work with them to provide access to dental care and education for many people in need. Dental hygienists should instruct social workers in proper oral hygiene and serve as a liaison between the social worker, patient, and dental home.

Did You Know?

Social workers are great resources for dental hygienists. They have invaluable information about local and state dental services that are available to the people they serve.

Dental Hygienists and Their Target Populations

The relationship of oral health to overall health is most important to remember in working with these population. A patient afflicted with a medically compromising condition such as cardiovascular disease, respiratory disease, metabolic and endocrine disease, immune-compromising diseases including HIV infection, liver and kidney disorders, arthritis, physical disabilities, joint prostheses, or cancer may also present with many symptoms, conditions, and diseases in the oral cavity.[4] Table 10-1 ■ provides specific information about oral health and systemic diseases and conditions.

Table 10–1 Medical Conditions and Their Descriptions, Oral Manifestations, and Preventive Strategies

Condition	Description	Oral Manifestations	Preventive Strategies
Alcohol abuse	Excessive consumption of ethanol	Oral cancer Poor oral hygiene Xerostomia Petechiae Ecchymoses Increased bleeding Candidiasis Tooth erosion	Individualized oral hygiene instruction Saliva stimulants and substitutes Self-care fluoride treatments Antifungal agent Diphenhydramine rinse
Arthritis	Group of diseases that damage joints	Poor oral hygiene Temporomandibular joint disorder (TMJ) issues	Individualized oral hygiene instruction Short appointment times Oral appliance Alternative positioning during appointments
Asthma	Abnormal function of the lungs	Candidiasis Increased caries Increase gingivitis	Antifungal agent Diphenhydramine rinse
Bulimia	Binge eating followed by purging	Tooth erosion Increased caries and periodontitis Tooth sensitivity	Individualized oral hygiene instruction Self-care fluoride treatments
Cancer	Out-of-control growth of abnormal cells	Mucositis Candidiasis Xerostomia Loss of taste Trismus Cervical caries Sensitive teeth Excessive, spontaneous bleeding Poor healing Increased susceptibility to infection	Antifungal agent Individualized oral hygiene instruction Saliva stimulants and substitutes Self-care fluoride treatments Antimicrobial rinse Mouth exercises Tongue depressors to open mouth
Cardiac arrhythmias	Abnormal heartbeat or rate	Xerostomia Ulceration Petechiae	Diphenhydramine rinse Saliva stimulants and substitutes Self-care fluoride treatments

Table 10–1 Medical Conditions and Their Descriptions, Oral Manifestations, and Preventive Strategies *(continued)*

Condition	Description	Oral Manifestations	Preventive Strategies
Cocaine use	Use of addictive stimulant drug	Ulceration of mucosa Palatal perforation Necrosis of gingiva Bruxism Cervical tooth abrasion Tooth erosion	Individualized oral hygiene instruction Mouth guard Diphenhydramine rinse
Congestive heart failure	Inability of heart to pump enough blood to the body's other organs	Infection Bleeding Petechiae Ecchymoses Xerostomia	Saliva stimulants and substitutes Self-care fluoride treatments
Depression	Illness of mind, body, and thoughts	Poor oral hygiene Xerostomia Damage to tissues due to overcleaning	Saliva stimulants and substitutes Self-care fluoride treatments
Diabetes	Metabolic disorder resulting in abnormal blood glucose levels	Impaired healing Increased susceptibility to infections Candidiasis Accelerated periodontal disease Xerostomia Ulcerations Numbness/burning/pain of oral tissues	Antifungal agent Diphenhydramine rinse Baking soda and water rinse Saliva stimulants and substitutes Self-care fluoride treatments
Epilepsy	Neurologic disorder causing seizures	Gingival hyperplasia Fractured teeth Injury to lips and tongue	Individualized oral hygiene instruction Surgical reduction of gingiva
Hemophilia	Bleeding disorder	Spontaneous bleeding Prolonged bleeding Hematomas	Individualized oral hygiene instruction
HIV/AIDS	Immune system failure	Candidiasis Kaposi sarcoma Hairy leukoplakia Linear gingival erythema NUG/NUP	Antifungal agent Individualized oral hygiene instruction Antibiotics Corticosteroid therapy
Hypertension	Elevated blood pressure	Xerostomia Ulceration Lichenoid reactions Decreased healing Increased bleeding Gingival hyperplasia	Diphenhydramine rinse Saliva stimulants and substitutes Self-care fluoride treatments
Hyperthyroidism	Excessive release of thyroid hormone	Progressive periodontal disease Extensive caries Tumors on tongue Osteoporosis of alveolar ridge Premature loss of teeth Early eruption patterns Burning sensation	Baking soda and water rinse Individualized oral hygiene instruction

(continued)

Table 10–1 Medical Conditions and Their Descriptions, Oral Manifestations, and Preventive Strategies *(continued)*

Condition	Description	Oral Manifestations	Preventive Strategies
Hypothyroidism	Thyroid failure	Increased tongue size Delayed eruption of teeth Delayed wound healing	Individualized oral hygiene instruction
Liver disease	Inflamed liver	Bleeding, lichenoid eruptions	Individualized oral hygiene instruction
Marijuana use	Smoking plant *Cannabis sativa*	Xerostomia Oral cancer Poor oral hygiene Candidiasis Increased gingivitis and periodontitis	Individualized oral hygiene instruction Antifungal agent Saliva stimulants and substitutes
Methamphetamine use	Addictive stimulant drug use may cause rapid weight loss, carelessness, mental impairment, and rapid tooth decay	Poor oral hygiene Xerostomia Rampant decay	Individualized oral hygiene instruction Saliva stimulants and substitutes Self-care fluoride treatments
Organ transplants	Solid organ/tissue or hematopoietic cell transplantation	Candidiasis Herpes (simplex and zoster) Hairy leukoplakia Kaposi sarcoma Aphthous stomatitis Spontaneous bleeding Increased infection Ulceration Petechiae Ecchymoses Gingival hyperplasia Salivary gland dysfunction Xerostomia	Individualized oral hygiene instruction Antifungal agent Saliva stimulants and substitutes
Renal disease	Complete or near failure of the kidneys	Mucosal pallor Xerostomia Metallic taste Ammonia breath Stomatitis Loss of lamina dura Bone radiolucencies Increased bleeding Ulcerations Candidiasis	Antifungal agent Diphenhydramine rinse Saliva stimulants and substitutes Self-care fluoride treatments Individualized oral hygiene instruction
Tobacco use	Use of plants in the genus *Nicotiana* compromises the immune system	Oral cancer Leukoplakia Xerostomia Alveolar bone damage Gingival damage Hairy tongue Nicotine stomatitis Increased caries	Saliva stimulants and substitutes Self-care fluoride treatments

Source: Aboytes D. In: Harris NO, Garcia-Godoy F, Nathe C. *Primary Preventive Dentistry.* 8th ed. Upper Saddle River, NJ: Pearson; 2013.

PEOPLE WITH MEDICAL CONDITIONS/DISEASES Dental education for patients with a systemic disease can be complicated but help to alleviate many infections and also may improve overall health. When making presentations to groups with systemic diseases or their caregivers, dental hygienists should have information available on oral manifestations of the disease, specific drugs that are commonly prescribed and their effects on dental health, and premedication coverage information.

PEOPLE WITH DEVELOPMENTAL DISABILITIES Developmental disabilities are either present at birth, occur during the developmental period, or may appear years later. The major disorders in this category are intellectual disability, autism spectrum disorder, cerebral palsy, down syndrome and attention deficit hyperactive disorder.[5] Education directed to this group may consist of interventions aimed at reducing high rates of periodontal diseases and caries as well as the care of teeth that may be rotated and/or crowded. Specific drug interactions and appointment scheduling issues common to this group should be assessed.

PEOPLE WHO HAVE MENTAL HEALTH DISORDERS Mental health is an integral dimension of overall health. Depression is the most common mental health illness, affecting more than 26% of the population in the United States.[6] Mental health can include emotional, psychological, and social health; and many times mental health issues coexist with other health issues and disease.[7] The dental hygienists should educate this population on medication side effects and dental care scheduling.

PEOPLE WHO ARE HEARING IMPAIRED Hearing impairment is hearing that is functional but not effective, and hearing aids may be utilized to improve it. *Deafness* refers to an inability to understand speech even with the use of a hearing device. Please see the Web site that accompanies this text for figures that illustrate sign language to use when educating this population. The use of technology and hands-on learning in which the entire group participates can be particularly helpful.

PEOPLE WHO HAVE VISUAL IMPAIRMENTS Education for individuals who are blind or visually impaired should focus on descriptions. When speaking to this group, dental hygienists can utilize technology and aids, allowing individuals to feel the teeth, brush, and floss while discussing proper oral hygiene care. Few resources are available for blind individuals regarding dental health. Therefore, it may be helpful to work with an individual who is blind when creating teaching aids for a presentation.

PEOPLE WHO OPPOSE PREVENTIVE MEDICINE Importantly, dental hygienists should realize that many individuals and populations within society do not share beliefs in preventive dental measures, such as routine dental hygiene treatment, fluoride, and sealants, to name a few. Many dental hygienists have been told by well-intended patients that *cleanings only make teeth loose* and *fluoride or sealants cause systemic diseases*. Dental hygienists can provide evidence-based information to the patient, but ultimately it is the patient's decision to consent to dental hygiene treatments. Remaining positive, yet open to listening, is important for the dental hygienist, whether presenting a talk or planning treatment options with a patient. Understanding where to find and how to evaluate evidence is important to all dental hygienists and will be discussed in detail in Unit 3.

INDIVIDUALS WHO LIVE WITH POVERTY In the United States, poverty affects more than 14.5 percent of the population, and children are consistently considered to be the age group it most afflicts.[8] A significant amount of public funding is spent on health care and safety net programs for those in need. Some researchers believe that the growth of an urban underclass locked in a cycle of welfare dependency, joblessness, crime, and out-of-wedlock birth has contributed to the persistence of poverty.[9] However, some researchers propose that the culture of poverty, which can be explained as individuals living in poverty and assuming their own culture, has not developed in the United States.[9] An important role for dental hygienists is to help these individuals gain access to their care and find dental providers who accept Medicaid insurance as payment. Dental hygienists may need to work with a social worker or case manager to locate funding for dental care if the individual or group is not enrolled or eligible for Medicaid insurance. Barriers to care for this population may include transportation, address changes, and language issues. As with all groups, this population needs to become aware of dental diseases and dental disease prevention.

INMATES This target population lives in a state or federal prison. In the United States, inmates have a right to health care, thus creating the need for dental hygiene services. Basically, dental hygienists working in a correctional institution can help decrease dental diseases and restorative and emergency dental conditions and subsequently decrease dental and overall health care costs within this group. Many inmates previously have had minimal if any prior dental hygiene treatment, so dental hygienists working with them need to focus on the etiology of dental disease and oral health behaviors designed to prevent or control disease. During the time they spend in prison, many inmates live a healthier lifestyle than they had previously and do not practice substance abuse and unhealthy behaviors. This is the ideal time to emphasize the value of optimum oral health on general health.

SPECIFIC AGE GROUPS Dental hygiene care for particular age groups differs. A table on the Companion Website describes age-specific competencies, which are summarized here.

DENTAL HYGIENIST SPOTLIGHT ··

Public Health Column: Tammy Keller, RDH, BS

Tammy Keller, recipient of a 2008 RDH Sunstar Award of Distinction, went to dental hygiene school at Northcentral Technical College for her associate's degree and graduated with a bachelor of science degree from the University of Minnesota. She currently works as a dental hygienist with the Menominee Indian Reservation in northern Wisconsin. In this role, she not only provides dental care to patients but also coordinates the school-based fluoride rinse program, is the health promotion/disease prevention representative, and is a member of the Menominee County AIDS Task Force, and Diabetes Committee.

In addition to her RDH Sunstar Award, Ms. Keller has received an outstanding Service Award from the Menominee Tribal Clinic and an Award for Excellence in Dental Hygiene from the Indian Health Service Division of Oral Health.

Her answers to a number of career-related questions follow.

Why did you decide to go into dental hygiene?

I chose dental hygiene because I loved the health field, and I found the dental profession to be very interesting. I have always enjoyed working with and helping others.

How did you get into the dental public health? Did you need additional education?

After five years of clinical hygiene in private practice I accepted a full-time clinical hygiene position on the Menominee Indian Reservation. Realizing the oral health needs of the population, I wanted to be able to improve their oral health. I enrolled in the Community Dental Health Certificate program at Northeast Wisconsin Technical College in Green Bay. The program was phenomenal in teaching me how to develop evidence-based oral health programs and how to effectively assess the community's needs, cultural diversity, and more. I strongly recommend this program.

What are your current positions?

I am the school-based mouth rinse and sealant program coordinator. I serve as the oral health representative on the AIDS task force, Tobacco Coalition, Health Promotion/Disease Prevention Committee, Head Start Health Advisory Board, and the Indian Health Service Bemidji Area Dental Hygiene Mentor. I currently work three days a week doing clinical hygiene and devote two days to community oral health programs. I am part of the diabetes team, seeing patients in the medical department and offering oral health education. I work with the Women, Infants and Children (WIC) Program and Head Start programs applying fluoride varnish four times per year. I have written a maternal child health grant working with pregnant women and infants using xylitol products to reduce tooth decay.

Can you discuss any particularly interesting experiences you have had in your dental public health position?

The most interesting thing to me in public health is the significant impact that you can make on a community. Community oral health prevention programs work! The most rewarding experiences in my life are seeing the significant oral health disparities in the native population and knowing that over the past ten years, there has been a documented decrease in tooth decay in native children.

What type of advice would you give to a practicing hygienist who is thinking of doing something different?

Think outside the box. Dental hygiene is not a job; it is a passion. It is a lot of work but very rewarding. I saw the opportunity to make changes and make a difference to better oral health in the community. I created my position, and others can too.

Source: Christine Nathe writes the Public Health Column in *RDH* magazine published by Pennwell Publishing. For more public health spotlights please see RDH magazine online at http://www.rdhmag.com/index.html.

- **Prenatal:** Women who are pregnant present with a variety of oral health needs. They may suffer from periodontal conditions exacerbated by hormonal fluctuations. Pyogenic granulomas and pregnancy-induced gingivitis occasionally occur during pregnancy. These conditions can be prevented by meticulous oral hygiene and professional dental hygiene care,

information about which dental health educators provide.
- **Infancy:** Periodontal disease in the mother has been associated with preterm births and babies with low birth weights.[10] Many infants are fed milk in bed or sugary drinks from a bottle, which causes early childhood caries, sometimes referred to as *nursing (baby*

bottle) tooth decay. In addition, many parents have questions about teething, the functions of the primary dentition, when to begin regular dental hygiene visits, and home care regimens. Dental hygienists who serve as dental health educators, promoters, or clinicians can refer infants and parents to dentists as needed.

- **Preschool:** Preschoolers are interested in learning and are busy striving for independence. They are impressionable, and therefore their education is vital for a lifetime of good oral hygiene. Early childhood caries is a preventable disease. In particular, in this stage of development, children rapidly assume a positive dental role model and respond to education. It is important to discuss with them the role of dental hygienists and other dental care providers as well as basic dental and nutrition information. Interactive learning with coloring and other hands-on methods is effective. (See Box 10-1 ■.)
- **Elementary Age Children:** This population is interested in obtaining knowledge and continuing to strive for independence. It is important for dental hygienists to discuss a detailed concept of dental health care and the use of preventive interventions such as fluoride and dental sealants. Dental hygienists can easily schedule educational presentations for children through their school or their teachers. Teachers

influence this age group, so dental educational materials integrated with the math, reading, and social sciences curricula are helpful for this age group. (See Box 10-2 ■.)

- **Teenagers:** This population generally strives for total independence and prefers presentations on dental health without parental supervision. Moreover, many teens are concerned with their looks or basic presentation. Discussing halitosis or tooth color may be effective for them. In addition, teens look for positive reinforcements, which can take the form of rewards such as T-shirts and hats for a job well done in oral home care. Because many teenagers are involved in athletics, a discussion about mouth guards with them is critical. (See Box 10-3 ■.)
- **Adults:** This population tends to be more cooperative in the oral health learning process if they are aware of the benefits. They focus on time constraints and want to learn only what is practical for them. Moreover, adults may have issues such as fear and anxiety concerning dental care. To treat them, dental hygienists must understand the individual's capabilities and values. Individuals who have no value for oral care will have little interest in its education. Dental hygienists must determine how to make oral health of real value to them. The presentation of information about

Box 10–1 Recommendations for Providing Dental Treatment to Early Childhood Patients

- Develop rapport with children and their parents as a foundation for cooperation and trust
- Regard parents as partners in the children's oral health care
- Maintain a calm, slow, reassuring voice that does not intimidate children
- Explain all procedures in simple, concrete terms
- Clarify what the children's role is during treatment, and set acceptable rules for behavior
- Demonstrate the use of equipment, and involve the children in the dental care as much as possible
- Use substitution words (e.g., refer to the *suction* as a *straw, handpiece* as a *tooth cleaner,* and *x-ray procedures* as *using a camera to take pictures of the teeth*)
- Give simple instructions and directions one at a time
- Use gestures and facial expressions
- Use a confident manner and positive voice when inviting children to sit in the dental chair independently
- Consider allowing children to sit on the parent's lap, depending on parental attachment
- Allow children to explore the environment through smell, taste, touch, sight, and sound (e.g., smelling the

fluoride, tasting prophylactic paste, handling a mirror, seeing the mask and gloves donned, or listening to the compressed air)
- Do not lie to children about pain; describe exactly what the procedure will feel like
- Allow children to make choices whenever possible, and give them a way to interrupt treatment, such as raising a hand to signal discomfort
- Answer questions and encourage curiosity
- Avoid overdirecting very cooperative children
- Be aware that negativism (saying "no") may be the only way children know for control and that temper tantrums are a possibility
- Teach parents and children appropriate oral hygiene care according to their specific needs
- Offer suggestions and/or recommendations to parents concerning risk factors and ways to assist children to perform oral hygiene activities
- Ignore inappropriate behaviors, but praise appropriate behaviors and cooperation
- Reward good behavior with a tangible gift (e.g., toothbrush, sticker, toy)

Source: Donald T. Pediatrics. In: Harris NO, Garcia-Godoy F, Nathe C. *Primary Preventive Dentistry.* 8th ed. Upper Saddle River, NJ: Pearson; 2013.

Box 10–2 Recommendations for Providing Dental Treatment to School-Age Children

- Develop rapport with children as a foundation for cooperation and trust
- Talk with children about their friends, school, and outside interests
- Direct questions to children first
- Develop rapport with the parents, and consider them partners in children's oral health care
- Clarify what children's role is during treatment, and set acceptable rules for behavior
- Encourage questions and give straight answers
- Explain procedures using simple vocabulary
- Describe the operation of equipment and reasons for its use
- Give clear explanations of what children will experience in terms of pain or discomfort; do not lie to or mislead them
- Help children retain control by including them in decision making, soliciting their help, giving them the opportunity to make choices involving their care

- when possible, and providing them a way to interrupt treatment, such as raising a hand to signal discomfort
- Introduce children to routine care of their teeth and gums, including regular brushing, flossing, and reductions in sugar consumption (e.g., candy, sodas)
- Teach parents to monitor their children's oral hygiene activities and offer suggestions to parents who struggle with their children regarding these issues
- Be positive to and supportive of the children; avoid making judgments and causing embarrassment
- Be aware that children at this age can have difficult-to-control temper tantrums and their behavior can be unpredictable, from cooperative to obstructive to withdrawn to enthusiastic
- Distinguish between emotional crying (pain, fear) and crying used to manipulate the environment (tantrums); handle emotional crying with patience and empathy; use behavior management techniques with tantrums
- Use praise as positive reinforcement and rewards (not necessarily tangible) for appropriate behaviors

Source: Pediatrics. In: Harris NO, Garcia-Godoy F, Nathe C. *Primary Preventive Dentistry.* 8th ed. Upper Saddle River, NJ: Pearson; 2013.

Box 10–3 Recommendations for Providing Dental Treatment to Adolescents

- Develop rapport with adolescents as a foundation for cooperation and trust
- Talk with the adolescents about friends, school, interests, and hobbies
- Reassure adolescents about confidentiality and privacy issues
- Set reasonable limits and standards for cooperation and behavior
- Help these patients retain control by including them in decision making, soliciting their help, giving them the opportunity to make choices involving their care when possible, and providing them a way to interrupt treatment, such as raising a hand to signal discomfort
- Allow self-expression and avoid being judgmental
- Listen and be attentive
- Be supportive and an available resource

- Set goals for oral hygiene activities and future appointments
- Appeal to the impact of their oral health on social interactions (e.g., plaque and oral bacteria can cause bad breath)
- Treat all questions seriously and provide full explanations
- Discuss oral health in terms of disease and infections; give explanations and consequences, especially physical consequences
- Give clear explanations of what the patient will experience in terms of pain or discomfort; do not lie to or mislead the patient
- Include dietary habits and tobacco, alcohol, and drug use in health education messages
- Strive for a positive dental hygiene experience, allowing the adolescents to gain more self-esteem

Source: Pediatrics. In: Harris NO, Garcia-Godoy F, Nathe C. *Primary Preventive Dentistry.* 8th ed. Upper Saddle River, NJ: Pearson; 2013.

dental care delivery in general and their children's oral health is interesting to adults.

- **Older Adults:** Many older adults remain independent, but others may have limited independence. Understanding this group's capabilities is necessary.

A number of normal but significant changes occur during aging. Fortunately, few of them cause oral diseases. Instead, the cumulative effects of both oral and systemic diseases result in the prevalence of oral disease among elderly people. Interestingly,

increasing numbers of well elderly are able to retain their natural teeth and enjoy normal oral function.[11] Furthermore, this group most likely is without dental insurance. Therefore, it is important for dental hygienists to serve as liaisons between older adults and the dental care delivery system. This population may also be interested in information about dental caries, periodontal diseases, oral cancer, disease etiology and prevention, nutrition, holistic health care, and specific dental services such as tooth bleaching and cosmetic dentistry.

made during a clinical appointment. A comprehensive overview of the target population that includes specific descriptions is termed a **target population profile** or community profile.

Areas to be assessed in creating a target population profile include the population's location, available resources, and partnerships. Dental hygienists may gather this information by conducting surveys, attending community meetings, and reviewing existing data. Numerous government agencies provide baseline data that can be used to profile a target population. (See Table 10-2 ■.)

Target Population Profiles

Researching the target population is necessary for dental hygienists to determine a profile much like the initial health history, educational assessment and charting that is

Demographic Information

Dental hygienists must include demographic information when profiling a target population. *Demographic information* includes such factors as age, gender, and

Table 10–2 Government Resources for Target Population Data

Agency/Survey	Function	Web Site
Agency for Health Care Research and Quality (AHRQ)	Collects data on the utilization of health and dental care services throughout the country through the Medical Expenditure Panel Surveys (MEPS)	http://www.ahrq.gov/
Bureau of the Census	Conducts the US Census	http://www.census.gov
CDC, Behavioral Risk Factor Surveillance System (BRFSS); CDC, Youth Risk Behavior Survey (YRBS)	Collects ongoing state-based data to measure behavioral risk factors among adults and youth	http://www.cdc.gov/brfss/ http://www.cdc.gov/healthyyouth/ data/yrbs/index.htm
CDC, DATA 2020	Tracks data for *Healthy People 2020*	http://www.healthypeople .gov/2020/tools-and-resources/ program-planning/Track
CDC, National Notifiable Diseases Surveillance System	Lists and collects national data on diseases required by law to be reported to official health authorities	http://wwwn.cdc.gov/nndss/
CDC, National Oral Health Surveillance System (NOHSS)	Monitors dental health, disease, and use of dental services within states for a collaboration between the CDC and the Association of State and Territorial Dental Directors	http://www.cdc.gov/nohss
CDC, National Health and Nutrition Examination Survey (NHANES)	Collects data on health and nutrition	http://www.cdc.gov/nchs/nhanes.htm
CDC, Health Interview Survey (NHIS)	Uses household interviews on the health of noninstitutionalized, civilian adults in the United States	http://www.cdc.gov/nchs/nhis.htm
CDC, National Nursing Home Survey	Performs continuing series of national sample surveys of nursing home staff and residents	http://www.cdc.gov/nchs/nnhs.htm
CDC, National Vital Statistics System (NVSS)	Collects data on births, deaths, fetal deaths, etc.	http://www.cdc.gov/nchs/nvss.htm

(continued)

Table 10–2 Government Resources for Target Population Data (continued)

Agency/Survey	Function	Web Site
CDC, Pregnancy Risk Assessment Monitoring System (PRAMS)	Collects data on maternal attitudes and experiences	http://www.cdc.gov/prams/
CDC, School Health Policies and Program Study (SHPPS)	Conducts national survey to assess school policies and programs	http://www.cdc.gov/HealthyYouth/shpps/index.htm
CDC, Water Fluoridation Reporting System	Monitors public water fluoridation	http://www.cdc.gov/fluoridation/factsheets/engineering/wfrs_factsheet.htm
Centers for Medicare and Medicaid (CMS)	Collects data on Medicaid utilization	https://www.cms.gov/
Health Resources and Services Administration (HRSA)	Collects data on the dental workforce and patients with special needs	http://www.hrsa.gov/index.html
National Institutes of Dental and Craniofacial Research (NIDCR)	Provides resources for dental diseases and oral manifestations of disease	http://drc.nidcr.nih.gov
National Cancer Institute (NCI)	Collects information on cancer rates, trends, etc., through its SEER program	http://seer.cancer.gov

ethnicity, which are important to describe when discussing a population's dental health. Other areas to address include family lifestyles, living arrangements, cultural backgrounds, religious beliefs, social attributes, social structure, social networks, community stability, and values of dental health.

Of course, the location of the target population is assessed and its boundaries determined. Important factors are community size, geographic isolation, physical conditions of its neighborhoods, and community infrastructure. Organizational facilities should be described, including their equipment and maintenance.

Because it is important to always "target" the population during program planning, the dental hygienist should assess geographic locations. Communities frequently can be defined as metropolitan, urban, suburban, rural, or frontier. They are defined based on all territory, persons, and housing units within an incorporated area that met the population threshold. A metropolitan area may have a population of over 100,000 whereas an urban area may have a population from 2500 to over 50,000. Suburban is loosely used to define a community bordering a major urbanized city. A rural area would have less than 2500 population. Frontier areas are the most remote and geographically isolated areas in the United States. These are usually sparsely populated, and in addition to extreme weather, they often face extreme distances and travel time to services of any kind.[12–15]

So, there can be differences when developing programs for different communities. For instance, in a metropolitan area, readily available, public transportation decreases barriers to get to a clinic for treatment, whereas, even in many urban communities, with less available and affordable public transportation options, arriving to a clinic even a mile away can present problems. Many times, cultural influences can occur within communities, because since its inception, America has been diversified in cultural influences. This diversity continues today. Funding opportunities such as grants or donations as well as the history of previous dental or health endeavors should be assessed. Local government structure and community organizations of the population should be described.

The ability to develop or strengthen partnerships is paramount to serving a target population. Too often dental hygienists develop programs without enough support. Community and political leaders, organizations, and other health providers are potential partnerships with dental hygienists to improve the community.

Did You Know?

Collaborative efforts that are multidisciplinary in nature in public health initiatives tend to last longer and be more effective than stand-alone dental programs because they have more *owners* of the initiative.

Faith-Based Initiatives

Many religious groups play significant roles in health care. Many religious leaders have great influence on health care beliefs, and many leaders work diligently to help those in

need. In 2001, the federal government created the Center for Faith-Based and Community Initiatives (CFBCI), an agency that ensures collaboration between the government and religious groups or community groups to improve life for people in need. CFBCI's mission is to create an environment within the Department of Health and Human Services (HHS) that welcomes **faith-based initiatives** and the participation of community-based organizations as valued and essential partners to assist Americans in need (Figure 10-1 ■). An example of a faith-based organization could be a local church group that raises funds for a dental clinic that provides care to the underserved populations, specifically those populations that have difficulty accessing dental care.[16]

Formal partnerships between the faith-based and public health sectors encompass activities in the fields of health behavior and health education, health policy and management, epidemiology and biostatistics, and environmental health.[17] These partnerships are instrumental for achieving both domestic and global health promotion priorities.[17] Many faith-based organizations are trusted entities within communities. This societal trust can be a huge asset when developing collaborations that impact health care and health care delivery.

Barriers to Dental Care

Many populations within a society face restrictive barriers to obtaining dental hygiene and dental care. **Barriers to care** can be defined as anything that limits an individual's ability to receive dental services. Barriers can include age, cultural variances, language difficulties, lack of information, disabilities, transportation issues, and financial limitations as well as laws preventing registered dental hygienists from providing dental hygiene care in a school setting. (See Box 10-4 ■.) Some barriers are easily overcome; for example, a state program offering rides to medical and dental appointments can address transportation problems. Addressing others, such as laws preventing practice in specific locations, is more complicated.

An individual's values may also be a barrier to care. For example, a teenage boy may believe that his teeth are invulnerable to the effects of periodontal disease. He may

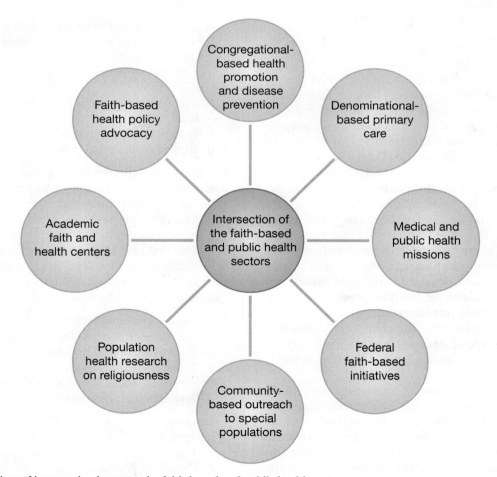

FIGURE 10–1 Points of intersection between the faith-based and public health sectors

Source: Levin, J Faith-based partnerships for population health: challenges, initiatives, and prospects. *Public Health Rep.* 2014 Mar-Apr;129(2):127–31.

Box 10–4 Possible Barriers to Obtaining Dental Hygiene and Dental Care

- Age
- Language
- Habit(s)
- Culture
- Financial situation
- Lack of confidence in treatment
- Education
- Lack of understanding
- Fear
- Transportation
- Values
- Safety of treatment
- Attitudes
- Denial of disease
- Unavailability of dental providers
- Sense of invulnerability
- Inconvenience
- Social issues
- Provider conflicts
- Inconvenient office hours
- Requirements for supervision of dental hygienists

not understand that keeping his teeth for a lifetime takes a commitment to home care as well as professional care. Consequently, he may not respond to information presented about the periodontal condition of his mouth, which could limit the services sought from a dental hygienist. Dental hygienists can alleviate this barrier by gearing the educational therapy toward the teenager's values. For example, the dental hygienist may be able to discuss the effect of periodontal disease on halitosis, which could interest him.

Barriers to care are often combinations of factors. For instance, a two-year-old child with Medicaid insurance who has severe stages of early childhood caries may receive no care if pediatric or qualified general dentists in the area are unwilling to provide treatment. The providers' reluctance could be caused by the child's age, severity of the disease, or the type of insurance to pay for the services. For this child, access may be limited by one factor or several.

Many barriers create missed appointments with the dental provider. With the increased use of technology, texting and e-mailing to confirm appointments or presentations may be one solution. Professional dental hygienists assume the responsibility for increasing access to quality dental hygiene and dental care. This responsibility requires understanding the barriers to them and working to alleviate them.

Summary

For dental health initiatives to be effective, it is vital that dental hygienists learn about a target population before treating or providing education. The first step in understanding what needs must be addressed is to identify a target population profile.

Dental hygienists should understand basic community demographics and their impact on dental health status. The importance of health-literate populations on health status cannot be underscored. Faith-based initiatives and their role in community health should be explored when developing dental health initiatives. Dental hygienists practicing in community settings must be aware of the barriers some populations face when trying to access dental hygiene care.

Self-Study Test Items

1. A group from a local church youth group could be considered a
   a. Target population
   b. Target population profile
   c. Faith-based initiative
   d. Community agency

2. It is important not to frighten child patients. It is better not to tell the truth if a procedure could involve some discomfort.
   a. The first statement is true; the second statement is false.
   b. The first statement is false; the second statement is true.
   c. Both statements are true.
   d. Both statements are false.

3. Faith-based initiatives are funded by the federal government. This funding does not generally include health care reimbursement.
   a. The first part of the statement is true, but the second is false.
   b. The first part of the statement is false, but the second is true.
   c. Both parts of the statement are true.
   d. Both parts of the statement are false.

4. Social workers and dental hygienists can work together during programs for target populations
   a. To provide dental hygiene care
   b. To assess dental health
   c. To ensure social services for the population
   d. To implement periodontal treatment

5. Inconvenient office hours of a dental practice can become a
   a. Target population profile technique
   b. Faith-based issue
   c. Barrier to care
   d. Long-term strategic plan

References

1. Diringer J, Phipps K, Carsel B. Critical trends affecting the future of dentistry: Assessing the shifting landscape. Prepared for the American Dental Association. San Luis Obispo, CA: DA Diringer and Associates; May 2013.
2. Horn J. *Osteoporosis Prevention and Screening: Potential Role for Oral Health Professionals?* Grand Rounds in Oral-Systemic Medicine, Vol. 2, No 2. 2007.
3. Zastrow C. *Introduction to Social Welfare Institutions.* 3rd ed. Chicago, IL: Dorsey Press; 1986.
4. Aboytes DB. Medically Compromised Populations. In: Harris NO, Garcia-Godoy F, Nathe C. *Primary Preventive Dentistry.* 8th ed. Upper Saddle River, NJ: Pearson; 2014.
5. Gonzalez E. Populations with Developmental Disabilities. In: Harris NO, Garcia-Godoy F, Nathe C. *Primary Preventive Dentistry.* 8th ed. Upper Saddle River, NJ: Pearson; 2014.
6. Kessler RC, Chiu WT, Demler O, Walters EE. Prevalence, severity, and comorbidity of 12-month DSM-IV disorders in the National Comorbidity Survey Replication. *Arch Gen Psychiatry* 2005;62:617–627.
7. CDC. Mental Health Basics. Retrieved from http://www.cdc.gov/mentalhealth/basics.htm on August 6,2015.
8. US Census Bureau. Poverty Highlights. 2013. Retrieved from http://www.census.gov/hhes/www/poverty/about/overview/index.html on August 5, 2015.
9. A Culture of Poverty Develops When the Poor Are Left Behind. Retrieved from http://www.poverty.smartlibrary.org/newinterface/segment.cfm?segment=1566. on September 12, 2008.
10. Saini, R Saini, S and Saini, S. Periodontitis: A risk for delivery of premature labor and low-birth-weight infants. *J Nat Sci Biol Med.* 2010 Jul–Dec; 1(1): 40–42. Retrieved from http://www.ncbi.nlm.nih.gov/pmc/articles/PMC3217279/ on August 6, 2015.
11. Tatlock CD. Geriatrics. In: Harris NO, Garcia-Godoy F, Nathe C. *Primary Preventive Dentistry.* 8th ed. Upper Saddle River, NJ: Pearson; 2014.
12. US Health and Resources Administration. How is rural defined? Rockville, MD: HRSA, 2015. Retrieved from http://www.hrsa.gov/healthit/toolbox/RuralHealthITtoolbox/Introduction/defined.html on June 2, 2015.
13. US Census Bureau. Current Lists of Metropolitan and Micropolitan Statistical Areas Delineations. Suitland, MD: US Census Bureau, 2015. Retrieved from http://www.census.gov/population/metro/data/metrodef.html on June 2, 2015.
14. US Census Bureau. Urban and Rural Areas. Suitland, MD: US Census Bureau, 2015. Retrieved from http://www.census.gov/history/www/programs/geography/urban_and_rural_areas.html on June 2, 2015.
15. Defining frontier. Silver City, NM: National Center for Frontier Communities, 2015. Retrieved from http://frontierus.org/defining-frontier/ on June 2, 2015.
16. Center for Faith-Based & Community Initiatives. Retrieved from http://www.hhs.gov/fbci/ on September 12, 2013.
17. Levin, J. Faith-based initiatives in health promotion: history, challenges, and current partnerships. *Am J Health Promot.* 2014 Jan–Feb;28(3):139–141.

Visit www.pearsonhighered.com/healthprofessionsresources to access the student resources that accompany this book. Simply select Dental Hygiene from the choice of disciplines. Find this book and you will find the complimentary study tools created for this specific title.

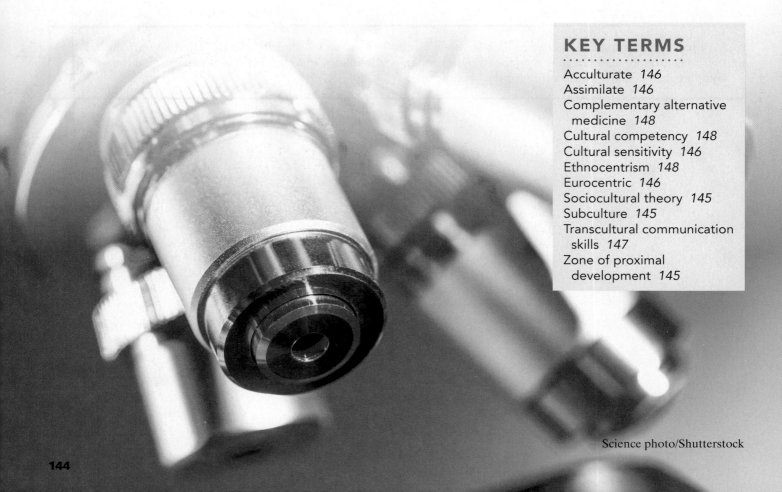

11

Cultural Competency

OBJECTIVES

After studying this chapter, the dental hygiene student should be able to:

- Describe how cultural values regarding health care can affect oral health habits
- Identify how culture influences people
- Describe cultural diversity in the United States
- Define cultural competency and its significance in treating for a culturally diverse population

COMPETENCIES

After studying this chapter and participating in accompanying course activities, the dental hygiene student should be competent to do the following:

- Communicate effectively with diverse individuals and groups, serving all persons without discrimination by acknowledging and appreciating diversity
- Initiate a collaborative approach with all patients when developing individualized care plans that are specialized, comprehensive, culturally sensitive, and acceptable to all parties involved in care planning
- Respect the goals, values, beliefs, and preferences of patients

KEY TERMS

Acculturate 146
Assimilate 146
Complementary alternative medicine 148
Cultural competency 148
Cultural sensitivity 146
Ethnocentrism 148
Eurocentric 146
Sociocultural theory 145
Subculture 145
Transcultural communication skills 147
Zone of proximal development 145

Science photo/Shutterstock

"Culture is a complex and multifaceted social phenomenon that has powerful influences on all aspects of modern life."[1] Culture encompasses attitudes, values, and beliefs. On a grand scale, culture influences global business dealings, trade agreements, and negotiations. Often, cultural history is the reason for continued conflict between groups of people as is evident around the world today. In fact, most critical events facing the world today result from cultural differences. The subject of culture can include differences in ethnic background, socioeconomic standing, gender, religion, beliefs, language, and all aspects of work and family life.[2] An individual raised in one culture never completely understands another culture because the person did not internalize values and traditions of the other culture during childhood.

Traditional descriptors of a population such as *race* no longer reliably distinguish a population, since many races are mixed with populations from many different countries. For example, cultural groups such as the Irish and the Germans living within the "white" population may display entirely different characteristics.

Did You Know?

In general, the Census Bureau defines ethnicity or origin as the heritage, nationality group, lineage, or country of birth of the person or the person's parents or ancestors before their arrival in the United States.

The 2010 Census reported 308.7 million people in the United States, a 9.7 percent increase from the 2000 Census population of 281.4 million. The Asian population saw the largest increase in the 2010 census for race, from 4 percent to 5 percent of the population and for ethnic group, the Hispanic population grew the fastest from approximately 13 percent to 16 percent of the population.[3] Knowledge of various cultures can enhance communication efforts between health care providers and the population they serve.

Theories of Cultural and Development of Self-Awareness

The **sociocultural theory** proposed by educational psychologist Lev Vygotsky suggests that an individual's social interaction as a child leads to continuous changes in thought and behavior that can vary greatly from culture to culture. This theory explains why, as stated earlier, fully understanding a culture that is not a person's own is difficult. Vygotsky's theory suggests that development depends on interaction with people and the tools that the culture provides to help form a view of the world. He theorized that there are three ways for cultural tools to pass from one person to another: (1) *imitative learning* by which a person tries to imitate or copy another, (2) *instructed learning,* which involves remembering the instructions of the teacher and then using these instructions to self-regulate, and (3) *passing along cultural tools* through collaborative learning, which refers to a group of peers striving to understand each other and working as a unit to learn a specific skill.[4]

Educator and researcher Barbara Rogoff elaborated on the relationship of Vygotsky's theory of zone of proximal development to culture. The **zone of proximal development** is the difference between a child's actual level of development displayed by unassisted performance and the child's potential level as indicated by assisted performance. Rogoff suggests that children actually seek assistance of adults around them to guide them through the process of problem solving until they are experienced to do it themselves. Through this guidance, children are expected to adapt to their specific cultural surroundings, and the zone of proximal development is where culture and cognition meet.[5]

Experts agree that the first step in effectively dealing with diverse populations is for people to be aware of their own cultural habits and values.[2,4] This is not an easy task. One way to become self-aware is to read books about one's culture as viewed from the perspective of someone outside one's culture. Another way is to ask a colleague or friend from another culture to frankly describe the person's culture.

Cultural competence begins with an honest desire not to allow biases to keep us from treating every individual with respect. This requires an honest assessment of our positive and negative assumptions about others. Again, this is not easy, no one wants to admit that they suffer from cultural ignorance, or in the worst case, harbor negative stereotypes and prejudices. Learning to evaluate our own level of cultural competency must be part of our ongoing effort to provide better health care.[6]

Culture-general training, which seeks to enhance receptiveness and sensitivity to cultural differences, is another venue for learning about a culture. Culture-general training helps promote adaptation and effective functioning in any type of culture. Please see the Companion Website for several links to Web sites that provide such training. Courses such as this can increase awareness about the limitations of one's own culture.

Professional Culture

Professional groups such as dental care providers have their own culture. For instance, dental hygienists share similar values regarding the importance of good oral health and the bidirectional relationship to total health. It could be said that dental providers belong to a subculture based on a professional and occupational affiliation.[7] **Subculture** refers to a group of people with a culture that differentiates them from the larger culture to which they belong.

Did You Know?

Many dental hygienists are prevention-oriented individuals in many matters of life, not just health care.

Instructors of dental hygiene students introduce a new value system regarding oral health, and over time, the student is assimilated into the culture or mores of the professional health care subculture.[1,5,7] Although dental hygienists and dentists internalize these values, many populations, including other health care providers, may place little importance on them and see no connection between oral health and total health.

Cultural Diversity in the United States

Historically, the population of the United States evolved from the immigration of people from a variety of countries. This influx of immigrants has brought cultures that are vastly different than those from one particular country, which makes the United States somewhat different than many countries because a variety of cultures have created the "American culture." Immigrants embrace different religions, diets, dress, beliefs, and values.[2]

Immigrants, such as those who came in the 1850s and the decade 1900–1910, arrived in the United States with **Eurocentric** beliefs, those reflecting a tendency to interpret the world in terms of European values and experiences. Some theorize that they strove to **acculturate,** or **assimilate,** or adapt to another culture by assuming its practices and beliefs to become part of the great "melting pot." However, research shows that while outward behavior might indicate acceptance of the dominant culture, these changes rarely take place in the inner self.[5] People rarely achieve complete assimilation because culture is an inseparable part of their being and is the foundation from which they form their values and beliefs.[1]

In reality, immigrants to the United States may choose to preserve their cultural heritage and belief systems, including dress, customs, language, and religious beliefs.[1] This may suggest that immigrants are less likely to aspire to completely assimilate into what is considered the mainstream, which is the reason America is sometimes described as a "salad bowl" and not a "melting pot." This signifies the uniqueness within the population, while highlighting the unification of the population as well. Many people in the United States now embrace pluralism instead of assimilation, or maybe a little of both. Maybe this partial assimilation, with the preservation of cultural values, should be termed *culturization.*

Did You Know?

Pluralism exists when numerous distinct ethnic, religious, or cultural groups are present and tolerated within a society.

Although not falling into the category of immigrants, Native American populations, including Native American Indians, Alaska Natives, and Native Hawaiian and Pacific Islanders have cultures that differ from each other and from that of "mainstream" populations. In some regions, dental hygienists have many opportunities to serve this population. See Figure 11-1 ■ for locations of Native Americans in the United States. A culturally sensitive clinician taking into account the Native American's respect for tradition will garner more credibility and success with health education than one who views traditional remedies or ceremonies as being unimportant. People display **cultural sensitivity** when they are aware of and respect cultural differences during interactions with people.

When discussing cultural diversity, traditional categories, including racial/ethnic, cultural, age, gender, and socioeconomics generally occur. Many do not think of nontraditional categories such as one's mobility, oral/facial piercings, tattoos, and anti-fluoridation philosophies. Yet, these are important categories, which may influence one's values and beliefs.

Cross-Cultural Communication

Practice management courses identify poor communication between patients and health care providers as the leading cause of lawsuits. Clear, concise communication can be difficult to achieve between people of the same culture; imagine the difficulties practitioners without preparation for cultures vastly different from the practitioner's own experience. Communication difficulties can cause barriers to health care, including the inability to explain health problems and the failure to understand outcomes of preventive measures.

Did You Know?

Race is usually defined as a population with shared physical characteristics, many times from a specific county, but race can also loosely be used to define a group of individuals from the same religion or political affiliation or a group from a specific geographic location.

Stereotyping refers to members of one group holding a common standardized mental picture that represents an oversimplified opinion or prejudice of that group. Stereotyping a population can quickly shut down communication and understanding for its concerns. Communication is more than verbal; it encompasses gestures, eye contact, physical proximity, and formal versus informal speech. Failure to understand these nonverbal cues can impair effective communication. As an example, many people in American society consider eye contact to be important, and avoiding it could be interpreted by some groups as having something to hide or being dishonest. However, other ethnic groups view direct eye contact as being disrespectful or rude. A culturally insensitive oral health professional may view avoidance of eye contact as lack of interest when it is actually communicating a cultural sign of respect.

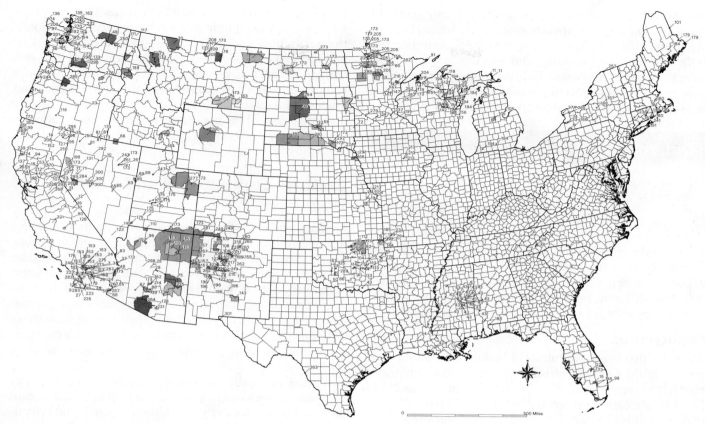

FIGURE 11–1 Geographic Location of Native American Reservations
Source: http://www.nps.gov/nagpra/documents/reserv.pdf

Effective communication is always the key to any successful transaction or interaction between people or groups of people. A diverse population urgently needs health care professionals to develop **transcultural communication skills,** or the ability to interpret and transmit information to someone from a different culture. Good communication is often considered the cornerstone of effective health care practice.[8] Successful communication with other cultures requires time, patience, caring, and dropping assumptions. (See Box 11-1 ■.)

Beware of the *cultural blind spot syndrome.* This is the belief that because a patient or population looks and behaves much like the provider, there are no cultural differences or potential barriers to care. Remember, all individuals regardless of race and ethnicity have a variety of cultural influences and are uniquely developed. This can be seen in family siblings.

Box 11–1 Processes to Develop Cultural Sensitivity

- Assess one's own cultural beliefs and values.
- Recognize one's culture influences affecting communication.
- Recognize one's own cultural biases.
- Be knowledgeable of the patient's belief system.
- Be sensitive to gestures, concerns, and questions.
- Be able to collect culturally relevant data concerning the population's health background and level of understanding of the presenting problems.
- Listen and observe.
- Be aware and respectful of cultural differences.

Culture Issues in Health Care

The continually changing demographics of the United States require the adaptation of cultural skills to communicate and interact successfully in all aspects of life, especially business, education, and health care. The constructs of culture, health, and disease are so interrelated that experts in the field

maintain that lack of cultural sensitivity can lead to invalid diagnosis. Inability to recognize health care–related cultural differences can result in treatment failure, frustration for both providers and patients, and withdrawal of patients from the health care system. Health care practitioners have a major responsibility to be culturally sensitive in a society of increasingly interdependent cultures and people.[1]

Did You Know?

Culture plays an important role in health care because beliefs and values concerning wellness, disease, and illness are culturally determined.

Dental hygienists are not responsible for knowing all details of the values, language, character, and behavior expectations of different populations, but they must recognize how different populations perceive disease, health, and the dental hygienist as a health care provider.

Ethnocentrism

The belief that one's own culture or traditions are better than other cultures is **ethnocentrism.** Although many Americans may fail to recognize or deny ethnocentrism, it does exist. Many health care providers practice from the point of view that their culture is the privileged culture.[2] For example, a practitioner in the United States who values traditional Western medicine may fail to value the use of acupuncture and acupressure to control pain or discomfort.[8]

The provider who is ethnocentric tends to antagonize and alienate patients from other cultures. To avoid cultural biases that distort perceptions of other people's values and behavior, which damage the ability to communicate, a person must first acknowledge that ethnocentrism exists.[1, 7]

Complementary Alternative Medicine

The use of herbs, *natural* products, and practices such as massage or yoga is referred to as **complementary alternative medicine (CAM)** in health care. Their use often comes from cultural practices that differ from those used in Western medicine. Many people who use alternative therapies do not discuss it with health care providers, which can lead to problems.

Clinicians should always question their patients about the use of such products. People frequently use herbs as prophylactic measures to prevent disease and/or maintain good health, and dental hygienists should be aware of how their use can impact treatment options. Some supplemental herbs can be contraindicated with use of Western medicines. For instance, some in various populations use ginseng as a panacea, which could be contraindicated for people with high blood pressure.

Cultural Representation in Health Professions

Although many health care providers may have been born outside the United States, minority populations may be underrepresented in the health professions. Many programs have been initiated to improve minority representation in the health professions. Importantly, health care providers must grasp the focus on cultural sensitivity, realize their own cultural beliefs and values, and strive to provide culturally competent health care regardless of their own background. The need for culturally competent health care providers to meet the needs of the underserved, who are often culturally diverse, is tremendous.

Cultural Competency and Dental Hygienists

Dental hygienists who desire to achieve culturally sensitive attitudes while serving in community programs and public health to provide care to diverse populations must consider cultural diversity as an important factor in every encounter with every person. **Cultural competency** is defined as the awareness of and respect for an individual's or a population's cultural differences, the recognition of how these differences impact a specific group, such as health care providers, and the ability to communicate effectively and work cross-culturally.

Being culturally competent when treating patients of different cultures can help the dental hygienist deliver care and education effectively. In addition, when dental providers understand values and perspectives of different cultures, they are more likely to respond to oral health disparities in an appropriate manner.

In a very diverse society, dental hygienists must be able to disseminate oral health care information and treatment while recognizing populations' cultural differences. In collaborative practice and community-based settings, dental hygiene care must meet the needs of these populations. There is no particular "way" to treat a specific racial or ethnic population; rather, dental hygienists should instead develop a plan that is individualized for a patient or population.

Professional Policies

The importance of cultural competence is reflected in the ADHA's recently revised National Dental Hygiene Research Agenda. This document, generated by the ADHA Council of Research, identifies areas of research needed in dental hygiene.[9] Threaded throughout this document are references to cultural diversity specifically when related to health promotion and disease prevention in diverse populations. (See Box 11-2 ■.)

The 84th Annual Session of the ADHA emphasized the need for cultural competency in the field of dental hygiene.[10] Its House of Delegates adopted the following definitions pertaining to cultural and linguistic competencies:

Cultural competence

Awareness of cultural differences among all populations, respect of those differences, and application of the knowledge to professional practice.

Box 11–2 Health Promotion/Disease Prevention for Diverse Populations

- Validate and test assessment instruments/strategies/mechanisms that increase health promotion and disease prevention among diverse populations.
- Investigate how diversity among populations impacts the promotion of oral health and preventive behaviors.
- Investigate the effectiveness of oral self-care behaviors that prevent or reduce oral diseases among all age, social, and cultural groups.
- Investigate how environmental factors (e.g., culture, socioeconomic status, education) influence oral health behaviors.

Linguistic competence

The ability to communicate effectively and respond appropriately to the health literacy needs of all populations.

The generation and adoption of these definitions clearly recognize and emphasize the need for dental hygienists to be aware of individual or population cultural differences, have respect for these differences, and understand how these cultural differences impact oral health. The ADHA encourages hygienists to expand their knowledge of diverse populations so they have the ability to communicate and work effectively in cross-cultural situations. Additional policy adopted by the 2007 House of Delegates stated the American Dental Hygienists' Association advocates cultural and linguistic competence for health professionals.

Educational Challenges

Health care educators have a major responsibility to prepare culturally sensitive health care practitioners for a world of increasingly interdependent cultures and people. Student dental hygienists should be prepared to serve all patients and populations without discrimination and to appreciate the diversity of the populations for whom they provide care. When addressing cultural competency, the American Dental Association's Commission on Dental Accreditation called for all graduates to be competent in interpersonal and communication skills to effectively interact with diverse population groups.[11]

To meet this challenge, educational institutions often require students to treat a specific number of culturally diverse individuals in the clinical environment. However, community/public health courses afford students the best opportunities to be involved with diverse populations. The ability of the educational institution to make these opportunities available to the students depends largely on the cultural makeup of the community in which the school is located.[12]

Barriers to Oral Health Care

Barriers to oral health care for diverse populations exist in the United States, a fact that the Surgeon General's landmark oral health report emphasized. The first of its kind, this national report on oral health revealed that members of ethnic minority groups experienced a disproportional amount of oral health problems. The following are excerpts from the report's Executive Summary.[13]

What Is the Status of Oral Health in America?

Despite improvements in oral health status, profound disparities remain in some population groups as classified by sex, income, age, and race/ethnicity. For some diseases and conditions, the magnitude of the differences in oral health status among population groups is striking.

What Is the Relationship Between Oral Health and General Health and Well-being?

Cultural values influence oral and craniofacial health and well-being and can play an important role in care utilization practices and in perpetuating acceptable oral health and facial norms.

As the Surgeon General's report emphasized, obvious disparities in access to oral health care for certain ethnic populations exist.[13] These barriers can include financial limitations, language differences, perceptions of good oral health, and lack of access to professionals qualified to provide oral health care services. Continuing to educate dental providers on the fundamentals of cultural competence should help alleviate access to qualified professionals.

A language barrier may also deter people from seeking care or reduce the effectiveness of care that they receive. Use of family members to interpret is not recommended because of privacy concerns and emotional involvement. Utilizing a trained interpreter may prove helpful, but establishing rapport with the patients or populations in this situation is difficult. The use of visual aids, repetition, clarification, and open-ended questions rather than questions calling for yes or no answers is a practical technique to overcome the language barrier.[7] Learning all languages and customs is not logical or practical, but dental hygienists should strive to learn as much as they can to communicate with, educate, and motivate populations they serve to achieve good oral health.

Did You Know?

Practicing the Golden Rule, which is to treat people as one would like to be treated, will help the dental hygienist in patient communication and decision making.

When working with diverse cultures, the dental hygienist should realize that the tradition of some cultures do not emphasize oral health and preventive dental care. Members

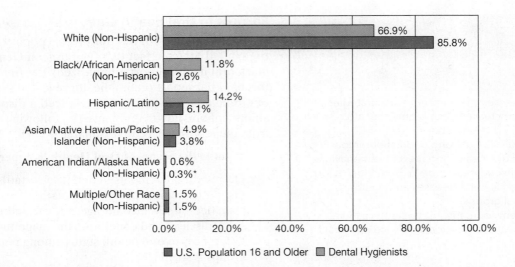

FIGURE 11–2 Race/Ethnicity of Dental Hygienists According to US Population Percentage, 2013

Source: Bureau of Labor Statistics, American Dental Association, Bureau of the Census. http://www.bls.gov/cps/cpsaat11.pdf

of these cultures may fail to understand the financial impact of poor oral health care and may not realize how disruptive and costly missed appointments are. Realize that dental hygiene has been practiced in America much longer than any country in the world, and so many populations recently immigrating or second-generation Americans will not have the same experiences with the evolution of dental hygiene like many Americans. Keep in mind that the majority of countries still do not have dental hygienists.

The fact that only a small number of some ethnic populations working in the oral health care professions may be considered a barrier to oral health care. A previous study of the racial and ethnic composition of the health care workforce reveals that the dental workforce is the least diverse of all the health professions.[12] Further investigation reveals that of all those included in the dental health care providers category—dentists, dental hygienists, dental assistants, and dental laboratory technicians—the dental hygiene profession is a more diverse workforce. (See Figure 11-2 ■.)

Value of Dental Hygiene

People from other cultures do not always share the American belief that present action can change future events. Americans tend to measure the success or failure of prevention by the statistical rate of disease occurrences over time, and they generally believe that improvements in public health result from prevention. However, many people from other cultures may not see the value of prevention if no disease is evident. If there is no pain or discomfort, why be subjected to periodontal scaling? Why fluoridate the water when caries may not occur? How could dietary changes affect already formed and erupted teeth? Concerns such as these must be acknowledged before public health dental hygienists can educate a culturally diverse population.

Cross-cultural dental hygiene is the effective integration of a patient's or population's socioethnocultural background into the dental hygiene process of care. See Table 11-2 ■ for basic guidelines for delivering oral health education and care to diverse populations.

Table 11–2 Guidelines for Delivering Oral Health Care to Diverse Populations

To Develop Cultural Awareness	To Deliver Culturally Competent Care
• Recognize how your culture influences your values, behavior, beliefs, and decision making. • Become a lifelong learner of diverse cultures, particularly those whose population you serve. • Know about your population's cultural background. • Assess your population's values, beliefs, and knowledge of oral and total health. • Consider the effects of religious beliefs on oral and total health. • Investigate cultural dietary practices and how they affect total health.	• Incorporate cultural practices into education and treatment when appropriate, but sensitively discourage harmful practices. • Incorporate culturally competent communication into oral health education. • Deliver dental hygiene services in a culturally sensitive manner and environment. • Develop relationships with health professionals from other ethnic and minority groups to promote a collaborative effort to improve the groups' oral health.

Source: Management Sciences for Health (MSH), US Department of Health and Human Services, Health Resources and Services Administration and the Bureau of Primary Health Care. The provider's guide to quality and culture. http://erc.msh.org. Accessed March 13, 2009. University of Michigan Health System. Program for multicultural health. http://www.med.umich.edu/Multicultural. Accessed March 13, 2009.

DENTAL HYGIENIST SPOTLIGHT ·····································

Public Health Column: Meg Zayan, RDH, MPH, EdD

Meg Horst Zayan, RDH, MPH, EdD, is the current dean of Fones School of Dental Hygiene in Bridgeport, Connecticut, the original dental hygiene school. Fones recently added a graduate degree in dental hygiene and opened a remodeled state-of-the-art dental hygiene clinic.

In addition to her teaching and management experience, Dr. Zayan has worked for the US State Department in Niger, Africa, as a volunteer to help in the treatment of dental disease, and as a dental hygienist in the Colorado migrant health program. She continues to teach students about the integral relationship between dental public health and dental hygiene. Not surprisingly, she has received numerous honors, including membership in Sigma Phi Alpha, the national dental hygiene honor society, and Phi Kappa Phi, the nation's oldest, largest, and most selective all-discipline honor society. Dr. Zayan has been awarded the Outstanding Teacher Award at Fones School of Dental Hygiene.

I recently asked her some questions about her career.

Why did you decide to go into dental hygiene?

As a child, I frequently visited the dentist and dental hygienist for routine appointments and restorations. I also experienced extractions of four primary and four permanent noncarious teeth to prevent crowding and the need for orthodontia.

These experiences allowed me to understand the dental office personnel and the advantages of serving the public and providing education. As I was in the decision-making process to choose a college major, it seemed beneficial to combine health care with education, and I chose dental hygiene. My grandfather always remarked that "a trade and an education will get you far and allow you to be financially stable." His words helped direct me into the dental hygiene profession.

How did you get into dental public health? Did you need additional education?

After graduating with a BS degree in dental hygiene education, I taught for one year. During that year, I realized the need for an advanced degree if I wanted to pursue a career in academia. I thought of various options that would allow me to obtain a dental hygiene "specialty" and expand my job opportunities in venues other than academia.

I was not particularly fond of dental public health as a dental hygiene student, but as I became aware of the many opportunities a degree in public health created, I began to read more and ask questions, and my interest flourished. As a clinician, I understood what it meant to serve the private sector. I wanted to learn more about serving the public sector.

I was fortunate to have received a scholarship the first year I applied for a master's degree in public health. The curriculum I chose required eighteen months of education to earn an MPH. For my minor, I chose health care administration. In retrospect, going into public health was one of the best decisions I made in regard to my education.

What are your current positions?

My current position is dean of Fones School of Dental Hygiene, Bridgeport, Connecticut. I also hold the positions of director of graduate studies and associate professor there.

Can you discuss any particularly interesting experiences you have had in your dental public health positions?

Two experiences come to mind.

First, I had the opportunity to work a summer in the Colorado migrant health program. This gave me insight to the benefits of a state-run oral health care initiative. Dental hygienists, dentists, nurses, doctors, and nutritionists collaborated to provide education and health services to the migrant farmers and their children. We were dispersed by team throughout the state of Colorado based on need and access. During the summers, these elementary school-aged children attend school while older siblings and parents farm. Our responsibility as dental hygienists was to provide classroom education, screenings, oral prophylaxes, fluoride treatments, and sealants to the children in the schools. If dental work was indicated, we scheduled transportation to local dental offices. During the evenings, we worked in dental offices providing services to the older children and the adults. We all worked together to improve health care, and the rewards were outstanding.

The second experience was living in Niger, West Africa, for two years. My husband, as a public health physician, was hired to work in Niger to help in the program to prevent blindness and eye diseases. I came on board as a volunteer to help in the treatment of dental disease. Due to the lack of integration of preventive dental hygiene in Niger, my role was small. However, I worked with dentists, assisting them in providing treatment and at times used my

own dental hygiene instruments to remove calculus. Because Niger is a French-speaking country, I was forced to improve my French so that communication when providing education was positive. This experience instilled a long-term interest in international dental hygiene in me.

What type of advice would you give to a practicing hygienist thinking of doing something different?

I would encourage everyone to always consider the various job opportunities we have in the dental hygiene profession. We have chosen a career for which there will always be a public need in the foreseeable future. I foresee the job opportunities for dental hygienists increasing in number and type. Clinical dental hygiene is the core of who we are. Anyone considering other opportunities will continually utilize their clinical knowledge to maintain and improve oral health care. I encourage dental hygienists to periodically search the various career options available to them. It is not so much that we need to change, but that if we want to change, we can. A dental hygienist who knows the options will have a better chance of job satisfaction with the choice made.

Source: Christine Nathe writes the Public Health Column in *RDH* magazine published by Pennwell Publishing. For more public health spotlights please see RDH magazine online at http://www.rdhmag.com/index.html.

Summary

Dental hygienists have been challenged to respond to current and projected demographic changes in the United States. Cultural competency in health care refers to the ability to provide care to populations that have beliefs, values, and behaviors that differ from those of the provider. Consideration must be given to the health beliefs and values as well as disease prevalence and incidence in each particular group. Although dental hygienists are educated to treat people equally, it is important to recognize that people do have differences and to respect them.

Self-Study Test Items

1. The fact that only a small number of minorities work in the oral health care professions may be considered a barrier to oral health care. A study of the racial and ethnic composition of the health care workforce reveals that the dental workforce is the least diverse of all the health professions.
   a. The first statement is true; the second statement is false.
   b. The first statement is false; the second statement is true.
   c. Both statements are true.
   d. Both statements are false.

2. Which of the following could prevent a patient from seeking care or reduce effectiveness of care?
   a. Unhealthy behaviors
   b. Severe pain
   c. Language barrier
   d. None of the above

3. A country in which people strive to acculturate into a new society and make valiant attempts to change their cultural patterns to those of their host society is colloquially called
   a. A melting pot
   b. A salad bowl
   c. Jello
   d. Amalgam

4. Which of the following is or are guidelines to effective communication?
   a. Assess one's own cultural beliefs and values
   b. Recognize those culture influences that affect communication
   c. Understand a patient's belief system
   d. All of the above

5. Cross-cultural dental hygiene is the effective integration of a population's socioethnocultural background into the process of care. Recognizing how your culture influences your values, behaviors, beliefs, and decision making is part of cross-cultural dental hygiene.
   a. The first statement is true; the second statement is false.
   b. The first statement is false; the second statement is true.
   c. Both statements are true.
   d. Both statements are false.

References

1. Kreps GL, Kunimoto EN. *Effective Communication in Multicultural Health Care Settings.* Thousand Oaks, CA: Sage Publications; 1994.
2. Connolly IM, Darby ML, Tolle-Watts L, Thomson-Lakey E. Cultural adaptability of health science faculty. *J Dent Hyg.* 2000;74(II):102–109.
3. US Department of Commerce, Economic and Statistics Administration, US Census Bureau. 2010. Retrieved from http://www.census.gov/prod/cen2010/briefs/c2010br-02.pdf on August 10, 2015.
4. Gallagher C. *Lev Semyonovich Vygotsky.* Retrieved from http://www.muskingum.edu/~psych/psycweb/history/vygotsky.htm on February 4, 2015.

5. Rogoff B. *The Cultural Nature of Human Development*. New York, NY: Oxford University Press; 2003.

6. Evaluating Oneself. The Provider's Guide to Quality and Culture. Retrieved from http://erc.msh.org/mainpage.cfm?file=2.2. htm&module=provider&language= September 28, 2015.

7. Stewart EC, Bennett MJ. *American Cultural Patterns: A Cross-Cultural Perspective*. Boston, MA: Intercultural Press; 1991.

8. Darby, ML, Walsh MM. *Dental Hygiene Theory and Practice*. 4th ed. St. Louis, MO: Elsevier; 2015.

9. American Dental Hygienists' Association. *National Dental Hygiene Research Agenda*. Retrieved from https://www.adha .org/resources-docs/7111_National_Dental_Hygiene_ Research_Agenda.pdf on February 4, 2015.

10. American Dental Hygienists' Association, 84th Annual Session, New Orleans, LA; 2007.

11. *Accreditation Standards for Dental Hygiene Education Programs*. Chicago, IL: Commission on Dental Accreditation, American Dental Association; 2014.

12. Mertz E, O'Neil E. The growing challenge of providing oral health care services to all Americans. *Health Affairs*. 2002;21(5):65–77.

13. US Department of Health and Human Services. *Oral Health in America: A Report of the Surgeon General—Executive Summary*. Rockville, MD: US Department of Health and Human Services, National Institute of Dental and Craniofacial Research, National Institutes of Health; 2000.

Note

The author wishes to thank Irene Connolly for her contribution of the original chapter in the third edition.

Visit www.pearsonhighered.com/healthprofessionsresources to access the student resources that accompany this book. Simply select Dental Hygiene from the choice of disciplines. Find this book and you will find the complimentary study tools created for this specific title.

Program Planning

OBJECTIVES

After studying this chapter, the dental hygiene student should be able to:

- Define the dental hygiene process of care program planning paradigm
- Describe the various program planning paradigms
- Describe various dental public health programs
- Develop a dental public health program plan

COMPETENCIES

After studying this chapter and participating in accompanying course activities, the dental hygiene student should be competent to do the following:

- Promote positive values of oral and general health and wellness to the public and organizations within and outside the profession
- Assess the oral health needs and services of the community to determine action plans and availability of resources to meet the health care needs
- Provide screening, referral, and educational services that allow patients to access the resources of the health care system
- Provide community oral health services in a variety of settings
- Facilitate patient access to oral health services by influencing individuals or organizations for the provision of oral health care
- Advocate for effective oral health care for underserved populations

KEY TERMS

Dental hygiene process
  of care *155*
Paradigm *155*
Prevention program *157*
Program planning *155*

Dental hygienists frequently provide dental health presentations to target populations. Before planning can begin for a dental health program, the dental hygienist must review past programs, identify a **paradigm,** and develop a program. A paradigm is an outstandingly clear framework that explains a concept or theory. Although many different paradigms are available, all possess common threads necessary in developing programs of all types. These common threads are described later in the section on dental hygiene program planning paradigm.

Program planning encompasses the **dental hygiene process of care,** including the assessment, diagnosis, implementation and evaluation stages of a dental public health program and documentation throughout. This chapter discusses paradigms and the process of planning a new dental health program following a paradigm.

Did You Know?

A *paradigm* is a model of a specific concept such as the development and operation of a public health program.

Common Dental Health Program Planning Paradigms

One of the reasons that dental public health may be difficult for students to grasp is that so many paradigms exist for developing public health programs.

Dr. A. C. Fones actually developed the first program planning paradigm or model in 1927.[1] (See Figure 12-1 ■.) It reflected the efforts at that time to include dental hygiene in existing systems to prevent and cure disease. Fones was a staunch believer in prevention, and when presenting this model, emphasized the fact that very few elementary schools had a well-defined health program. Everything in the paradigm on the health side represented efforts to prevent disease. He then defined the ways that those who became ill, chiefly from preventable disease, convalesced and needed treatment. Everything below the line represented mortality.

The logic model has been used as a method to help guide the program planning process (Figure 12-2 ■). The logic model, interestingly, was originally used as a program evaluation tool for identifying performance measures. Since that time, the tool has been adapted to program planning, as well.[2]

The PRECEDE-PROCEED model is another logic model planning paradigm that focuses on a change process that focuses on outcome, not merely the activity (Figure 12-3 ■). PRECEDE and PROCEED are acronyms (words in which each letter is the first letter of a word). PRECEDE stands for Predisposing, Reinforcing, and Enabling Constructs in Educational/Environmental Diagnosis and Evaluation. As the name implies, it represents the process that precedes, or leads up to, an intervention.[3] PROCEED spells out Policy, Regulatory, and Organizational Constructs in Educational and Environmental Development, and true to its name as well, describes how to proceed with the intervention itself.

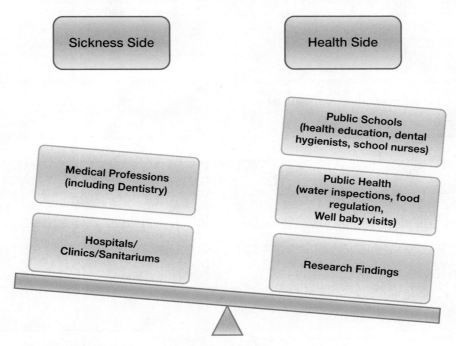

Fones' Model for Prevention of Disease Efforts

FIGURE 12–1 Prevention Program Planning Model

Source: Data from Fones AC *Mouth Hygiene*. 3rd edition. Lea and Febiger; 1927.

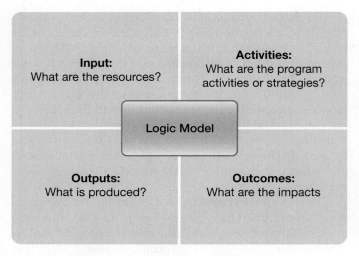

FIGURE 12–2 Logic Model Dental Hygiene Paradigm

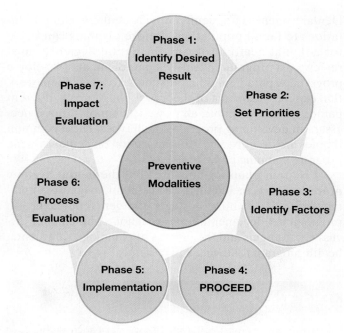

FIGURE 12–3 PRECEDE-PROCEED Model

Another model, the *planning and implementation strategy flowchart,* emphasizes the necessity for making ongoing needs assessments and revisions as well as the importance of assessment and planning. The emphasis on having an ongoing needs assessment and implementing revisions as needed are important functions in public health program operation. The Association of State Territorial Dental directors proposed a seven-step model for assessing oral health needs and developing community

plans. (See Figure 12-5 ■.) The comprehensive plan addresses existing state infrastructure and policies and emphasizes quality assurance.[4] To find more program planning models, please visit the Web site.

PRECEDE has four phase, which we'll explore in greater detail later in the section:

Phase 1

Identifying the ultimate desired result.

Phase 2

Identifying and setting priorities among health or community issues and their behavioral and environmental determinants that stand in the way of achieving that result, or conditions that have to be attained to achieve that result; and identifying the behaviors, lifestyles, and/or environmental factors that affect those issues or conditions.

Phase 3

Identifying the predisposing, enabling, and reinforcing factors that can affect the behaviors, attitudes, and environmental factors given priority in Phase 2.

Phase 4

PROCEED has four phase (also to be discussed in more detail later) that cover the actual implementation of the intervention and the careful evaluation of it, working back to the original starting point – the ultimate desired outcome of the intervention.

Phase 8

Outcome evaluation. Is the intervention leading to the outcome (the desired result) that was envisioned in Phase 1?

Phase 7

Impact evaluation. Is the intervention having the desired impact on the target population?

Phase 6

Process Evaluation. Are you actually doing the things you planned to do?

Phase 5

Implementation – the design and actual conducting of the intervention.

Identifying the administrative and policy factors that influence what can be implemented.

FIGURE 12–4 Precede Proceed

Source: Seven-Step Model for Assessing Oral Health Needs and Developing Community Plans. Guidelines for State and Territorial Oral Health Programs. July 1997.

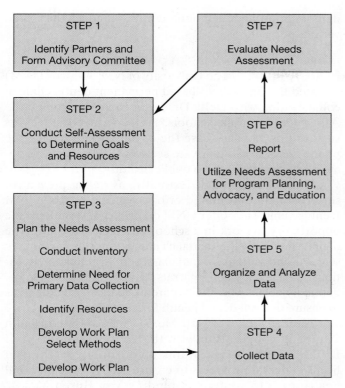

FIGURE 12–5 Assessing Oral Health Needs and Developing Community Needs

Source: Seven-Step Model for Assessing Oral Health Needs and Developing Community Plans. Guidelines for State and Territorial Oral Health Programs. July 1997.

Core Program Planning Functions for Government Agencies

The Institute of Medicine (IOM) in Washington, DC, has identified core functions to be conducted by government public health agencies: assessment, policy development, and assurance to ensure effective dental care delivery. These core functions can be critical to program planning and evaluation. *Assessment* involves monitoring communities and populations at risk to identify their health needs and to set priorities for meeting them. It includes monitoring public health, collecting and interpreting data, examining case findings, and evaluating outcomes of programs and policies. *Policy development* is the process by which society makes decisions about problems, chooses goals and strategies to reach them, and allocates resources. Public policy formulation usually occurs through collaboration between the community, private sector, and government. *Assurance* involves making certain that all populations have access to appropriate and cost-effective services to reach agreed on public health goals. In addition to treatment services for individuals, assurance activities include promoting health promotion and disease prevention. *Serving all functions* describes the research for new insights and innovative solutions to health problems.[5]

Dental Hygiene Public Health Programs

Program planning and implementation are quite possibly the most exciting areas of public health. Studying a population's needs and creating dental programs to meet them are motivating and intriguing. This first part of this section discusses general program types, and the final section describes specific private and publicly funded programs.

General Prevention Programs

A health **prevention program** is designed to prevent disease in a target population. Prevention programs can occur in a wide range of settings, including communities, schools, long-term care facilities, health care support groups, and day care facilities. As discussed in Chapter 10, communities can be defined as metropolitan, urban, suburban, rural, or frontier. There can be differences when developing programs for different communities. For instance, in a metropolitan area, readily available, public transportation decreases barriers to get to a clinic for treatment, whereas, even in many urban communities, with less available and affordable public transportation options, getting to a clinic even a few miles away can present problems.

Many times, cultural influences can occur within communities. America, since its inception, has continued to become diversified in cultures and language. Many newer immigrants may be from countries without dental hygiene and therefore may not value preventive dental medicine. Or language barriers may exist within communities, so health literacy can become an issue, with those populations not fluent in English.

Dental health educational programs seek to provide preventive dental health tools to large populations. Many programs instituted in schools, such as a program consisting of a dental hygienist visiting a third-grade class to present twenty minutes of dental health education, are often sporadic and have no measurable outcome assessment.

A widely recognized and successful prevention program supports the use of community water fluoridation to prevent caries. Historically, localities fluoridated their school water supplies, but now many local areas across the country implement a school fluoride mouth rinse program instead. In this program, students take time out to "swish and spit," as it is sometimes called. Dental hygienists coordinate the program and instruct the teachers in administering it. This is an example of public health service linking people to necessary health interventions, which was discussed in the first chapter.

Did You Know?

School fluoride mouth rinse programs represent a great preventive alternative for areas that have no public water supplies, such as those using well water without naturally occurring fluoride.

Dental sealant programs are also common in schools. Dental hygienists (and dentists when required) travel to schools placing sealants on children's teeth and providing them with oral hygiene instruction. This type of program enables students who may not visit the dental office to have the preventive benefits of dental interventions. This is an inexpensive program to prevent dental caries, especially for the 50 percent of the population who do not receive dental care via private dental offices.

Programs to promote dental health include having dental hygienists develop and implement a dental hygiene association–sponsored poster-designing contest for students during dental health month. The introduction of public health interdisciplinary programs is vital to the success and effectiveness of dental programs.

Through another program, dental hygienists in a school fabricate athletic mouth guards for all sports teams. Programs of this type are designed to prevent oral trauma and concussions because young athletes are often prone to dental trauma. This program type is frequently offered in middle and high schools because the number of school-sponsored athletics is larger in the upper grades.

In a nonschool setting, long-term care facilities, commonly referred to as *nursing homes*, often hire dental hygienists to coordinate and provide a dental care program as a cost-effective way for their residents to obtain oral care. Such programs provide preventive services on a routine basis to help residents maintain their quality of life and dignity. Many dentists are unable to visit long-term care facilities as frequently as dental hygienists and are therefore limited to providing urgent or restorative dental services. Facilities benefit from the resulting family satisfaction and enhanced reputation for providing total care to residents.

Collaborative dental programs are generally the most effective ones. For example, the collaborative relationship between dentist and dental hygienist long-term care facility programs benefits dental hygienists by providing a career option beyond private practice, and it allows dentists working in private practice to increase job satisfaction and care for the people who are underserved. Collaboration between teachers, social workers, case managers, and other health care providers in the operation of dental programs helps to integrate oral health into general health and promotes oral health as a valued service.

Did You Know?

Oral health screenings are mandated in all nursing facilities that receive Medicare or Medicaid funding, but many nursing facilities do not hire dental hygienists or dentists.

Existing Public Health Programs

One of the first practice settings for dental hygienists was in the Bridgeport, Connecticut, public school system. Since then, numerous organizations have offered preventive dental clinics and/or mobile dental practices that serve various populations.

UNIVERSITY OF NEW MEXICO SCHOOL-BASED DENTAL HYGIENE CLINICS The University of New Mexico (UNM) initiated the first school-based permanent dental clinic in collaboration with Delta Dental of New Mexico and the Albuquerque public schools.[6-7] Cooperative endeavors such as this one showcase the advantages of having the public sector and the private sector work together to create a program to improve public health.

These clinics provide restorative as well as preventive services in a coordinated effort with the nearby UNM Dental Clinic. They offer UNM dental hygiene students the opportunity to work in a school-based environment. The dental clinic provides dental cleanings, fluoride treatments, sealants, individualized and classroom oral health education, dental exams, and referrals for needed treatment. The dental hygienist works with parents, teachers, and dentists to ensure optimal dental health for all students.

The University of New Mexico School-Based Health Center in cooperation with the UNM Department of Dental Medicine maintains a coordinated group of licensed dental providers to ensure access to quality oral health care to students attending Van Buren Middle School. The goal is to improve the overall health of Van Buren Middle School students by striving to meet established program goals. (See Box 12-1 ■.)

Did You Know?

Many states have mobile prevention programs that travel to schools providing dental hygiene services to increase access for all children.

COLLABORATIVE ORAL PREVENTION PROGRAM AT SANDOVAL COUNTY, NEW MEXICO, HEALTH COMMONS The New Mexico Department of Health, Sandoval County Government, Women with Infants and Children (WIC) and the UNM Division of Dental Hygiene collaborated on a program at the Sandoval County Health Commons that provided an innovative dental hygiene clinical management program targeting pregnant women and their children. Oral health teams from UNM composed of a dental hygienist, dentist, and dental assistant focused on preventive dental hygiene services to pregnant women and children. They provided local oral health care management assessment, preventive service and practice as outreach workers, and serve as a referral resource for the WIC program and county health department for restorative dental care for patients in need. Sandoval County Health Commons provides UNM dental hygiene students "real-life" dental practice experience in an interdisciplinary setting.[8]

Additionally, UNM initiated a pilot program consisting of dental hygienists within a pediatric care clinic operation by UNM entitled Young Children's Health Center.

Box 12–1 Program Goals, University of New Mexico School-Based Dental Clinic

1. **Patient Care.** Provide preventive care and coordinate comprehensive dental care with neighboring clinics that are in the best interest of the patient.
2. **Education.** Inform students of the significance of high-quality personal oral hygiene, proper diet and nutrition, diagnoses and maintenance of systemic diseases, and avoidance of addiction-forming substances in order to maintain a state of health.
3. **Oral Hygiene Instruction.** Evaluation of student's initial oral hygiene level and subsequent verbal and mechanical demonstration of oral hygiene measures including, but not limited to, tooth brushing, flossing, and pertinent oral hygiene adjuncts based on individual patient needs.
4. **Increase Access to Dental Care.** Raise the overall number of students that seek and receive preventive dental hygiene care by providing an environment that is readily available on site within the school setting.
5. **Non-traditional Practice Setting.** Generate a group of qualified oral health care practitioners who will provide oral health care in a non-traditional practice setting.
6. **Promote Oral Health Needs of Children.** Create a network of participating oral health care practitioners, school administrators and educators, and allied health care professionals that will serve as advocates for the oral health needs of school aged children.

Source: UNM School-Based Dental Clinic Goals. Albuquerque: University of New Mexico, Division of Dental Hygiene. June 19, 2009.

MATTHEW 25 DENTAL CLINICS Approximately forty years ago, a dream of helping those in need became a reality for a group of parishioners from St. Mary's Catholic Church in Indiana who wanted to exemplify the verses from Matthew 25, a biblical call to care for the poor.[9] The program Matthew 25 is a faith-based initiative. The clinic goals are to provide direct health care to those in need and promote health through education and screenings. The medical clinic opened in 1976 and a dental clinic two years later. Matthew 25 provides dental care for individuals with low income who are not eligible for Medicaid. Services include dental exams, cleanings, simple extractions, and restorations, and it provides dentures made by Indiana University dental lab students in the clinic's lab. Matthew 25, which does not rely on government grants for funding, continues to grow.

OPERATION SMILE'S INTERNATIONAL DENTAL HEALTH EDUCATIONAL PROGRAM Operation Smile (OS) is a private, nonprofit, volunteer medical service organization that provides free dental work, reconstructive surgery, and related health care to indigent children and adults in the United States and developing countries. Dr. William Magee, a plastic surgeon and dentist, and his wife Kathy, a nurse and clinical social worker, founded OS in 1982.[10–11] The Magees traveled to the Philippines with a group of American physicians and nurses in 1981, where they provided surgery to children with cleft lip and palate deformities. Their frustration on realizing that more children needed treatment than could be seen during one visit led to the founding of OS. (See Box 12–2 ■.)

OS volunteer health care teams travel to various locations to provide surgeries for disfigurements such as cleft lip and palate deformities, tumors, orthopedic

DENTAL HYGIENIST SPOTLIGHT

Public Health Column: Tammi Byrd, RDH

Tammi Byrd is a wonderful inspiration for showing how many lives a dental hygienist can touch by reaching out! She is an excellent example of public health dental hygienists reaching out to the dentally underserved population—and she is an entrepreneur! She started the successful school-based dental program Health Promotion Specialists, which treats thousands of children every year in South Carolina. Many of these children would not be treated without her tireless efforts to operate the program. Ms. Byrd also teaches at Midland Technical College in South Carolina and has held numerous officer and council positions with the American Dental Hygienists' Association, including her tenure as president of the ADHA. She is the recipient of the ADHA Distinguished Service Award,

the South Carolina Dental Hygienist of the Year Award (twice), and the South Carolina American Association of University Women/Women of Distinction Award.

I asked some questions about her career.

Why did you decide to pursue a dental hygiene degree?

A very close family friend who was a grandfather figure to me inspired me to want to serve others in the health care field. He was a physician, a family practitioner, who was always on the cutting edge. He designed the first neck brace, invented numerous "burn" creams and ointments used to this day, and dabbled in acupuncture yet always had time to attend medical association meetings, paint, travel,

and spend time with his family. I knew I didn't want to work hospital hours; dental hygiene intrigued me, and my dental visits had always been pleasant.

How did you get into dental public health?

That's a good question. If you had asked me ten years ago if I'd be working in public health, I would've said no. I loved private practice periodontics and was a good clinician. But since my graduation, I've always been very active legislatively. When I graduated, dental hygienists in South Carolina were not able to work in schools and provide the same services my current program offers. Organized dentistry strongly opposed the original program, which allowed dental hygienists to work in schools, to the point that our state oral health division was shut down. I had seen the benefits of having dental hygienists provide preventive care in schools and become involved in the lobbying efforts to allow dental hygiene services to be delivered again with or without the division. To make a long story short, twenty years later, passage of new statutes to allow dental hygienists to deliver services without an exam by a dentist was imminent. Dental hygienists would again be able to work in school settings. I met with the policy adviser for the South Carolina Department of Health to discuss restarting our state public health dental hygiene division, but I was told that the state was not interested in being involved with the delivery of services. I asked how the law could be implemented without such a program.

The Department of Health understood the need for the program but did not know how it would come about. I left there feeling bewildered. After much soul searching and prayer, I knew it had to be done and that I, with God's help and the support of my husband, would make it happen.

Did you need additional education?

I had researched the supporting evidence for public health programs and saw how they operated when preparing to provide testimony to the legislature. Hindsight tells me that having a better understanding of business prior to starting one would have been beneficial. However, with the wealth of friends and colleagues that I have developed throughout my membership in ADHA, I had wonderful mentors I could count on for advice.

Can you discuss any particularly interesting experiences you have had in your dental public health position?

The entire experience has been interesting. I'm still amazed that even after seven years, a ruling by the South Carolina administrative law judge in our favor, a civil suit settlement with the South Carolina Dental Association, and an FTC ruling against the South Carolina Board of Dentistry, I'm still having to defend the merits of dental sealants to school board members, principals, and school nurses because the "local" dentists have told them that dental hygienists are sealing in cavities and the children will end up with "blown-up" teeth. It can be frustrating. But, one by one and group by group, we are educating the masses about the benefits of prevention.

When I see the smiles of the children we treat and hear the school nurses say there are fewer dental problems now, I know we're making a difference. We now have some dentists calling and asking our school-based program to add them to our referrals list.

What Type of Advice Would You Give Us?

Understand cash flow, that being a boss can ruin friendships, that you must have the passion to stick with it, and you must have the desire to continue climbing the ladder of lifelong learning. Dental hygienists are in the best position ever to make a difference in the oral health of this nation. Consumers are going to demand increased access to services. We need to be prepared to deliver.

Source: Christine Nathe writes the Public Health Column in *RDH* magazine published by Pennwell Publishing. For more public health spotlights please see RDH magazine online at http://www.rdhmag.com/index.html.

problem cancrum oris, and burn scars. Cancrum oris, or noma, a commonly seen disease, is an acute, necrotizing process involving the mucous membrane of the mouth. Cancrum oris is characterized by rapidly spreading and painless destruction of bone and soft tissues. The condition is most commonly seen in children with poor oral hygiene, malnutrition, and debilitating disease. Healing frequently occurs but often with disfiguring effects, and OS physicians perform reconstructive surgeries on patients affected by cancrum oris. Dental hygienists have an important role in preventing and controlling this disease.

Operation Smile provides education and training to achieve a long-term self-sufficiency dental hygiene program. It focuses on training teachers and health care workers to prevent and control oral disease and to promote dental health through an organized effort.

Dental hygienists are crucial in facilitating dental care in the countries OS serves. They implement the program in conjunction with a dental counterpart from the host country and secure funding for the program's dental care and educational supplies. Their primary role, however, is to plan and implement two-week training programs to educate

Box 12–2 Operation Smile

Operation Smile (OS), headquartered in Norfolk, Virginia, is a worldwide children's medical charity.

Operation Smile is an international children's medical charity that performs safe, effective cleft lip and cleft palate surgery, and delivers postoperative and ongoing medical therapies to children in low and middle income countries.

OS is the largest volunteer-based children's medical charity providing free cleft surgeries. Since 1982, Operation Smile—through the help of dedicated medical volunteers—has provided 220,000 free surgical procedures for children and young adults.

As one of the most prominent charities for children in the world, OS works in over 60 countries, and thousands of health care professionals have been trained globally.

Source: Operation Smile. Norfolk, VA. Retrieved from http://www.operationsmile.org. on February 19, 2015.

Box 12–3 Dental Hygiene Program Planning Paradigm

Assessment

Assess via surveys, existing data, or dental screenings

Population's dental needs

Population's demographics

Facility availability and state

Workforce needed and available

Existing resources

Funding needed

↓

Dental Hygiene Diagnosis

Prioritize needs

Diagnose to provide goals and objectives for blueprint

↓

Planning

Develop blueprint

Identify methods to measure goals

Address constraints and possible alternatives

↓

Implementation

Begin program operation

Revise and make changes identified

Identify workforce and operation management

↓

Evaluation

Measure to determine success in meeting goals via surveys and dental indexes

Make qualitative and quantitative evaluation

Make ongoing revisions as needed

Documentation

Document all data and information throughout all stages

---

teachers and health care providers on dental hygiene fundamentals. The training program presents basic lectures on oral anatomy, oral pathology, oral hygiene techniques, fluoridation, nutrition, dental screenings, dental emergencies, and teaching strategies. At the end of the didactic portion of the program, the participants present an oral health lesson to local schoolchildren and provide oral screenings under the supervision of OS dental hygienists. More important, these individuals serve the community as dental hygiene consultants when dental health concerns arise.

Many developing countries often place a low priority on dental conditions because they experience tremendous health issues. One way to improve the quality of life and challenge the exhausting health issues is through prevention. For this reason, dental hygiene plays a critical role in these countries.

Dental Hygiene Public Health Program Planning Paradigm

The dental hygiene program planning paradigm in Box 12-3 ■ uses the steps of the dental hygiene process of care model in program planning. *Assessment, dental hygiene diagnosis, planning, implementation, evaluation,* and *documentation* woven throughout all steps are its basic elements. Refer to Chapter 9 for a detailed discussion of these steps.

Assessment

During the assessment phase, the dental hygienist assesses the population's needs, facility needs, resources, and funding. Population needs can be assessed by administering surveys or performing dental screenings using specific dental indexes to measure dental health/disease. Dental indexes will be discussed in detail in the next chapter on program evaluation. Additional assessment data often can be found in documentation from the facility, community, or existing grant applications. Surveys or personal interviews aid in gathering information about demand, perceived needs, the population's approximate knowledge level, and existing problems and issues.

The assessment phase should identify facilities (public school, nursing home, or other organization) involved, specifically regarding available space, equipment, and dental and educational materials as well as workforce needs, sometimes referred to as *labor force planning*. In regard to this, it is essential to determine whether dental hygienists are allowed to work without supervision of dentists, which would decrease personnel needs. Dental coordination should be addressed for a program combined with a larger one.

Did You Know?

Ensuring an interdisciplinary approach to care using nurses, teachers, social workers, and other health care providers in addition to dental health providers enhances a program's value to the public.

Dental Hygiene Diagnosis

A dental hygiene diagnosis basically identifies needs, which is the natural conclusion to the assessment phase. Dental hygienists must prioritize these diagnoses in order of severity and offer care following that order.[12] An example of a dental hygiene diagnosis based on an assessment follows. The majority of prison inmates diagnosed using two dental indexes had moderate to advance periodontal diseases and heavy calculus. While analyzing this information, the dental public health planner noted that most inmates had not had their teeth cleaned for more than fifteen years and then made the dental hygiene diagnosis of periodontal disease associated with no regular dental hygiene care.

Remember, just as in lesson planning, a dental hygiene diagnosis is implemented to follow the dental hygiene process of care. The step that entails diagnosis development may occur within the planning model in different models.

Planning

Planning involves reviewing the target population assessment that was used in making the diagnosis. This information provides the basis for formulating program operations. The first step is to draw a dental program blueprint identifying the goals, objectives, and methods to measure the program's effectiveness; activities planned; possible constraints and detailed strategies to address them; and funding for the program. A program's effectiveness can be measured both quantitatively by using pretest/posttest exams and dental indexes and qualitatively by conducting surveys and interviews and obtaining personal statements from those who participated.

Implementation

The dental hygiene program actually begins to operate at the implementation stage. It can be revised as necessary during this stage. Most programs require revisions as a result of unforeseen difficulties or needs not originally assessed.

Did You Know?

Implementation includes managing the program and the people working in the program. Effective communication results in a more effective team.

Evaluation

The program must be evaluated to determine its success and to ensure that it functions at the optimum level. The methods used to evaluate the program are determined in the planning phase. Program evaluation is discussed in more detail in Chapter 13.

Documentation

This component of the paradigm includes complete and factual recoding of all collected data, assessments, and planned and implemented program attributes. Accurate and comprehensive documentation should be intertwined in all stages of the program.

Summary

Dental hygienists working in public health typically develop dental programs for target populations. These programs assess a population's needs and then plan an appropriate intervention directed at the needs identified. During the needs assessment, evaluative mechanisms should be identified.

Effectively planning and implementing a dental public health program can be challenging and exhausting. It is important to remember the dental hygiene process of care at each stage. A helpful reminder is to think of program planning in the already comfortable mode of developing a treatment plan in clinic. Public health program planning simply parallels that process used in treating an individual patient for population-based care.

Self-Study Test Items

1. Which of the following is part of the planning phase of program development?
   a. Identify methods to measure goals
   b. Assess the population's dental needs
   c. Begin program operation
   d. Revise program as needed

2. Dr. Fones's original paradigm for the school dental hygienist program focused on
   a. Restoration
   b. Utilization of a case manager
   c. Prevention of disease
   d. All of the above

3. Which school program is particularly advantageous for middle school athletes?
   a. Sealant program
   b. School fluoridation
   c. Case management
   d. Athletic mouth guard program

4. During which stage of the program paradigm planning should the target population's needs be identified?
   a. Assessment
   b. Dental hygiene diagnosis
   c. Planning
   d. Evaluation

5. A dental hygienist employed in a nursing home could provide routine preventive care. In addition, the dental hygienist could have a collaborative relationship with a dentist so that restorative and urgent care is provided as needed.
   a. The first statement is true; the second statement is false.
   b. The first statement is false; the second statement is true.
   c. Both statements are true.
   d. Both statements are false.

References

1. Fones AC. *Mouth Hygiene.* 3rd ed. Philadelphia, PA: Lea and Febiger; 1927.

2. McCawley, PF. The logic model for program planning and evaluation. Moscow, ID: University of Idaho Extension. Retrieved http://www.cals.uidaho.edu/edcomm/pdf/CIS/CIS1097 .pdf on August 10, 2015.

3. The Community Tool Box. Preceed Precede-Proceed. Retrieved from http://ctb.ku.edu/en/table-contents/overview/ other-models-promoting-community-health-and-development/ preceder-proceder/main on September 28, 2015.

4. *Seven-Step Model for Assessing Oral Health Needs and Developing Community Plans.* Guidelines for State and Territorial Oral Health Programs. July 1997. http://www .astdd.org/docs/Introduction.pdf. Accessed June 19, 2009.

5. Institute of Medicine. The Future of the Public's Health in the 21st century. Washington, DC: National Academy Press; 2003.

6. Nathe CN. Back to school. *RDH.* July 2008.

7. Nathe CN. School-based dental clinics: collaboration and partners. *RDH.* April 2008.

8. Nathe CN. UNM Clinical Programs. *Educ Update.* January 2008.

9. Matthew 25 Health/Dental Clinic. Retrieved from http://www .matthew25online.org/services.html on February 19, 2015.

10. Nathe C. Operation Smile: dental hygiene program. *Den Hyg News.*1994;7:9–10.

11. Operation Smile: Our story. Retrieved from http://www .operationsmile.org/vision/our-story/. on August 10, 2015.

12. Darby ML, Walsh MM. *Dental Hygiene Theory and Practice.* 4th edition. St Louis, MO: Elsevier; 2015.

13

Program Evaluation

OBJECTIVES

After studying this chapter, the dental hygiene student should be able to:

- Describe the mechanisms of program evaluation
- Compare qualitative and quantitative evaluation
- Identify various dental indexes and define their purposes
- List the governmental evaluation resources for oral health

COMPETENCIES

After studying this chapter and participating in accompanying course activities, the dental hygiene student should be competent to do the following:

- Assess the oral health needs of the community and the quality and availability of resources and services
- Provide screening, referral, and education to bring individuals into the health care delivery system
- Evaluate the outcomes of community-based programs and plan future activities

KEY TERMS

Clinical evaluation *165*
Dental index *166*
Formative evaluation *165*
Measurement *165*
Nonclinical evaluation *165*
Summative evaluation *165*

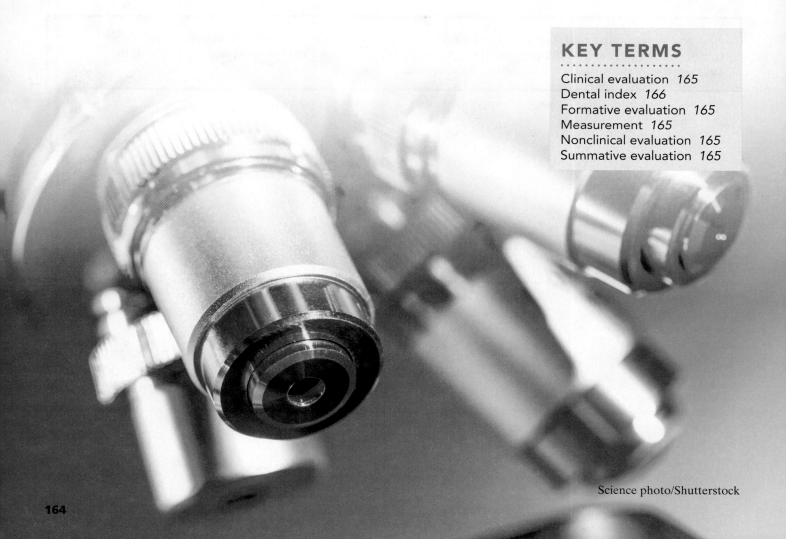

During a dental public health program and at completion, the program planner must use scientific techniques to ascertain effectiveness. Without evaluations, dental health programs cannot be promoted as effective tools in preventing and/or treating dental diseases.

When planning a program, including those addressing the health needs of a target population and to formulate meaningful content, planners identify the methods that will measure how well goals are being met. Planners also identify the strengths and weaknesses of the program's workforce, strategies, and organization. Evaluations of the perceptions and attitudes of the target population should serve as guidelines for discussion and recommendations related to specific problems and their solutions. Formal and informal results of the evaluation, which is ongoing during all program phases and activities, are regularly reported. The process involves obtaining and interpreting baseline data. Baseline data refers to the information collected during the assessment phase, before a program has been started, and can be used to identify needs and subsequently evaluate program outcome.

Qualitative and quantitative documentation of the program must be reported to administrators, funding agency, target population, and the general public on an ongoing basis. See Box 13-1 ■ for questions to ask when planning a program's evaluation. *Qualitative evaluation* involves non-numerical data such as perceptions and attitudes of the population from observations, survey results, and interviews to determine how well a goal is being accomplished. Although not reported numerically, a numerical coding system for qualitative data should be developed in order to summarize the results. *Quantitative evaluation* identifies measures expressed as a quantity or amount, often on a numerical scale. **Measurement** refers to the process of using a particular method to gauge or evaluate something; counts, proportions, ratios, rates, prevalence, and incidence are all quantitative measures. An evaluation enables planners to revise the program as needed to improve outcomes.

Did You Know?

Both qualitative and quantitative measures are equally important when evaluating a program because each provides a unique perspective of the program.

Formative evaluation is an internal examination of a program's process and is usually conducted while planning the program. **Summative evaluation** is an examination of a program's merit after it has been implemented. *Performance management* refers to the systematic process by which an organization involves employees as individuals and members of a group in improving program effectiveness in accomplishing its mission.

Box 13–1 Questions to Ask When Planning a Program

- What should be evaluated?
- Whom should be evaluated?
- Who should administer the evaluation?
- When should the evaluation be conducted?
- How should the evaluation be conducted?

Evaluation Techniques

Many methods are available to evaluate a dental public health program's effectiveness. They are grouped into two areas: nonclinical and clinical. (See Table 13-1 ■.) **Nonclinical evaluations** are methods employing questionnaires, individual or group interviews, telephone interviews, focus groups, direct observations, document analysis, and surveys. **Clinical evaluations** are measurements supported by clinical data such as basic screenings and epidemiological examinations that utilize dental indices. *Basic screenings* can be performed quickly using a tongue blade and dental mirror. In contrast, *epidemiological examinations* consist of detailed visual-tactile assessment of the oral cavity with dental instruments, a dental mirror, and a dental light. When conducting an oral health survey, the public health practitioner must communicate the limitations of the examination. When disease is identified during an oral health survey, the practitioner has a responsibility to provide a referral for treatment. Refer to Box 13-2 ■ for different areas of dentistry to be evaluated. These areas can be indicators such as disease status of a population, modalities used to prevent disease, or use of dental care by a population.

Table 13–1 Methods Used to Evaluate the Effectiveness of Dental Public Health Programs

Nonclinical Methods	Clinical Methods
Face-to-face personal interviews	Basic screenings
Telephone interviews	Epidemiological examinations
Surveys	
Document analysis	
Focus groups	
Observation	

Box 13–2 Dental Indicators to Evaluate

- Access to care
- Dental caries
- Dental care delivery
- Dental hygiene treatment
- Dental fluorosis
- Dental treatment needed
- Dental sealants
- Occlusion
- Oral cancer
- Oral and craniofacial diseases and conditions
- Oral disease disparities
- Oral health and quality of life
- Oral trauma
- Periodontal diseases
- Social impact of oral health
- Tooth loss
- Community water fluoridation

Box 13–3 Classification of Dental Caries Examinations

Type 1—Complete Examination
Comprehensive including all tests, it is the least commonly used in public health and is not required for epidemiological studies.

Type 2—Limited Examination
Performed with a mouth mirror, explorer, and adequate illumination and exposed posterior bite-wing radiographs and selected periapicals, this is useful for a public health treatment program but is not required for oral health surveys.

Type 3—Inspection
The most common type used in public health programs employs a mouth mirror, explorer, and adequate illumination.

Type 4—Screening
The least valid type uses a tongue depressor and available illumination and produces the largest number of false negatives.

Did You Know?

Oral health screenings provided during health fairs are least likely to yield usable data, especially when they are performed without adequate illumination.

Dental caries examinations are classified according to the comprehensiveness of the examination. Type 1 is the most comprehensive, and Type 4 is the basic, or least comprehensive. An epidemiological examination is Type 3. (See Box 13-3 ■.) Because neither basic nor epidemiological examinations constitute a thorough dental examination for diagnostic and treatment purposes, a Type 1 or Type 2 examination must be performed when treatment is planned. However, if treatment will not be provided by a dental program, the comprehensiveness of Type 1 and Type 2 examinations is unnecessary, costly, and unethical due to the radiographic exposure. Technological advances in dental caries diagnosis should continue to improve assessment options.

Dental Indexes

A **dental index** is a standardized quantitative method for measuring, scoring, and analyzing oral conditions in individuals and groups. During a program's planning stage, the planner identifies the index to be used in the implementation phase. A dental index score is used to educate, motivate, and evaluate a patient and can serve as a legal record. A comparison of index scores from an initial exam during a follow-up exam can indicate the effects of personal daily care and/or a program or specific treatment. Characteristics

of a dental index include clarity, simplicity, objectivity, validity, reliability, and that it is relatively easy and quantifiable. See Table 13-2 ■ for a definition of these desirable characteristics.

Did You Know?

A dental index used during program evaluation or research can be compared to a dental examination of a patient, which is then evaluated for outcomes at subsequent appointments.

Indexes can be described as simple, cumulative, irreversible, and reversible. A *simple index* measures the presence or absence of a condition; a *cumulative index* measures all past and present evidence of a condition. An *irreversible index* measures conditions that will not change, such as dental caries, whereas a *reversible index* measures those that can be changed, such as the presence of plaque. (See Figure 13-1. ■)

Many index types screen only a few teeth or tooth surfaces. Usually these teeth are the six teeth numbered 3, 9, 12, 19, 25, and 28 as shown in Figure 13-2 ■, referred to as *Ramjford teeth*. The Ramjford teeth are six teeth that are representative of all the teeth; in other words, these teeth can be generalized to the entire dentition. When applying these Ramjford teeth to the dental index, the term modified or simplified is added to the index. See the interactive Companion Website created specifically to accompany this textbook for more information on the labeling of tooth surfaces and teeth numbers. A few frequently used indexes are described next.

Table 13–2 Desirable Characteristics of a Dental Index

Characteristic	Definition
Clarity	Criteria are understandable
Simplicity	Results are easily measured
Objectivity	Results are not subject to individual interpretation
Validity	Index measures what is intended
Reliability	Examiner consistency and calibration are reproducible
Quantifiability	Statistics can be applied
Sensitivity	Small degrees of difference can be detected
Acceptability	Subjects experience no pain and index expense is minimal

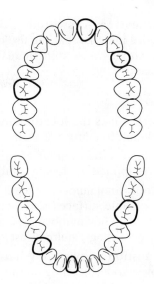

FIGURE 13–2 Ramjford Teeth

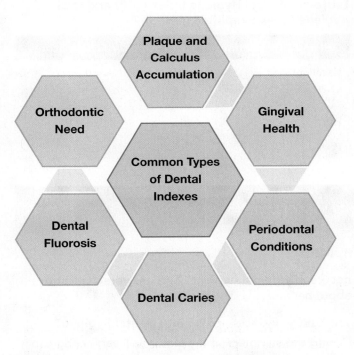

FIGURE 13–1 Common Types of Dental Indexes

Table 13–3 Patient Hygiene Performance (PHP) Rating Scale

Rating	Scores
Excellent	0
Good	0.1–1.7
Fair	1.8–3.4
Poor	3.5–5.0

Procedure: Divide each tooth numbered 3, 8, 14, 19, 24, 30 into five subdivisions (two in interproximal portion) and direct lingual and facial areas into thirds (cervical, middle, and coronal). After application of disclosing solution, score each area retaining plaque and/or debris up to 5 points per tooth (basically, the tooth is divided into 5 subsections). Divide total points given to all teeth by total number of teeth assessed.

Example Question Answered: Will the use of dental plaque charting during oral hygiene instruction result in adolescent motivation to improve oral hygiene as measured by this index?

PLAQUE CONTROL RECORD (PCR)

Purpose: Records presence of bacterial plaque on individual tooth surfaces.

Procedure: After application of disclosing solution, examine gingival margins for plaque.

Scoring: Count and record number of surfaces with retained plaque; calculate the index by dividing the number of plaque-containing surfaces by the total number of available surfaces.[1,3]

Common Dental Indexes for Plaque, Debris, and/or Calculus

PATIENT HYGIENE PERFORMANCE (PHP) AND PATIENT HYGIENE PERFORMANCE MODIFIED (PHP-M) (TABLE 13-3 ■)

Purpose: Assesses extent of plaque and debris over facial surfaces of incisors and maxillary molars and lingual surface of mandibular molars; PHP-M used for Ramjford teeth with same scoring process.[1,2]

Example Question Answered: Does the Plaque Control Record indicate that the use of a mouth rinse prior to toothbrushing significantly reduces the amount of plaque?

PLAQUE-FREE SCORE

Purpose: Determines the location, number, and percentage of plaque-free areas of teeth.

Procedure: Record the number of surfaces of plaque marked by the applied disclosing solution.

Scoring: Multiply total number of teeth by 4 to calculate number of available surfaces; subtract number of surfaces with plaque to find number of plaque-free surfaces. To determine percentage, multiply last number by 100.[1,3]

Example Question Answered: What are the clinical effects of power toothbrushing on the presence of gingivitis and supragingival dental plaque as measured by the Plaque-Free Score?

PLAQUE INDEX (PLI)

Purpose: Assesses thickness of plaque in gingival area in evaluating each of four tooth surfaces—distal, facial, lingual, and mesial—for plaque retention.

Procedure: Use a periodontal probe to identify the plaque level on each tooth evaluated.

Scoring: Plaque levels: free = 0, small amount = 1, moderate amount visible to the naked eye = 2, large amount in the sulcus or at the gingival margin = 3. Add scores for all teeth and divide by number of teeth assessed.[1,3]

Example Question Answered: Which is more effective in improving a patient's oral health, the recognition of gingival bleeding as infection or the use of disclosing tablets to see dental plaque?

ORAL HYGIENE INDEX (OHI) AND ORAL HYGIENE INDEX SIMPLIFIED (OHI–S) (TABLE 13-4 ■) The OHI has two components, the debris index and the calculus index; either or both can be evaluated.

Applied to: Tooth numbers 3, 8, 14, 24; lingual surfaces of tooth numbers 19, 30 (both OHI and OHI–S).[1,3]

Purpose: Measures existing plaque and calculus as oral cleanliness indication.

Procedure: Select one tooth with the most debris or calculus from each sextant; use periodontal probe or explorer to estimate the amount of its debris or calculus and assign a score.

Scoring: Add all scores for all sextants, and divide by the number of sextants evaluated.

Example Question Answered: What is the state of oral cleanliness of schoolchildren at age 10 as measured by the Oral Hygiene Index?

Table 13–4 Oral Hygiene Index (OHI) and Oral Hygiene Index Simplified (OHI-S)

OHI and OHI-S Ratings	OHI Scores	OHI-S Scores
Excellent	0.0	0.0
Good	0.1–0.6	0.1–1.2
Fair	0.7–1.8	1.3–3.0
Poor	1.9–3.0	3.1–6.0

DENTAL HYGIENIST SPOTLIGHT ·······················

Public Health Column: Lynn Bethel, RDH, BSDH, MPH

Lynn Bethel, RDH, BSDH, MPH, is a dental hygienist who has a wealth of experience in public health. Currently, she serves as Interim Director of the Office of Health in Massachusetts. In addition, she is the Association of State and Territorial Dental Directors (ASTDD) liaison to the ADHA. She also mentors other dental hygienists as an adjunct faculty member at the Department of Dental Hygiene of Mount Ida College, Massachusetts. She has lectured and published articles pertaining to public health in various venues. She also has served as the program coordinator for school oral health programs in Massachusetts and has been very active in various dental organizations, including service as president of the Massachusetts Dental Hygienists' Association.

What is so amazing about Ms. Bethel is the way she became interested in dental public health—not necessarily dental hygiene. She answered questions about her story.

Why did you decide to go into dental hygiene?

During the summers of my junior and senior years in high school in the late 1970s, I worked as a teacher's assistant in a Head Start program. A woman would come in and talk to the children about their teeth, look at their teeth, and so on. I decided from that experience that I wanted a job like that. My goal for my life at that point was to drive from school to school to teach toothbrushing and check teeth. It wasn't until my senior year of high school that I learned that the woman who visited the Head Start programs was a dental hygienist; so I then decided I was going to be a dental hygienist. The funny thing was that I had no idea that the "red-haired lady" who cleaned my

teeth every six months was also a dental hygienist. It wasn't until the first week of hygiene school when the mirrors and explorers are passed out that I had any knowledge that dental hygienists worked in dental offices. A dental office was not where I wanted to work; I wanted to work in schools, but I stuck it out for the next eighteen months to get to the fourth semester when community dental health was in the curriculum.

How did you get into dental public health?

I don't think I got into dental public health. I think dental public health was always in me, and dental hygiene was the path I took to express it.

Did you need additional education?

After graduating from hygiene school with my associate's degree in 1983, I transferred to Old Dominion University in Norfolk, Virginia, for my bachelor's degree. I received a bachelor's degree in dental hygiene with a minor in sociology in 1984. While I was there, I volunteered to spend some of my summer on the Delmarva Peninsula providing dental treatment to the migrant workers on the Eastern Shore. During the day, I would go into the schools and provide oral health education to the children, and at night I would work on a mobile dental van where the workers who had come directly from the fields would receive both preventive and restorative treatment. I always knew I wanted a master's degree in public health (MPH), so in 1991, I began working toward that part-time by attending the Boston University School of Public Health. I was the only person with a dental background. The other students worked in medicine or law, for large companies, nonprofits, and so on, which made it a great educational experience. I wasn't learning about dental public health, but public health and, in that, I learned how to apply the principles of public health to my interests in dental hygiene. I graduated in 1995 with my MPH.

What are your current positions?

I am the Interim Director in the Office of Oral Health, a consultant for the Massachusetts Department of Public Health, and I serve on the Massachusetts Coalition for Oral Health. In addition, I am a clinical dental hygienist (part-time) in the same pediatric practice I have worked in since 1987. I teach dental hygiene as a faculty member at Mount Ida College. I also serve as editor of *Prevention Matters*.

Do you have any exciting experiences to share?

Every day is a learning experience for me both professionally and personally. I have learned so much (and am still learning) about fluoride and fluoridation issues. One day, I might be consulting with local water operators, a dental professional, or listening to a resident of the state who has a question or concern about fluoridation. Another day, I could be meeting with partners on a program we are developing, writing a grant, or working with dental hygiene students on a school-based sealant program. I can tell you honestly that I have never left work wishing I wasn't doing what I was doing or wishing that I wasn't a dental hygienist.

What advice would you give to a practicing hygienist who is thinking about doing something different?

These are my five recommendations in order:

1. Stop thinking and do!
2. Go back to school! If you have an associate's degree, go get a bachelor's degree. If you have a BS, go get a master's degree. Education opens not only doors but also your mind. From one degree to the next, you learn so much beyond your normal scope of thinking, and you experience yourself in different situations. Education is invaluable.
3. Consider every opportunity offered to you. It may be to join an oral health coalition or assist with a fluoridation campaign or a sealant program. But with each opportunity, you'll network with other professionals in public health and gain a lot of knowledge and experience.
4. Don't let money be your guide. I noticed a few years ago that I always have just what I need. It may not be everything that I think I want, but it has always been what I have needed.
5. Remember that dental hygiene isn't just about scaling.

Source: Christine Nathe writes the Public Health Column in *RDH* magazine published by Pennwell Publishing. For more public health spotlights please see RDH magazine online at http://www.rdhmag.com/index.html.

Common Dental Indexes for Gingival Bleeding

GINGIVAL BLEEDING INDEX (GBI)

Purpose: Records presence or absence of gingival inflammation as determined by bleeding from interproximal gingival sulci.

Procedure: Pass unwaxed dental floss interproximately into the gingival sulcus on both sides of the interdental papillae alternately using new length of clean floss for each interproximal unit. Then evaluate floss and site for bleeding and reevaluate nonbleeding sites after 30 seconds for delayed bleeding.

Scoring: Add number of all bleeding points.[1,4]

Example Question Answered: Does use of a power flosser positively enhance oral hygiene status?

Table 13–5 Sulcular Bleeding Index (SBI) Scoring Criteria

Score	Criteria
0	Healthy appearance of gingiva, no bleeding upon probing
1	Healthy appearance of gingiva, no change in color, no swelling or bleeding upon probing
2	Bleeding upon probing, change of color, no swelling
3	Bleeding upon probing, change of color, slight swelling
4	Bleeding upon probing, change of color, obvious swelling
5	Bleeding upon probing, spontaneous bleeding, change of color, marked swelling

SULCULAR BLEEDING INDEX (SBI) (TABLE 13-5 ■)

Purpose: Locates areas of gingival sulcus bleeding upon gentle probing.

Procedure: Evaluate four gingival areas (marginal from the facial and lingual aspects, mesial and distal papillary) per tooth for bleeding. After probing, wait 30 seconds before scoring.

Scoring: Divide sum of all surfaces scored by 4.[1,4]

Example Question Answered: Is there a significant reduction in the amount of bleeding when a chlorhexidine rinse is used as an adjunct to normal oral hygiene practices?

EASTMAN INTERDENTAL BLEEDING INDEX (EIBI)

Purpose: Measures papillary bleeding after interproximal stimulation as indicator of inflammation in papillary gingiva.

Procedure: Depress the papilla with wooden interdental cleaner inserted horizontally between the teeth from the facial aspect 1–2 mm and then remove cleaner; repeat four times. Record presence or absence of bleeding within 15 seconds.

Scoring: Divide sum of the interdental spaces that bled by total number of spaces evaluated.[1,5,6]

Example Question Answered: Does the addition of a flossing aid to a toothbrushing regime decrease interproximal bleeding as measured by the Eastman Interdental Bleeding Index?

Common Dental Indexes for Gingival Changes

GINGIVAL INDEX (GI) (TABLE 13-6 ■)

Purpose: Assesses severity of gingivitis of facial, lingual, mesial, and distal aspects of each tooth based on color, consistency, and bleeding when probed.

Procedure: To evaluate one tooth or more or all teeth, insert probe into sulcus 1–2 mm, gently press against gingiva to determine firmness, and move probe circumferentially in horizontal stroke along soft tissue side of the pocket.

Scoring: Give each tooth assessed a score of 0–3 and divide score for each tooth by 4. For multiple teeth, total all scores and divide by total number of teeth.[1,7,8,9]

Example Question Answered: Is brushing with a hydrogen peroxide-sodium bicarbonate paste as effective as brushing with fluoridated toothpaste in reducing gingival inflammation and bleeding in patients with periodontitis?

Common Dental Indexes for Periodontal Diseases

PERIODONTAL INDEX (PI) (TABLE 13-7 ■)

Purpose: Measures periodontal disease in populations based on the clinical exam alone or combined with radiographic evaluation.

Procedure: Perform a clinical examination with periodontal probe and diagnostic radiographs.

Scoring: Give each tooth assessed score of 0–8 and then average scores to determine index (for a population, average all individual scores). The higher the score, the higher is incidence of periodontal disease.[3,10]

Example Question Answered: What are the effects of having lifelong access to free dental care on the periodontal disease status of adults?

Table 13–6 Gingival Index Criteria for Scoring Facial, Lingual, Mesial, and Distal Aspects of Each Tooth Assessed

Points	Appearance	Sulcular Bleeding	Inflammation
0	Normal	None	None
1	Slight color change, mild edema, slight texture change	None	Mild
2	Redness, hypertrophy, edema, glazing	Bleeding on probing	Moderate
3	Marked Redness, Hypertrophy, Edema, Ulceration	Spontaneous Bleeding	Severe

Table 13–7 Criteria for Scoring Periodontal Index

Score	Criteria for Field Study	Additional Radiograph Criteria
0	Negative	Normal appearance
1	Mild gingivitis	None
2	Gingivitis	None
4	Not used in field study	Early resorption of the alveolar crest
6	Gingivitis with pocket formation	Horizontal bone loss involving the entire alveolar crest and up to half of the length of the root
8	Advanced destruction of bone	Advanced bone loss involving more than half of the length of the root

GINGIVAL PERIODONTAL INDEX (GPI)

Purpose: Combination of Gingival Index and Periodontal Index discussed previously to assess gingivitis and pocket depth in dentition. This index can be used to provide detail regarding both gingivitis and periodontitis.

PERIODONTAL DISEASE INDEX (PDI) (TABLE 13-8 ■)

It is a modified version of the Periodontal Index (PI) for Ramjford teeth.

Purpose: Assesses prevalence and severity of gingivitis and periodontitis and shows the periodontal status of an individual or a group.

Procedure: Perform a clinical examination of the tissues, including use of the periodontal probe.

Scoring: Give each Ramjford tooth assessed a score of 0–6 and average them (for a population, average all individual scores).[3,10] Tissue is graded based on inflammation, redness, bleeding, ulceration, and loss of attachment.

Example Question Answered: Is prevalence of periodontal diseases greater in elderly patients as opposed to the general population as measured by the Periodontal Disease Index?

COMMUNITY PERIODONTAL INDEX OF TREATMENT NEEDS (CPITN) AND PERIODONTAL SCREENING AND RECORDING (PSR) (TABLES 13-9 ■ AND 13-10 ■)

Purpose: CPITN classifies individual or group periodontal treatment needs quickly and efficiently. Gingival recession does not result in a higher score.

Procedure: Probe each sextant to determine deepest pocket depth using specially designed probe for CPITN and PSR.

Scoring: Use classification from 0–III (for a population, average all individual scores or compile frequency data).[1,11,12]

Example Question Answered: Are marked periodontal probe depth changes found when comparing advanced periodontal patients on three-month recalls with those on six-month recalls following scaling and root planing?

Table 13–8 Criteria for Scoring Periodontal Disease Index

Score	Appearance
0	Absence of inflammation
1	Mild to moderate inflammatory gingival changes not extending completely around tooth
2	Mild to moderately severe gingivitis extending completely around tooth
3	Severe gingivitis, characterized by marked redness, tendency to bleed, and ulceration
4	Periodontal loss of attachment on any portion of tooth extending no more than 3 mm
5	Periodontal loss of attachment on any portion of tooth extending 3–6 mm
6	Periodontal loss of attachment on any portion of tooth extending more than 6 mm

Table 13–9 Criteria for Scoring Community Periodontal Index of Treatment Needs (CPITN) and Periodontal Screening and Recording (PSR)

CPITN Status	Score	PSR Status
Healthy periodontal tissues	0	Colored area of probe completely visible
Bleeding after probing	1	Colored area of probe completely visible with bleeding after probing
Supra- or subgingival calculus present, or a defective margin found on a restoration	2	Colored area of probe completely visible with supra- or subgingival calculus present, or a defective margin found on a restoration
4–5 mm pocket	3	Colored area of probe partially visible
6 mm or deeper pocket	4	Colored area of probe not visible
Not used	*	Furcation involvement, mobility, a mucogingival problem or recession

Table 13–10 Criteria for Classifying Community Periodontal Index of Treatment Needs (CPITN)

Classification	Criteria
0	No need for treatment
I	Oral hygiene instruction given
II	Oral hygiene instruction with scaling and root planing and removal of defective margins
III	I+II and any recommended complex periodontal therapy such as surgery

Common Dental Indexes for Dental Caries

DECAYED, MISSING, OR FILLED PERMANENT TEETH OR SURFACES (DMFT OR S) (TABLE 13-11 ▪)

Purpose: Determines status of dental caries activity of decayed, missing, or filled teeth or surfaces of permanent dentition.

Procedure: Evaluate twenty-eight teeth, excluding third molars, by clinically examining five surfaces of each posterior tooth (occlusal, lingual, facial, mesial, and distal) and four surfaces of each anterior tooth (facial, lingual, mesial, and distal) and record using stated criteria.[1, 3, 13] DMFT stands for total number of teeth, whereas DMFS stands for total number of surfaces and can only be completed with the use of radiographs. Because DMFS accounts for all surfaces, it is much more detailed. The totals are calculated per each indicator including decayed, missing, and filled (D, M, or F).

Scoring: Sum totals within each category scored D, M, or F.

Example Question Answered: What effects does exposure to a dental health fair have on the total caries rate of attendees as measured with the DMFT preattendance and three-year postattendance?

DECAYED, EXTRACTED, FILLED PRIMARY TEETH OR SURFACES (Deft OR s)

This index is always written in lowercase letters as opposed to uppercase DMFT because it is used for the primary dentition.

Purpose: Determines status of decay, extractions, and filled primary teeth or tooth surfaces.

Procedure: Evaluates twenty primary teeth using same procedure as DMFT or S index.[1, 3]

Scoring: Use same scores as DMFT or S index.

Example Question Answered: Is there increased risk of developing nursing bottle caries in children in day care facilities?

ROOT CARIES INDEX (RCI)

Purpose: Calculates ratio of teeth with carious lesions of the root and/or restorations of the root to teeth with exposed root surfaces.

Procedure: A clinical examination is conducted by counting the number of root caries in the dentition.

Scoring: Add numbers of caries and root restoration together, divide sum by total number of teeth showing gingival recession, and multiply this number by 100. 0 = minimum score; 100 = maximum score; the higher the score, the more diffuse is the caries.[14]

Example Question Answered: What are the effects of fluoride varnish on root caries development?

Common Dental Index for Malocclusion

TREATMENT PRIORITY INDEX (TABLE 13-12 ▪)

Purpose: Measures malocclusions according to the Malocclusion Severity Estimate (MSE) and records

Table 13–11 Criteria for Recording a Decayed, Missing, or Filled Permanent Teeth or Surfaces (DMFT or S) Score

Score	Criteria
D	Dental carious lesion is present
	Dental caries and a restoration are present
	A tooth is broken because of caries
	Third molars with dental carious lesions are not counted
	Supernumerary teeth with dental carious lesions are not counted
	Teeth restored for reasons other than dental carious lesions such as esthetic purposes or use as an abutment tooth are not counted
M	Tooth has been extracted or is not restorable and indicated for extraction
	Teeth that have been extracted for orthodontic purposes or impactions are not counted as missing
	Third molars that have been extracted are not counted as missing
	Unerupted teeth are not counted as missing
	Congenitally missing teeth are not counted
F	Permanent or temporary restoration is present
	Third molars with restorations are not counted
	Supernumerary teeth with restorations are not counted

Table 13–12 Ratings for the Treatment Priority Index

Rating	Description
0	Virtually classic normal occlusion
1–3	Minor manifestations of malocclusion and treatment
4–6	Definite malocclusion, but treatment is elective
7–9	Severe handicap, treatment highly desirable
>10	Very severe handicap, treatment mandatory

results; mesio-, neutro-, and disto-occlusion measured keeping neutro-occlusion constant.

Procedure: Perform a clinical examination of the occlusions, measuring occlusal defects.

Rating: Malocclusion is assessed according to the rating of the scale shown in Table 13-12: 0 to >10.[15, 16]

Example Question Answered: What are the types of malocclusions found in a group of Argentinean primary school children and what is the need for orthodontic treatment in relation to age by using the Treatment Priority Index?

Common Dental Indexes for Dental Fluorosis

DEVELOPMENTAL DEFECTS OF DENTAL ENAMEL (DDE)

Purpose: Scores enamel opacities regardless of origin of opacities to avoid any bias.

Procedure: Examine entire mouth for any enamel mottling and select two worst teeth for evaluation. If two teeth have unequal amounts of mottling, choose the one less affected. Dry tooth for two minutes and then score it.

Scoring: 0 = no fluorosis present, 1–2 = mild fluorosis, 3–9 = advanced changes to enamel.[17, 18]

Example Question Answered: What is the prevalence of caries and developmental defects of enamel in nine- to ten-year-old children living in areas in Mexico with different water fluoride amounts?

DEAN'S INDEX OF FLUOROSIS (TABLE 13-13 ■)

Purpose: Rates fluorosis within a population; is sensitive to mild through severe cases.

Procedure: Same as for DDE index.

Table 13–13 Criteria for Classifying Dean's Index of Fluorosis

Classification	Description
Normal	Smooth, glossy, pale creamy-white translucent surface
Questionable	Few white flecks or white spots
Very mild	Small opaque, paper white areas covering less than 25% of tooth surface
Mild	Opaque white areas covering less than 50% of tooth surface
Moderate	All tooth surfaces affected; marked wear on biting surfaces; brown stain may be present
Severe	All tooth surfaces affected; discrete or confluent pitting; brown stain present

Criteria: Normal to severe.[10, 19]

Example Question Answered: What is the estimated prevalence and level of fluorosis attributable to fluoridation using Dean's Index of Fluorosis?

FLUOROSIS RISK INDEX

Purpose: Assesses fluorosis, particularly the specific time of enamel formation.

Procedure: Divide enamel surfaces of permanent dentition into two developmentally related surface zones: classification I for enamel formation begun during first year of life, and classification II for enamel formation begun in years 3–6.

Scoring: Give each zone a negative for fluorosis or positive for mild to moderate fluorosis. Zone with more than 50% display of pitting, staining, or deformities indicates severe fluorosis.[20]

Example Question Answered: Is there an association between enamel fluorosis and infants given formula?

TOOTH SURFACE INDEX OF FLUOROSIS (TSIF) (TABLE 13-14 ■)

Purpose: Rates fluorosis within a population more sensitively than Dean's Index.

Procedure:

Scoring: Give separate score 0–7 (0 = no fluorosis evidence, 7 = missing enamel surface large areas of enamel with altered tooth anatomy, dark brown stain) to each facial and lingual surface of anterior teeth and buccal, occlusal, and lingual surface of posterior teeth.[11]

Example Question Answered: What fluorosis effects are seen in people living in a community with four times the optimal concentration of fluoride?

Other Common Dental Indexes

Several other indexes are calculated as rates or proportions that describe a portion of a whole that possesses a particular characteristic. Two of the most commonly used are incidence and prevalence rates, which typically refer to the occurrence of an attribute, for example a disease, in a population. *Incidence rates* refer to how many new cases are seen, and *prevalence rates* refer to the total number of cases at a given time. Some examples of dental conditions that may use rates for description are cleft lip or palate cases and oral cancer. An example question might be this: What is the prevalence rate of oral cancer diagnoses in New Mexico?

Table 13–14 Criteria for Scoring Tooth Surface Index of Fluorosis (TSIF)

Score	Description
0	No evidence of fluorosis appears
1	Parchment white fluorosis involves < 33% of visible tooth surface
2	Parchment white fluorosis involves ≥ 33% but < 66% of visible tooth surface
3	Parchment white fluorosis involves ≥ 66% of the visible tooth surface
4	Enamel staining occurs in conjunction with any of preceding findings
5	Discrete pitting of enamel surface occurs without staining of intact enamel
6	Discrete pitting of enamel surface and staining of intact enamel occur
7	Enamel surface shows confluent pitting, large areas of enamel may be missing with altered tooth anatomy, and dark brown stain is usually present

Governmental Evaluation of Oral Health

The oral health goal of *Healthy People 2020* is to prevent and control oral and craniofacial diseases, conditions, and injuries and to improve access to preventive services and dental care.[21] All oral health objectives in *Healthy People 2020,* managed by the Office of Disease Prevention and Health Promotion of the US Department of Health and Human Services, include a way to measure each objective. See Table 13-15 ■ for specific objectives and evaluation mechanisms.

The National Oral Health Surveillance System (NOHSS), a collaborative effort between the Centers for Disease Control and Prevention and The Association of State and Territorial Dental Directors, is based on a set of oral health indicators from *Healthy People 2020.*[22] NOHSS is designed to aid public health programs in monitoring

Table 13–15 *Healthy People 2020*: Oral Health Objectives

Oral Health of Children and Adolescents

OH 1: Reduce the proportion of children and adolescents who have dental caries experience in the primary or permanent teeth.

OH 2: Reduce the proportion of children and adolescents with untreated dental decay.

Oral Health of Adults

OH 3: Reduce the proportion of adults with untreated dental decay.

OH 4: Reduce the proportion of adults who have ever had a permanent tooth extracted because of dental caries or periodontal disease.

OH 5: Reduce the proportion of adults aged 45–74 with moderate or severe periodontitis.

OH 6: Increase the proportion of oral and pharyngeal cancers detected at the earliest stage.

Access to Preventive Services

Access to Preventive Care

OH 7: Increase the proportion of children, adolescents and adults who used the oral health care system in the past year.

OH 8: Increase the proportion of low-income children and adolescents who received any preventive dental service during the past year.

OH 9: Increase the proportion of school-based health centers with an oral health component.

OH 10: Increase the proportion of local health departments and Federally Qualified Health Centers (FQHCs) that have an oral health component.

OH 11: Increase the proportion of patients who receive oral health services at Federally Qualified Health Centers (FQHCs) per year.

Oral health interventions

OH 14: Increase the proportion of adults who receive preventive interventions in dental offices.

OH 15: Increase the number of States and the District of Columbia that have a system for recording and referring infants and children with cleft lips and cleft palates to craniofacial anomaly rehabilitative teams.

OH 16: Increase the number of States and the District of Columbia that have an oral and craniofacial health surveillance system.

OH 17: Increase the health agencies that have a dental public health program directed by a dental professional with public health training.

Source: http://www.healthypeople.gov. Retrieved from http://www.healthypeople.gov/2020/topicsobjectives2020/objectiveslist.aspx?topicId=32 on February 19, 2015.

System	Acronym	Description
Behavioral Risk Factor Surveillance System	BRFSS	Continuous health survey conducted by telephone. An example question from BRFSS would be how many sugar-sweetened drinks are you consuming daily
National Health and Nutrition Examination Survey	NHANES	Program of studies designed to assess the health and nutritional status of adults and children in the United States. The survey is unique in that it combines interview and physical examinations
National Health Interview Survey	NHIS	The U.S. census Bureau has been the data collection agent for the NHIS and the survey results have been instrumental in providing data to track health status, health care access, and progress toward achieving national health objectives
Youth Risk Behavior Surveillance System	YRBSS	National school-based survey conducted by CDC and state, territorial, tribal, and local surveys conducted by state, territorial, and local education and health on • Behaviors that contribute to unintentional injuries and violence • Sexual behaviors that contribute to unintended pregnancy and sexually transmitted diseases, including HIV infection • Alcohol and other drug use • Tobacco use • Unhealthy dietary behaviors • Inadequate physical activity • Obesity and asthma
Behavioral Risk Factor Surveillance System	BRFSS	State-based, ongoing data collection program that measures behavioral risk factors in the noninstitutionalized population eighteen years of age or older
Basic Screening Survey	BSS	Standardized set of cross-sectional and descriptive surveys that collect information on the observed oral health of participants; self-reported or observed information on age, gender, and race and Hispanic ethnicity; and self-reported information on access to care for preschool, school-age, and adult populations. The health care worker or dental provider records the presence of (1) untreated cavities and urgency of need for treatment for all age groups, (2) early childhood caries and caries experience for preschool children, (3) sealants on permanent molars and caries experience for school-age children, and (4) edentulism (no natural teeth) for adults.
2006 Fluoridation Census		Record of the fluoridation status for each state. It identifies each state's fluoridated water system and the communities each system served; the status—adjusted, consecutive, or natural—of fluoridation; the system from which water was purchased, if consecutive; the population receiving fluoridated water; the date on which fluoridation started; and the chemical used for fluoridation, if adjusted. Adjusted means that fluoride is added or removed, whereas natural means that the fluoride was naturally present.
Pregnancy Risk Assessment Monitoring System	PRAMS	State-specific, population-based data on maternal attitudes and experiences prior to, during, and immediately following pregnancy. The sample participants are taken from the state's birth certificate file.
Synopses of State Dental Public Health Programs		The Synopses of State Dental Public Health Programs is a collection of oral health program information provided to the Association of State and Territorial Dental Directors (ASTDD) annually by each state's dental director or oral health program manager. ASTDD, in conjunction with CDC's Division of Oral Health, includes that information with data from standard sources (U.S. Census, Department of Education, Bureau of Labor Statistics, etc.) on the State Synopses Web site. Each state's synopsis contains information specific to it on demographics and oral health infrastructure, program administration, and activities. An interactive national trend table aggregates that information to track changes over time. Maps indicate which states conduct each of twelve types of oral health activities and which have full-time dental directors.

FIGURE 13–3 National Oral Health Surveillance System

the prevalence of oral diseases, the dental care delivery system, and the use of fluoridation. (See Figure 13-3 ∎.) The oral health indicators include the list in Box 13-4 ∎.

Did You Know?

The specific oral health disease patterns or dental rates for each state can be found at http://www.cdc.gov/nohss/.

Box 13–4 Specific National Oral Health Surveillance System Indicators

- Caries experience
- Complete tooth loss
- Dental sealants
- Dental visits
- Fluoridation status
- Oral and pharyngeal cancer
- Teeth cleaning
- Untreated caries

Summary

Evaluation is a mandatory phase of any type of dental hygiene program. A variety of evaluation mechanisms can be utilized during all phases of program planning. Dental indexes are frequently used to determine effectiveness of program planning.

The government has developed indicators to be used in evaluation. These are great resources to use when developing and evaluating programs. Using existing evidence helps the dental hygienist create programs that are evidence-based. Additionally, many government publications exist to report on research findings.

Self-Study Test Items

1. Program goals should be evaluated based on
   a. Measurement tools
   b. Baseline data
   c. National guidelines
   d. State surveillance records

2. During which phase of program planning should evaluation be started?
   a. Assessment
   b. Dental hygiene diagnosis
   c. Planning
   d. Evaluation

3. Which type of evaluation refers to the internal evaluation of a program?
   a. Formative
   b. Summative
   c. Quantitative
   d. Qualitative

4. Which type of evaluation is a basic screening?
   a. Nonclinical
   b. Clinical
   c. Provider driven
   d. Educational

5. An index that measures a condition that will not change, such as dental caries, is termed a(n)
   a. Clinical index
   b. Nonclinical index
   c. Irreversible index
   d. Reversible index

References

1. Wilkins E. *Clinical Practice of the Dental Hygienist.* 11th ed. Philadelphia, PA: Lippincott Williams and Wilkins; 2012.
2. Darby M. *Mosby's Comprehensive Review of Dental Hygiene.* 11th ed. St. Louis, MO: Elsevier; 2011.
3. Darby M, Walsh M. *Dental Hygiene Theory and Practice.* 3rd ed. St. Louis, MO: Elsevier; 2015.
4. Tomko P. *Kaplan National Dental Hygienist Licensure Exam.* New York, NY: Simon and Schuster; 2005.
5. Caton J, Polson A. The interdental bleeding index: a simplified procedure for monitoring gingival health. *Compendium Continuing Educ Dent.* 1985;6:88–92.
6. Caton J, Polson A, Bouwsma O, Blieden T, Frantz B, Espeland M. Associations between bleeding and visual signs of interdental gingival inflammation. *J Perodont.* 1988;59:722–727.
7. Bollmer BW, Sturzenberger OP, et al. A comparison of 3 clinical indices for measuring gingivitits. *J Clin Periodont.* 1986;13:392–395.
8. Loe, H. The Gingival Index, the Plaque Index, and the Retention Index. *J Periodont.* 1967;38:610–616.
9. Marks RG, Magnusson I, et al. Evaluation of reliability and reproductivity of dental indices. *J Clin Periodont.* 1993;20:54–58.
10. Dentistry and Oral Medicine. *The Medical Algorithms Project.* Houston, TX: Institute for Algorithmic Medicine; 2006–2007.
11. Ainamo J, et al. Development of the World Health Organization (WHO) Community Periodontal Index of Treatment Needs (CPITN). *Int Dent J.* 1982;32:281–291.
12. Periodontal Screening and Recording (PSR) Index: precursors, utility and limitations in a clinical setting. *J Lebanese Dent Assoc.* 2002;40(2):81–87.
13. Caries Prevalence: DMFT and DMFS from the World Health Organization: Switzerland. www.whocollab.od.mah.se/expl/orhdmft.html. Accessed June 17, 2009.
14. Katz RV. Assessing root caries in populations: the evolution of the root caries index. *J Public Health Dent.* 1980 Winter; 40(1):7–16.

15. Ugur T, Ciger S, Aksoy A, Telli A. An epidemiological survey using the Treatment Priority Index (TPI). *Eur J Orthod.* 1998;20:189–193.

16. Ununcu N, Ertugay E. The use of the Index of Orthodontic Treatment Need (IOTN) in a school population and referred population. *J Orthod.* 2001;28:45–52.

17. Wozniak K. Changes in developmental defects of dental enamel within the space of centuries. *Durham Anthropol J.* 2005;12(2–3).

18. Clarkson J. Review of terminology, classifications, and indices of developmental defects of enamel. *Adv Dent Res.* 1989;3(2):104–109.

19. Pereira A, Moreira B. Analysis of three dental fluorosis indexes used in epidemiological trials. *J Dent Braz.* 1999;10:1–60.

20. Pendrys DG. The Fluorosis Risk Index: a method for investigating risk factors. *J Public Health Dent.* 1990;50:291–298.

21. US Department of Health and Human Services. *Healthy People 2020.* Rretrieve from http://www.healthypeople.gov/2020/default.aspx on February 19, 2015.

22. National Oral Health Surveillance System. CDC: Atlanta, GA. Retrieved from on February 19, 2015.

Visit www.pearsonhighered.com/healthprofessionsresources to access the student resources that accompany this book. Simply select Dental Hygiene from the choice of disciplines. Find this book and you will find the complimentary study tools created for this specific title.

Dental Hygiene Research

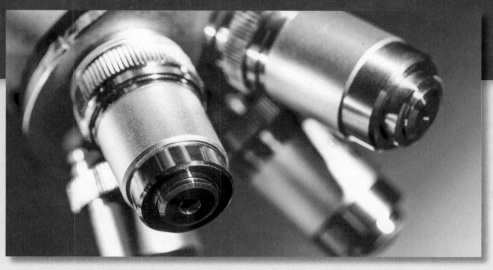

Science photo/Shutterstock

Dental hygiene practice is based on published research, meaning that practitioners derive decisions from documented evidence rather than anecdotal tradition. This is commonly referred to as **evidence-based practice.** Moreover, dental hygienists share the responsibility not only to practice science-based modalities but also to increase the scientific body of knowledge that encompasses the dental hygiene sciences.

Although many dental hygienists choose to practice in the clinical field, those working in other settings also incorporate research into their daily practice. It is imperative for the practitioner to fully understand basic research principles. Additionally, dental hygienists must be able to critically evaluate scientific literature and dental care products and modalities and subsequently communicate accurate information to the public whom they serve.

Research in Dental Hygiene

OBJECTIVES

After studying this chapter, the dental hygiene student should be able to:

- Explain the purpose of dental hygiene research
- Describe the role of research in dental hygiene
- Discuss the use of evidence-based practice in dental hygiene
- Explain the connection between research and private practice
- Describe the role of research in professional development

COMPETENCIES

After studying this chapter and participating in accompanying course activities, the dental hygiene student should be competent to do the following:

- Use evidence-based decision making to evaluate emerging technology and treatment modalities to integrate into patient dental hygiene care plans to achieve high-quality, cost-effective care
- Assume responsibility for professional actions and care based on accepted scientific theories, research, and the accepted standard of care
- Continuously perform self-assessment for lifelong learning and professional growth.
- Integrate accepted scientific theories and research into educational, preventive and therapeutic oral health services
- Pursue career opportunities within health care, industry, education, research, and other roles as they evolve for the dental hygienist

KEY TERMS

Discipline *184*
Evidence-based practice *181*
Field of study *184*
Occupation *184*
Scientific method *181*

Dental public health seeks to prevent or control disease through evidence-based programs that are cost-effective to administer. Conducting research is necessary to develop new programs that meet these criteria and to ensure entrenched programs have not become obsolete. To accurately interpret research and incorporate these findings, dental hygienists must understand basic research principles.

Much of dental hygiene practice exists within the confines of a private clinical setting in which the practitioner is concerned with a single patient at any given time. Dental hygienists' ability to assess an individual's condition, plan and carry out an intervention, and expect predictable results from treatment is predicated on a much larger sphere in which the study of dental disease and the creation of dental practices originate: the world of public health research.

The number of dental professionals who practice research full-time is small, yet the volume of information generated by medical, dental, and pharmaceutical researchers is more than the average practitioner has time to review thoroughly. Conducting research often can seem distant and unrelated to a practitioner's daily concerns; however, practice is based on this same research. The encounter of a dental hygienist with a single patient bears many commonalities to the structure of research methodology. (See Table 14-1 ■).

Research and Dental Public Health

Throughout history, astute practitioners have made many observations about the occurrence of disease in specific populations. Some illnesses seem to run in families. Others seem confined to specific ethnic groups, and other diseases are rarely seen in certain populations or specific locations. The study of disease in populations is accomplished by conducting research using the **scientific method,** which is a body of techniques using observation, reason, and experimentation to gather empirical and measurable evidence. (See Box 14-1 ■.) The accuracy of the research determines the usefulness of the information obtained and the conclusions that can be drawn. Good research is the foundation for understanding why disease occurs and how to prevent and control disease.

EVIDENCE-BASED PRACTICE   If dental hygiene advice and treatment are to be based on known methods with predictable results rather than anecdotes, scientific research is crucial. The requirement for using evidence-based dental hygiene means students can be taught the practice of dental hygiene based on independent research done by practitioners and scientists as reported in peer-reviewed health-related and dental hygiene journals. Emphasis should be placed on equipping future dental hygiene providers with the tools necessary to understand published research so this knowledge can be put into practice. For example, the standard treatment modality for a patient with incipient periodontal disease might be periodontal

Table 14–1 Analogy Between Private Practice and Research Methodology

Private Practice Methodology	Research Methodology
Identifies chief complaint	Takes survey or makes observations about a population
Takes health history	Conducts literature review
Makes diagnosis	Develops research question or hypothesis
Determines treatment plan	Writes research proposal
Obtains informed consent for treatment	Obtains informed consent
	Obtains research funding
Initiates treatment intervention	Conducts research
Recalls or Reevaluates Patient	Analyzes and publishes research results

Box 14–1 Steps of the Scientific Method

1. Name the problem or question
2. Form an educated guess (hypothesis) of the cause of the problem and make predictions based on the hypothesis
3. Test hypothesis by doing an experiment or study (with proper controls)
4. Check and interpret results
5. Report results to the scientific community

debridement, more commonly referred to as nonsurgical periodontal therapy. A return to health and normal probing depths would be expected in a reliable percentage of cases treated in this fashion.

Evidence-based practice also considers patient preferences. (See Figure 14-1 ■.) This would include what treatment option the patient is interested in receiving as well as patient compliance. Simply put, without the patient's interest or motivation in attaining periodontal health, so daily plaque biofilm removal is practiced, no nonsurgical or surgical treatment will be effective in the long-term.

Dental hygienists who graduated from school several decades ago were more likely to base their practices on what their instructors had learned from trial and error and

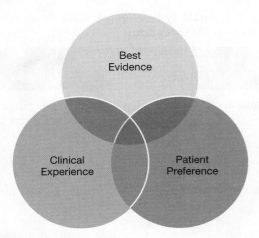

FIGURE 14–1 Evidence-Based Practice

anecdotal reports from other dental hygienists, the proverbial "what worked for them." Although this anecdotal approach has frequently been the basis for treatment, this approach is not the most scientific or reliable method. Clinicians are not the only people who are frequently swayed by anecdotal tales. Dental hygienists encounter patients daily who have selected an oral care product because of an advertisement or because the product worked for a friend.

Dental hygiene practice has changed as the result of research. For many years, instructors taught that fluoride treatments should be provided only after scaling and polishing. Likewise, patients were instructed to brush and floss at home prior to rinsing with fluoride. The prevailing argument was that the plaque biofilm needed to be removed for the fluoride to be effective. These practices

DENTAL HYGIENIST SPOTLIGHT ·····················

Public Health Column: Gayle McCombs, RDH, MS

Gayle McCombs, RDH, MS, is a dedicated researcher with a public health agenda who helps broaden the science on which dental hygiene practice is built. She currently is an associate professor and the director of the Old Dominion University Dental Hygiene Research Center. She is the author of several published research papers and has spoken on numerous topics. Professor McCombs has also won numerous research awards. She exemplifies a dental hygiene scholar with a focus on building the knowledge base of the profession and practice.

She answered the following questions about her career.

How did you decide to pursue dental hygiene as a career?

After working as a dental assistant for many years and observing the dental hygienist in the office, I decided that I wanted to advance my career. While in dental hygiene school, one of my instructors was very instrumental in formulating my life's goals. Unfortunately, after graduation, she became very ill with cancer. One day while I was visiting her in hospice, she made me promise that I would continue my education and become a teacher.

For the next ten years, while working in private practice, I pursued my bachelor's degree, and I ended up teaching in the Florida and South Carolina community college systems. As time went by, I wanted to broaden my professional options. I decided to press on for a master's degree at the University of North Carolina-Chapel Hill. It was during graduate school

that I was introduced to clinical research. Throughout the program, the mentorship and support I received from professors Rebecca Wilder and Steven Offenbacher, in addition to the experience I gained, shaped my career.

Did you need additional education or credentials for dental hygiene research?

I acquired my research foundation in graduate school; however, most of my practical experience is a result of working as a research faculty member at UNC-CH. Learning how to manage and coordinate clinical trials involves a great deal of organizational skill. In addition to sponsor and governmental regulations, there are professional and ethical responsibilities that must be adhered to.

Agencies such as the National Institutes of Health (NIH), the Food and Drug Administration (FDA), the pharmaceutical industry, local universities, and private clinical research training organizations such as the Society of Clinical Research Associates (SoCRA) offer numerous continuing education courses and workshops in clinical trial management. There are also various online training opportunities to become certified or obtain specialty training in topics such as monitoring, regulatory affairs, and clinical trial design and management.

What is the most valuable piece of advice you can give?

Be adaptable, self-motivated, and have the capability to be a leader, as well as a team player.

What do you think the future holds for this field?

I believe it is wide open for those individuals who are interested in research. When our graduate students complete the program, they have no problem finding employment. I think one of the most rewarding aspects of my job is getting students energized about research. I mentor students who are fearful of the process and then watch as they become excited about research once they realize they can be successful.

Do you have any suggestions for others who may be considering research as a career?

My suggestion to those who would like to follow this path would be start out simple. Volunteer for a study, take a course, shadow someone in research, search the Internet, and read your professional journals. Seek out someone who is involved in clinical research and observe for a day or two to see whether this is something that sparks your interest.

Source: Christine Nathe writes the Public Health Column in *RDH* magazine published by Pennwell Publishing. For more public health spotlights please see RDH magazine online at http://www.rdhmag.com/index.html.

remained the standard of care for many years until one day a researcher questioned them, and discovering a lack of evidence to support them, conducted a research study to test their effectiveness. The research study revealed fluoride can indeed penetrate plaque.[1,2] Dental hygiene practice based on documented evidence from critically reviewed research is referred to as evidence-based practice.[3] However, many dental hygienists continue to remove all plaque with prophy paste prior to applying fluoride. In this case, the anecdotal method and the method based on scientific research differ widely.

The importance of conducting dental hygiene research is to establish a scientifically based standard of care for the practice of dental hygiene. Understanding something about research methods benefits any dental hygienist whether directly involved in conducting research or only occasionally reading about it to be able to critically decide whether the research has scientific merit and should be applied in daily practice.

Did You Know?

Dental hygienists need to conduct dental hygiene research to validate current methods of practice and to investigate new ones.

Because of what is now known about the multifactorial nature of disease, which will be discussed in more detail in Chapter 18, using the same anecdotal treatment that met with success on patient A does not guarantee that patient B will obtain the same results.

The Role of Research in Dental Hygiene

Research, surprisingly, has had a cornerstone role in dental hygiene since the inception of the practice. Dr. Fones actually developed and implemented a research study using his first trained class of dental hygienists within the Bridgeport Public School setting. Unfortunately, after the initial study, dental hygienists did not routinely conduct research in the early years, although dental hygiene did benefit from results obtained from other health and dental research focused on preventive modalities.

Historical Aspect of Research in Dental Hygiene

Dental hygiene was promoted in the early days by research conducted by Dr. Alfred C. Fones, the founder of dental hygiene.[4] As soon as he was able to get permission to begin the first class of dental hygienists, within the Bridgeport Public Schools, he began the first documented study on the impact of dental hygienists on schoolchildren.

The first school-based dental clinic began operation in 1914, and the research results yielded by the practice were published in 1921. Before implementing the preventive dental clinics, Dr. Fones interestingly pointed out a major health issue that affected schoolchildren:

> If otherwise, a ten year old boy's body appears normal we ask him open his mouth. Here we find teeth covered with green stain; temporary and permanent teeth badly decayed, possibly fistulas on the gum surface showing an outlet for pus from an abscessed tooth or teeth and decomposing food around and between the teeth. Here at the gateway of the system is a source of infection and poison that would contaminate every mouthful of food taken into his body, no wonder that the child suffers from an auto-intoxication which produces eye-strain, anemia, malaise, constipation, headaches, fevers and many other ailments.[4]

In order to show if placing dental hygienists in schools was effective in preventing and reducing disease, Fones implemented an evaluation method. The dental hygienists collected data on the condition of the mouths of children and also included a control group of older children who had never had a school-based dental clinic in younger years. Data showed a reduction of 34 percent of dental decay in permanent teeth. Additionally, Fones noted the excessive consumption of sugar as an issue, which resulted in the dental decay and thereafter mentioned malocclusion as a secondary issue. One especially engaging statistic was

that Fones found only three children out of a hundred with teeth that were entirely free from dental caries. He also noted the relationship between bacterial infections and communicable diseases to oral infection.[4] In 1926, an article published in the *Journal of the American Dental Hygienists' Association* (now titled *Journal of Dental Hygiene*) presented information on research that documented the effectiveness of dental hygiene.[5]

In fact, the preventive oral health services provided by dental hygienists have been supported by research, and the practice of dental hygiene expanded as a result of research findings since the inception over 100 years ago.[5] However, most research in dental hygiene did not commence until the 1960s. The most compelling reason for this was that this was the era the first Master's Degree in Dental Hygiene began. As witnessed in most disciplines, research is conducted by dental hygienists with terminal degrees.

Did You Know?

A terminal degree typically refers to the highest degree available in a discipline. In most disciplines this is a doctoral degree, but in dental hygiene a master's degree is the terminal degree. This may be changing because Idaho State University is in the process of developing a doctoral degree program in dental hygiene.

The ADHA appointed the first Committee on Research in the 1970s followed by the creation of the ADHA Foundation, now called the ADHA Institute of Oral Health, which provides funding for the educational and research activities of dental hygienists.[6] The Committee on Research became the Council on Research in the 1980s, further emphasizing the importance of dental hygiene research to the profession. The first text book on research in dental hygiene was written by Darby and Bowen in 1980, which is also the decade the national research conferences began being conducted regularly.[7] By the 1990s, ADHA had established a research division within the headquarters in Chicago. By the turn of the century, the MSDH programs grew in number, dental hygiene publications increased, and dental hygienists frequently conducted and disseminated their results in dental and dental hygiene periodicals and venues.[8]

Did You Know?

If dental hygiene is to evolve as a specific scientific discipline, a research base solely generated by the profession must be established.

Currently, the National Research Agenda includes the following the priorities, health promotion, disease prevention, health services research, professional education and development, clinical care and occupational health and safety. The National Center for Dental Hygiene Research and Practice supports dental hygienists conducting

research and educators' teaching research. For more information about this please see the companion website.

Dental Hygiene: A Developing Discipline?

Undoubtedly, the most profound goal of dental hygiene research should be to improve the public's oral health. Another compelling reason for dental hygienists to conduct and promote dental hygiene research is to advance and promote the profession of dental hygiene, which should subsequently improve the public's oral health.

In landmark reports, dental hygiene has been described as a developing discipline by some and a field of study by others.[9–11] Essentially, the term **field of study** represents a subdiscipline or an area of emphasis within the larger context of a **discipline.**[9] Although the terms discipline and field of study are used differently in some professions, they have been defined by the dental hygiene profession in terms of the following indicators, a relevant theoretical body of knowledge, possessing a societal need and demand and lastly learning by a master in the field.

In order for dental hygiene to be viewed as a discipline and not merely a field of dentistry, it is imperative that dental hygiene has a unique knowledge base that focuses on the scientific basis of dental hygiene practice and that this knowledge base is driven by dental hygiene research conducted by dental hygienists.

Dental hygienists can be involved in basic research, but the majority of dental hygienists will conduct translational research. Translational research simply defined is when scientific discoveries are translated into practical applications.[12] Scientists discover phenomena when conducting basic research. Translational researchers then apply this new found knowledge to clinical care and evaluate the outcome.

Secondly, dental hygiene must have a societal need and demand. Society must have a need for dental hygiene treatment and the population must be demanding that the care is being provided by a dental hygienists and not some other provider. Lastly, dental hygienists must be trained by experts in their area. Namely, dental hygiene professors with their terminal degrees in dental hygiene.

Whether conducting research or providing care, the ability to comprehensively work as a team is important in all aspects. Although a profession may strive to be scientific discipline, it is vital that all disciplines are multidimensional and interprofessional in nature. Importantly, a discipline although unique is still dependent upon research and practice with an interprofessional team. And, although dental hygiene may be considered a developing discipline, there is much advancement to be attained, which is why dental hygienists must continue to conduct research phenomenon germane to the dental hygiene sciences.

Walsh and Ortega proposed the scholarly identity of the dental hygienist as professional will continue advancing practice.[13] (See Box 14-2 ■.)

The definition of a professional depicts one who possesses a distinct body of knowledge, utilizes a specialized

Box 14–2 Definition of a Scholarly Identity

- Has a sense of the dental hygiene discipline as a whole
- Has a lifelong commitment to the development of the dental hygiene discipline's knowledge base by asking and answering research questions central to the discipline
- Uses evidence to support one's viewpoint
- Considers the related work of other dental hygiene scholars as well as that of other disciplines
- Reports one's own results in the context of those of others in the field and beyond
- Disseminates the findings of one's work through scientific publication

Source: Walsh MW, Ortega EO. Developing a scholarly identity and building a community of scholars. Special Commemorative Issue. 100th. *Journal of Dental Hygiene.* 2013:15–19.

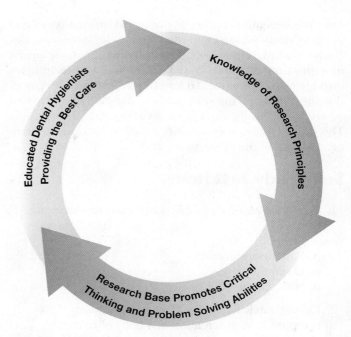

FIGURE 14–2 The Professional Model

skill set to earn a livelihood, conducts himself by a code of ethics unique to his discipline, acts autonomously to formulate decisions, and is regulated by his own profession.[14–16] Bowen has described term "profession" as linked to prestige, credibility, and image as much as it is to autonomy, service, and a scientific theoretical base.[9] In essence a professional should be knowledgeable in a specialized area, ethical and self-directed. Further, a health care professional should try to help patients, prevent further harm or disease and work to advance the particular health care science.[13,14]

Darby and Walsh discussed the conceptual model of the Occupational versus the Professional dental hygienist.[14] This model is significant for multiple reasons. The model operationalizes the dental hygienist's functioning paradigm; addresses the responsibility of the dental hygienist to one's self, the patient, and other professionals; and provides a potential solution to the crisis of access to dental care.[13] While personality and experience are contributing factors, the formal training a dental hygienist receives will chiefly influence one's tendency towards a specific paradigm.[17]

The Occupational Model, as defined by Darby and Walsh, is a conceptual model based on technical competence.[14] The dental hygienist focuses mechanical abilities on disease management as defined and delegated by the supervising dentist.[10] Procedural care is routine, uncomplicated, and considered trivial; recall appointments are predictable; and perspectives toward the patient are paternalistic because the dentist is responsible for oral health outcomes.[14] The practice of dental hygiene is deemed risky if unsupervised; therefore, organized dentistry assumes responsibility for close regulation and influence on the private and public practice of dental hygiene.[10] Ultimately, dental hygienists have little to no ownership of the actions of their care or responsibility to the patients they are serving.[17]

The opposite of a dental hygiene technician is a dental hygiene professional, the second component of Darby and Walsh's theory (See Figure 14-2 ■.) The Professional

Model is grounded in the belief everything a dental hygienist does is derived from a solid, scientific research base.[14] A research base promotes critical thinking and problem-solving abilities as the dental hygienist uses a process of care system to seek the overall wellness of the client.[14] The focus then shifts to a proactive risk assessment and prevention strategy instead of a reactive disease management approach.[14] Because the dental hygienist assumes personal responsibility to the patient, prevention-oriented care is highly valued and appointments become personalized, based on the need of the patient.[14] The oral health care professional is considered to be a co-therapist member of the primary care team, and thus is not limited to private clinical practice as the only venue for employment.[14] By looking beyond clinical practice as the only answer to populations accessing care, the dental hygienist assumes a visionary, proactive role in providing a solution instead of compounding the problem.[17]

The role research can play in the professional is pivotal to the advancement of the profession. Further development of a body of dental hygiene research will help position the profession alongside other academically reconized health care disciplines.[18] Although many dental hygienists will not engage in basic, clinical, or translational research during their careers, all dental hygienists need to understand basic research concepts. Moreover, the dental hygienists should have the skills to communicate research results to patients and the public as needed.

Summary

Dental public health has been an important component in the creation of a body of research that impacts dental hygiene practice. Every dental hygienist, whether or not directly involved in research, should be familiar with basic

research design, including hypotheses, various types and merit of study designs, and the uses and limits of statistics. Each individual clinician supports a scientific discipline by incorporating evidence-based knowledge and techniques into his or her practice. To be effective in initiating, conducting, and applying research, the dental hygienist must be able to critically analyze the existing body of literature. This crucial link allows scientific study to become the standard of care in the profession.

Self-Study Test Items

1. Evidence-based decisions come from research, practice, and
   a. Science
   b. Patient preferences
   c. Disciplines
   d. None of the above

2. Dental public health has been an important component in the creation of a body of research that impacts dental hygiene practice. Every dental hygienist, whether or not directly involved in research, should be familiar with basic research design.
   a. The first statement is true; the second statement is false.
   b. The first statement is false; the second statement is true.
   c. Both statements are true.
   d. Both statements are false.

3. An occupational dental hygienist provides care based on
   a. Dentists' recommendations
   b. Evidence-based knowledge
   c. Sales representatives' advice
   d. Internet search and clinical knowledge

4. In clinical practice, the dental hygienist completes a health history on a patient. In research, the dental hygienist would complete a parallel function called
   a. Research proposal
   b. Informed consent
   c. Literature review
   d. Reference check

5. Dental hygiene research began two decades ago, after the MSDH programs were created.
   a. The first statement is true; the second statement is false.
   b. The first statement is false; the second statement is true.

c. Both statements are true.
d. Both statements are false.

References

1. Ripa LW. Open questions and form. In: Wei S, ed. *Clinical Uses of Fluoride.* Philadelphia, PA: Lea and Febiger; 1985.
2. ADHA position paper on polishing procedures. Retrieved from http://www.adha.org/profissues/prophylaxis.htm. on June 22, 2009.
3. Fourth national research conference agenda. Chicago, IL: American Dental Hygienists' Association; 1999.
4. Fones AC. *Report of Five Years of Mouth Hygiene in the Public Schools of Bridgeport, Connecticut.* Documents Division. Library of Congress: Washington DC, April 18, 1921.
5. Booker PD. Oral hygiene as an exact science. *J Dent Hyg.* 1926; 11(2): 14–22.
6. Bowen DM. History of dental hygiene research. *Journal of Dental Hygiene.* Special Commemorative Issue. 100th. 2013:5–14.
7. Darby ML, Bowen DM. *Research Methods for Oral Health Professionals.* St. Louis, MO: CV Mosby; 1980.
8. Nathe CN. Advancing dental public health and dental hygiene research. *RDH.* 2013. Retrieved from http://www.rdhmag.com/articles/print/volume-33/issue-3/columns/advancing-dental-public-health-and-dental-hygiene-research.html February 13, 2014.
9. Bowen, DM. Dental hygiene: a developing discipline? Dental Hygiene, Volume 62, number 1: 1988.
10. Karlsson, IB. Dental hygiene: field of study. Dental Hygiene, Volume 62, number 1: 1988.
11. Cobban SJ. Edgington EM. Compton SM. An argument for dental hygiene to develop as a discipline. Int J Dent Hygiene 5, 2007; 13–21 2007
12. Nathe, CN. The use of translational research in dental hygiene. RDH. Retrieved from http://www.rdhmag.com/articles/print/volume-27/issue-9/columns/the-use-of-translational-research-in-dental-hygiene.html on August 24, 2015.
13. Walsh MW, Ortega EO. Developing a scholarly identity and building a community of scholars. Special Commemorative Issue. 100th. *Journal of Dental Hygiene.* 2013:15–19.
14. Darby ML, Walsh MM. A proposed human needs conceptual model for dental hygiene. *J Dent Hyg.* 1993;67(6):326–334;
15. Merriam-Webster Dictionary. Definition of *Professional.* 2013. Retrieved on http://www.merriam-webster.com/dictionary/professional on August 25, 2015
16. Ozar DT. Professionalism: challenges for dentistry in the future. *Journal of Forensic Odontostomatology.* 2012;30(1):72–84.
17. Beatty C. *Evaluation of Curricula for the Dental Hygiene Occupational and Professional Models [thesis].* University of New Mexico. Retrieved from http://repository.unm.edu/handle/1928/24234 on October 13, 2015.
18. Lyle, DM, Dental hygiene and research: irrevocably connected. *J Evid Base Dent Pract* 2014;14S:227–234.

15

Ethical Principles in Research

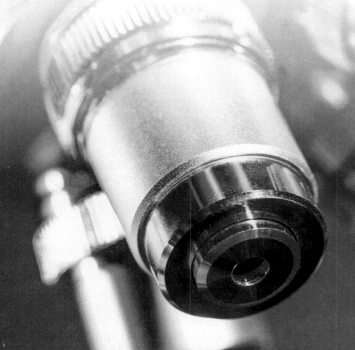

OBJECTIVES

After studying this chapter, the dental hygiene student should be able to:

- Describe the evolution of ethics in research
- Define common ethical principal terminologies
- Describe the role of ethics in research
- Identify the role of government and private entities in research

COMPETENCIES

After studying this chapter and participating in accompanying course activities, the dental hygiene student should be competent to do the following:

- Apply a professional code of ethics in all endeavors
- Adhere to state and federal laws, recommendations and regulations in the provision of oral health care
- Use critical thinking skills and comprehensive problem-solving to identify oral health care strategies that promote patient health and wellness
- Assume responsibility for professional actions and care based on accepted scientific theories, research, and the accepted standard of care
- Continuously perform self-assessment for lifelong learning and professional growth.
- Integrate accepted scientific theories and research into educational, preventive and therapeutic oral health services

KEY TERMS

Autonomy *188*
Beneficence *188*
Bioethics *188*
Health Information Portability and Accountability Act (HIPAA) *191*
Informed consent *190*
Institutional review board (IRB) *190*
Justice *188*
Misconduct *190*
Nonmaleficence *188*
Paternalism *188*
Veracity *188*

The participation of individual subjects in research studies has the potential to improve clinical care and health outcomes. Ultimately, research can improve the quality of life for many. Although results can yield new modalities, it is important to not cause harm to individual subjects participating in research. Researchers and clinicians should understand and appreciate ethical dimensions associated with research projects and be able to describe the history of ethics in research and the ethical principals involved in the conduction of research.

Ethical Considerations in Research

Bioethics, an important aspect of conducting research, refers to the inherent role of ethics in health care and the established norms that distinguish between morally acceptable and unacceptable research practices. The field of ethics has its origins with the father of modern medicine, Hippocrates, who developed an oath of medical ethics in 400 BC. Hippocrates is long remembered as the individual who helped create the distinct profession of medicine.

As depicted in Box 15-1 ■, the Hippocratic Oath, which is widely regarded for its moral construct, clearly defines ethical standards for a physician. Since then, the definition of what constitutes ethical research has continued to evolve. Relevant terms are important for the dental hygienist to understand when making ethical decisions in practice or research. For instance, **nonmaleficence** means that a health care provider's first obligation to the patient is to do not harm. Further, the provider should not to inflict harm, should prevent harm, remove harm, and do or promote good.

This leads to the next term, **beneficence,** which actually requires that existing harm be removed. The premise of beneficence is to provide quality health care, which is a benefit to the patient.

Autonomy is the ability to govern one's profession and to basically be self-determined and directed as a profession. Additionally, autonomy is based on respect for others–sometimes referred to as respect for persons–which emphasizes the belief that patients have the power to make decisions about issues that may affect their health. Actually, respect for the individual was the guiding principle for the development of the Declaration of Helsinki, which was written by the World Medical Association to define the ethical principles that would serve as a standard for human subject research.

Paternalism involves that dental hygienist or dental hygiene researcher doing what he or she thinks is best for the patient according to his or her ability and judgment. Although autonomy and paternalism seem to be contradictory in definition, the dental hygienist will use both of them for the evidence-based research and treatment.

Justice refers to providing patients, test subjects, or populations with what is owed, due, or deserved. Justice is trying to promote fairness during treatment or research. And lastly, **veracity** can be defined simply as being honest.

Box 15–1 Hippocratic Oath

I swear by Apollo the physician, and Asclepius, and Hygieia and Panacea and all the gods and goddesses as my witnesses, that, according to my ability and judgment, I will keep this Oath and this contract:

- To hold him who taught me this art equally dear to me as my parents, to be a partner in life with him, and to fulfill his needs when required; to look upon his offspring as equals to my own siblings, and to teach them this art, if they shall wish to learn it, without fee or contract; and that by the set rules, lectures, and every other mode of instruction, I will impart a knowledge of the art to my own sons, and those of my teachers, and to students bound by this contract and having sworn this Oath to the law of medicine, but to no others.
- I will use those dietary regimens which will benefit my patients according to my greatest ability and judgment, and I will do no harm or injustice to them.
- I will not give a lethal drug to anyone if I am asked, nor will I advise such a plan; and similarly I will not give a woman a pessary to cause an abortion.
  In purity and according to divine law will I carry out my life and my art.
- I will not use the knife, even upon those suffering from stones, but I will leave this to those who are trained in this craft.
- Into whatever homes I go, I will enter them for the benefit of the sick, avoiding any voluntary act of impropriety or corruption, including the seduction of women or men, whether they are free men or slaves.
- Whatever I see or hear in the lives of my patients, whether in connection with my professional practice or not, which ought not to be spoken of outside, I will keep secret, as considering all such things to be private.
- So long as I maintain this Oath faithfully and without corruption, may it be granted to me to partake of life fully and the practice of my art, gaining the respect of all men for all time. However, should I transgress this Oath and violate it, may the opposite be my fate.

Translated by Michael North, National Library of Medicine, 2002.

Source: Greek Medicine. History of Medicine Division, National Library of Medicine. Bethesda, MD: National Institutes of Health. Retrieved on January 22, 2014 from http://www.nlm.nih.gov/hmd/greek/greek_oath.html

Did You Know?

Integrity or veracity have similar meanings and many have theorized that honesty is a personal characteristic that can permeate a researcher's persona.

After World War II, the Nuremberg War Crimes trials brought to light examples of medical research that had clearly exploited human beings. Crimes had been committed that involved unethical research on humans that were

Box 15–2 The Nuremberg Code

1. The voluntary consent of the human subject is absolutely essential. This means that the person involved should have legal capacity to give consent; should be so situated as to be able to exercise free power of choice, without the intervention of any element of force, fraud, deceit, duress, over-reaching, or other ulterior form of constraint or coercion; and should have sufficient knowledge and comprehension of the elements of the subject matter involved, as to enable him to make an understanding and enlightened decision. This latter element requires that, before the acceptance of an affirmative decision by the experimental subject, there should be made known to him the nature, duration, and purpose of the experiment; the method and means by which it is to be conducted; all inconveniences and hazards reasonably to be expected; and the effects upon his health or person, which may possibly come from his participation in the experiment.
2. The duty and responsibility for ascertaining the quality of the consent rests upon each individual who initiates, directs or engages in the experiment. It is a personal duty and responsibility which may not be delegated to another with impunity.
3. The experiment should be such as to yield fruitful results for the good of society, unprocurable by other methods or means of study, and not random and unnecessary in nature.
4. The experiment should be so designed and based on the results of animal experimentation and a knowledge of the natural history of the disease or other problem under study, that the anticipated results will justify the performance of the experiment.
5. The experiment should be so conducted as to avoid all unnecessary physical and mental suffering and injury.
6. No experiment should be conducted, where there is an *a priori* reason to believe that death or disabling injury will occur; except, perhaps, in those experiments where the experimental physicians also serve as subjects.
7. The degree of risk to be taken should never exceed that determined by the humanitarian importance of the problem to be solved by the experiment.
8. Proper preparations should be made and adequate facilities provided to protect the experimental subject against even remote possibilities of injury, disability, or death.
9. The experiment should be conducted only by scientifically qualified persons. The highest degree of skill and care should be required through all stages of the experiment of those who conduct or engage in the experiment.
10. During the course of the experiment, the human subject should be at liberty to bring the experiment to an end, if he has reached the physical or mental state, where continuation of the experiment seemed to him to be impossible.
11. During the course of the experiment, the scientist in charge must be prepared to terminate the experiment at any stage, if he has probable cause to believe, in the exercise of the good faith, superior skill and careful judgment required of him, that a continuation of the experiment is likely to result in injury, disability, or death to the experimental subject.

Source: "Trials of War Criminals before the Nuremberg Military Tribunals under Control Council Law No. 10", Vol. 2, pp. 181–182. Washington, D.C.: U.S. Government Printing Office, 1949.] Retrieved on January 22, 2014 from http://www.hhs.gov/ohrp/archive/nurcode.html.

held in concentration camps, such as researching the effects of and treatments for high altitude conditions; freezing; malaria; poison gas; sulfanilamide; bone, muscle, and nerve regeneration; bone transplantation; saltwater consumption; epidemic jaundice; sterilization; typhus; poisons; and incendiary bombs.[1] Box 15-2 ■ defines standards developed after the Nuremberg trials.

The United States had its own sad chapter in unethical research practices from 1932 to 1972 in the Tuskegee study of syphilis. Men of African-American descent had agreed to be examined and treated in a US Public Health Service (US PHS) study on syphilis, but the men were not informed about the real purpose of the study and had been misled. Even more troubling, when penicillin became the drug of choice for syphilis in 1940s, researchers did not offer it to the subjects nor did they give the subjects the option to quit the study.[2]

As a result of these exploitations, medical research became a slow, laborious process with many checks and balances to protect human subjects. In the 1990s, activists

for persons with AIDS complained to Congress about the long time required to obtain approval for new treatments and drugs. People with AIDS were willing to take some personal risk to get treatments on the market faster. As a result of their lobbying efforts, some of the protections in human research were changed to permit the Food and Drug Administration (FDA) to implement a fast-track approval process for drug companies. More recently, the Ebola outbreak in Africa reiterated the need for safe and effective research protocols to reduce the chance of a communicable disease pandemic.

ETHICS AND THE LAW Ethics "in a nutshell" is about doing what is the right thing. In a research setting, ethics also involves ensuring that the organizational mission and goals are upheld. Ethical behavior in research may be described as what is right, legal, and fair. What sometimes makes it more difficult is that what is right, legal, or fair is not always obvious, which can make for an ethical dilemma. Making good ethical decisions in research can help

an institution, researchers, and society as a whole. On the other hand, poor ethical choices tend to accumulate or snowball and can sometimes become unethical habits, which can affect all of us.

Ethics in medical research goes beyond what the law requires. A course of action may be legal but not ethical. Large institutions including the Food and Drug Administration (FDA), Environmental Protection Agency (EPA), National Institutes of Health (NIH), and all major universities have their own code of ethics. Institutions that conduct medical research usually have an entity known as the **institutional review board (IRB)** charged with reviewing the ethical implications of every research study. The IRB has two responsibilities.

Did You Know?

Most college IRB boards have unique titles and acronyms. For instance, at the University of New Mexico, the Human Research Review Committee (HRRC) serves as the IRB.

First, it must ensure that the rights and safety of the research subjects are respected and protected. Second, it must protect the institution and the researchers against lawsuits and help to ensure that the research results will not be flawed because the study was ethically unsound. The IRB holds the researchers accountable to the public. A research proposal may have to pass the scrutiny of more than one IRB. The institution funding the research and the institution where it is actually conducted may each have its own board.

ETHICAL ISSUES OF RESEARCH   The *Belmont Report: Ethical Principles and Guidelines for the Protection of Human Subjects of Research, Report of the National Commission for the Protection of Human Subjects of Biomedical and Behavioral Research*, commonly referred to as the Belmont Report, was developed by the National Commission for the Protection of Human Subjects of Biomedical and Behavioral Research. The Belmont Report describes ethical principles and guidelines for research involving human subjects. Three principles are identified: respect for persons, beneficence, and justice. Also included are informed consent, assessment of risks and benefits, and selection of subjects.

A number of ethical considerations involved in doing research are common to all institutions. The first is research **misconduct.** This includes plagiarism, copyright or patent infringement, falsifying or fabricating data, misrepresenting data, and conflict of interest. Like malpractice, research misconduct must be intentional. Bias, unintentional negligence, or disagreement about the meaning of the results does not constitute misconduct. Animal research has ethical guidelines that usually include such things as making

sure the animals do not suffer needlessly, are euthanized for no reason, prohibiting frivolous research, and requiring proper care for the animals during the course of the studies. (See Box 15-3 ■.)

Informed consent, another ethical consideration, requires educating a subject in a research study about the study's purpose, duration, experimental procedures, alternatives, risks, and benefits. Informed consent requires information to be presented so that prospective research subjects can voluntarily decide whether or not to participate; it is a fundamental mechanism to ensure respect for persons by having them give thoughtful consent for a voluntary act. Human study participation must always be voluntary. In the past, research projects conducted at closed institutions, such as prisons, were often coercive in recruiting subjects. Participants must be free to participate or not and to withdraw at any time for any reason.

The procedures used in obtaining informed consent should be designed to educate the subject population in terms that they can understand. Therefore, informed consent language and documentation must be written in "lay language" (ie, understandable to the people being asked to participate) and written in a language understood by the subject. The written presentation of information is used to document the basis for consent and for the subjects' future reference. The consent document should be revised when deficiencies are noted or when additional information would improve the consent process.[3] Informed consent for research involves presenting the research information orally and obtaining written consent prior to a subject's entering into a study and documenting the consent process in the subject's medical record or research file.

When research involves human subjects, an informed consent must be obtained except in one circumstance: If the research uses survey methodology, such as a questionnaire or an interview, the subjects' willing participation in answering the questions is their informed consent. They can decline to participate or can refuse to answer specific questions. However, if the study participant is a minor, a non-English-speaking person, or someone not competent to give consent (such as a person with Alzheimer's disease), a valid informed consent becomes an extremely important ethical piece of the research.

Federally established guidelines regulate research conducted on people. An outline for an informed consent and a sample document are presented on the interactive Companion Website created specifically to accompany this textbook. Other ethical considerations in human research involve confidentiality. Research subjects are never identified when research is published. However, the researcher may ask for a subject's consent to use photographs in an article. In clinical research, dental hygienists–investigators often stand in dual roles to the subject: as a practicing dental hygienist and as a researcher. For the practicing dental hygienist, the responsibility of confidentiality has long been established under well-known legal

Box 15–3 Radium Girls: Another Public Health Disaster

In the early 1900s, [a] US Radium Corporation['s] factory in New Jersey that made timepieces for the military, employed young women to paint the faces of the watch dials with luminescent paint made from radium, a radioactive substance. The work was too delicate to be done by machine. The girls used very fine sable brushes to trace the numbers on the dial, which they often moistened with their tongues. In addition they often used the glow-in-the-dark substance for more fun endeavors such as painting their fingernails. Radium was invisible, odorless, tasteless, and—according to the employer—completely harmless.

It was not long before a number of girls fell ill with bone pain, loose teeth, anemia, jaw tumors, and necrosis of the jaw. Joseph Knef, a dentist who treated several of the girls, suspected the radium exposure as a cause of their illness. He devised an ingenious method to ascertain a crude measurement of the radioactivity by wrapping extracted teeth and pieces of jaw in dental x-ray film for several days and then developing the film. It is likely that the medical and dental x-rays of the time exposed the women to significant additional radiation exposure.

One woman, Grace Fryer, decided to sue. It took several years to find a lawyer but her case was finally taken up by the Consumer League of New Jersey, and she was joined in the lawsuit by four other women who also worked at the factory.

The company denied accusations that radium was to blame for the women's illness. Company doctors who knew of the dangers and monitored the women produced advertisements of the time indicating radium was a curative for cancer, and suppressed the women's company medical files. Doctors insisted the women were in perfect health. Company owners attempted to smear the women's reputation by insisting their illnesses were the result of syphilis or diphtheria. The company refused to pay for the women's medical expenses. Company lawyers used delaying tactics to avoid a trial until the women were dead or too sick to assist in the prosecution. Marie Curie was even called in to give an expert deposition.

As the women began to die, an out-of-court settlement was reached. The company agreed to pay the women's medical expenses and each woman was awarded $10,000 in damages.

The first article on the association of radium and jaw necrosis was published in the *Journal of the American Dental Association* in 1924. By the mid-1930s all five of the women were dead. The total number of women affected by the radium is unknown, but the plant employed thousands of workers in plants throughout the country. Additional lawsuits followed in Illinois and other states. As a result of this case, new legislation was enacted that improved industrial safety standards and gave workers the right to sue for damages. The cleanup of the factory sites, local water, soil, and subsequent buildings erected on the sites have cost the Environmental Protection Agency millions of dollars. Some towns still have radium "hotspots" to this day.

Source: Based on Clark C. *Radium Girls: Women and Industrial Health Reform, 1910–1935.* Chapel Hill, NC: University of North Carolina Press; 1997.

and ethical standards. The **Health Information Portability and Accountability Act (HIPAA)** adds to these standards in practice and research. When a covered entity conducts clinical research involving protected health information (PHI), dental hygienists–investigators must understand the HIPAA privacy rule's restrictions on the use and disclosure of patient's PHI, such as information from a patient's medical chart or test results, as well as an individual's billing information for medical services rendered, when that information is held or transmitted by an entity. PHI also includes identifiable health information about subjects of clinical research gathered by a researcher who is a health care provider.

Another issue related to human research is the participant's right to receive treatment, as was the case with research into new AIDS treatments in the 1990s. Many prospective research studies rely on a control group who does not receive treatment to prove efficacy. Studies now offer most control groups access to the experimental treatment at the end of the study if they so choose. In contrast, participants need to be protected from experimental treatments or tests that might cause harm.

Did You Know?

Not too long ago, studies at the NIH on hormone replacement therapy was stopped early because the treatment was shown to be harmful and continuing the study could not be ethically justified.

Without a doubt, the worst ethical chapter in American research history was the aforementioned Tuskegee study. In 1932, the Public Health Service recruited close to six hundred African-American men from Alabama to do a historical study on the progression of syphilis and its presentation at autopsy. Many believed that this prospective study on African-American men could be compared to an earlier retrospective study conducted in Norwegian men. At the onset of the Tuskegee study, there was no cure for the disease. The men were given free medical care for their participation and additional monetary benefits, which was adequate incentive because the men were poor farmers. In the late 1940s, penicillin was discovered and became the

standard treatment for syphilis, but the men were never told about this cure. As the study continued into the 1970s, the men began dying. Some of them had passed syphilis to their wives and children. The ethical misconduct of the research was leaked to the media. A class action lawsuit awarded the surviving men, wives, and children free medical care for life in addition to a large cash settlement. The Belmont Report actually was created as a result of this horrendous violation.

Another ethical research dilemma is the increased use of repeat, normal volunteers as research subjects.[4] In 2001, eighty thousand clinical trials were conducted in the United States with an estimated 20 million people enrolled as research subjects, three times the number a decade ago.[5] A 24-year-old normal, healthy volunteer who died as part of a challenge study examining asthma at Johns Hopkins University in June 2001, was a repeat volunteer.[6] Zink (2001) suggests traditional categories of the paid research subject: students, who participate for extra spending money; low-income unskilled workers, who participate for the small financial remuneration; and professional "guinea pigs" who chose to participate as a way of maintaining a marginal lifestyle.[7] In other words, an ethical dilemma in research is paying subjects as a way to make a living. This involves the ethical dilemma about doing harm, but also focuses on the dilemma, if these subjects are repeats in numerous drug studies, what type of wash-out period is involved and is the drug being tested on a randomized population. One would theorize that repeated use of numerous study drugs would create side effects that would bring extraneous variables— those variables that are not being tested, but in fact bias study results—into a research project.

Research Roles of Government and Private Entities

The federal government has always been at the center of medical research. It has a dual role of promoting research while protecting the public. The government primarily is involved in setting standards for conducting research and ethics. Government entities such as the FDA review research conducted in the private sector. This government oversight provides strict controls on what treatments, medicines, and medical devices can be sold and on what health claims may be made regarding these products. Government oversight also prevents the intrusion of less standardized research from other countries. The government often provides funding for research; in theory, it is an ideal mechanism through which to provide grants because it neither manufactures nor profits from the development of new products. The federal government also conducts research, mostly at the NIH through the Public Health Service and the military.

Local governments, such as public health departments, may serve as research centers for studies and may be able to tap a minority population of interest to the research (eg, people with type 2 diabetes). In addition, local governments may benefit from grant money or medical equipment resulting from the research study. Local governments also provide tax incentives to attract private research companies to work in their area.

Private institutions design and carry out the bulk of medical research in the United States. They can do so more quickly and cost effectively than other entities. Their funding for research may come from federal government grants, from the institution itself, from private companies, or through philanthropy. Competition for grant money is usually great, which theoretically should stimulate better research ideas. Large institutions can contribute multiple perspectives on a single topic. For example, two dental schools in different areas of the country might conduct the same study using two different populations.

Research conducted by private companies also has a negative side. Some researchers, in an effort to conduct studies more quickly and less expensively, have turned to developing countries to find participants. These researchers may pay a private institutional review board to approve the study although ethical controls over it can be poor and the research results of questionable quality.

DENTAL HYGIENIST SPOTLIGHT ·······················

Public Health Column: Christine Stephan, RDH, MS

This month the spotlight in public health is focused on a dental hygienist who works with in an interprofessional faith-based initiative. Christine Stephan is an accomplished clinician, educator, and presenter. She obtained her associate's, bachelor's and master's degrees in dental hygiene. She has really developed an expertise for all of these roles. She has also published research and has been awarded the Gloria H. Huxoll Award. Not surprisingly, she has maintained an active role in her local and state dental hygiene associations. Recently, I asked Christine some questions about her career.

Why did you decide to go into dental hygiene?

Honestly? When I was 14, my parents told me I needed to start thinking about a career. So, I went to the school counselor and got the Occupational

Outlook Handbook. This was before internet research! I thumbed through it and landed on dental hygiene. I thought, "Cool. It is only two years of school and they make good money. I can do this!" My adventure started as a quest for a job, but has become so much more than that and little did I know I would actually spend many, many more years furthering my education!

How did you get into public health? Did you need additional education?

I had been working in private practice for 16 years and have worked at the local university, part-time, as a clinical instructor for eight years. My plan—and I plan everything— was to go into dental hygiene education, full time. That plan did not work out as I had anticipated. When the position at Matthew 25 became available, I contemplated, I sought the advice of friends and family, and then I prayed. I knew I was ready for something different in my career, but I did not know what that "different" should be. When I accepted the position, I was excited, but still unsure. I told my nine-year-old son that I was leaving my job to start a new adventure. He said, "Mom, this is why you did not get that teaching job. God already had a plan for you. This is your plan!" My eyes welled up with tears, my heart swelled, and I knew my son was right. This is the best career decision I have made. I love it, every single minute of it. The position required a master's degree because part of the responsibilities included clinical instruction of students; however, since I already had my master's, I did not need any additional education.

What is your current position?

I have an awesome job. I am the dental hygiene coordinator,which entails overseeing and scheduling the dental hygiene schedule as well as recruiting and coordinating our dental hygiene volunteers. I also conduct dental and health education appointments, which are 30-minute appointments focusing on necessary home care regimens, healthy eating habits, and discussions regarding smoking cessation. Additionally, I coordinate schedules, supervise, and instruct senior dental hygiene students from Indiana Purdue University, Fort Wayne, when they come to Matthew 25 for their clinical rotations. When I am not in an office or instructing students, I get to do what I love—provide direct care to patients.

Can you discuss any particularly interesting experiences you have had in your dental public health positions?

After having worked in private practice, serving mostly middle to upper class patients for 16 years, every day in public health provides interesting experiences. We see patients from every ethnicity, nationality, and walk of life—no two days are ever the same. I find myself seeing and saying things I would have never imagined I would and I am no longer surprised by anything I encounter. What I find most interesting is the gratitude expressed by our patients. During my entire career, I have never had patients who are so grateful for any and all care we provide, even down to giving anesthesia and doing scaling and root planing. Patients thank us over and over again. They bring us homemade goodies. They offer to volunteer at the clinic, and they go out of their way to find ways to thank us. It is amazing and so incredibly rewarding. What type of advice would you give to a practicing hygienist that is thinking of doing something different? You have to be willing to get a little uncomfortable. Change is not easy. It can be scary, unpredictable, and usually not in the plans. However, if you are not happy, you need to keep an open mind and pray. You will never experience anything different if you never leave your comfort zone continue to do the same thing every day. My dad once told me, "Opportunities do not come often; but when they do, do not let them pass you by." Go. Explore. You will not regret it. I promise.

As felt in this interview, Christine has definitely found her niche in dental hygiene. Another interesting note that is seen often in the dental hygienists who are profiled in this column, stay positive and keep moving forward. This can-do attitude is the most important part of advancing a career forward, which benefits the profession, and ultimately patients benefit too.

Source: Christine Nathe writes the Public Health Column in *RDH* magazine published by Pennwell Publishing. For more public health spotlights please see RDH magazine online at http://www.rdhmag.com/index.html.

Summary

The public's health has been an important component in the creation of ethical standards for use in dental hygiene research. Every dental hygienist, whether or not directly involved in research, should be familiar with basic ethical principles, guidelines, and practices. Further, dental hygienists should continually evaluate benefits and risks when reviewing research reports. To be effective in initiating, conducting, and/or applying research, the dental hygienist must be able to critically analyze the bioethics of all studies conducted. This crucial link allows scientific study to become the standard of care in the profession.

Self-Study Test Items

1. A dental hygiene researcher's first obligation to the patient is to do no harm, which is termed
   a. Nonmaleficence
   b. Beneficence
   c. Autonomy
   d. Veracity

2. Which principle is based on respect for others and the belief that patients have the power to make decisions about things that may affect their health?
   a. Autonomy
   b. Beneficence
   c. Justice
   d. Nonmaleficence

3. Informed consent is an ongoing process that is initially obtained at the first step of the research process. It should be discussed in a group setting.
   a. The first statement is true; the second statement is false.
   b. The first statement is false; the second statement is true.
   c. Both statements are true.
   d. Both statements are false.

4. Private institutions design and carry out the bulk of medical research in the United States. Their funding for research may come from federal government grants, from the institution itself, from private companies, or through philanthropy.
   a. The first statement is true; the second statement is false.
   b. The first statement is false; the second statement is true.
   c. Both statements are true.
   d. Both statements are false.

5. Research misconduct includes intentional plagiarism and falsifying data. For this reason, research bias, or disagreement about the meaning of the results, does not constitute misconduct.
   a. Both the statement and reason are correct and related.
   b. Both the statement and reason are correct but NOT related.
   c. The statement is correct, but the reason is NOT.
   d. The statement is NOT correct, but the reason is correct.
   e. NEITHER the statement NOR the reason is correct.

References

1. Introduction to NMT Case 1 U.S.A. v. Karl Brandt et al. Harvard Law School Library. Retrieved from http://nuremberg.law.harvard.edu/php/docs_swi.php?DI=1&text=medical on March 3, 2015.
2. US PHS Syphilis Study at Tuskegee Timeline. Atlanta, GA: CDC. Retrieved from http://www.cdc.gov/tuskegee/timeline.htm. on August 26, 2015.
3. Office for Protection from Research Risks. Tips on Informed Consent. Retrieved from http://www.hhs.gov/ohrp/policy/ictips.html. on August 26, 2015.
4. Participation among normal healthy research volunteers: professional guinea pigs in clinical trials? Tishler CL, Bartholomae S. *Perspectives in Biology and Medicine*. Autumn 2003;(46)4:508–520 [article]. Published by The Johns Hopkins University Press. DOI: 10.1353/pbm.2003.0094. Retrieved from http://muse.jhu.edu/journals/perspectives_in_biology_and_medicine/v046/46.4tishler.pdf on August 26, 2015.
5. Lemonick MD, Goldstein A. Human guinea pigs. *Time*. 22 April, 2002.
6. Bor J, Pelton T. Hopkins faults safety lapses. *Baltimore Sun*. 17 July, 2001. Retrieved from http://www.baltimoresun.com/bal-te.md.hopkins17jul17-story.html. on August 25, 2015.
7. Zink S. Maybe we should pay them more. *Am. J. Bioethics*. 2001;1:88–89.

16

The Research Process

OBJECTIVES

After studying this chapter, the dental hygiene student should be able to:

- Describe and compare various research approaches
- Describe various research designs used in oral epidemiology
- Describe methods used to conduct research studies
- List the parts of a research design

COMPETENCIES

After studying this chapter and participating in accompanying course activities, the dental hygiene student should be competent to do the following:

- Use critical thinking skills and comprehensive problem-solving to identify oral health care strategies that promote patient health and wellness
- Use evidence-based decision making to evaluate emerging technology and treatment modalities to integrate into patient dental hygiene care plans to achieve high-quality, cost-effective care
- Assume responsibility for professional actions and care based on accepted scientific theories, research, and the accepted standard of care
- Continuously perform self-assessment for lifelong learning and professional growth
- Integrate accepted scientific theories and research into educational, preventive, and therapeutic oral health services

KEY TERMS

Data *197*
Descriptive approach *199*
Double-blind study *202*
Experimental approach *201*
Historical approach *199*
Hypothesis *196*
Literature review *197*
Pilot study *197*
Placebo *201*
Quasi-experimental approach *204*
Research approach *198*
Research design *197*
Research proposal *196*
Retrospective approach *198*
Sampling techniques *204*
Variable *197*
Washout period *204*

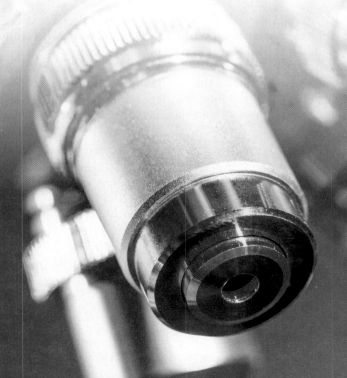

Science photo/Shutterstock

The process of research flows much like the dental hygiene process of care, with the exception of beginning with a question. In fact, research always begins with a question. Someone wonders why something is so. Why do 25 percent of the children in the United States have 80 percent of the caries? Why is the survival rate for oral cancer so low? Why are communities becoming more resistant to water fluoridation? If milk were fluoridated, would it work as well as water to prevent caries? Does having soda in school vending machines affect caries rates?

Hence, the research process has been set in motion. The basic components of the research process depicted in Figure 16-1 ■ include, importantly, the question to be posed, why the question is so significant, what is already known about the question and/or broad topic, and how do we propose to answer the question. Once the decision is made on what approach will best answer the question, a design is developed and implemented. Data can then be analyzed and results discussed.

THE RESEARCH QUESTION OR HYPOTHESIS The first step in the planning process is the development of a **hypothesis,** which is a question to be answered by a study. Hypotheses are the result of asking a question *that can be researched.*

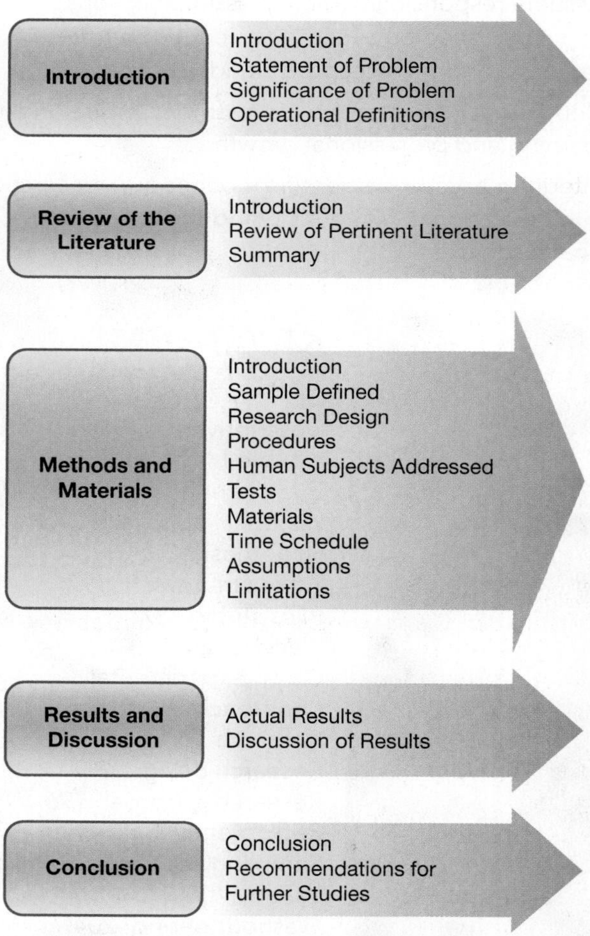

Introduction
Introduction
Statement of Problem
Significance of Problem
Operational Definitions

Review of the Literature
Introduction
Review of Pertinent Literature
Summary

Methods and Materials
Introduction
Sample Defined
Research Design
Procedures
Human Subjects Addressed
Tests
Materials
Time Schedule
Assumptions
Limitations

Results and Discussion
Actual Results
Discussion of Results

Conclusion
Conclusion
Recommendations for
Further Studies

FIGURE 16–1 Dental Hygiene Research Study Components

After answering the research question, a hypothesis can be stated in terms of a positive outcome (a research or positive hypothesis) or in terms of a negative outcome, as a null hypothesis (a statistical hypothesis to be tested and rejected in favor of an alternative).

Question: Which means of instrumentation is superior in periodontal debridement?

Research (Positive) Hypothesis: Ultrasonic instrumentation is significantly more effective than hand scaling during periodontal debridement.

Null Hypothesis: Ultrasonic instrumentation is not significantly more effective than hand scaling during periodontal debridement.

Question: Does brand X toothpaste really whiten teeth?

Research (Positive) Hypothesis: Brand X significantly whitens teeth.

Null Hypothesis: There is no statistically significant difference between brand X and a placebo when comparing the whitening of teeth.

Often the questions arise from researcher observations and observed occurrences. They may also come from questions arising out of previous research projects and from colleagues' experiences. In order for a hypothesis to be considered researchable, it must possess the characteristics in Box 16-1 ■. Hypotheses are usually stated in the null form. If the researcher finds that a significant difference does exist, the null hypothesis is rejected, thereby stating that a difference does exist.[1]

BASICS OF RESEARCH Once a valid hypothesis is stated, the researcher must write a detailed plan for the study called a **research proposal** or protocol. Writing a research proposal involves several steps. The proposal is often used not only to validate the significance of the research, but also to secure funding. Smaller studies not involving the manipulation of human subjects may be funded by grass

---

Box 16–1 Hypothesis Characteristics

A researchable hypothesis must be:
 Ethical to all participating subjects
Necessary research, that has the possibility to
 Improve clinical practice
 Improve health policy
 Confirm or change previous theories
 Recommend future research directions
Fundable research that
 Includes an adequate number of subjects
 Is cost effective
 Is manageable in terms of the project scope
 Involves professional expertise

roots organizations or local health care coalitions. Funding for major research studies is highly competitive and awards are based, in part, on how well the proposal is written. Funding can come from private industry or the governmental sector as discussed in Chapters 3 and 5.

After formulating a workable hypothesis, the second step is to conduct a **literature review,** which is a review of all pertinent reports and studies to determine what is currently known about the issue. The researcher may find that the question has already been answered, or may find little information on the subject. Literature reviews should include all issues associated with the research topic.

Reviewing the literature used to require many hours of library time looking through card catalogs and journal indexes. Thanks to the technological advances of computers and the Internet, literature reviews can now be conducted online. Any clinician can conduct a literature review to find the most current information about a disease or a treatment. The largest volume of online literature in the United States is at the National Library of Medicine.[2, 3] Begun in the 1800s, it now contains over 17 million citations online going as far back as the 1950s. New journal references are added monthly. Searching for information on a subject is now remarkably easy and will bring up a plethora of information on almost any subject. However, Web sites are not regulated as to the quality of information they provide, so researchers should carefully and critically view scientific information that does not come from legitimate and trusted sources.

The third step in writing a proposal is to design the research project. Box 16-2 ■ includes questions to ask when deciding on the research design.

All these questions, and likely others as well, need to be carefully thought out and planned before the researcher recruits the first subject or sends out the first questionnaire. For this reason, research is often time-consuming and requires months or years to conduct. (Teaching actual methodology of research is beyond the scope of this textbook; for more detailed information, the reader is referred to specific textbooks on research and/or a separate class on the subject.)

Developing the methods of a study depends on the research approach chosen. If a descriptive approach is chosen, for example, the researcher will likely develop a survey. Designing historical approaches and retrospective studies should be done at the same time the statistical method for analyzing the data is chosen. Experimental approaches are frequently clinical, laboratory, or epidemiological in nature and tend to employ specific, well-validated designs. These three main components—the research question, the review of the literature, and the research study design—make up the research proposal.

Up until this point the research project may have been conducted entirely by one researcher who is called the *principal investigator.* At the point of implementation of the study, research most often takes on a team approach. It generally takes a group of people working in concert to successfully conduct a research project.

Research Approaches and Designs

Dental hygiene research can be conducted using a variety of approaches. It also can focus on a variety of topics: One study might focus on dental hygiene providers' comparative status of educational level versus annual salary; another might focus on patients' compliance with daily flossing regimens.

Because understanding research-related terminology is crucial, we define some of the most important ones before our discussion begins. To gather **data,** or information collected, a researcher may use various methods from questionnaires to clinical testing. Some research makes no intervention, or experimental manipulation, of a variable in a study. A **variable** is a treatment, a drug, or an educational component whose value may change over the course of a research study.

Before the research process begins, a **pilot study,** which is a version of a proposed study, is conducted on a small, sometimes intentionally chosen sample. It is a trial run to work out unforeseen errors in the overall plan for a study, which is called the **research design.** In addition, the pilot study conserves valuable and limited research funding for the actual study. After conducting a pilot study, revisions may be made in the research design to obtain results with a higher degree of accuracy.

Box 16–2 Questions to Ask When Writing a Research Proposal

How will the research question be answered?
What method will be used to gather data?
Will human subjects be needed?
Will the project require any manipulation of subjects?
Will additional collaborators be needed to conduct the research?
How will the researchers be calibrated?
Will funds and/or supplies be needed?
How will they be purchased?
Will human subjects be compensated?
Have the data collection instruments been used before and are they valid?
Can the resulting data be statistically analyzed?
What statistical methods will be used?
How many subjects are needed?
Will a control group be used?
How will the sample groups be selected?
Does a pilot study need to be conducted first?
Who will fund the research?
How much money will be needed?

Did You Know?

Many times, pilot studies must be conducted before research funding can be obtained for complete studies.

Various research approaches may be utilized for dental hygiene research. A **research approach** is the type of research used to obtain information. All approaches observe, describe, measure, analyze, and interpret occurring phenomena.

Research approaches may be classified as historical, descriptive, experimental (prospective), quasi-experimental, and **retrospective** (ex post facto). (See Table 16-1 ■ for examples.)

Table 16–1 Research Approaches

Approach and Subtype	Definition/Purpose	Methods	Limitations	Application Examples
Historical	To determine the meaning of past events	Records review Interviews Literature reviews	Location of accurate data Gaps in knowledge No ability to replicate Biased reports Distortion of events	Development of ADHA community water fluoridation program 1945–2005 The evolution of dental hygiene degree programs in the United States.
Descriptive	To describe and indentify current events or situations			
Survey To gather broad information about status quo; usually involves large sample size		Questionnaires Opinionnaires Interviews Indices	Lack of depth	Use of pit and fissure sealants by dental hygienists Caries experience of high school sophomores
Case Study To conduct in-depth report on a single person, group, event, or situation		Interviews Observation Testing Records review	Uniqueness Replication not possible Subject to bias	Orthodontic case report Apthous ulcer case report in three patients using three different toothpastes
		Dental Indexes Questionnaires	Unrecognized chance variables might exist because of the number of samples	Periodontium assessment of children in grades 1-10
Cross-Sectional To study cross section of population in limited period of time				
Cohort or Longitudinal To study same population over extended period of time			Time-consuming process Extended financial commitment Loss of subjects	Changes in the children's periodontium over time
Document or Content Analysis To analyze documents themselves		Examination of records or documents for specific information or presentation style	Subjectivity in evaluation	Evaluation of dental journals for types of articles printed Gender biases in dental hygiene text books
Trend Combines descriptive and historical research to establish patterns from the past and present in order to predict future occurrences		Records review Review of the literature Interviews Observation Surveys	Long-range prediction less valid and reliable than short-range prediction	ADHA actions 1968–2008 regarding expanding scope of dental hygienists Use of sugar substitutes in carbonated beverages

(continued)

Approach and Subtype	Definition/Purpose	Methods	Limitations	Application Examples
Correlational Measure the relationship between variables	Comparison of two sets of data	No indication correlation indicates cause-effect relationship between variables Plausible rival hypotheses	Frequency of flossing and periodontal disease Predental hygiene grades and clinical dental hygiene grades
	Retrospective (causal-comparative or ex post facto) To investigate existing differences to determine possible causes. (Reverse of experimental approach)	Reverse of experimental approach Independent variable is not manipulated	Cannot determine causal relationship Can only determine functional relationship Independent variable cannot be manipulated	Periodontal disease (study adults over 40 with periodontal disease and adults over 40 without periodontal disease) Oral cancer (similar methodology)
Experimental (prospective)	To investigate cause-and-effect relationships Involves manipulation of variables	Manipulation of one or more independent variables Control of extraneous variables Measurement of dependent variable(s) Use of a control group	Artificiality due to amount of control Decreased external validity	Effect of intraoral sodium bicarbonate rinses versus the standard rinse on the periodontal ligament of dental patients The effectiveness of calculus removal with hand instrumentation versus magnetostrictive ultrasonic instrumentation.
Quasi-Experimental	Approximates true experimental approach but lacks control of true experimentation	Same as experimental except lacks the control of a true experimental design	Decreased internal validity Lack of control of extraneous variables	Effect of intraoral sodium bicarbonate rinses on the periodontal ligament of dental patients. The effectiveness of calculus removal with magnetostrictive ultrasonic instrumentation.

Source: Darby M, Bowen D. *Research Methods for Oral Health Professionals: An Introduction.* St. Louis, MO: C.V. Mosby; 1980.

Dental hygiene research can be categorized in numerous ways and with a plethora of titles. This chapter discusses the wide array of research approaches and designs used in dental hygiene to enable the dental hygienist to understand scientific studies and research reports.

Research may be descriptive or analytic in nature. Descriptive research is characterized as the attempt to identify and describe the topic being researched whereas analytic research attempts to establish why something is the way it is and how it came to be that way.[4] For example, descriptive research may identify the magnitude or distribution of a disease. Analytical research may test a hypothesis about the relationship of an exposure to a disease.[5]

Historical Approach

The purpose of studies using the **historical approach** is to determine the meaning of past events by reviewing records and literature and conducting interviews. It is one of the approaches that does not study interventions. Historical studies can lead to new insights and subsequent recommendations for the future.

Descriptive Approach

The **descriptive approach** uses a variety of methods, including surveys, case studies, developmental studies, document or content analysis, trend studies, and correlational studies. Descriptive studies use the survey method

to measure and describe the presence and distribution of a disease or health condition in a population or sample[5] at one point in time.

DESCRIPTIVE APPROACH TYPES A *survey* is a type of descriptive approach that involves collecting data using written or oral questionnaires or dental indices but does not perform interventions. The larger the representative sample for a survey, the more valid are the results. Descriptive surveys can be used to measure knowledge, attitudes, and values related to disease and health conditions, all of which can be used to determine needs for public health programs. For example, knowledge of the effectiveness of fluoride can be measured in a sample of the patient population of a community children's clinic to determine whether further fluoride education is needed. This information can be obtained by surveying parents and children by having them complete questionnaires when they come to the clinic.

A *case study* is research about a specific incidence of a disease in one person. It is an excellent way to discover possible treatment options for a variety of conditions or diseases. A case study entails assessing or diagnosing a specific patient or community population and planning, implementing, and evaluating treatment. A famous case study mentioned in a previous chapter involved Dr. Jenner's patient explaining her fortune of contracting cowpox as a way to protect her against smallpox. The incentives and rewards for conducting clinical research from a simple case study were never more apparent.[6] This example clearly demonstrates an effective, practical treatment that began as a case study.

A case series reports on a small group of people but cannot be generalized to the overall population; however, it often is interesting to read and frequently contributes to practical ideas for clinical practice.

A developmental study, simply looks at events as they exist but performs no intervention. Like a natural history study, a developmental study attempts to describe a condition or situation comprehensively. It observes growth, development, maturation, or change over a period of time. Many developmental studies are classified as *cross-sectional* or *cohort/longitudinal.*

A *cross-sectional study* measures the outcome and the exposure at the same time to determine the association between the two.[7] By measuring outcomes and exposures at the same time, a correlation or noncorrelation between the outcome and exposures could be identified. Such a study would be conducted on a sample across the population as its name indicates. The sample is measured only once. A descriptive survey can be expanded into a cross-sectional study by going beyond simply measuring the presence of a condition. For example, a cross-sectional study could identify the characteristics of parents' return of consent forms for their children to participate in a school-based dental sealant program. A sample of the school population is studied to measure parents' socioeconomic status, dental knowledge, dental history, and other traits. Parents' attributes (suspected characteristics) and compliance (condition) are measured only one time in only one group for associations.

A *cohort (group) study* examines one population group or subset with a common characteristic (for example, age, gender, special needs classification) over a specified time period to measure the change or progress of a disease or condition.[8] The study starts with a group of individuals who do not have the disease or condition but are at risk for it and then collects information regarding exposure to that risk. The group is observed to identify members who do or do not eventually develop the disease or condition. This requires at least two measurements on the same group of people at different times.

A cohort study can be described as a *longitudinal study* (measured over time).[8] The most well-known and comprehensive longitudinal study could be the Harvard Nurses' Health Study.[9] Begun in 1976 to determine any relationship between the use of oral contraceptives and smoking, the study has followed 100,000 nurses over the three decades and has resulted in more than 400 publications on numerous health topics. Another longitudinal cohort study has tracked the use of tobacco products in the US population for more than a century to determine prevalence of smoking, incidence of new smokers each year, characteristics of the population that use tobacco, and events related to increases and decreases in use, such as the free distribution of cigarettes to US troops in World War I and the more recent policy to control the sale of cigarettes.[8]

A *document* or *content analysis* study analyzes documents to understand phenomena. One example of a document analysis is a detailed review of the content of a college course, such as reviewing all topics that have been covered. Another example is the review of dental records of a dental practice to determine its payer mix.

A *trend study* combines descriptive and historical research to establish patterns or phenomena from the past and in the present to predict future occurrences. Reviewing the consumption of sports drinks over the past two decades to predict their future use is an example of a trend study. Cross-sectional studies are often compared over time to determine trends, such as oral health surveys conducted as part of an oral health surveillance system.

A *correlational study* is exploratory in nature and attempts to establish a link between two variables or conditions but does not provide evidence for a cause-and-effect relationship between them. It can consider a population's past, present, and future as well as study specific occurrences of a disease. It is followed by an experimental study to determine whether a cause-and-effect relationship actually exists. This research approach may use indices, survey methodology, and clinical testing.

In recent years, a large number of correlation studies have linked oral health with overall systemic health. They have linked periodontal disease with heart disease, osteoporosis, obesity, Alzheimer's disease, pancreatic cancer, and preterm births.[10] This research approach is often misinterpreted to infer that having periodontal disease causes heart disease or vice versa—an erroneous extrapolation. When a research study has identified a possible relationship, additional prospective controlled cohort or experimental studies may be needed to determine cause and effect. Identifying causality requires repeating several such studies over several different populations that obtain the same results.

Retrospective (Ex Post Facto) Approach

A **retrospective study** looks backward (**ex post facto,** or after the fact) to investigate a group of people with a particular disease, usually via medical records. For example, one retrospective study examined the impact of dental interventions before organ transplants. Persons undergoing bone marrow transplants to treat advanced cancer often receive preoperative dental evaluation and periodontal therapy as a standard of care to reduce the chance of septicemia after the transplant. For example, a retrospective study in a public health hospital with a dental clinic examined medical records to compare patients who did and did not have dental intervention prior to transplant. Contrary to expected results, no septicemia was observed for either group.[11]

One type of retrospective study is a case–control study; its purpose is to compare two groups to identify factors in the history of the group associated with a specific disease or condition. One group has a disease or condition (called a case) but the second group does not. Cases are compared to controls, hence its name.[7] Case–control studies investigate the outcome (presence or absence of a disease) and then probe for information about exposure to factors that could be associated with it.[12] The computation of risk from a case–control study is called odds ratio.[13] Case–control studies are sometimes referred to as case history or ex post facto studies.[14] The relationships they establish are called functional relationships.[14]

During the early stages of research on fluorosis, researchers conducted a case–control study by comparing two naturally occurring groups, one of people with severe fluorosis and the other without fluorosis. The researchers measured each group only once to identify the common exposure or factor(s) related to the condition's presence

and then attempted to relate common exposure(s) to the presence of fluorosis (outcome). In this case, their drinking water was the common factor.[15]

An ecologic study also attempts to relate outcome with exposure to a suspected risk factor but does so using existing data for the population to identify any correlations rather than measuring the exposure and the outcome in the same group.[7, 8] The ecologic study forms no groups and does not measure variables but uses data that had previously been recorded for another purpose. Ecologic studies, which can be useful in establishing associations, have the advantages of being low cost and quick to conduct because they do not require data collection. Their weakness is the use of existing data. Because the data are collected at different times for different purposes, the groups being compared may be different. To relate exposure and outcome, they both must be measured on the same individuals. In other words, the exposure data may come from one group and the outcome data from another group, producing what is called an ecologic fallacy.[13] Because of the ecologic fallacy, ecologic studies are not definitive in identifying risk factors or even risk indicators. Results of ecologic studies are sometimes reported using correlations. Measures of risk that are established with cross-sectional, cohort, and case–control studies provide more information about association for comparisons than ecologic studies.[7] Health recommendations should not be based on ecologic studies alone. These studies should be followed with analytic studies to more closely examine the risk of an exposure resulting in the disease or condition.

Antifluoridationists have conducted ecologic studies to try to implicate fluoridation as a risk factor for conditions such as cancer, Down syndrome, and infant mortality. These researchers used existing data measured at different times to demonstrate invalid relationships. Closer scrutiny using well-controlled cohort and case–control studies have disproved antifluoridationists' claims.[16]

Experimental (Prospective) Approach

The **experimental approach,** also known as a clinical trial, is probably most familiar to a layperson. This research studies an experimental treatment or intervention using a *dependent variable* whose value or outcome is determined by that of one or more other variables. An independent variable is the variable that is being manipulated. The dependent variable may be a new drug or surgical procedure; its effectiveness is the outcome being studied. See Box 16-3 ■ for requirements of an experimental research.

PLACEBO EFFECT Experimental research frequently uses placebos and control groups. The control group is the group with the disease/condition being studied that does not receive experimental treatment. The **placebo** is a control. It is not the factor being studied but can be a nontreatment or sometimes a "sugar pill." It is more likely

Box 16–3 Requirements for Conducting Experimental Research

- Use a control group for comparison with the experimental group
- Control extraneous variables
- Randomize study participants
- Control errors in measurement
- Directly manipulate one or more independent variables
- Observe and measure the dependent variable
- Ensure occurrence of independent variable before dependent variable in the design

however, to be either the standard drug of choice for a disease or the standard treatment procedure against which the experimental one is being compared, called an active control. Even in carefully controlled studies with a placebo drug or treatment, a proportion of the participants, typically 15–35 percent receiving the placebo actually improve, a phenomenon known as the *placebo effect.* First described in detail in 1955, the placebo effect is testimony not only to the multifactorial nature of illness and healing but also to the human mind's ability to provoke physiological change.[17, 18]

Did You Know?

Interestingly, the research that led to the description of the placebo effect was found in the 1970s to be significantly flawed by researchers doing retrospective studies.[18]

Sometimes subjects in a study are affected simply by being subjects in it. This phenomenon, known as the Hawthorne effect, was discovered as a result of a study held in the late 1920s and early 1930s. Investigators at the Western Electric Company's Hawthorne plant in Chicago found that because factory workers knew they were participating in a study, anything the researchers did caused the workers' productivity to change. This theory suggests that when subjects are singled out for a study of any kind, they may improve their performance or behavior not because of any specific condition being tested but simply because of the perception of being observed.

DOUBLE-BLIND STUDIES   Most experimental research is conducted using a **double-blind study,** that is, a research project in which neither the subjects nor the investigators know who is in the control (or placebo) group and who is in the other (independent variable) group that receives the experimental treatment. This type of study is considered to be highly reliable because it eliminates a great deal of the researcher's bias. An investigator who does not know which treatment a subject is receiving could not make any suggestive comments to the participant, and the data collection can be done without any preconceived expectations.

Suppose, for example, a dental hygienist who was providing services in a correctional facility wanted to evaluate the relative merits of rinsing with chlorhexidine over a commercially available mouth rinse. A pharmacist could dispense two rinses: both blue and mint flavored in identical unmarked bottles. The pharmacist kept a record of which subjects received which rinse, but neither the dental hygienist nor the subjects knew. Therefore, the hygienist could not inadvertently suggest to the patients that one rinse is superior, and any indices would be scored without the preconceived expectation that the subjects on chlorhexidine "should" be healthier than the control subjects. The dental hygienist could not bias the results of the study. The subjects also would be less likely to bias the results because people who know they are getting a placebo are less likely to comply with study protocol.

INDEPENDENCE OF RESEARCHERS   Because bias may also be introduced through the funding source of a research study, it is important that clinical trials be conducted by independent researchers. If a pharmaceutical company produces mouthwash G, its efficacy should be confirmed by independent studies that are not funded by the manufacturer. In most studies, the principal investigator is usually required to disclose that there is no financial conflict of interest.

EXPERIMENTAL RESEARCH DESIGNS   An experimental study can be a pretest-posttest design or a posttest only design.[19] These and other designs appear in Figure 16-2 ■. Pretest-posttest designs are a common type of repeated measures because the same test is given at least twice: before the independent variable is introduced and after the independent variable is introduced.[20] A *pretest-posttest* study measures the dependent variable—the treatment or intervention being studied—before and after introducing the independent variable—the placebo. The advantage of the pretest-posttest design is having the pretest for comparison. Also, the pretest is used to check for equivalent groups before introducing the intervention.

A *posttest-only* design introduces the independent variable and then measures the dependent variable. This study is conducted when administering a pretest is impractical. For example, a study could be conducted in a school-based oral screening program to compare the percentage of compliance with two referral systems. Although randomization would be possible, no pretest could be administered, so a posttest-only design would be appropriate for this experimental study.

Posttest-only designs are used also to control the effect of a pretest on the dependent variable in a study.

One-Group Time Series Design

Repeated Pretest Measures	Independent Variable	Repeated Post-Test Measures
Y_1 Y_2 Y_3	X	Y_4 Y_5 Y_6

Control Group Time Series Design

Group	Repeated Pretest Measures	Independent Variable	Repeated Post-Test Measures
E	Y_1 Y_2 Y_3	X	Y_4 Y_5 Y_6
C	Y_1 Y_2 Y_3	—	Y_4 Y_5 Y_6

Randomized Subjects Pretest/Post-Test Design

Group	Pretest	Independent Variable	Post-Test
(R) E	Y_1	X	Y_2
(R) C	Y_1	—	Y_2

Randomized Subjects Post-Test Only Design

Group	Independent Variable	Post-Test
(R) E	X	Y_2
(R) C	—	Y_2

Randomized Matched Subjects Post-Test Only Design

Group	Independent Variable	Post-Test
(RM) E	X	Y_2
(RM) C	—	Y_2

Solomon Four-Group Design

Group	Pretest	Independent Variable	Post-Test
(R) E	Y_1	X	Y_2
(R) C_1	Y_2	—	Y_2
(R) C_2	—	X	Y_2
(R) C_3	—	—	Y_2

FIGURE 16–2 Quasi-Experimental and Experimental Study Designs

Source: Adapted from Darby ML, Bowen DM. *Research Methods for Oral Health Professionals: An Introduction.* St. Louis, MO: C.V. Mosby; 1980. Reprinted by J. T. K. McCann Co., Pocatello, ID, 1993.

This effect is called pretest sensitization.[14] For example, in educational research studies, conducting an exam to measure knowledge prior to evaluating the effectiveness of various teaching methodologies could in and of itself bring about learning. A *Solomon four-group design* can be used to determine whether the pretest affects the dependent variable.[19] The Solomon design (see Figure 16-2 ■) combines a pretest/posttest design with a posttest only design. For example, a study of four groups using the Solomon design would place two of them in an experimental and control group with a pretest-posttest design. The other two would be an experimental and control group with a posttest-only design. The change in the dependent variable is compared across groups to determine whether the control group or pretest affects the outcome. Solomon designs are infrequently used because they are difficult to implement.[19]

Using the example of educational research, four groups would be tested to determine the effectiveness of an educational method to improve fluoride knowledge of clients in a public health program. Two would be an experimental and control group with a pretest-posttest. The other two would be an experimental and control group using a posttest only. Knowledge would be measured at pretest and posttest with a questionnaire consisting of questions about fluoride. The Solomon design would be used to determine whether completing the fluoride questionnaire results in learning about fluoride. The two experimental groups would be exposed to the

educational program being evaluated, but the two control groups would not be. To determine the learning in each group, the results for two pretest groups are compared with those of the posttest-only groups. If the outcome is higher in the pretest groups, some of the learning could be attributed to the pretest questionnaire rather than the educational program. A variation of this design that eliminates the control posttest-only group is used for the same purpose and is called the Solomon three-group design.[19]

Sometimes the dependent variable is measured several times over a specific period, either at pretest or posttest to determine whether the effect of the independent variable on the dependent variable holds over time. This is called *time series design*.[21] It can be applied to a one-group, before-and-after trial but is most valid when applied to an experimental study. Its measurement of the dependent variable at posttest is its most valid use. Figure 16-2 ■ represents the measurement of the posttest three times in a randomized pretest-posttest design. The pretest-posttest study of hypersensitivity described earlier would likely be conducted as a time series study. The reduction in hypersensitivity would be measured at posttest repeatedly over several weeks or months to make sure that the hypersensitivity did not return.

A *factorial design* is used to study two or more independent variables in combination.[14] For example, this design could compare the effectiveness in removing plaque of a power toothbrush to a manual toothbrush at the same

Table 16–2 2 × 2 Factorial Design

Manual brush	Manual brush
Traditional floss	Tufted floss
Power brush	Power brush
Traditional Floss	Tufted floss

time it compares a tufted floss to a traditional floss to determine whether they interact. Two levels of two independent variables are involved: toothbrush and dental floss, referred to as a 2 × 2 factorial design. (See Table 16-2 ■.) Four groups are formed with various possible combinations of these two levels of the two independent variables. This design can be applied with more independent variables and/or more levels of each independent variable for factorial designs that are 2 × 3, 3 × 3, 3 × 4, and so on. In a factorial design, the effect of each independent variable is tested on the dependent variable, referred to as a *main effect,* and the combined effect of the independent variables is tested on the dependent variable, referred to as an *interaction effect.*[14]

CONTROLS   Two types of studies in which participants serve as their own control are crossover and split mouth. Participants are assigned randomly to a study and a control group in a *crossover design.* After a specified length of time, participants are switched ("crossed over") to the opposite group. Then the participants in both groups experience a period of time with no treatment, called a **washout period.** In drug trials, this is the period allowed for all of any administered drug to be eliminated from the body. It reduces the effect of the first treatment on the second. After the washout period, each group receives the opposite treatment it had earlier received. This crossover design is not appropriate for regimens that have a permanent effect that the washout period cannot eliminate.

The crossover design could be applied to a study of a new power toothbrush. A sample is randomly assigned to a test group that will use a new power toothbrush or to an active control group that will use the best-selling power toothbrush currently on the market. After three weeks, all study participants are told to return to using their regular manual toothbrush for three weeks, and then those participants who were in the test group for the first three weeks are now in the control group for three weeks, and vice versa. Thus, all participants use both toothbrushes for a three-week period with a three-week washout period between.

In a *split mouth design,* one side of the mouth is used for the test treatment, and the other side of the mouth is used for the control treatment.[22] This design is common in testing treatment regimens in dentistry because it is very effective to control subject-relevant variables.

A split mouth and crossover design can be combined so that the sides of the mouth are switched. In the crossover toothbrush study discussed earlier, participants could be asked to brush with the new power toothbrush on the right side of the mouth and with the standard power brush (active control) on the left side, making it a split mouth design. In this case, the brushing should be done under supervision to ensure that the correct toothbrush is used on the proper side. The participants could then return for another supervised brushing session during which they switch sides with each toothbrush. Another example of a split mouth design is related to the earlier hypersensitivity study. The new treatment could be used to treat hypersensitive teeth on one side, and the placebo used to treat hypersensitive teeth on the other side. In this example, use of a crossover design would not be appropriate because the test treatment could have a carryover and possibly permanent effect. A final example of a split mouth design is a test of the retention rate of a new dental sealant product by using it on one side of the mouth and using the standard sealant product (active control) on the other side of the mouth. Again, a crossover design would not be suitable for this study.

An advantage of using participants to serve as their own control is that they can provide near perfect group similarity.[5] Crossover and split mouth trials control for subject-relevant variables because results are not affected by variations in response among participants. Therefore, they have increased validity. Another advantage is that they can be conducted with small samples because each study participant is a member of both the test group and the control group. Of course, having participants serve as their own control is not feasible in all studies.

Quasi-Experimental Approach

A **quasi-experimental approach** is used in an experimental study that lacks inherent control. Results may be used when planning other studies. This approach is employed because the use of a control is not practical or necessary. For instance, when studying the use of a mandibular advancing oral appliance to treat obstructive sleep apnea, a researcher could not replace the appliance with a control that did not advance the mandible, especially when the intervention is medically necessary.

Did You Know?

A quasi-experimental study could use a historical finding as a control.

DENTAL HYGIENIST SPOTLIGHT ·······································

Public Health Column: Irene O'Connor Navarre, RDH

The spotlight person this month is very near and dear to my heart, because it is pioneer dental hygienist Irene O'Connor Navarre who, through her teaching, practice, service, and policy-changing roles has had a significant impact in advancing the profession of dental hygiene. This, in my opinion, translates into improving society's oral health. Irene O'Connor Navarre graduated from the University of Minnesota in 1938.

She practiced dental hygiene in Minnesota and California and taught dental practice management at the University of Southern California before moving to New Mexico to help start the University of New Mexico's dental hygiene program, which, by the way, recently celebrated the 50–year landmark! She was instrumental in starting the New Mexico, Arizona, and Nevada Dental Hygienists' Associations, and has always been active in the American Dental Hygienists' Association, serving as a trustee as well as president in 1964–1965. I recently had the opportunity to ask Irene some questions, which I know you'll find inspiring.

Although Minnesota had one of the first dental hygiene programs in 1920, there still were not many dental hygienists when you were young, so how did you decide to go into dental hygiene?

I had a very good experience when I was a child in the care of a dentist. My father took me to his dentist's office to have a deciduous tooth extracted, and after the dentist extracted it, my father paid the bill, which was $1. Dr. Acheson took the dollar bill and handed it to me, and instructed me to save it! The kindness that the dentist showed me was instilled in me. When I was older in Minneapolis, I fortunately was sent to a progressive dental office, and the dental hygienist gave me the full treatment. I just knew I could learn to do that! From then on I wanted to become a dental hygienist.

What are the most exciting changes you've witnessed in dental hygiene?

That's easy. I worked with the dental hygiene associations to change the scope of practice to include subgingival scaling. This is most definitely the premier

change that enabled dental hygienists to further attain optimal oral health for patients.

What advice do you have that could help dental hygiene continue to advance?

I think we need to stay focused on the core of dental hygiene, which includes the essential skills of prevention through educational and clinical practices. We need to remember Dr. Fones' original intention, which was to prevent dental disease and improve health, with a focus on children. I remember the quote that was printed at the bottom of ADHA stationery for quite a while — For the health of the community, especially the children.

I also feel that as a profession we need to emphasize public relations, specifically educating the public on dental hygiene and the importance of optimum oral health. In addition, we need to strive to improve professional relations within dentistry to promote the importance of dental hygiene science and practice, and the importance of a dental hygienist within the dental team.

My interview with Irene was very inspirational and particularly poignant since the profession has hit its centennial year. So to hear about the beginnings of dental hygiene was insightful, and it clarified for me that we have, in the past 100 years, advanced our science and practice. Irene Navarre is truly a pioneer dental hygienist. She worked effortlessly to ensure the growth of dental hygiene science and practice by changing our practice so that we could adequately prevent and treat dental disease. She empowered patients in her practice, taught students how to become professional dental hygienists, mentored practicing dental hygienists, encouraged state dental hygiene associations, presided over the ADHA in the mid '60s and, of course, worked in many different roles in the ADHA, and promoted dental hygiene all over the world!

Her motto is "Be the best dental hygienist you can be." Irene Navarre embodies just that. Irene, we do appreciate what you have done for the profession, and we will strive to keep promoting and advancing dental hygiene. Thank you for your service to our profession, Irene Navarre, a true pioneer dental hygienist!

Source: Christine Nathe writes the Public Health Column in *RDH* magazine published by Pennwell Publishing. For more public health spotlights please see RDH magazine online at http://www.rdhmag.com/index.html.

SAMPLING TECHNIQUES Generally, it is impossible for a researcher to study an entire population that may be affected by a particular disease. The logistics and cost of such research would be prohibitive. Therefore, the researcher selects a sample population to study. To generalize research results to the whole population, the researcher must be sure that the sample is a representative subset.

A sample can be large or small depending on the type of research. A large sample is the most accurate representation of the population. This is especially important for descriptive studies, where the larger the sample, the better to produce valid results. It is easier to demonstrate statistical significance of differences when larger sample sizes are used in experimental studies.

Individuals have the right to participate or to not participate in a study. This volunteer participation can result in loss of subjects from longitudinal studies. Attrition must be planned for by selecting an initial sample size adequate to accommodate for loss of study participants. Otherwise, resulting group sizes will be too small to produce valid results.

TYPES OF SAMPLES When a dental hygiene researcher is conducting a descriptive study, such as a survey, the sample can be easily defined. If the researcher is studying dental hygiene curricular options in the United States, the sample of dental hygiene program directors is readily available via email. When deciding on an experimental approach, it is necessary to understand the types of sampling techniques available.

Did You Know?

The term research subjects or participants can be used when discussing the individuals being studied in research.

Different types of techniques can be used to select a sample from a population to study depending on the research approach. These **sampling techniques** vary in how well they represent the population and in how easy they are to employ. Random, stratified, systematic, judgmental, convenience, and cluster samples are all sampling techniques.

The best way of ensuring adequate representation is to take a *random sample*. Every possible subject is selected independently and has an equal chance of being selected. Selection may be done by lottery for a small sample or by computer selection for a large sample.

Random sampling is also important to employ once subjects have been chosen and it is necessary to place them in experimental or control groups. Randomly selecting subjects for participation in either group increases validity.

Did You Know?

Stratifying a sample provides additional data from studies by breaking the sample into populations.

Systematic technique samples every "n^{th}" subject, which can be determined by dividing the total population size by the desired sampling size. For example, if a researcher was studying all 8000 residents in state nursing homes, a sample of 800 residents could be chosen. The "n^{th}" term would then be computed by diving 8000 by 800, which equals ten. It is important to ensure that there are no hidden patterns that could threaten randomness.

A *convenience sample* is a sample of individuals who are most readily available to be selected for the study.[14] If the researcher wants to study the prevalence of oral cancer at a nursing home, the researcher may be able to study the "whole" population. However, results could not be applied to other nursing homes because in essence a convenience sample was studied. For the study to be generalized, a sample of residents in multiple facilities would be needed.

Intact groups and volunteers are used because of the impracticality of using random and other samples. The problem with the use of intact groups and volunteers is that they do not represent the population in many ways and, therefore, their use introduces bias. Volunteers may be inherently different from non-volunteers. An intact group is a convenient group of subjects that is already together, such as a classroom of children, an orphanage, or a Head Start program. The advantage of using intact groups is their convenience, especially for certain types of research.

If a clinician selects a sample of patients through personal judgment of who would be typical patients to include in the sample based on an understanding of the purpose of the research, this would be called a *judgmental,* or *purposive,* sample. A great deal of bas is introduced with this type of sample. The bias resulting from the sample selection is called selection bias. Judgmental samples are effective for action research, although not appropriate for experimental research studies.

Action research in relation to health care involves the reflective evaluation of programs in place in the community that are designed to improve health practices and behaviors by changing them. Another type of study benefiting from this technique is if the researcher would like to study specific populations such as individuals with comorbidity issues such as diabetes and hypertension and advanced periodontal disease. The researcher would need to purposely look for individuals who meet this criterion.

In summary, the technique that results in the most representative samples is random sampling. Judgmental and convenience samples result in selection bias. Many

clinical trials in oral health research use convenience samples and are replicated in different samples. Even when samples are large and selected randomly, research can never predict the effects on the whole population with complete accuracy. This is seen most frequently in new drugs that are taken off the market when serious side effects show up in widespread use that did not appear in the testing phases.

Research should ideally represent a cross section of the population with regard to gender, age, race, and ethnicity. Much research has come under criticism recently because certain groups are not well represented in the study populations. Sometimes this can make a difference when trying to apply the information to other groups. For example, if a drug is tested only on men, do women and children need similar dosing? If a drug for hypertension is tested only in males, will it work the same way in females? Often research is not feasible in some populations—for example, pregnant women are not typically thought of as good candidates for drug studies.

On one hand, public health is ideal for recruiting subjects that provide an adequate cross section of the population. This is true because public health tends to serve a wide variety of target populations. On the other hand, public health serves people who are typically socioeconomically disadvantaged, and they should not be targeted as research subjects. Death rates from oral cancer are higher for African Americans than for other races, even when adjusting for later diagnosis.[23] Suppose a researcher wished to study a new treatment for oral cancer. A good way to recruit patients might be through a state sponsored program that conducts community oral cancer screenings funded by tobacco restitution money. Patients who qualified for and enrolled in the study would receive their treatment for free. Would those candidates be more likely to participate in the research study because it is the only way they can afford to get treatment?

DATA ANALYSIS AND INTERPRETATION Once the study has been completed, or perhaps at prescribed intervals in a longer study, the data are collected for statistical analysis. The analysis method is selected prior to the inception of the study. Often not all the data collected are useful for analysis. Subjects withdraw or are lost from studies for many reasons. Unless the researcher is experienced at statistical analysis, a biostatistician is often called in to do the mathematics. Fortunately, there are several computer programs available now that make this task simpler. Chapter 17 provides more detail on data analysis and interpretation. For an amusing look at how statistics can be misinterpreted and misused, read Mark Clifton's "The Dread Tomato Affliction" (Box 16-4 ■).

The skeptic of apocryphal statistics, or the stubborn nonconformist who will not accept the clearly proved conclusions of others, may conduct his own experiment. Obtain two dozen tomatoes—they may actually be purchased within a block of some high schools, or discovered

---

Box 16–4 The Dread Tomato Addiction by Mark Clifton

Ninety-two point four percent of juvenile delinquents have eaten tomatoes.

Eighty-seven point one percent of the adult criminals in penitentiaries throughout the United States have eaten tomatoes.

Informers reliably inform that of all known American communists, ninety-two point three percent have eaten tomatoes.

Eighty-four percent of all people killed in automobile accidents during the year 2000 had eaten tomatoes.

Those who object to singling out specific groups for statistical proofs require measurements within a total. Of those people born before the year 1850, regardless of race, color, creed, or caste, and known to have eaten tomatoes, there has been one hundred percent mortality!

In spite of their dread addiction, a few tomato eaters born between 1850 and 1900 still manage to survive, but the clinical picture is poor—their bones are brittle, their movements feeble, their skin seamed and wrinkled, their eyesight failing, hair falling, and frequently they have lost all their teeth.

Those born between 1900 and 1950 number somewhat more survivors, but the overt signs of the addiction's dread effects differ not in kind but only in degree of deterioration. Prognostication is not hopeful.

Exhaustive experiment shows that when tomatoes are withheld from an addict, invariably his cravings will cause him to turn to substitutes—such as oranges, or steak and potatoes. If both tomatoes and all substitutes are persistently withheld—death invariably results within a short time!

---

growing in a respected neighbor's back yard!—crush them to a pulp in exactly the state they would have if introduced into the stomach, pour the vile juice and pulp into a bowl, and place a goldfish therein. Within minutes the goldfish will be dead!

Those who argue that what affects a goldfish might not apply to a human being may, at their own choice, wish to conduct a direct experiment by fully immersing a live human head into the mixture for a full five minutes.

RESEARCH CONCLUSIONS AND PUBLICATION No single research study can prove a hypothesis. Hence, most research articles end with the caveat that more research is warranted in the area. No single research study can be applied beyond the population that was studied. Each bit of information gathered from a well-designed research study contributes to the overall body of knowledge and suggests further questions for study.

For research to make the leap from the scientist's bench to evidence-based practice, it must be published. Peer-reviewed journals allow a panel of professionals from the same (or similar) discipline to assess the merits of the research and access the largest volume of readers. Without the distribution of this information, the dental hygienist in private practice will not be able to incorporate new knowledge and techniques into daily practice that will benefit both clinicians and patients. Oral health and dental hygienists' occupational health can and do suffer as a result. Through professional journals, the science of the laboratories becomes the art of patient care.

Summary

Dental hygienists need to understand different research approaches and designs. Research approaches are varied and are based and conducted on the specific phenomenon or phenomena the researcher wishes to study. Understanding this enables dental hygienists to critically review scientific literature and make evidence-based decisions during dental hygiene treatment.

Self-Study Test Items

1. Which of the following is a descriptive approach to research?
   a. Case study approach
   b. Experimental approach
   c. Retrospective approach
   d. Prospective approach

2. Which studies combine descriptive and historical research to establish patterns from the past and present to predict future occurrences?
   a. Document analysis studies
   b. Correlational studies
   c. Trend studies
   d. Prospective studies

3. In a split mouth study, one side of the mouth is used for the test treatment. The other side of the mouth is used for the control treatment.
   a. The first statement is true; the second statement is false.
   b. The first statement is false; the second statement is true.
   c. Both statements are true.
   d. Both statements are false.

4. A quasi-experimental study is designed as an experimental study but lacks inherent control. However, results from a quasi-experimental study may be used when planning further studies.

   a. The first statement is true; the second statement is false.
   b. The first statement is false; the second statement is true.
   c. Both statements are true.
   d. Both statements are false.

5. Studying the relationship between obesity and oral health is an example of which type of study?
   a. Experimental
   b. Quasi-experimental
   c. Correlational
   d. Analytic

References

1. Burns N, Grove S. *The Practice of Nursing Research.* 2nd ed. Philadelphia, PA: W. B. Saunders; 1993.
2. US National Library of Medicine. www.nlm.nih.gov.
3. PubMed. www.ncbi.nlm.nih.gov/pubmed.
4. Ethridge, DE. *Research in applied economics: organizing, planning and conducting economic research.* Malden, MA: Blackwell Publishing; 2004.
5. Burt BA, Eklund SA. *Dentistry, Dental Practice, and the Community.* 6th ed. St. Louis, MO: Elsevier; 2005.
6. Berg AO, Gordon MJ, Cherkin DC. *Practice-Based Research in Medicine.* Kansas City, MO: American Academy of Family Physicians; 1986.
7. Koepsell TD, Weiss NS. *Epidemiologic Methods: Studying the Occurrence of Illness.* New York, NY: Oxford University Press; 2003.
8. Friis RH, Sellers TA. *Epidemiology for Public Health Practice.* 3rd ed. Boston, MA: Jones & Bartlett; 2004.
9. Nelson NJ. Nurses health study: nurses helping science and themselves. *J Natl Can Inst.* 2000;92(8):597–599.
10. Oral and Whole Body Health. *Sci Am.* 2006 (special publication).
11. Akintoye SO, Brennan MT, Graber CJ, et al. A retrospective investigation of advanced periodontal disease as a risk factor for septicemia in hematopoietic stem cell and bone marrow transplant recipients. *Oral Surg, Oral Med, Oral Path.* 2002;94(5):581–588.
12. Morabia A. Epidemiology: An epistemological perspective. In: Morabia A. *A History of Epidemiologic Methods and Concepts.* Boston, MA: Birkhauser Verlag; 2004:3–125
13. Gerstman BB. *Epidemiology Kept Simple: An Introduction to Traditional and Modern Epidemiology.* 2nd ed. Hoboken, NJ: Wiley-Liss; 2003.
14. Darby M, Bowen D. *Research Methods for Oral Health Professionals: An Introduction.* St. Louis, MO: C.V. Mosby; 1980.
15. National Institute of Dental and Craniofacial Research, National Institutes of Health. The Story of Fluoridation. Retrieved from http://www.nidcr.nih.gov/oralhealth/Topics/Fluoride/TheStoryofFluoridation.htm. on August 28, 2015.
16. American Dental Association. Fluoridation facts. Retrieved from http://www.ada.org/en/public-programs/advocating-for-the-public/fluoride-and-fluoridation/fluoridation-facts. on August 28, 2015.

17. Beecher HK. The powerful placebo. *JAMA*. 1955;159(17): 1602–1606.
18. Kienle GS, Kiene H. The powerful placebo effect: fact or fiction? *J Clin Epid*. 1997;50:1311–1318.
19. Cottrell RR. *Health Promotion and Education Research Methods*. Boston, MA: Jones & Bartlett; 2005.
20. Minke A. Conducting repeated measures analyses: experimental design considerations. Paper presented at Southwest Educational Research Association. 1997. Austin, TX. Ericae. net Clearinghouse on Assessment and Evaluation. Retrieved from http://ericae.net/ft/tamu/Rm.htm. on August 28, 2015.
21. Last JM. Time series. *Encyclopedia of Public Health. Retrieved from* http://www.Answers.Com/. Updated 2008. on January 13, 2008.
22. Hackshaw A, Paul E, Davenport E. *Evidence-Based Dentistry: An Introduction*. Hoboken, NJ: John Wiley; 2007.
23. Shiboski CH, Schmidt BL, Jordan RC. Racial disparity in stage at diagnosis and survival among adults with oral cancer in the US. *Comm Dent Oral Epid*. 2007;Jun 35(3):233–40.

17

Biostatistics

Christine French Beatty, RDH, PhD

Connie E. Beatty RDH, MS

OBJECTIVES

After studying this chapter, the dental hygiene student should be able to:

- Define and describe data analysis and interpretation
- Identify data by their type and scale of measurement
- Define and describe descriptive, correlation, and inferential statistics
- Select and compute appropriate measures of central tendency and measures of dispersion for various types of data
- Describe and construct frequency distributions and graphs for various types of data
- Identify and describe a study's research (alternate) hypothesis, null hypothesis, and the process involved with making a statistical decision
- Interpret correlation statistics
- Select appropriate inferential statistical tests for various types of data
- Interpret research results

COMPETENCIES

After studying the chapter and participating in accompanying course activities, the dental hygiene student should be competent to do the following:

- Use critical thinking skills and comprehensive problem-solving to identify oral health care strategies that promote patient health and wellness
- Use evidence-based decision making to evaluate emerging technology and treatment modalities to integrate into patient dental hygiene care plans to achieve high-quality, cost-effective care
- Assume responsibility for professional actions and care based on accepted scientific theories, research, and the accepted standard of care
- Integrate accepted scientific theories and research into educational, preventive, and therapeutic oral health services

KEY TERMS

Science photo/Shutterstock

The subject of **biostatistics,** the use of data analysis and interpretation in health care research, is a course unto itself, and fortunately for the dental hygienist in the twenty-first century, computer programs are available to do the computations.[1] Nevertheless, the dental hygienist must have a working knowledge of statistics to use these computer programs and interpret research results (See Table 17-1 ■ Statistical Symbols and Their Meanings).

Upon completion of a research project or program evaluation, data must be analyzed in preparation for interpreting the results. Data analysis involves the application of statistical tests to the data in order to organize, describe, summarize, and analyze it to answer a research question or test a hypothesis.[2] When the data have been analyzed, the researcher must interpret these results. Interpretation, which is the explanation of results, requires that critical thinking be used to explain the meaning and application of the findings, identify possible factors that could have influenced the results, and draw inferences to the population.[3,4] Biostatistics is used to demonstrate response to dental hygiene therapy; to test products and treatment regimes used in dental hygiene therapy; to determine the needs of target populations; to evaluate oral health treatment, prevention, and educational programs; and to complete a variety of other purposes in relation to oral health care. (See Table 17-2 ■).[4] Although not every dental hygienist will conduct research studies or evaluate community programs, each and every dental hygienist must understand the research process, including data analysis and interpretation, to be able to critically analyze the results of published studies and understand the epidemiology of disease. This is essential for the dental hygienist to be able to practice therapies and implement programs that are based on scientific evidence.[5]

Did You Know?

A foundation in biostatistics helps the dental hygienist understand literature and research reports.

Students of research often reflect a bias that statistics are undependable because they can be used to "say whatever you want them to say."[4] However, the appropriate application of the sound principles of biostatistics will produce valid results and interpretations.[4] For the researcher who is not familiar with statistical analysis, consultation with a statistician experienced in this field is highly recommended when planning a research project to avoid errors in research design and misinterpretation of results. If the number of participants in a study is insufficient, the study is not long enough in duration, incorrect measurement instruments or procedures are used, or the wrong statistical tests are used to analyze the data, the resulting conclusions will be invalid.[5] Repeating the research study due to statistical errors is frustrating for the principal investigator and highly aggravating to the financial sponsors. A

Table 17–1 Statistical Symbols and Their Meanings

Symbol	Meaning
α	Greek letter, alpha, for the level of significance set in a study
p	p-value: the level of statistical significance
H_o	Null hypothesis
α error	Type I error
β error	Type II error
N	Population size
n	Sample size
f	Frequency
μ or M	Greek letter, *mu*, for population mean
x or $\bar{x}$	x-bar, the sample mean
σ	Greek letter, *sigma*, for population variance
σ^2	Greek letter, *sigma*, squared for population standard deviation
s	Sample variance
s^2 or SD	Sample standard deviation
df	Degrees of freedom
χ^2	Greek letter, *chi*, squared to represent the statistical test appropriately named "chi squared"
ρ	Greek letter, *rho*, for population correlation coefficient
r	Sample correlation coefficient

*Adapted from Munro BH. Mathematical symbols in statistics, taken from *Statistical Methods for Health Care Research*. 6th ed. Philadelphia, PA: Lippincott; 2013.

Table 17–2 Why Does Biostatistics Matter?

- A clinician determines the correct dental hygiene therapy for any given condition from statistically significant research results.

- A health care professional recommends a safe and effective product by correctly understanding biostatistics.

- A dental hygienist prioritizes the needs of the client and community by utilizing statistically significant assessment outcomes.

- An oral health professional uses statistics to evaluate the effectiveness of a treatment plan, community intervention, and oral health educational program.

statistician also can be very helpful in interpreting the results and making inferences to the population.

Data Categorization

Data are the information that a researcher collects.[6] The word *data* actually is the plural term; the singular term is *datum.* Each piece of information is called an *item of data,* and a group of all data items collected is called a *data set.* Data can be quantitative or nonquantitative, sometimes referred to as *qualitative. Quantitative data* are numerical representations. For example, pocket depths, number of sealed teeth, and number of communities with water fluoridation can be expressed as counts, percentages, and means. Information that reflects the quality or nature of variables that cannot be measured numerically is referred to as *qualitative data.* The values of qualitative data are expressed as outcomes or states and can be counted for reporting. These variables can often be rank ordered as well.[7] An example is a list of clients' responses to what they liked most and least about their treatment visits to a dental clinic.

Variables are classified as continuous or discrete. A *continuous variable* is made up of distinct and separate units or categories and can be expressed by a large or infinite number of measures along a continuum.[7] These variables can be expressed in fractions and are considered quantitative. For example, height, weight, and time are continuous because they fall on a continuum and have value when expressed as fractions.

A *discrete variable* is also made up of distinct and separate units or categories, but it is counted only in whole numbers[7] and is quantitative because these data are represented numerically. An example of a discrete variable is the number of children. Logically, there cannot be fractions of children, although reports might refer to having a mean of 2.3 children per family. The dental index, decayed, missing, and filled teeth (DMFT) is also a discrete variable because it is not possible to have a fraction of a tooth. However, sometimes the distinction between discrete and continuous variables is unimportant in application because many discrete variables, especially those that have a high number of possible scores, can be treated meaningfully as continuous for statistical analysis.[8] For example, it is meaningful to express a mean of 2.5 on a DMF index, plaque index, gingival index, number of sealants, most other dental indices, and many rating scales.

A variable that has no numeric representation is a *categorical variable.*[7] Gender (male/female), color (red/blue/yellow), or rating (excellent/fair/poor) are examples of this type of variable. Religious preference and socioeconomic status (SES) are also categorical variables. Although categorical variables can be arranged logically and numbered accordingly, there is no meaning to the numeric representation. For example, an average religious preference or SES of 1.8 makes no sense. A *dichotomous variable* is a categorical variable that places data into only two groups, such as male/female, pass/fail, yes/no, or true/false.[6] Categorical and dichotomous variables are qualitative in nature.[6]

Data are also classified by the use of **scales of measurement.**[6] See Table 17-3 ■ for an illustrated reference. Four scales of measurement exist: nominal, ordinal, interval, and ratio. The higher the level of data, the more information it conveys about the differences among values. The scale of measurement is important because it determines which statistics and graphs can be used to represent and analyze the data.

The *nominal* scale of measurement organizes data into mutually exclusive categories, but the categories have no rank order or value, and there is no numeric relationship between the different classifications.[7] Ethnic group membership is an example. African American; American Indian and Alaska native; Asian; Hawaiian and other Pacific Islander; and White are five categories of ethnic group.

The *ordinal* scale of measurement organizes data into mutually exclusive categories that are rank ordered based on some criterion, but the difference between ranks is not necessarily equal in value.[6] An example is the classification of level of difficulty of patients' needs in a dental hygiene clinic: Class 0, 1, 2, 3, and 4. The higher classes reflects more difficulty, but the difference between class 1 and class 2 is not numerically equivalent to the difference between class 2 and class 3, and so on. Also, a class 4 is not necessarily twice as difficult as a class 2. Another common example is a five-point scale of ordered responses that range from strongly agree to strongly disagree to statements that evaluate the value of a program.

The *interval* scale of measurement has the characteristics of the ordinal scale, but in addition, the distance between any two adjacent units of measurement is equal. However, there is no meaningful zero point.[6] In other words, the zero point is arbitrary, not determined by nature. An example is the Fahrenheit measurement scale. Scores on an interval scale can be added and subtracted meaningfully but not multiplied and divided. A one-degree difference is numerically equal all along the scale. However, because of the arbitrary zero point, it cannot be said that 90°F is twice as hot as 45°F, although it is appropriate to state that 90°F is warmer than 45°F. There are no examples of oral health variables for the interval scale of measurement.

The *ratio* scale of measurement contains all characteristics of the preceding scales and has an absolute zero point determined by nature.[6] Therefore, all arithmetic procedures can be applied. Blood pressure, height, weight, number of teeth, and number of sealants are examples of ratio variables. A person who weighs 150 pounds is twice as heavy as a person who weighs 75 pounds. Four sealants is twice as many as two sealants, and it is possible to have no sealants (absolute zero point).

In general, categorical and dichotomous variables use the nominal and ordinal scales of measurement, and discrete and continuous data use the interval or ratio scales of measurement. However, several important points are necessary to understand that sometimes the rules vary for treating the various scales of data statistically. One point is that discrete and continuous data can be converted to nominal or ordinal data.[8] For example, study participants can be placed in nominal categories of "controlled BP" or

Table 17–3 Scales of Measurement

Measurement	Purpose	Dental Hygiene Example	Pictorial Example
Nominal	Data are grouped into **categories only** with no numerical value.	Dental Hygiene degree possessed (AAS, AS, BS, MS)	
Ordinal	This **ranks data** according to attributes.	Shades of whiteness of teeth (A1, A2, B1, B2 etc)	
Interval	Distances between scores are equal; **no absolute zero is present.**	N/A	
Ratio	Distances between scores are equal <u>with</u> an absolute zero point. **The absence of a score (a "zero" score) indicates the absence of the variable.**	Number of teeth; Number of participants enrolled in a community oral health program	

Source: Based on Munro BH. Mathematical symbols in statistics. In: *Statistical Methods for Health Care Research.* 6th ed. Philadelphia, PA: Lippincott; 2013. Tape measure image retrieved September 2, 2013 from http://s629.photobucket.com/user/jheath16407/media/bddef0a4.jpg.html; other graphics are Microsoft Office online clip art.

"uncontrolled BP" according to their blood pressure, which is a continuous variable. An additional example is to categorize study participants' gingivitis as mild, moderate, or severe (ordinal scale) according to the number of bleeding points (discrete variable). Another point discussed previously is that when ordinal data consist of many ranks or categories, the data are customarily treated as continuous rather than discrete.[6,8] For example, ordinal attitude scales (eg, very satisfied, satisfied, neither satisfied nor dissatisfied, dissatisfied, very dissatisfied) are commonly treated as interval data.[6] A third point is that the distinction between interval and ratio data is insignificant. Both types of variables are handled the same way when analyzing data.[9]

Descriptive Statistics

Statistics are divided into two major categories: descriptive and inferential. **Descriptive statistics** consist of the procedures that are used to summarize, organize, and describe quantitative data.[7] Data are generally presented by describing and summarizing them with the use of descriptive statistics and tables and graphs rather than presenting all of the raw data. **Inferential statistics,** on the other hand, are used to make inferences or generalizations about a population based on data taken from a sample of

that population.[6] This process is also called *making statistical decisions*. The application of descriptive statistics to a data set always precedes the use of inferential statistics. A data set can be summarized numerically with a measure of central tendency, a measure of dispersion, and a sample size. Data can be displayed in tables and graphs to further enhance the understanding of the nature of the variable. Descriptive statistics include measures of central tendency, measures of dispersion, frequency distribution tables, and graphing techniques.

Measures of Central Tendency

The term **measures of central tendency** refers to statistical methods that describe the clustering of the numerical values in a distribution of data within a research study. When describing statistics, the term *average* is rarely used. Instead, one of the three measures of central tendency (*mean, median,* or *mode*) is used, depending on the type of data the researcher is describing.[10] A summary of the measures of central tendency is presented in Table 17-4 ∎.

The *mean* is what is commonly called the *average*. It is the arithmetic average of the data set. The symbol used to denote the mean is x; the symbol M is also commonly used in journal articles.[8] To arrive at the mean, one would add

Table 17–4 Measures of Central Tendency

Measure	Description	Appropriate Use
Mean	Arithmetic average	Ratio and interval data
		Ordinal data that are treated as continuous
Median	Middle score	Ordinal data
Mode	Most Frequently Occurring Score	Nominal data

all scores and divide by the total number. The formula for the mean is $\Sigma x/n$. The uppercase Greek letter sigma (Σ) means "the sum of." If the letter x represents a single value in the distribution, then Σx means "the sum of all the values." The letter n represents the sample size or number of observations. For example, to compute the mean of the numbers 2, 3, 3, and 4, $\Sigma x/n = 12/4 = 3$. The mean is appropriate to use with interval and ratio data. It is also commonly used with ordinal data when they are treated as continuous data as previously described.

Did You Know?

The mean cannot be used to describe nominal data.

The *median* is the midpoint of the data, in other words, the point at which exactly half of the values are above and half are below.[10] The median of the scores 2, 2, 3, 4, and 5 is 3. If we have only the scores 2, 2, 3, and 4, the median is the average of the middle two scores, which in this case is 2.5. Note that the scores must be placed in ascending or descending order (called an *array*) to be able to determine the median manually. The median can be used to describe ratio, interval, or ordinal data, but not nominal data because they cannot be rank ordered.

The *mode* is the value that occurs most often in the distribution.[10] The mode of the scores 2, 3, 3, and 4 is 3. Some distributions may have more than one mode, which would be referred to as *bimodal* (two modes) or *multimodal* (more than two modes). The mode can be used to describe all types of data. When analyzing nominal data, such as gender and SES, the mode is the only measure of central tendency that can be used.[7]

Measures of Dispersion

A **measure of dispersion,** also called a *measure of variability,* communicates how much variation is present in a group of data.[11] It describes the distribution of data within a research study. Two distributions of data can have the same measure of central tendency and vastly different measures

of dispersion. For example, a distribution could have a mean of 90 with a low score of 80 and a high score of 97, while another distribution could have a mean of 90 with a low score of 88 and a high score of 94. The distribution with the wider spread of scores has a higher measure of dispersion. Because of this, to report a measure of central tendency without a measure of dispersion can misrepresent the data.

The measures of dispersion are the range, variance, and standard deviation. The *range* is determined by subtracting the lowest score from the highest score. It is the simplest and least useful measure of dispersion because it is based only on the lowest and highest scores.[11] Sometimes the range is reported as the distance between the lowest and highest scores, for example, a range of 80 to 97 for a set of test scores. The range is usually reported with the median.[4]

Did You Know?

At all times, it is important to look not only at the average or mean but also at the dispersion of the data.

The *variance* represents the average distance of each score from the mean, and the *standard deviation* (SD) is the square root of the variance. Because they are based on the average squared distances of values around the mean, these are the most common and useful measures of dispersion.[12] The variance or SD is usually reported with the mean. When analyzing normally distributed data, standard deviation can be used in conjunction with the mean in order to calculate data intervals.

The steps for computing a variance and SD are presented in Box 17-1 ■. Although it is no longer necessary to compute these values manually, understanding the computation helps to understand the significance of the values.[12] Notice that each score in a distribution is used to compute the variance and SD. This makes them more accurate and

Box 17–1 Steps to Compute the Variance and Standard Deviation (SD)

1. Calculate the mean for the distribution of scores.
2. Subtract the mean from each score (individual score – mean). This is called the *deviation*. When the mean is larger than the score, the result is a negative value.
3. The sum of the deviations always equals zero. Add the deviations to check this.
4. Square each deviation ([individual score – mean]^2).
5. Add the squared deviations to determine the sum of squares (Σ[individual score – mean]^2).
6. Divide the sum of square by N – 1 (number of scores – 1). This resulting value is called the *variance*.
7. Take the square root of the variance. This resulting value is the *standard deviation*.

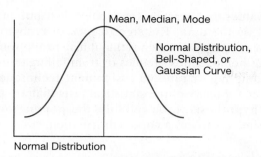

FIGURE 17–1 Standard Normal Distribution

useful measures of dispersion than the range. In the previous example of two distributions with a mean of 90, the distribution with a high score of 97 and a low score of 80 would have a wider variance and SD than the distribution with a high score of 94 and a low score of 88. In this way, the value of the variance or the SD in relation to the mean depicts the distribution of scores.

The Normal Distribution

Most occurrences in this world theoretically fall into a bell-shaped curve, called the **normal distribution** or *Gaussian distribution*.[7] Generally, the majority of scores fall under the large part of the middle of the curve with a few low and high outliers. Grades are a good example of this tendency. If one looked at a group of people from the general population of college students who took a class in principles of chemistry, most of them would receive a grade of C with a

few getting Bs and Ds and an even fewer receiving As and Fs. When researchers want to know whether an intervention has made a difference, they cannot just look at pure numbers. It is not enough that a group's mean score improved; the improvement also must be *statistically significant*. The normal distribution forms the theoretical foundation for these comparisons and in making statistical decisions.

This theoretical normal distribution yields a symmetrical, unimodal, bell-shaped curve.[6] This shape explains why random variables tend to be normally distributed.[11] The mean, median, and mode of the normal distribution are of equal value. The curve's extreme ends (called *tails*) do not touch the abscissa (*x*-axis). See Figure 17-1 ■ for an example of standard normal distribution.

Use of the *empirical rule* estimates the spread of the data given the mean and the standard deviation of a data set that follows the standard normal distribution.[13] According to this empirical rule, for a normal distribution, approximately 68 percent of the data fall within 1 SD of the mean, 95 percent within 2 SD, and 99.7 percent within 3 SD.[11] See Figure 17-2 ■ for a graphic presentation of the empirical rule.

The normal distribution is also the foundation of the *central limit theorem*. Based on this statistical proposition, less sampling error will occur with a larger sample, and a sample size of thirty or more will estimate the population mean with reasonable accuracy.[10] The normal distribution can be used to study a wide variety of statistical problems.[10] According to the central limit theorem, if an infinite number of randomly selected samples are drawn from a

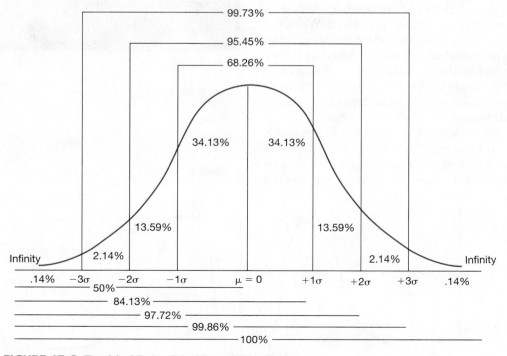

FIGURE 17–2 Empirical Rule of the Normal Distribution

Source: Darby ML, Bowen DM. *Research Methods for Oral Health Professionals: An Introduction.* St. Louis, MO: C. V. Mosby; 1980. Reprint. Pocatello, ID: McCann; 1993.

population, the means of the samples tend to be normally distributed, and the average of the sample means is very close to the actual population mean. The SD of these sample means is called the *standard error of the mean*.[10] To calculate it, the SD is divided by the square root of the sample size; hence, a larger sample size significantly reduces the standard error. The term *error* here does not signify an error made but indicates the fact that each sample mean is likely to vary somewhat from the population mean.[6]

Did You Know?

In oral health research studies it is important to have at least thirty study participants in a clinical trial.

In contrast to a normal distribution, when a distribution of scores is asymmetrical, the curve is said to be distorted, or skewed, and the study is said to have a **skewed distribution**.[11] (See Figure 17-3 ■.) The skew is caused by a few extreme scores in the distribution. A skewed curve can be identified by the curve's appearance resulting from plotting the data. A skewed distribution also can be identified by comparing the mean and median of the distribution.[14] In a positively skewed (or upward or right-skewed) distribution, the infrequent or extreme scores are on the right side of the *x* axis, the mean is larger than (to the right of) the median, and the tail is in a positive direction. In a negatively skewed (or downward or left-skewed) distribution, the infrequent or extreme scores are on the left side, the mean is smaller than (to the left of) the median, and the tail is in a negative direction. Vogt suggests a method to remember which skew is which.[6] Remember that a skewer is pointed. When the point is on the right, it is right skewed; when the pointed end is on the left, it is left skewed.[6] Because of the relative position of the mean and median, the skew of a curve can also be determined by examining the values of the mean and median of the distribution in relation to each other without seeing a curve that represents the plot of the data.

The mean is highly affected by extreme scores and is pulled in their direction; therefore, the median and mode more accurately represent central tendency in a skewed distribution.[11] For this reason, it is wise to examine all

three values to determine the type of distribution represented by the data. The significance of recognizing a skewed sample distribution is that it may result from using small or homogenous samples or from failing to use random sampling or random assignment techniques.[10] In addition, for many of the statistical tests that are used to test a hypothesis to be reliable, the population must approximately follow a normal distribution.[10]

Graphing Data

Data can be presented pictorially in graphs. The advantages of using graphs and tables include effective and economic communication of data, easier and quicker understanding and interpreting of data, and the ability to compare multiple distributions visually.[2]

Frequency Distribution Tables

A *frequency distribution table* presents data in a way that shows the number of times each score occurs in the group of scores.[7] For nominal and ordinal variables, the categories are listed in a natural order and then the frequency for each category is tabulated. Table 17-5 ■ illustrates a frequency distribution table for ordinal data, that is, age category of patients treated in a dental hygiene clinic.

For interval and ratio data, the values are first arranged in an array, which is an ordered display of a set of

Table 17–5 Frequency Distribution Table of Nominal Data

Number of Patients Treated in Dental Hygiene Clinic in Fall 2006 by Age Category		
Patient Type	**Number**	**Percentage**
Child	55	11%
Adolescent	62	12
Adult	173	34
Geriatric	216	43
Total	506	100%

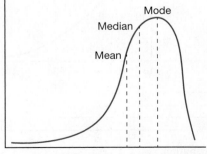

Negatively skewed distribution

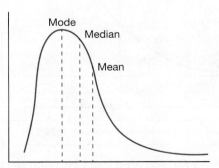

Positively skewed distribution

FIGURE 17–3 Skewed Distributions

observations.[6] For these types of data, the frequency can be expressed in four ways:

1. The actual frequency or count for the category
2. The relative frequency or percent calculated by dividing the frequency by the total number in the data set
3. The cumulative frequency, which is the total up to and including that value
4. The cumulative relative frequency, or cumulative percent, which is also known as the percentile rank

Frequency distribution tables can be ungrouped or grouped.[7] An *ungrouped frequency* distribution includes all the scores in the distribution. It is recommended for small samples with less than 30 observations. With a large data set (more than 30 observations), a grouped frequency distribution can be constructed by grouping the data into class intervals. Also, if the difference between the maximum and minimum values is more than 15, a grouped frequency distribution is recommended.[6] However, it is important to note that when the scores are widely dispersed, grouping the data can cause loss of detail in the scores reported.

To construct a *grouped frequency distribution,* group a set number of scores into mutually exclusive intervals called *class intervals,* also known as *collapsing the data.*[6] It is important to choose an interval and a starting point that are divisible by 5. To determine the number of intervals, the total number of measurements is considered. It is equally inappropriate to have just one or two measurements in several intervals and to have a large number of measurements in only a few intervals. About 5–10 intervals are appropriate for most distributions.[10] See Table 17-6 ■ for an ungrouped frequency distribution for ratio data and Table 17-7 ■ for a grouped frequency distribution for the same data. Note how much easier it is to understand the data in the grouped frequency distribution table. Relative frequency or percent and cumulative relative frequency or percent columns could be added if desired. Sometimes, these tables present a frequency column and a relative frequency or percent column with no cumulative column.

Types of Graphs

A frequency distribution can also be displayed in a graph, which is a diagram showing the variation of a variable in comparison with one or more other variables; it is also called a *chart.* A graph showing a frequency distribution is usually constructed by representing the variable on the horizontal (x) axis and the frequency on the vertical (y) axis, although the axes can be reversed. The vertical axis should have a height of one-half to three-fourths the width of the graph.[8] This prevents expanding or collapsing the x and y scales and minimizes misrepresentation and misinterpretation of the data.[15] Computers have facilitated the construction of graphs. Some computer programs, for example Excel, label graphs as charts. Some of the most commonly used graphs are the bar graph, histogram, polygon, frequency polygon, scattergram, and pie chart.

Table 17–6 Ungrouped Frequency Distribution for Ratio Data

X	f
100	0
99	2
98	1
97	1
96	0
95	1
94	3
93	1
92	1
91	1
90	0
89	4
88	2
87	2
86	0
85	0
84	3
83	4
82	2
81	1
80	0
79	1
78	3
77	1
76	4
75	1
74	2
73	0
72	0
71	0
70	0
69	1
68	0
67	0
66	0
65	0
64	1
63	0
62	0
61	0

Table 17–7 Grouped Frequency Distribution

Class Interval	f	Cumulative f
95–99	5	45
90–94	6	40
85–89	8	34
80–84	12	26
75–79	10	14
70–74	2	4
65–69	1	2
60–64	1	1

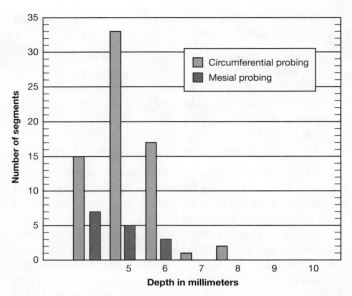

FIGURE 17–5 Cluster Bar Graph

A *bar graph* (or bar chart) is used to present categorical data.[6] A space separates the bars to emphasize the discrete nature of the data. The length of each bar corresponds to the frequency of the value it represents. See Figure 17-4 ■ for an example of a bar graph. Each bar represents a reason for a missed appointment. Two or more distributions can be compared by using a cluster bar graph (Figure 17-5 ■) .

A *histogram* is similar to a bar graph, but the bars appear side by side, that is, touching. It is appropriate for showing interval or ratio variables and sometimes ordinal variables that are treated as continuous data.[7] Both ungrouped and grouped frequencies can be represented in a histogram. Computer programs are handy for experimenting with the number and height of bars and the width of the intervals to help meet the goal of constructing a graph with a smooth appearance that accurately represents the data. See Figure 17-6 ■ for an example of a histogram.

A *frequency polygon* is a line graph that represents frequency data that are continuous in nature and drawn by connecting the midpoints of the bars of a histogram and then extending the line at both ends to imaginary midpoints at the right and left of the histogram. This extension of the line ensures that the total areas of both graphs are

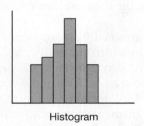

Histogram

FIGURE 17–6 Histogram

equivalent.[8] As with histograms, frequency polygons can be used to represent ungrouped or grouped frequency distributions and can present frequency, percent, cumulative frequency, or cumulative percent. They are especially useful for comparing two or more distributions visually by superimposing them in one graph as in Figure 17-7 ■.

A line graph can also be used to plot a variable over time.[15] Refer to Figure 17-8 ■ for an illustration of such a polygon that depicts the change in mean plaque scores over a series of periodontal therapy appointments.

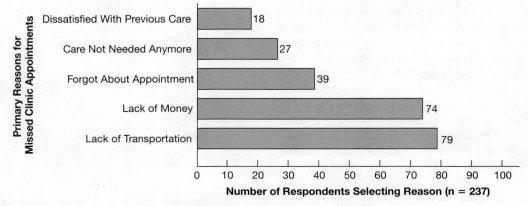

FIGURE 17–4 Bar Graph of Reasons for Missed Clinic Appointments

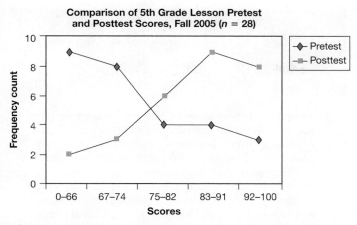

FIGURE 17–7 Frequency Polygon Comparing Two Distributions

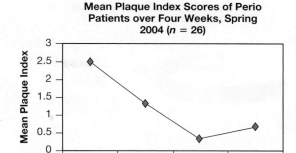

FIGURE 17–8 Polygon

A *scattergram* shows the relationship between two variables. For each subject, the level of one variable is plotted on the *x* axis against the level of the other variable on the *y* axis.[11] The resulting scattergram shows how the level of one variable varies as the level of the other variable changes. See Figure 17-9 for scattergrams that depict different relationships between variables.

A *pie chart* represents parts of a whole. Its use is more acceptable with lay audiences than in scientific or technical publications and presentations. When used, the percentage represented by each part of the pie should be labeled for clarity.[16] See Figure 17-10 ■.

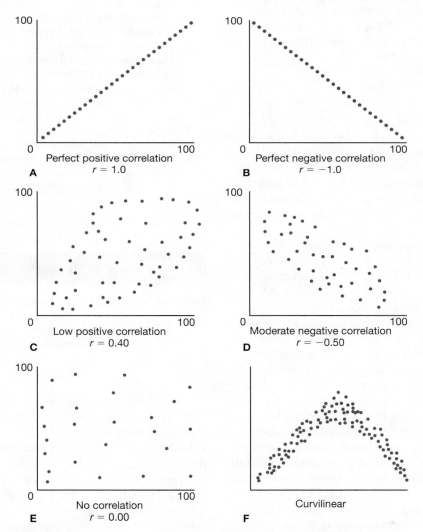

FIGURE 17–9 Scattergrams Demonstrating Relationships of Data

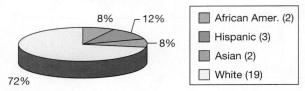

Ethnic Groups Represented in Dental Hygiene Class of 2004

- African Amer. (2)
- Hispanic (3)
- Asian (2)
- White (19)

8% — 12%

8%

72%

FIGURE 17–10 Pie Chart

Did You Know?

Pie charts are helpful to use when describing the demographics of study participants.

Tables and graphs facilitate our understanding and interpretation of the data. They help us quickly spot the shape of the distribution, where the data cluster, and how the data scatter around the clustering points, outliers, and gaps in the data.[8] Data presented in tables and graphs should be understandable even without the written discussion of the data. See Box 17-2 ■ for characteristics of effective tables and graphs and appropriate ways to achieve them.[6,8,15]

Correlation

Correlational techniques are used to study relationships among variables. The term correlation is used in everyday language to mean relationship. In statistics, **correlation** refers to a relationship or association between variables that can be measured mathematically.[11] The null hypothesis in a correlation analysis is one of no association between the variables. Correlation statistics are a form of inferential statistics.

The statistic used to measure correlation is the *correlation coefficient*, signified by *r*, which is expressed as a number between −1 and +1. The value of *r* communicates both the direction and strength of the association.[11] The sign (+ or −) determines the direction of the relationship. In a positive relationship, both variables vary in the same direction. In other words, as one increases in value, the other also increases in value. In the same way, as one decreases in value, the second also decreases in value. An example is the relationship between periodontal disease and heart disease. Heart disease and periodontal disease increase and decrease together in the population. In a negative relationship, the variables vary in opposite directions, so as one variable increases in value, the other decreases, and vice versa. This is also described as an *inverse relationship*. An example is the relationship between oral hygiene and gingivitis. As the frequency and effectiveness of oral hygiene practices increase, gingivitis decreases; as the frequency and effectiveness of oral hygiene decrease, gingivitis increases.

Box 17–2 Characteristics of Effective Tables and Graphs and Ways to Achieve Them

1. **Accuracy.** Enter data carefully. Follow basic principles for construction of tables and graphs. Select the type of table or graph considering the type of data being presented. Construct graphs that will not be misleading or open to misinterpretation. Begin the vertical axis at zero with a break drawn in, if necessitated by a high frequency of scores. Make the height of the vertical axis one-half to three-fourths of the horizontal width of the graph.
2. **Simplicity.** Present data in a straightforward manner. Highlight only the major points of information. Minimize the use of grid lines, tics, unusual fonts, and showy patterns.
3. **Clarity.** Make data easy to understand and self-explanatory. Use brief but clear titles and headings, and label all axes and variables including type of frequency (count, percent, cumulative). Carefully choose intervals. Include information on when and where data were collected, if appropriate, and the size of the groups. Communicate exclusions of observations from the data set including the reasons and criteria for their exclusion. Include the basis for the measurement of rates. Use textbooks on statistics and graphing, scientific writing style manuals, and samples of tables and graphs in journal articles to guide your construction.
4. **Appearance.** Pay attention to the construction so that the final result is neat and appealing.
5. **Well-Designed Structure.** Emphasize the important points visually. Use dark bars and light grid lines and horizontal lettering when possible.

Did You Know?

Another example of inverse relationship would be that as the consumption of fluoridated water increases in a population, the caries rate decreases, and as the consumption of fluoridated water decreases in a population, the caries rate increases.

The value of *r* indicates the strength of the relationship. As the value moves closer to +1.0 or −1.0, it indicates a stronger relationship; as it moves closer to 0, it indicates a weaker relationship. This means that a value of +0.90 is just as strong as a value of −0.90. A value of +1.0 or −1.0 indicates a perfect relationship, and a value of zero indicates no relationship. Refer to Table 17-8 ■ for a general interpretation of *r*. In oral health when two variables are associated, the relationship generally is not perfect because other variables are also associated with the variables being

Table 17–8 Guide to Interpretation of *r*

Value of *r*	Strength of Association
0.00–0.25	Little if any
0.26–0.49	Weak
0.50–0.69	Moderate
0.70–0.89	High
0.90–1.00	Very high

Source: Based on Munro BH. *Statistical Methods for Health Care Research*. 6th ed. Philadelphia, PA: Lippincott; 2013.

correlated. For example, the association between fluoride and dental caries is not perfect because of the role of diet and plaque bacteria in the development of caries.

Several correlation techniques are available. The selection is based on the number of variables to be correlated, the nature of the variable (discrete or continuous), the measurement scale, and the linearity of the relationship between the variables,[17] which is depicted by the scattergram. (See Figure 17-9 ■.)

The most common correlation coefficient is the *Pearson product moment correlation coefficient*. Pearson *r* is used when both variables are continuous, are at least interval scaled, and have a linear relationship.[11] The linearity of the relationship is determined by plotting the scores on a scattergram. In Figure 17-9, scattergrams A, B, C, and D demonstrate linear relationships, E demonstrates no relationship, and F demonstrates a curvilinear relationship.

The *Spearman rank-order correlation coefficient* (also called *Spearman rho*) is a variation of *r* used to correlate two ordinal variables.[11] Other correlation techniques are available for data that are nominally scaled, for data with curvilinear relationships, for relating more than two variables, and for other purposes.[8] Correlation techniques are also used to determine reliability of data collection instruments, intrarater reliability, and interrater reliability.[11] Statistical significance of correlation can also be determined to rule out the possibility that the observed correlation is due to chance alone.

Regression analysis, like correlation, can be used to quantify the relationship of two variables. However, unlike correlation, it expresses the functional relationship between the variables.[13] It is used to predict the score of one variable (dependent variable referred to as *y*) based on the score of another (independent variable referred to as *x*).[11] For example, regression can be used to predict an individual's score on the National Board based on GPA in the program. Multiple regression analysis goes a step further to provide a mathematical model that gives the strength of the ability of two or more variables (independent variables) to predict another variable (dependent variable). For example, the strength of the ability of GPA,

Scholastic Aptitude Test scores, and other factors to predict success on the National Board could be tested with multiple regression analysis.

Results of correlation statistics and regression analysis do not necessarily equal causality, otherwise known as a *cause-and-effect relationship*.[11,18] Simply, **causality** means that a certain exposure will result in a particular outcome. Correlation and regression statistics provide information about how variables relate and can be predicted, but do not provide evidence of causality.

However, causality can sometimes be inferred from results of epidemiological studies that apply correlation and regression statistics. Inferred causality in epidemiology depends on the strength of the association of the variables, the consistency of their association in repeated observations, the specificity of the relationship (not dependent on other factors), the occurrence of the causal factor at a point in time prior to the outcome, evidence of a dose-response curve in the relationship, plausibility of causality, agreement with current knowledge of the disease or condition, and analogy to causal relationships previously established.[19] Correlation provides much of the evidence in oral epidemiology because it establishes risk, which is the probability that a specified event will occur but not necessarily through a causal chain.[17] In other words, a strong significant correlation between two variables does not mean that one necessarily has caused the other. For example, caries and fluorosis are highly correlated, but fluorosis is not the cause of caries and caries does not cause fluorosis. Fluoride is the causal factor for both fluorosis and low caries rates. It is also a mistake to think that two correlated variables cannot be causally related or that correlation provides no evidence whatsoever for cause.[6] Remember that the first evidence of a cause-and-effect relationship between caries and fluoride was correlation. Additional research demonstrated that there was indeed causation. When correlation techniques indicate that two variables are associated, further longitudinal observational research and/or experimental research are indicated to be able to establish or infer causality.[17] (See Chapter 18 for a more detailed discussion of risk and causality.)

Did You Know?

Research does not "prove" anything! Research demonstrates cause-and effect relationships (causality) by describing characteristics, suggesting associations, and predicting risk.

Statistical Decision Making

The null hypothesis is an initial negative statement of belief about the value of a population parameter, for example, that two groups do not differ for a variable.[11] Basically, a null hypothesis is accepted unless the statistical test indicates it should be rejected. The research (alternative) hypothesis, also called the *positive hypothesis,* is the logical

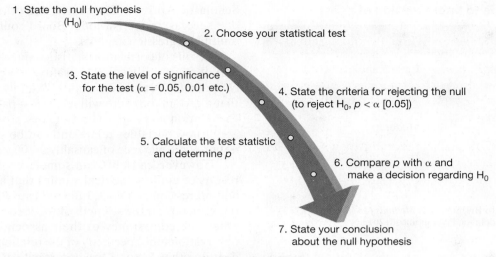

FIGURE 17–11 Seven-Step Process for Hypothesis Testing

Source: Adapted from Nichols D. Seven step procedure for hypothesis testing. [PowerPoint]. 2013.

opposite of the null hypothesis and can indicate a direction of difference. (See Chapter 16.) For example, the null hypothesis is that the retention rate of one brand of sealants does not differ from the retention rate of a second brand. The accompanying research hypothesis can be that the retention rates differ (no direction of difference specified) or that the first brand has a higher retention rate than the second (directional hypothesis). See Boxes 17-3 ■ and 17-4 ■ for examples of hypotheses. The object of hypothesis testing is to decide whether it is reasonable to continue believing that the null hypothesis is true or to reject this belief in favor of the research hypothesis. See Figure 17-11 ■ for a depiction of the Seven-Step Process for Hypothesis Testing.

A statistical decision is made about the null hypothesis based on the results of inferential statistics.[10] Remember that inferential statistics (more later) is the category of statistics used to make inferences or generalizations about a population based on data taken from the sample. These statistics are used to test a hypothesis or to estimate a population parameter based on the sample data, for example, to estimate the mean satisfaction score of dental hygienists in the United States based on the mean satisfaction score of a representative sample surveyed.

The statistical decision to reject or accept the null hypothesis is based on probability at a set significance level, also known as the *alpha* α *level*. It is expressed as a probability value or p **value,** or the probability that the findings from a study are due to chance. The *p* value commonly accepted as statistically significant in oral health research is equal to or smaller than 0.05 ($p \le .05$).[11] We see *p* values of .05, .01, and .001 in research reports. A low *p* value signifies greater statistical significance of the result. When the *p* value is larger than .05, the results are said to be not statistically significant, or NS. Simply stated, a result of hypothesis testing reported as $p = .05$ means that the probability of this result occurring by chance alone equals

5 percent. The *p* value is the final arithmetic solution obtained by using the calculated test statistic, the sampling distribution of the test statistic, and the size of the sample. Regardless of the inferential statistic used, the statistical decision is made this same way by using the *p* value to determine statistical significance.

A caution regarding the interpretation of a *p* value is appropriate at this point. A *p* value is not simply the probability that the null hypothesis is true. Rather, the *p* value is the probability that the data have a sampling error and the null hypothesis is true. When reacting with disbelief about the null hypothesis because the *p* value is small, it does not necessarily mean that a false null hypothesis has been detected. There is a possibility of error when either rejecting or accepting a null hypothesis because the statistical decision is based on probability.[10]

A Type I error (also called *alpha* α *error*) occurs when the null hypothesis is rejected but it is actually true and should have been accepted.[10] (See Table 17-9 ■.) The probability of a Type I error is the same as the alpha α level. For example, in a study comparing the retention rates of two sealants, a Type I error would be made if the statistical decision indicated that one sealant had a better retention rate than the other when in actuality their retention rates were equivalent. Setting an alpha level at .05 denotes a

Table 17–9 Type I and Type II Errors Made When Rejecting and Accepting the Null Hypothesis

	Decision About the Null Hypothesis	
	Accepted	Not Accepted
True	No error made (Correct decision)	Type I error (α)
Not True	Type Ii Error (β)	No error made (Correct decision)

willingness to take a 5 percent chance of making an alpha error. A large sample size can lead to a Type I error,[6] but a randomly selected representative sample and a good study design help to avoid making it.[14] The researcher can also control a Type I error by setting the alpha level low.

A Type II error (also called *beta β error*) occurs when the null hypothesis is accepted, but it is actually false and should have been rejected.[10] (See Table 17-9 ■.) Using the same example of a study to test the retention of sealants, a Type II error would be made if the statistical decision was that the retention rates of the two sealants did not differ when in fact one had better retention than the other. Unlike the probability of a Type I error, the exact probability of computing a Type II error is generally unknown. Using too small a sample, unreliable measuring devices, or imprecise research methods increases the probability of making a Type II error.[9]

The *power* of a test is its ability to reject a false null hypothesis or to detect relationships among variables. By increasing power, we decrease the Type II error rate. A power of .80 is considered reasonable.[6] Power can be improved by increasing the sample size, improving the measuring device, increasing the α level, or choosing a different study design.[9,10] Power is critically important in clinical trials using a positive control because the differences in the groups are likely to be slight.[10] For example, if a test fluoride dentifrice is compared with a positive control of a standard fluoride dentifrice, differences in caries rates between the two groups will likely be small. In this case, group sizes have to be extremely large. A power analysis is a technique used to determine the appropriate sample size considering the statistic being used, the α level, and characteristics of the data.[8]

The probability of Type I and Type II errors is inversely related; that is, the smaller the risk of one, the greater the risk of the other (See Box 17-3 ■). However, if the sample size is large enough, the researcher has the ability to decrease the risk of making a Type II error at the same time the risk of a Type I error is small.

Committing a Type I error can be more costly than a Type II error.[14] Type I errors lead to unwarranted change while Type II errors maintain status quo. For example, with a Type I error, a participant could receive incorrect treatment, but with a Type II error, a participant could not receive treatment that could have been helpful, even life saving. The degree of risk of a Type I or Type II error relates directly to the level of significance. When planning a research project, the Type I and Type II error rates should be considered regarding the particular research problem and which error type is more serious for the situation.[14] Because it is not possible to know whether a Type I or Type II error has occurred, it is important to conduct replication studies to increase the confidence that results are valid.[14] This is why the hierarchy of evidence for evidence-based decision making places multiple randomized clinical trials above a single randomized clinical trial. (See Chapter 18 for a description of the hierarchy). Guidelines for the conduct of oral research should be followed to avoid both Type I and Type II errors.[20]

Degrees of freedom (*df*) refers to the number of values or observations that are free to vary when computing a statistic, that is, the number of measurements taken minus 1 for each population parameter estimated.[17] The number is necessary to interpret inferential statistical tests. Degrees of freedom is based on the sample size so the larger the *df*, the easier it is to obtain a statistically significant result.

Did You Know?

Statistics text *books* contain clear rules for calculating and using *df* to interpret a statistic.

Box 17–3 Example Hypothesis 1

In the population, individuals who floss more than 3 times per week have a significantly lower Gingival Index score than individuals who do not floss at all. A sample is randomly selected from each population and GI scores are compared between the two samples (α = 0.05). The resulting *p* value for this comparison is *p* = 0.12.

- *What is the null hypothesis?* There is no difference in GI scores between those who floss 3 times per week and those who don't floss at all.
- *What is the decision about the null?* $p > α$, so the null is retained
- *Does this decision have the potential for a Type I or Type II error? Why?* Type II error (null is accepted) if the mean is actually different in one population compared to the other

Box 17–4 Example Hypothesis 2

In the population, individuals consuming high amounts of coffee have the sample DMFT scores as individuals consuming high amounts of soda. A sample is randomly selected from each population and DMFT scores are compared between the two samples (α = 0.05). The resulting *p* value for this comparison is *p* = 0.02.

- *What is the null hypothesis?* There is no effect on DMFT scores between those who consume high amounts of coffee versus those who consume high amounts of soda.
- *What is the decision about the null?* $p < α$, so the null is rejected
- *Would this decision have the potential for a Type I or Type II error? Why?* Type I error (null was rejected) if the null is actually true in the population and there is no difference between coffee drinkers and soda drinkers.

Inferential Statistics

The purpose of inferential statistics is to generalize between the sample being studied and the population that it represents.[7] Computing inferential statistics and analyzing the results require a more sophisticated understanding of statistics. Some of these are fairly easy to compute using a computer program. Others are more complex to compute and to interpret, and the use of computers and consultation with a statistician are advised when these statistics are used.

Confidence Interval

A *confidence interval* is a statistical technique used to infer the true value of an unknown population parameter, for example, the mean from the sample statistic.[7] Typically, 95 percent and 99 percent confidence intervals are used, and the standard error of the mean is used to calculate the intervals. The use of a 95 percent confidence interval is acceptable in oral health research. For example, if the 95 percent confidence interval for the mean Plaque index of 1.16 in a representative sample of school children is 1.08 to 1.24, we can be 95 percent certain that the mean Plaque index of the population is between 1.08 and 1.24.

Parametric Statistics

Inferential statistics used to test a hypothesis are classified as either parametric or nonparametric. (See Box 17-6 ■) Parametric statistics are used for hypothesis testing when the data meet certain assumptions.[7] (See Boxes 17-5 ■ and 17-6 ■.) One of these assumptions is that the data are classified as continuous. This includes ratio and interval data as well as ordinal data that approximate the continuous nature. Recall the previous discussion about continuous and discrete data. Discrete variables that have a large number of possible scores can be treated as continuous data, for example, DMF, Plaque index, Gingival index, most other dental indices, and many rating scales. The *t*-test and ANOVA will be discussed here.

STUDENT *t*-TEST The *t*-test is used to compare two mean scores to determine whether a statistically significant difference exists.[10] Formally known as the *Student* t-*test*, it is named after its inventor who published under the pseudonym Student. It is used to test a null hypothesis of

differences, for example, "the mean sealant retention rates for the two groups do not differ." There are two versions of the *t*-test. The t-*test for independent samples,* also called the *nonpaired* t-*test,* is selected when the mean scores are from two groups drawn independently from a population, that is, two different and unrelated groups of study participants.[10] For example, a dental hygienist might want to test the effectiveness of a new model of electric toothbrush compared with the existing older model of the same toothbrush. In this case, the dental hygienist would have one group of patients use the new model and have the second group use the older model. At the end of the study, the mean improvement of the two groups could be compared using the *t*-test for independent samples because the two data sets are drawn from two different groups of people. The statistical decision to reject or accept the null hypothesis is based on the resulting *p* value. Today, computers make the task easier for the statistical computation, comparison to the *t* distribution, and determination of the *p* value.

In this same study of a new electric toothbrush model, assume that the dental hygienist wanted to compare the pretest and posttest plaque scores for only the group that used the new model. In this case, the groups of data (pretest and posttest) are not mutually exclusive or independent, thereby violating one of the assumptions described earlier. To accommodate, the dental hygienist would use the t-*test for correlated samples,* also known as the t-*test for paired samples.* This *t*-test is used when the two mean scores are derived from the same group of study participants, as described, or when the experimental and control groups are matched on the basis of a variable known to be correlated with the independent variable.[10] For example, in fluoride dentifrice studies, the experimental and control groups are frequently matched for baseline DMF, age, and gender because these variables correlate with dental caries. The *t*-test for correlated samples would be used to compare the difference in caries improvement of the two groups. The results of the *t*-test for correlated samples would be interpreted the same way as the *t*-test for independent samples.

ANALYSIS OF VARIANCE (ANOVA) In this same example of the study testing the new model of electric toothbrush, a third group of patients using a manual toothbrush could be included for comparison purposes. In this case, three mean improvement scores would be compared. ANOVA is the parametric statistic used to determine whether statistically significant differences occur when comparing more than two mean scores.[10] Sometimes similar studies are reported in journals in which the data are analyzed using the *t*-test to perform multiple comparisons with different combinations of mean scores, two at a time. This is an incorrect application of the *t*-test because the Type I error rate will increase exponentially by the number of combinations of the *t*-test conducted.[8,10] When more than two mean scores are being analyzed, the ANOVA should be used. (See Figure 17-12 ■.)

Box 17–5 Assumptions Required for the Use of Parametric Statistics

- Data are continuous
- Adequate sample size is used
- Population distribution is normal
- Group variances are equal

Box 17–6 Parametric versus Nonparametric Data

Nonparametric Data	Parametric Data
Used to compare frequency counts	Used to compare means
Small sample sizes	Moderate to large sample sizes
Data are extremely skewed (extreme outliers)	Assume the data are normally distributed (bell-shaped curve)
Primarily nominal or ordinal data	Interval or ratio data
Compares observed frequencies from the sample data with expected frequencies	Compares observed data from the sample to known information about the population

Various forms of the ANOVA statistic are used according to the number of independent variables: one-way ANOVA for one independent variable and two-way ANOVA for two independent variables.[8] It can also be used as multivariate analysis of variance (MANOVA) to analyze the effects of the independent variable(s) on two or more dependent variables within the same test to increase power, limit Type I errors, and control for a relationship among the dependent variables. Analysis of covariance (ANCOVA) is another variation that controls for the effect of an extraneous variable that equally affects all groups, called a *covariate.*

ANOVA is used to analyze the differences within each group, the differences between or among groups, and the interactions. The data are presented in a complex table that describes these various comparisons. The result of the ANOVA test is an *F* ratio, which communicates whether a difference exists among the groups. However, it does not indicate which group mean significantly differs from the others. For example, when comparing the means of three groups, all three means could differ from each other significantly, or two means could be similar while the third mean differs significantly.[13] To determine which mean is significantly different, a post hoc analysis follows the ANOVA analysis by using one of a variety of available tests, including Tukey, Scheffe, Duncan, and Newman-Keuls.[6]

Using the previous example of the study testing the effectiveness of a new electric toothbrush model, the use of the ANOVA allows comparison of the mean improvement of plaque scores from the three groups: new model electric brush, older model electric brush, and manual brush. The *F* and corresponding *p* values suggest that the improvement of one group is statistically different from

the others, and the post hoc analysis tells us which group has the statistically different improvement. Now, assume that some of the participants are regular flossers while others are not. It is imperative to ensure that this extraneous variable does not affect the study results. In this case, ANCOVA could be used to control the effects of flossing on the outcome of the study. Finally, to measure the effect of the different brushes on plaque and gingivitis (two dependent variables that are correlated), the MANOVA is the test of choice.[10]

Nonparametric Statistics

When the assumptions for parametric statistics are not met (variables are discrete, sample size is small, population distributions are not normal, and/or group variances are not equal), nonparametric statistics should be used for hypothesis testing.[10] There is a variety of nonparametric statistics to test a range of null hypotheses from a question about relationships among variables to a question about group differences in outcome measures (see Figure 17-12).

CHI-SQUARE TEST   The chi-square test (χ^2), the most commonly used nonparametric statistic,[8] is utilized to determine whether a significant difference exists between frequency counts of nominal (categorical or dichotomous) data by comparing the observed frequencies to expected frequencies.[11] It can be used to compare two or more data sets from different sample groups (χ^2 test of the independence of categorical variables) or to compare the observed frequencies in one group to the expected frequencies

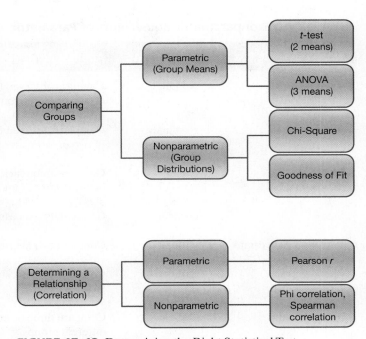

FIGURE 17–12 Determining the Right Statistical Test

Source: Adapted from Steinberg WJ. Selecting the appropriate analysis. In: *Statistics Alive.* 2nd ed. Thousand Oaks, CA: Sage Publications; 2011:509.

(goodness of fit). Use of the chi-square test requires that a group be composed of at least five.

This example illustrates two uses of chi-square for the same study of the new model electric toothbrush. The researcher crossed over the groups so that by the end of the study, all study participants had used each of the toothbrushes. Then each participant was asked which was the preferred brush to use. Thus, the three groups formed one group of 90 who scored their toothbrush preference. According to probability theory, the normal (or expected) preference frequencies would be equal for each toothbrush. With 90 participants in the study, 30 would be expected to prefer the new electric model, 30 to prefer the old electric model, and 30 to prefer the manual brush. The observed frequencies, which are the participants' reported preferences, are 40 for the new electric model, 30 for the old electric model, and 20 for the manual. The goodness of fit χ^2 test would reveal whether the observed preference for the new model is statistically significant compared with the expected preferences. Another example is to conduct the same study in two offices, one a family practice and the other a periodontal practice. The observed frequencies for the family practice clients are 40, 30, and 20 as in the previous example. The observed frequencies for the periodontal practice clients are 47 for the new electric model, 38 for the old electric model, and 5 for the manual brush. The χ^2 test of independence reveals whether the different preferences of the patients in the two offices are statistically significant.

OTHER NONPARAMETRIC TESTS Various other tests provide nonparametric equivalents to parametric statistics. The *Fisher test* is used for nominal data in place of the chi-square when group sizes are less than five.[10] The *sign test for paired comparisons* and the *Wilcoxon matched pairs signed-rank test* are used to compare ordinal or higher data from two paired measures and are considered to be nonparametric equivalents of the paired *t*-test.[7,10] The Wilcoxon matched pairs signed-rank test is more powerful than the sign test because it considers the magnitude of the differences between observations as well as the direction of the difference.[9,10] *McNemars's test* is used for the same purpose for nominal data, that is, to compare distributions of two paired data sets such as from the same sample.[10] The *Mann-Whitney rank-sum test* is used to test whether two independent groups have been drawn from the same population and is an alternative to the *t*-test for independent samples with ordinal variables.[10] The *Kruskal-Wallis* and the *Friedman matched-pairs tests* are nonparametric equivalents of two forms of ANOVA.[8] See Table 17-10 ■ for a summary of nonparametric equivalents to parametric tests.

Interpretation of Data and Research Results

When the research project has been concluded, the study participants dismissed, and the statistical analysis completed, the researcher must interpret the results and draw conclusions from the study. This requires the researcher to critically think and rethink about the meaning of the results in an unbiased manner. Interpretation should answer the questions presented in Box 17-7 ■.

Table 17–10 Nonparametric Equivalents of Parametric Tests

Nonparametric Test	Type of Data	Application	Equivalent Parametric Statistic
Chi-square	Nominal	Compare observed to expected frequencies of two or more groups of 5 or more	*t*-test for independent samples
Fisher	Nominal	Compare observed to expected frequencies of two or more groups of less than 5	*t*-test for independent samples
McNemar	Nominal	Compare frequencies of two or more measures from same group	Paired *t*-test
Sign	Ordinal	Compare two measures in same group	Paired *t*-test
Wilcoxon signed-rank	Ordinal	Compare two measures in same group	Paired *t*-test
Mann-Whitney rank-sum	Ordinal	Compare two measures from different groups	*t*-test for independent samples
Kruskal-Wallis	Ordinal	Compare three or more measures from different groups	ANOVA
Friedman	Ordinal	Compare three or more measures in same group	ANOVA

Box 17–7 Questions That Should Be Answered by Interpretation of Data

1. What could these results mean?
2. What factors might be contributing to these results?
3. Were these results expected based on the theoretical framework of the study and what is known in the field?
4. Do these results agree or disagree with other researchers' findings related to the same subject area?
5. Are there any known limitations or threats to internal and external validity that could have contributed to the results?
6. To what conclusions do these results lead?
7. How do the findings relate to, contribute to, advance, or have implications for the current knowledge or practice in the field?
8. In what populations, conditions, or settings would these same results hold true?
9. What additional research questions did these research results identify?
10. What additional research is needed to further answer this research question?

Source: Colorado State University. *Reliability and Validity*; 2013. Accessed August 31, 2013 from Writing @CSU Web site at http://writing .colostate.edu/guides/guide.cfm?guideid=66

Interpretation requires taking a close look at the course and events of the research project that could have impacted the results. Important factors to examine include study participants who dropped out and other unforeseen occurrences such as subject death, subject noncompliance, contaminated samples, and uncontrolled variables. These and other elements of the study must be scrutinized in regard to how they might have affected the study's internal and external **validity.** *External validity* means that the results of the study can be inferred to the general population and depends on how well the sample represents the population.[18] On the other hand, *internal validity* means that the study measured what it was supposed to measure. (See Chapter 18 for further discussion of internal and external validity.) Use of valid and reliable instruments, control of intra- and interrater reliability, standardization of procedures among groups, use of a control group, and randomization are examples of procedures that affect the study's internal validity.[3] A research study should be reliable and valid. **Reliability** refers to the degree to which the study would yield the same results within the same population each time the study is repeated. Reliability focuses on the consistency of the study. The replication of research study results by independent observers is critical so that researchers are able to draw conclusions from research studies, formulate further theories, or generalize results of a study to the population.

The researcher should avoid the temptation to make speculative deductions and conclude more than the numerical data indicate. Also, replications and effect size computations are more important than results from a single study that conclude only with a *p* value and a statistical decision about its statistical significance. A single research project rarely answers a question definitively but requires many types of studies with different sample populations over time to do so. These replication studies are necessary to provide results that can be used to make evidence-based practice decisions.[5] Results based on one sample do not provide enough evidence to warrant changes in practice.

Most often, research projects reflect the need for continued research and give rise to new questions.[10] Each carefully planned and executed research study is valuable because the additional scientific evidence can provide new insight into the results of previous studies and increase the overall understanding of this study's topic. Results of a study should be discussed in relation to those of previous studies conducted on the same or related topics.[5] In this way, much like a jigsaw puzzle, each bit of research provides a small clue to solving the big picture.

Did You Know?

If a clinician wants to make a recommendation from research, he or she must first make sure the reliability of a conclusion has been established. Reliability is determined through testing the same research question (or a similar one on the same topic) in multiple studies over time (replication).

It is possible that results of a study can have statistical significance but not have *clinical* or practical *significance.*[2] In other words, research that may or may not be inherent in the statistical results can have practical implications. When study groups are large, even trivial differences in disease increments can be statistically significant,[3] which can be misleading when they have no clinical importance. Also, the actual reductions in disease or health-related conditions should be scrutinized. One example of statistical versus clinical significance is a study comparing the time that it takes two tooth-bleaching products to whiten teeth. The statistical decision may reveal that one product whitens teeth in less time than the other product. However, the actual difference in time could be clinically meaningless or negligible. In this case, although the statistical significance is real, it is not useful in clinical application. Another example is the evaluation of an oral hygiene regime with a group of residents in a state mental health residential facility. If their baseline plaque score was 90 percent and was reduced throughout the program by one-fourth, at the end of the program the residents would still have 67.5 percent plaque score. Even if these results were

Table 17–11 What to Look for in a Research Report

Study design
Number of participants
Length of study time
Instrument or procedure utilized
Statistical test used

statistically significant, the remaining plaque biofilm status would still reflect compromised oral hygiene, which will likely lead to continuing oral disease. Although it may be worthwhile to continue the oral hygiene regimen tested, it would be wise also to seek other measures to further reduce the group's plaque biofilm status. Critically interpreting research results before applying them to dental hygiene practice is important for professionals. This is accomplished by carefully analyzing whether or not the ingredients of a successful investigation are reflected in the research being reviewed (see Table 17-11 ■).

One of the responsibilities of the ethical researcher is to disseminate research results to the profession and the appropriate public.[21] Without the distribution of research results, practicing dental hygiene professionals will not be able to fulfill their professional responsibility for continued competence and lifelong learning.[22,23] Incorporating

new knowledge and techniques into daily practice can benefit both the public's oral health and dental hygienists' occupational health. Reported research should include not only a description of the project and the results but also a candid discussion of the interpretation of the results including the study's limitations.[11,24] This allows the consumer of research to apply the results intelligently to professional practice.

Quality research is disseminated through peer-reviewed formats intended to provide reliable sources of quality research results.[25] The peer review process is designed to protect the consumer of research by controlling the quality of published research results. By depending on peer-reviewed publications and presentations to gain new knowledge, the practitioner can be more confident of the information's validity, which is necessary for evidence-based decision making. Evidence-based practice, by definition, requires the incorporation of research findings in combination with the clinician's personal expertise and the client's preference in order to make the best possible recommendations for care.[26] Laboratory science and epidemiology become the art of oral care through the practice of interpreting and applying peer-reviewed research results to evidence-based practice.[27]

Some examples of the interpretation of research studies are provided in Boxes 17-8 ■, 17-9 ■, and 17-10 ■. These will be helpful to provide practice relating the information in this chapter in terms of analyzing and applying research results to evidence-based practice.

Box 17–8 Example Research Study 1

A study sought to compare the effectiveness of a chlorhexidine varnish and a fluoride varnish in school-aged children in reducing *Streptococcus mutans* counts within plaque biofilm of occlusal pits and fissures. The children were randomly divided into 2 groups (Group 1 = chlorhexidine varnish; Group 2 = fluoride varnish) and received 3 applications of a varnish treatment over a six-month period. Plaque samples were collected at baseline, three months, and six months. $\alpha \leq 0.05$ and $\beta \leq 20$ percent. After statistical analysis, comparison of the 2 groups at six months revealed the following information: Comparison of mean plaque levels of Group 1 at baseline, three months, and six months revealed a *p* value of 0. 013. Comparison of mean plaque levels of Group 2 at baseline, three months, and six months revealed a *p* value of 0.065. Comparison of mean plaque levels between the 2 groups at six months revealed a *p* value of 0.005.

- *What is the null hypothesis?* There is no effect on *S. mutans* counts between those who receive a chlorhexidine varnish treatment and those who receive a fluoride varnish treatment.
- *What type of statistical test was used to compare the two groups?* t-test, which is classified as a parametric inferential test
- *What type of statistical test compared the measurements within the group (one, three, and six months)?* ANOVA
- *This type of study data could be classified as?* Continuous data; ratio scale of measurement
- *What can be concluded from the results of this study?* There was an effect on (reduction in) *S. mutans* counts by those who received the chlorhexidine treatment but not by those who received the fluoride varnish treatment.
- *Given these research findings, is this evidence conclusive enough to help a clinician make a recommendation for care? Why or why not?* No, according to the hierarchy of evidence-based practice,[28] a clinician should not make a clinical recommendation based on the results of only one study. Ideally, this study needs to be replicated multiple times, using a longitudinal design with a bigger sample size, to establish reliability and validity of the results.

Source: Adapted from Sajjan PG, Nagesh L, Sajjanar M, Reddy SKK, Venktesh UG. Comparative evaluation of chlorhexidine varnish and fluoride varnish on plaque *Streptococcus mutans* count—an *in vivo* study. *Int J Dent Hyg.* 2013;11:191–197.

Box 17–9 Example Research Study 2

The purpose of this study was to analyze relationships between subgingival colonies of yeast organisms, including *Candida albicans*, and the severity of chronic periodontitis. Fifty (50) patients with chronic periodontitis were compared against 50 healthy patients. Yeast organism samples were acquired from the periodontal pocket or sulcus with sterile paper points; the samples were cultured and analyzed for the association of yeast-positive individuals and periodontal disease status. Chi-square tests, in addition to Kruskal-Wallis and ANOVA tests, indicated a statistically significant association between the presence of *Candida albicans* organisms and deep periodontal pockets.

- *What is the research hypothesis?* The presence of *Candida albicans* will be positively associated with deep periodontal pockets.
- *Would this study be classified as descriptive, correlational, or experimental?* Correlational—it is studying the relationship between the two variables (yeast organisms and deep periodontal pockets)
- *A chi-square test compares what type of data?* Nonparametric, nominal data
- *Because a chi-square test compares observed to expected frequencies, what type of graphical representation would be used for the data?* A frequency table
- *Could a clinician conclude from these study results that the presence of yeast organisms causes chronic periodontitis?* No, these results suggest an increased risk for chronic periodontitis in the presence of yeast organisms, but they do not establish causality. In order to establish causality, this research needs to be replicated through additional longitudinal studies. (See Chapter 18 for further discussion of risk versus causality and longitudinal versus experimental studies.)

Source: Adapted from Canabarro A, Valle C, Farias MR, Santos FB, Lazera M, Wanke B. Association of subgingival *Candida albicans* and other yeasts with severity of chronic periodontitis. *J Periodont Res*. 2013;48:428–432.

Box 17–10 Example Research Study 3

A study that examined the association of coffee consumption and a reduced risk for oral/pharyngeal cancer had 500,000 participants enrolled. During the course of the 20-year study, 915 deaths from oral/pharyngeal cancer were noted. Cox regression statistical techniques estimated the participants' relative risk status as part of the statistical analysis. After controlling for other variables, a strong inverse linear association was noted between daily consumption of four cups or more of caffeinated coffee and oral/pharyngeal cancer. Researchers summarized that the antioxidant and polyphenol properties of coffee contribute towards a stronger immune response to the genetic mutations involved in the carcinogenesis process.

- *What is the research hypothesis?* A daily habit of coffee consumption will decrease one's risk for developing oral/pharyngeal cancer.
- *How would you describe the strength of the study design?* Very strong—this study represents a longitudinal cohort epidemiological study design (over 20 years with a very large sample size of 500,000).
- *Would the statistics used be classified as descriptive, correlational, or inferential?* Although it examines the relationship of variables, regression analysis is an inferential statistic. It goes beyond the simple examination of relationship done with correlation statistics and infers the results to the population at large through the use of prediction (regression) statistical techniques.
- *"A strong inverse linear association" between the two variables can be interpreted to mean what?* The greater the amount of coffee consumed, the lower the risk for oral/pharyngeal cancer.

How could a clinician relay this study information to a client who is at risk for oral cancer? These study findings suggest that if coffee consumption is already a part of someone's normal diet, there may be some beneficial properties that help reduce the risk of oral/pharyngeal cancer development. Although this is not an experimental research design, causality can be inferred by cohort studies. Even so, these findings need to be confirmed by additional studies before the conclusion can be drawn that coffee prevents cancer development (causality). Until confirmed, it is not advisable to recommend that a patient add coffee to the diet to prevent oral/pharyngeal cancer.

Source: Adapted from Hildebrand JS, et al. Coffee, tea, and fatal oral/pharyngeal cancer in a large prospective US cohort. *Am J Epidemiol*. 2013;177(1):50–58.

DENTAL HYGIENIST SPOTLIGHT ·····················

Public Health Column: Kim Poon, RDH

This month I am spotlighting a dental hygienist, Kim Poon, who has served our country first in military service and then continued to serve others by pursuing her career in dental hygiene. Additionally, she has continued to serve by practicing within public health and is coordinating an innovative public health position in the schools. She is a perfect example of figuring out ways to increase access to care for those most in need. Her career exemplifies the opportunities we all have as dental hygienists. This is what she had to say.

Why did you decide to go into dental hygiene?

During my childhood I was self-conscious of my teeth and my smile, which led me to being interested in dentistry. Growing up, my dental office was always a caring and friendly place, which allowed me to ask questions. I was able to observe the many tasks the dental hygienist did during my visits, and my interest in hygiene continued to grow. Growing up and seeing people who needed dental care, I knew this would be my career choice. My path to becoming a dental hygienist was using the GI Bill through the military that I earned while serving in the U.S. Army, which provided the financial support for my dental hygiene degree.

How did you get into dental public health?

I grew up in the Panhandle of Florida and the opportunities were mainly working for a private dental office. After working in dental hygiene for years and not having the option for health insurance with my employers, I decided to apply for dental positions that included health benefits. Additionally, I was interested in advancing my career into management. A job opportunity came up with the Florida Department of Health in Pasco County for a dental assistant supervisor that included health benefits that met my goals. I moved to Tampa, Fla., and started my new position in public health and have never looked back. Working in public health is an exciting area for a dental hygienist, and it allows many opportunities for career growth and public service to the community.

What are your current positions?

Currently, I am the senior human services program manager for the dental program at the Florida Department of Health in Pasco County. We have two fixed dental clinics, dental outreach programs, and, in the near future, a mobile dental van that I will manage and coordinate for the dental program. My responsibilities include supervising employees, dental operations, maintaining dental budget, working with insurance companies, clinical hygiene, coordinating with outside partners, and community outreach.

Each day brings new and challenging opportunities that as a dental hygienist in public health provides for a rewarding career.

Can you discuss any particularly interesting experiences you have had in your dental public health positions?

There have been many wonderful experiences since I have been in public health, but establishing our second dental clinic in an elementary school is most rewarding, because we have reached children on Medicaid who might not have received dental services. When I started at the health department, we had only one dental clinic location and the health department had discussed expanding to another location within the county that was in need of dental services for children.

With the support of the health department and the Pasco County School Board, we began the process of updating a full dental clinic located within a local elementary school. We have been at the elementary school for four years and now include two operatories, a sterilization room, and front office operating full-time. The dental clinic continues to grow each year with an increase in the number of patients. Since the school is familiar to the children and students in the community, it allows for ease of accessibility and comfort in coming to the elementary school for their dental care. Being a part of a program that continues to provide assistance to the community is very rewarding.

What type of advice would you give to a practicing hygienist who is thinking of doing something different?

I would ask what area(s) do you enjoy most about dental hygiene and encourage you to continue to pursue those area(s) within your career in dental hygiene. There are many other opportunities for dental hygienists to include sales, ownership, management, public health, military, and more that you could experience and excel in throughout a career in dental hygiene. For those dental hygienists who are feeling trapped in a certain setting, please realize there are many opportunities. I have been fortunate to be in this profession, and I have to admit, times are changing . . . gone are the days that dental hygienists had only one career option. Make changes if you feel that you have other skills to offer!

Source: Christine Nathe writes the Public Health Column in *RDH* magazine published by Pennwell Publishing. For more public health spotlights please see RDH magazine online at http://www.rdhmag.com/index.html.

Summary

Volumes have been written on research, biostatistics, and even various types of statistics and specific statistical tests. The information presented in this chapter is intended to serve as a guide for conducting research, assessing communities, evaluating community programs, and understanding the oral health literature. However, planning and interpreting complex research projects requires more information and consultation with a statistician.[28] In this way, solid research results will be disseminated to the professional and the appropriate public for the benefit of both.

Self-Study Test Items

1. Which variable is made up of distinct and separate units or categories but is counted only in whole numbers?
   a. Quantitative
   b. Qualitative
   c. Continuous
   d. Discrete

2. Which scale of measurement contains all of the characteristics of all scales and has an absolute zero point determined by nature?
   a. Interval
   b. Ordinal
   c. Ratio
   d. Numerical

3. Which type of correlational relationship would the following statement indicate? As the consumption of fluoridated water increases, the caries rate decreases.
   a. Positive
   b. Inverse
   c. Strong
   d. Weak

4. The research hypothesis, also called the *alternative* or *positive hypothesis,* is the logical opposite of the null hypothesis. The research hypothesis can indicate a direction of difference.
   a. The first statement is true; the second statement is false.
   b. The first statement is false; the second statement is true.
   c. Both statements are true.
   d. Both statements are false.

5. The chi-square test (χ^2) is the most commonly used non-parametric statistic. It is used to determine whether a significant difference exists between frequency counts of nominal (categorical or dichotomous) data by comparing the observed frequencies to expected frequencies.
   a. The first statement is true; the second statement is false.
   b. The first statement is false, the second statement is true.
   c. Both statements are true.
   d. Both statements are false.

References

1. Peng RD. *Computing for Data Analysis.* You Tube; July 16, 2012. Retrieved from http://www.youtube.com/watch?v=gk6E57H6mTs on August 31, 2013.
2. Faculty Development and Instructional Design Center. *Data Analysis.* University of Illinois; 2005. Retrieved from https://ori.hhs.gov/education/products/n_illinois_u/datamanagement/dmabout.html on August 31, 2013.
3. Katz DL, Wild D, Elmore JG, Lucan SC. *Jekel's Epidemiology, Biostatistics, Preventive Medicine, and Public Health.* 4th ed. Philiadelphia, PA: Elsevier Saunders; 2014.
4. Syracuse University. *Analyzing and Interpreting Data.* Retrieved from https://oira.syr.edu/assessment/assesspp/Analyze.htm on August 23, 2013.
5. Brunette DM. *Critical Thinking: Understanding and Evaluating Dental Research.* 2nd ed. Hanover Park, IL: Quintessance Publishing; 2007
6. Vogt WP. *Dictionary of Statistics and Methodology: A Nontechnical Guide for the Social Sciences.* Thousand Oaks, CA: Sage Publications; 2005.
7. Vincent WJ, Wier JP. *Statistics in Kinesiology.* 4th ed. Champaign, IL: Human Kinetics; 2012.
8. Munro BH. *Statistical Methods for Health Care Research.* 6th ed. Philadelphia, PA: Lippincott; 2013.
9. Gravetter FJ, Wallnau LB. *Statistics for the Behavioral Sciences.* 9th ed. Independence, KY: Cengage Learning; 2013.
10. Rosner B. *Fundamentals of biostatistics.* 7th ed. Boston, MA: Brooks/ Cole, Cengage Learning; 2011.
11. Kim JS, Dailey RJ. *Biostatistics for Oral Healthcare.* Ames, IA: Blackwell Munksgaar; 2008.
12. Gerstman BB. *Basic Biostatistics: Statistics for Public Health Practice.* Sudbury, MA: Jones & Bartlett; 2008.
13. Good PI, Hardin JW. *Common Errors in Statistics (And How to Avoid Them).* 3rd ed. Hoboken, NJ: Wiley/Jossey Bass; 2009.
14. Good PI, Hardin JW. *Common Errors in Statistics (And How to Avoid Them).* 3rd ed. Hoboken, NJ: Wiley/Jossey Bass; 2009.
15. Plonsky M. *Psychological statistics.* 2012. Retrieved from http://www.uwsp.edu/psych/stat/ on August 21, 2013; Lane DM (Rice University, Project Leader). *Online Statistics Education: A Multimedia Course of Study* (http://onlinestatbook.com/). In: University of Florida, *Biostatistics: Open Learning Textbook*; 2013. Retrieved from http://bolt.mph.ufl.edu/ on September 1, 2013.
16. North Carolina State University. *Graphing Resources.* Retrieved from LabWrite Resources Web site at http://www.ncsu.edu/labwrite/res/gh/gh-linegraph.html September 1, 2013.
17. Good PI, Hardin JW. *Common Errors in Statistics (And How to Avoid Them).* 3rd ed. Hoboken, NJ: Wiley/Jossey Bass; 2009.
18. Darby ML. Community oral health planning and practice. In: Darby ML. *Mosby's Comprehensive Review of Dental Hygiene.* 7th ed. St. Louis, MO: Mosby; 2012.
19. Friis RH, Sellers TA. *Epidemiology for Public Health Practice.* 4th ed. Boston, MA: Jones and Bartlett; 2009.
20. Dumitrescu AL. *Understanding Periodontal Research.* New York, NY: Springer; 2012.
21. Brunson D. Social responsibility. In: Geurink KV. *Community Oral Health Practice for the Dental Hygienist.* 3rd ed. St. Louis, MO: Elsevier Saunders; 2012.

22. Daniel SJ, Harfst SA, Wilder RS. *Mosby Dental Hygiene Concepts, Cases, and Competencies.* 2nd ed. St. Louis, MO: Mosby Elsevier; 2008.

23. Wilkins EM. *Clinical Practice of the Dental Hygienist.* 11th ed. Philadelphia, PA: Lippincott Williams & Wilkins; 2012.

24. Weil SA. Research. In: Geurink KV. *Community Oral Health Practice for the Dental Hygienist.* 3rd ed. St. Louis, MO: Elsevier Saunders; 2012.

25. Brunette DM. *Critical Thinking: Understanding and Evaluating Dental Research.* 2nd ed. Hanover Park, IL: Quintessance Publishing; 2007.

26. Clobban SJ, Edgington EM, Clovis JB. Moving research knowledge into dental hygiene practice. *J Dent Hyg.* 2008;82(2):1–10.

27. Williams KB. Overcoming the fear of statistics: survival skills for researchers. *J Dent Hyg.* 2012;86(1):21–25.

28. Howick J. *Levels of Evidence 1*; 2009. Retrieved August 31, 2013, from Oxford Center for Evidence-Based Medicine Web site at http://www.cebm.net/?o=1025

Visit www.pearsonhighered.com/healthprofessionsresources to access the student resources that accompany this book. Simply select Dental Hygiene from the choice of disciplines. Find this book and you will find the complimentary study tools created for this specific title.

18

Oral Epidemiology

Christine French Beatty, RDH, PhD

Charlene Dickinson, RDH, MS

OBJECTIVES

After studying this chapter, the dental hygiene student should be able to:

- Define oral epidemiology and describe the uses of epidemiology
- Relate epidemiology to evidence-based practice
- Define common epidemiologic terms
- Relate measurement to epidemiology
- List and describe various publications that report oral epidemiology in the United States
- Apply surveillance data to the planning of strategies to improve oral health
- Compare and contrast various types of epidemiologic studies and the usefulness of the results of the studies
- Describe ways to increase validity of epidemiologic research methods

COMPETENCIES

After studying this chapter and participating in accompanying course activities, the dental hygiene student should be competent to do the following:

- Use critical thinking skills and comprehensive problem-solving to identify oral health care strategies that promote patient health and wellness
- Use evidence-based decision making to evaluate emerging technology and treatment modalities to integrate into patient dental hygiene care plans to achieve high-quality, cost-effective care
- Continuously perform self-assessment for lifelong learning and professional growth
- Integrate accepted scientific theories and research into educational, preventive, and therapeutic oral health services

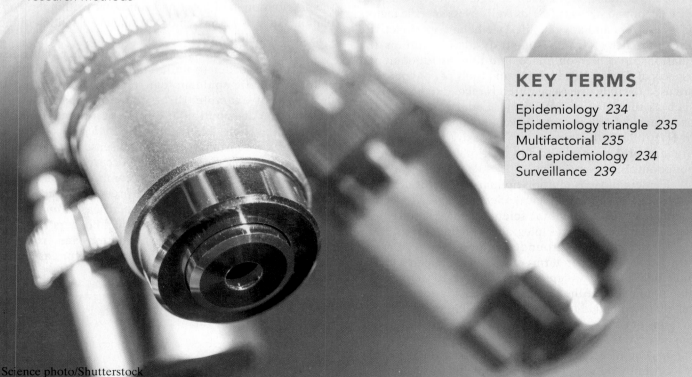

KEY TERMS

Epidemiology *234*
Epidemiology triangle *235*
Multifactorial *235*
Oral epidemiology *234*
Surveillance *239*

Science photo/Shutterstock

As Chapter 14 discussed, evidence-based practice combines the use of the best evidence available, clinical expertise, and patient preferences.[1] This evidence-based decision-making process requires skills in critically evaluating the evidence and accepting it or rejecting it as research without merit, applying research with merit to clinical practice, and evaluating the outcomes.[2] Understanding the importance of reliable evidence in the form of meta-analyses and randomized clinical trials and the role of analytic studies in identifying risk factors is critical to being able to participate in evidence-based practice.[2,3]

An understanding of oral epidemiology and the methodology used in epidemiologic research is essential to evidence-based practice.[4] This chapter presents an overview of the principles and methods of epidemiology and oral epidemiology so dental hygienists will be able to analyze the scientific literature to apply it to making evidence-based practice decisions. Sources of epidemiologic data and national oral health objectives are discussed in relation to oral health program planning.

Epidemiology Defined

Merrill has defined **epidemiology** as the study of the nature, cause, control, and determinants of the frequency and distribution of disease, disability, and death in human populations. Epidemiology also includes the application of this study to prevention measures that control health-related problems in the population.[5] The *population* can be as large as the entire globe or as small as a nursing home or elementary school. Epidemiology includes the process of characterizing the distribution of disease and various related factors, such as age, gender, race, and socioeconomic status (SES), as well as less specific factors such as stress and adverse lifestyle behaviors (inactivity and unhealthy diet).[6] This study also examines the relationship of person, place, and time as fundamental aspects of disease.[4] The science and tools of epidemiology are used to study disease and trends related to health care, such as the rates of oral diseases and conditions, the occurrence of oral opportunistic infections in relationship to HIV/AIDS, the success of Gardasil® vaccination to prevent oral cancer, and the link of heart disease to periodontitis, to name a few.

Epidemiology is multidisciplinary in that it draws on knowledge from the biological sciences, physical sciences, social sciences, behavioral sciences, and biostatistics.[6] Research methodology is integral to epidemiology.

Epidemiology is grounded in population thinking rather than thinking in terms of what will happen with the individual.[4] Epidemiologic methods are used to form reliable predictions at the population level; these predictions can then be applied to an individual within the population in terms of risk or probabilities that a disease or condition can occur in the individual.[7]

In general, epidemiology is used to describe the health status of populations, identify multiple factors associated

with disease and conditions to explain their etiology, predict the occurrence of disease and conditions, and control the distribution of diseases and conditions within the population.[4] Box 18-1 ■ has a more detailed explanation of the uses of epidemiology.[4,6,7,8]

Epidemiology uses a specific vocabulary that must be learned in order to understand it. Throughout this chapter, specific epidemiologic terms will be used and defined. For example, three common terms used to describe the distribution of disease in a population are endemic, epidemic, and pandemic.[6] *Endemic* is the relatively low but constant presence of disease in a particular geographic region. *Epidemic* is the occurrence of disease in excess of normal in a specific community or region, usually occurring suddenly and spreading rapidly; it is often referred to as an "outbreak" of disease. *Pandemic* is an epidemic that crosses international borders to affect several countries or continents. Definitions and examples of these terms are provided in Table 18-1 ■ for easy comparative reference.[8]

Box 18–1 The Uses of Epidemiology

- To study:
  - Trends of disease to help plan for health services and public health programs
- To assess:
  - Disease or health conditions within a population or community
  - Current public health policies, activities, and services
- To identify:
  - Risk factors that affect a population group to predict risk of disease
  - Cause-and-effect relationships of diseases and various factors to help in the diagnostic processes of disease identification
  - Syndromes from the distribution of clinical phenomena
- To control:
  - Causes of diseases, conditions, injury, disability, or death for prevention and/or elimination
- To evaluate
  - How well public health policies, activities, and services meet the priorities and needs of the population
- To research
  - The effectiveness of measures to prevent and control disease

Did You Know?

Oral **epidemiology** simply is epidemiology in relation to oral diseases and conditions.

Table 18–1 Commonly Used Epidemiologic Terms and Examples

Term	Definition	Example
Endemic	Usual presence of disease in a particular geographic region	Malaria continues to be a constant concern in parts of Africa.
Epidemic	Occurrence of an illness or condition in excess of normal expectance in a community or region, usually occurring suddenly and spreading rapidly	Nine (9) cases of measles occurred in Tarrant County, TX, in August 2013 compared to the normal rate of 0 to 2 each year.
Pandemic	Epidemic in which the disease may cross international borders to affect several countries or continents	Over 20 million people worldwide died from influenza in 1918–1919.

Sources: Merrill RM. *Introduction to Epidemiology.* 5th ed. Burlington, MA: Jones & Bartlett; 2010. Friis RH, Sellers TA. *Epidemiology for Public Health Practice,* 4th ed. Burlington, MA: Jones & Bartlett; 2009. Gerstman BB. *Epidemiology Kept Simple: Introduction to Traditional and Modern Epidemiology,* 2nd ed. Oxford, England: Wiley-Blackwell; 2013. Centers for Disease Control and Prevention. *Principles of Epidemiology in Public Health Practice.* 3rd ed; 2012. http://www.cdc.gov/ophss/csels/dsepd/SS1978/SS1978.pdf Accessed August 15, 2013. Mitchell M. Nine measles cases confirmed in Tarrant County, four more in North Texas. Fort Worth, TX: *Star-Telegram;* August 16, 2013. http://newsok.com/article/3873009 Accessed August 16, 2013.

What Is Oral Epidemiology?

Oral epidemiology is the only study within epidemiology that is specific to diseases confined to one component of the body, the oral cavity.[4] Without oral epidemiology, providers would not be aware of the associations of oral diseases and conditions to other diseases and conditions, nor would providers be aware of risk factors for various diseases and conditions. For example, oral epidemiology has clarified the relationship of periodontal diseases to other conditions such as heart disease, diabetes, and blood dyscrasias; the bacterial origin of dental caries and its association with sugar consumption, saliva quality, and many other factors; and how to prevent and control oral diseases and conditions.

The Multifactorial Nature Of Disease

Epidemiology attempts to understand the causes of disease and health conditions in a population. A key aspect of epidemiology is *determinants,* which is defined as a factor or event that can bring about a change in health.[7] At the turn of the nineteenth century with the discovery of bacteria, the cause of disease was generally considered in terms of exposure to an etiologic agent. A simple cause-and-effect mechanism was understood to be at work. Today, epidemiology is based on a **multifactorial** approach, which assumes that a disease or condition has multiple causes.[7] These factors—the host, the agent, and the environment—are organized by epidemiologists as the **epidemiology triangle** to demonstrate their interaction and interrelatedness in bringing about the disease or condition over time.[6,7,9]

Agent is the biologic or mechanical cause of a disease or condition, such as specific bacteria in relation to dental caries or brushing with a hard toothbrush in relation to abrasion. *Host* refers to an individual's genetic or social factors that contribute to the person's susceptibility or resistance, such as tooth morphology, salivary flow, salivary composition, and personal behaviors in relation to dental caries. *Environment* refers to the physical, social, sociocultural, sociopolitical, and economic circumstances required for the disease to thrive, survive, and spread, such as sugar in the diet and low SES in relation to dental caries as well as social norms and policies that control smoking in relation to oral cancer.[9,10] (See Table 18-2 ■.) Time issues include incubation periods, time periods of exposure to risk factors for a disease, life expectancy, duration of the course of an illness or condition, and the severity of the illness. Approaching the diagnosis, treatment, and control of disease from a multifactorial approach requires consideration of these different factors.[10] See Figure 18-1 ■ for an example of the application of the epidemiology triangle to the multiple causation of periodontitis.

Measurement In Epidemiology

Epidemiology involves the measurement of diseases, other health conditions, and death. Several terms relate to this measurement in epidemiology. *Morbidity* is the extent of disease, injury, or disability in a defined population, and *mortality* refers to the death rate resulting from a specific disease or condition.[6,7,11] The most common measures of morbidity and mortality are prevalence and incidence.[12] *Prevalence* is the numeric expression of all existing cases of a disease or health condition in a population measured at a given point or period of time.[12] This can be determined by case reports during the time period or surveying the population at a point in time. *Incidence* refers to the development of new cases of a disease or condition within a specified time period. Determining incidence requires measuring the same population at least twice, at the beginning and at the end of the specified time period.[12]

FIGURE 18–1 The Epidemiology Triangle in Relation to Periodontitis

Source: Based on Merrill RM. *Introduction to Epidemiology.* 5th ed. Burlington, MA: Jones & Bartlett; 2010. Genco RJ, Borgnakke WS. Risk factors for periodontal disease. *Periodontol 2000.* 2013;62(1):59–64.

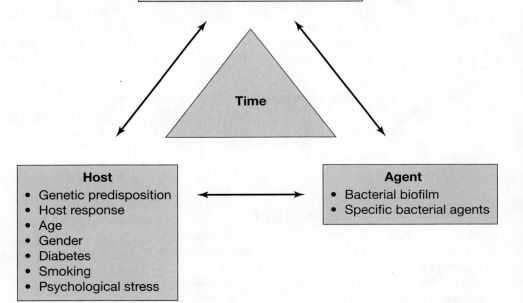

Environment
- Oral health self care
- Dental plaque
- Subgingival calculus
- Cultural factors
- Existing clinical attachment loss
- Protective factors (antimicrobials)

Time

Host
- Genetic predisposition
- Host response
- Age
- Gender
- Diabetes
- Smoking
- Psychological stress

Agent
- Bacterial biofilm
- Specific bacterial agents

Table 18–2 Terminology Related to Multifactorial Nature of Disease

Term	Definition	Example
Determinants	Factors or events capable of bringing about change in health; various factors that make up a multifactorial approach to a disease or health condition	Social and economic environment, physical environment, and a person's individual characteristics and behaviors
Multifactorial	Concept that more than a single cause must be present for a disease or health condition to occur; multiple causation	Bacteria present, genetics, chromosomal disorders, environmental factors, nutrient deficiencies, social and economic factors, health behaviors
Host	Organism housing the disease; the "who" factor of a disease or condition	Humans or animals
Agent	Microbial agent that causes the disease or mechanical cause of the condition; the "what" factor	Type of bacteria, parasite, virus, fungus, or protozoa, for example, plaque biofilm; or misuse of toothpicks to injure interdental papilla
Environment	External factors that contribute to disease transmission and severity; the "where" factor	Environments wherever disease factors occur such as dirty water, warm temperatures, seasons of the year, poverty, and stress, for example, the environmental conditions in the oral cavity and the social factors related to drug and tobacco use

Sources: Merrill RM. *Introduction to Epidemiology.* 5th ed. Burlington, MA: Jones & Bartlett; 2010. Friis RH, Sellers TA. *Epidemiology for Public Health Practice.* 4th ed. Burlington, MA: Jones & Bartlett; 2009. Gerstman BB. *Epidemiology Kept Simple: Introduction to Traditional and Modern Epidemiology.* 2nd ed. Oxford, England: Wiley-Blackwell; 2013. Centers for Disease Control and Prevention. *Lesson 1: Understanding the Epidemiologic Triangle through Infectious Disease,* n.d. http://www.cdc.gov/bam/teachers/documents/epi_1_triangle.pdf. Accessed August 15, 2013. World Health Organization. *The Determinants of Health.* Health Impact Assessment (HIA); 2013. http://www.who.int/hia/evidence/doh/en/. Accessed August 15, 2013.

Table 18–3 Terminology Related to Measurement in Epidemiology

Term	Definition	Example
Morbidity	Extent of disease, injury, or disability in a defined population	In the United States, 30,000 people are diagnosed with oral or pharyngeal cancer each year.
Mortality	Death rate resulting from a specific disease or condition	In India, 130,000 people die from oral cancer every year; this is estimated to be 14 deaths every hour.
Incidence	Rate of new cases of a disease during or over a given time period	Annually, tobacco users develop oral cancer lesions at a rate ranging from 5.2/1000 to 30.2/1000.
Prevalence	Numeric expression of the number of all existing cases of a disease or health condition in a population measured at a given point or period of time	Out of all adults with less than high school education, 28.4% are smokers.
Eradication	Elimination of an infectious disease agent through surveillance and containment; contrasted to control, which is to keep the disease at a minimum level so that it no longer poses a health problem	The eradication of polio in the United States through vaccination

Sources: Merrill RM. *Introduction to Epidemiology.* 5th ed. Burlington, MA: Jones & Bartlett; 2010. Friis RH, Sellers TA. *Epidemiology for Public Health Practice.* 4th ed. Burlington, MA: Jones & Bartlett; 2009. Gerstman BB. *Epidemiology Kept Simple: Introduction to Traditional and Modern Epidemiology.* 2nd ed. Oxford, England: Wiley-Blackwell; 2013. Oral Cancer Foundation. *Incidence and Prevalence*; 2012. http://ocf.org.in/professional/IncidenceAndPrevalence.aspx. Accessed August 16, 2013. Centers for Disease Control and Prevention. Current cigarette smoking prevalence among working adults—United States, 2004–2010. *Morbidity and Mortality Weekly Report.* Sept 30, 2011;60(38):1305–1309. Centers for Disease Control and Prevention. *Updates on CDC's Polio Eradication Efforts.* Global Health Polio; 2013. http://www.cdc.gov/polio/updates/. Accessed August 30, 2013.

Incidence requires three important elements: a numerator (the number of new cases), a denominator (the population at risk), and a time dimension (the time period during which the new cases occurred).[6] Prevalence is an indication of how widespread a disease is, whereas incidence expresses information about the risk of contracting the disease. (See Table 18-3 ■.)

Did You Know?

A good way to remember prevalence and incidence is that *prevalence* refers to all of a disease or condition in the population at the designated time, and *incidence* refers to only new cases identified during the specific time period.

Epidemiologists also express measures using counts, proportions, ratios, rates, and indexes.[6,7,8] (See Table 18-4 ■.) A *count* is the simplest form of measurement. It is simply the number of cases of the disease or condition in the population. It provides the least information because it does not communicate the size of the population.[7] An example is a statement that 20 patients presented in the community dental clinic for dental hygiene treatment with secondary oral herpetic lesions.

A count becomes a *proportion* when it is expressed relative to the size of the population. A proportion is a fraction and can be expressed as a percentage.[7] Expression of the frequency as a proportion rather than a count provides more information about the extent of the disease in the population. Using the preceding example, a proportion would be that 20 patients out of 200, or 10 percent, presented with herpetic lesions. This would be less significant if the 20 cases had been in a population size of 2000, thus representing only 1 percent. Use of a proportion versus a count communicates this information. A proportion is a type of *ratio*.[7] Prevalence is a proportion and should not be described as a rate, a commonly made mistake.[7]

Another type of ratio is a fraction that expresses the magnitude of one occurrence in relation to another.[6] One could refer to the ratio of the incidence of oral herpetic lesions in individuals who are under extreme stress in relation to individuals who are not experiencing stress. This would be expressed as a ratio, such as 5:1. This ratio is not a proportion because the numerator (those experiencing extreme stress) is not reflected in the denominator (those not experiencing stress). This 5:1 ratio can be translated to a relative risk of 5.0.[6,7,12]

A *rate* is the expression of disease in a population using a standardized denominator and including a time dimension.[7] The use of the common denominator allows for making valid comparisons across different populations or detecting trends within the same population. The value of the common denominator (eg, per 1000, per 100,000, or per 1,000,000) depends on the relation to the value being reported. For example, the mortality from oral cancer among African Americans in the year 2000 was 4.1 per 100,000 compared to 5.2 per 100,000 in 1988–1992.[13] Expression of these rates as 0.041 per 1000 and 0.052 per

Table 18–4 Terminology Related to Measures in Epidemiology

Term	Definition	Example
Count	Number of cases of disease or condition	42,000 Americans are expected to be diagnosed with oral or pharyngeal cancer in 2013.
Proportion	Type of ratio that expresses the amount of disease or health condition with a fraction that presents it in relation to the size of the population; can be expressed as a percentage	57% of those diagnosed with oral or pharyngeal cancer in 2013 are expected to die within 5 years (23,940 out of 42,000).
Ratio	Expression of the magnitude of one occurrence of disease exposure in relation to another with a fraction; in contrast to a proportion, not necessary to have a relationship between the numerator and denominator	Oral cancers account for 3% of cancers in men and 2% of cancers in women in the United States; the ratio of oral cancers in men versus women is 3:2.
Rate	Expression of disease in a population using a standardized denominator and including a time dimension; allows for valid comparisons	Rate of oral cancer in the United States in 2013 is expected to be approximately 13 cases per 100,000 people.
Index	Abbreviated, standardized measurement used to express severity of problems and aid in data collection.	The rates of oral or pharyngeal cancer are expressed in terms of how many are diagnosed at each stage of severity (Stages I, II, III, and IV).

Sources: Oral Cancer Foundation. *Oral Cancer Facts.* http://www.oralcancerfoundation.org/facts/;2013. Accessed August 17, 2013. American Cancer Society. *Cancer Facts & Figures 2009.* Atlanta, GA: ACS; 2009. http://www.oralcancerfoundation.org/facts/pdf/Us_Cancer_Facts.pdf. Accessed August 17, 2013. United States Census Bureau. *U.S. and World Population Clock.* http://www.census.gov/popclock/. Accessed August 17, 2013. National Cancer Institute. *Cancer Staging.* National Cancer Institute Fact Sheet. http://www.cancer.gov/cancertopics/factsheet/detection/staging; 2013. Accessed August 22, 2013.

1000 would be just as correct mathematically although more difficult to interpret.[7] Incidence is a rate.[7]

An *index* reports more detailed information than a count, proportion, and rate by providing an abbreviated, standardized measurement of the amount or severity of the disease or condition in the population.[14] An index usually involves a graduated numeric scale to measure the extent of the health problem and to aid in data collection and analysis. (See Chapter 13.)

Two clinical methods are used to measure disease in oral epidemiologic surveys: basic screening and epidemiologic examination. These clinical assessment methods in epidemiology differ from a clinical examination in that they do not involve a clinical diagnosis and corresponding treatment plan. They are non-diagnostic but aid in identifying unrecognized disease.

Basic screening is a rapid assessment accomplished in a short time by visual detection. Because it can be achieved with a tongue blade, dental mirror, and appropriate lighting, it is easy to implement in the community. It provides information about gross dental and oral lesions and is commonly used for assessment of oral disease in the population.

Epidemiologic examination differs from basic screening in that it provides a thorough visual-tactile assessment accomplished with dental instruments and a light source.

Thus, it provides more detailed information. Epidemiologic examination is used with most dental indexes.

Two properties of measurement in epidemiology are validity and reliability. *Validity* is the ability of a measure to accurately classify people with and without disease. Measurement of disease in epidemiology should be evaluated to ensure the validity of the study. Sensitivity and specificity of a measure refer to how the test performs related to the disease process. *Sensitivity* is the ability of a test or index to accurately identify the presence of a disease or condition when the disease is in fact present. *Specificity* is the capacity of a test or index to accurately identify the absence of a disease or condition. Together they measure what is required from a test. *Predictive value* is a mathematical expression of validity, which is a combination of sensitivity and specificity. If a test is both sensitive and specific, it will possess validity and predictive value.[4,6,13]

Reliability is the dependability or consistency of a measure to present the same result when it is repeated. The reliability of a test indicates that results of its measurement are similar when it is applied repeatedly. Reliability is also used to refer to the consistency of one or more examiners as they measure oral disease with a dental index. *Intra-rater reliability,* also referred to as intra-examiner reliability, is the degree of agreement within a single examiner when he or she measures a disease or condition on two or more

Table 18–5 Terminology Related to Validity and Reliability of Measurement in Epidemiology

Term	Definition	Explanation
Validity	Accuracy of a measurement; measurement results are true or accurate	The accuracy of a DMF to indicate caries experience in children
Reliability	Consistency or reproducibility of a measurement over time	The consistency of an examiner to get the same results when repeating the DMF on the same child
Sensitivity	The ability to identify all screened individuals who actually have the disease; influences validity	The ability of the DMF to identify caries when it is present
Specificity	The ability to identify only non-diseased individuals who actually do not have the disease; influences validity	The ability of the DMF to identify the absence of caries when the tooth has no carious lesion
Predictive value	Ability of a test to accurately measure a disease or condition	The ability of the DMF to measure caries with accuracy (without the use of other diagnostic tools)
Inter-rater reliability	Agreement among two or more examiners as they apply a test or index	Two examiners agree when they measure DMF on the same individual in a study
Intra-rater reliability	Consistency of a single examiner in the application of a test or instrument multiple times	One examiner is consistent when measuring DMF at several examinations on the same individual
Calibration	Standardization of examiners as they apply epidemiologic measurements	Training and standardization of the examiners on the use of the DMF to measure caries
Positive reversal	Change of the measurement made in error in a logical direction	Caries is absent when DMF is measured the first time and is present when DMF is measured the second time, if the second measure is inaccurate
Negative reversal	Change of diagnosis in an illogical direction over a period of time	Caries is present when DMF is measured the first time and is absent when DMF is measured the second time

Sources: Chattopadhyay A. *Oral Health Epidemiology: Principles and Practice*. Sunbury, MA: Jones and Bartlett; 2011. Friis RH, Sellers TA. *Epidemiology for Public Health Practice*. 5th ed. Sudbury, MA: Jones & Bartlett; 2013. Pine C, Harris R. *Community Oral Health*. 2nd ed. In: Scheutz F. *Principles and Methods of Oral Epidemiology*. New Malden, Surrey KT, United Kingdom: Quintessence; 2007:115–140.

occasions. *Inter-rater reliability*, also called inter-examiner reliability, refers to the degree of agreement between two or more examiners when they measure a disease or condition with a dental index. (See Table 18-5 ■)

The use of standardized tests, instruments, and measures such as dental indexes is important to ensure validity and reliability during epidemiologic measurement. *Calibration* is the process of standardizing these measures. It is also used to refer to the training and testing of agreement within and between examiners when they measure a disease or condition with an index or instrument. Failure to calibrate examiners can cause reversals. This means that the results of the measurement of a disease or condition change, although the status of the disease or condition is no different. A *positive reversal* is when the change is in a logical direction, and a *negative reversal* is when the change is in an illogical direction.[4,6,13]

Oral Epidemiology Surveillance and Reports

Various systems of epidemiologic surveillance are used to collect data to determine the presence of disease, injury, disability, and related factors. **Surveillance,** If an ongoing process, is the observation, persistent watching over, scrutiny, constant monitoring, and assessment of changes in populations related to disease, conditions, injuries, disabilities, or death trends.[6] It uses methods that are quick, simple, and practical, such as those discussed in Chapter 15, putting as little burden as possible on the health practitioners reporting the data.[15] Surveillance data are used to identify *trends*, which are the long-term changes or movements in disease patterns and health-related conditions.[6] Surveillance data are not as accurate as those collected under a strict protocol for research purposes, but this is

---

Box 18–2 Terminology and Examples of Surveillance Systems

Surveillance: The observation of the disease process in populations.

    Passive: Surveillance of data collected is voluntary
        Example: Youth Risk Behavioral Surveillance System (YRBSS)

    Active: Surveillance of data collected out in the field to identify cases of disease
        Example: Basic Screening Survey (BSS)

Trends: Long-term changes or movements in disease patterns and health-related conditions identified by examining surveillance data.

    Examples:

- Percentage of children ages 6–19 years with untreated dental caries: 15.6% (2007–2010) is higher than previous decades
- Percentage of children ages 2–17 with a dental visit in the past year: 81.4% (2011) is higher than previous decades

Source: Centers for Disease Control and Prevention. http://www.cdc.gov/nchs/fastats/dental.htm. Accessed August 25, 2013.

---

appropriate because the purpose of identifying these trends is primarily to initiate epidemiologic investigations and to develop public health prevention and control programs.[6,15] Oral health professionals can utilize these data in making evidence-based decisions to impact the oral health of the population.

The primary means of surveillance in the United States is *passive surveillance,* which involves voluntary reporting, even though this may be in response to laws that require reporting.[15] For example, some state dental boards require that HIV be reported by dental personnel who are carriers, but the authorities do not actively solicit the data. *Active surveillance* in which public health staff personnel go into the field to collect data is used to identify cases of disease that would be missed by passive reporting. For example, active surveillance was used when attempting to eradicate smallpox.[16] See Box 18-2 ■ for terminology and examples of surveillance systems.

In the United States, surveillance activities are conducted by various components of the Centers for Disease Control and Prevention (CDC) of the US Department of Health and Human Services (USDHHS). Except for oral cancer (and cleft lip and cleft palate in some states), oral health data have not been available through these traditional surveillance systems. The Surveillance, Epidemiology, and End Results (SEER) program is a system that provides a source for data of virtually all cancer, including oral cancer, in the United States.[17]

Surveys have been conducted to generate oral health data for other oral conditions for purposes of planning public health programs. These surveys, which are more similar to active surveillance, were originally conducted by the National Institute for Dental (and Craniofacial) Research and then by the National Center for Health Statistics, which is part of CDC.[18] The National Health and Nutrition Examination Survey (NHANES) is a continuous, national survey program consisting of questionnaires and clinical assessment. Conducted annually on different samples across the nation, it focuses on different populations as well as different health and nutrition measurements, including oral health, to meet emerging needs. The National Health Interview Survey (NHIS) has been used to track various oral health–related conditions reflected in *Healthy People 2020* objectives.[19] Another national survey is the Medical Expenditure Panel Survey (MEPS) conducted by the Agency for Healthcare Research and Quality of the USDHHS, which measures progress of the *Healthy People 2020* objectives related to dental events.[20]

National Oral Health Surveillance System

National surveys such as those just described provide valuable national data, but their information could not be separated into state-level data necessary for local public health program planning. (See Table 18-5 ■.) In response to that limitation, the National Oral Health Surveillance System (NOHSS) was established in the mid-1990s as a joint venture of the CDC and the Association of State and Territorial Dental Directors (ASTDD). The NOHSS was designed to monitor the burden of oral disease, utilization of the oral health care delivery system, and community water fluoridation on both national and state levels. The CDC assists states in collecting their specific survey data, and the CDC then reports the data in a national database. Data are collected for a set of nine oral health indicators: dental visits, (professional) teeth cleaning, complete tooth loss, loss of six or more teeth, fluoridation status, dental sealants, caries experience, untreated tooth decay, and cancer of the oral cavity and pharynx.[21]

Did You Know?

The Web site http://www.cdc.gov/nohss/ is an excellent resource for information about dental disease and dental services in your state. It can be particularly helpful for writing reports and planning and developing public health programs.

In addition to the national surveys listed above, several state-level surveys collect the surveillance data for the NOHSS. The Behavioral Risk Factor Surveillance System (BRFSS) and its companion Youth Risk Behavior Surveillance System (YRBSS) collect several indicators. Both surveys consist of core questions developed by the CDC that a state health agency can adapt to its local needs. Fluoridation status is monitored at local, state, and tribal levels for the NOHSS by using the Water Fluoridation Reporting System (WFRS), an interactive, real-time,

Web-based, surveillance system developed by the CDC in collaboration with the ASTDD.

Clinical data for other indicators are collected using the Basic Screening Survey (BSS) developed by the ASTDD. Its purpose is to collect valid although limited clinical data in an unobtrusive, efficient, and cost-effective manner.[22] Rather than measuring the total caries experience with a decayed, missing, filled tooth (DMFT) index, which was discussed in Chapter 13, the BSS uses the basic screening approach of oral surveying to assess the prevalence of untreated dental caries and dental caries experience on a per person basis using dichotomous (yes/no) measures. With this approach, individuals with a DMFT score of 1 or greater are classified as having caries experience; individuals with a DMFT of 0 are classified as caries free. Classification of treatment—no obvious problem, early treatment needed, or urgent treatment needed—can be utilized for referral purposes and surveillance.[23] (See Table 18-6 ■.)

Table 18–6 Epidemiologic Surveillance Systems

Surveillance System	Developed by	Data Surveyed	URL for Source
Basic Screening Survey (BSS)	Association of State & Territorial Dental Directors (ASTDD)	Clinical data with basic screening to assess the prevalence of dental caries experience and untreated dental caries	http://www.astdd.org/basic-screening-survey-tool/
Surveillance, Epidemiology, and End Results (SEER)	National Cancer Institute (NCI)	Collects and publishes cancer incidence and survival data from cancer registries	http://seer.cancer.gov/about/
National Institute for Dental and Craniofacial Research	N/A	Scientific research on oral, dental and craniofacial health and disease	http://www.nidcr.nih.gov/AboutUs/FastFacts.htm
National Health and Nutrition Examination Survey (NHANES)	National Center for Health Statistics (NCHS), which is part of the Centers for Disease Control and Prevention (CDC)	Designed to assess the health and nutritional status of adults and children in the United States	http://www.cdc.gov/nchs/nhanes/about_nhanes.htm
National Health Interview Survey (NHIS)	US Census Bureau and Centers for Disease Control and Prevention	Collects data on a broad range of health topics through personal household interviews	http://www.cdc.gov/nchs/nhis.htm
Medical Expenditure Panel Survey (MEPS)	US Department of Health & Human Services (USDHHS) and Agency for Healthcare Research and Quality (AHRQ)	The most complete source of data on the cost and utilization of health care and health insurance coverage	http://meps.ahrq.gov/mepsweb/about_meps/survey_back.jsp
National Oral Health Surveillance System (NOHSS)	Centers for Disease Control and Prevention (CDC) and Association of State and Territorial Dental Directors (ASTDD)	Monitors the burden of oral disease, use of the oral health care delivery system, and status of community water fluoridation on both a national and state level	http://www.cdc.gov/nohss/about.htm
Association of State and Territorial Dental Directors (ASTDD)	N/A	Formulates and promotes the establishment of national dental public health policy, assists state dental programs in the development and implementation of programs and policies to prevent oral diseases, builds awareness and strengthens dental public health professionals' knowledge and skills by developing position papers and policy statements, provides information on oral health to health officials and policy makers, and conducts conferences for the dental public health community	http://www.astdd.org/

(*continued*)

Table 18–6 Epidemiologic Surveillance Systems (continued)

Surveillance System	Developed by	Data Surveyed	URL for Source
Behavioral Risk Factor Surveillance System (BRFSS)	Centers for Disease Control and Prevention (CDC)	Used to collect prevalence data among adult US residents regarding their risk behaviors and preventive health practices that can affect their health status; conducted with randomly selected samples monthly at the state levels	http://www.cdc.gov/brfss/data_documentation/
Youth Risk Behavioral Surveillance System (YRBSS)	Centers for Disease Control and Prevention (CDC)	Monitors six types of health-risk behaviors that contribute to the leading causes of death and disability among youth and adults; anonymous and voluntary survey	http://www.cdc.gov/HealthyYouth/yrbs/index.htm
Water Fluoridation Reporting System (WFRS)	CDC in partnership with Association of State and Territorial Dental Directors (ASTDD)	Manages states' water fluoridation programs and describes the percentage of the US population on community water systems who receive optimally fluoridated drinking water	http://www.cdc.gov/fluoridation/factsheets/engineering/wfrs_factsheet.htm

Morbidity and Mortality Weekly Report

The CDC publishes current, relevant epidemiologic data in the United States weekly in the *Morbidity and Mortality Weekly Report* (*MMWR*). It compiles cogent health and health-related issues currently being studied. Its primary purpose has been to report events of public health interest and importance as well as a list of nationally notifiable diseases (diseases that must be reported to the CDC) to state and local health departments as quickly as possible.[4] The CDC receives case-report surveillance data that are voluntarily contributed electronically by states and then compiles the statistics for the nationally notifiable disease list. The CDC also summarizes these case counts annually.[15] Many of these health and health-related conditions and events, such as herpes, hepatitis, asthma, autism, health behaviors, fluoridation, immunizations, and use of tobacco, are of interest to those in dental hygiene. The *MMWR* is available online free or by subscription for a paper copy.

Healthy People 2020 Objectives

Oral health surveillance in the United States has resulted in the establishment of oral health objectives for the nation for the last three decades.[24] National publications have provided a statement of these objectives designed to identify the most significant preventable threats to health and to establish national goals to reduce them. Thus, these publications have set the prevention agenda for the United States. The most recent version, *Healthy People 2020,* has four overarching goals and consists of nearly 600 objectives encompassing 1200 measures and organized around 42 focus areas.[24,25,26] (See Table 18-7 ■.)

The vision of *Healthy People 2020* is to create a society where people live long, healthy lives. Four foundation health measures serve as a guide to measuring the attainment of these objectives: general health status, health-related quality of life and well-being, determinants of health, and disparities.[24] Leading health indicators are a set of fewer objectives that indicate high-priority health issues and actions that address these issues. There are 26 leading health indicators organized under 12 topics, one of which is oral health.[24] (See Box 18-3 ■.)

Oral health is a specific focus area of *Healthy People 2020*. It is also integrated into many of the other 42 focus areas, indicating the recognition of the importance of oral health.[26] (See Table 18-7 ■.) The goal for these areas is to prevent and control oral and craniofacial diseases, conditions, and injuries, and improve access to related services. The oral health objectives build on oral health initiatives over the last decades, including NOHSS surveillance data.[27] A summary of the oral health objectives is presented in Table 18-8 ■.

Box 18–3 *Healthy People 2020* Leading Health Indicator Topics[25]

- Access to Health Services
- Clinical Preventive Services
- Environmental Quality
- Injury and Violence
- Maternal, Infant, and Child Health
- Mental Health
- Nutrition, Physical Activity, and Obesity
- Oral Health
- Reproductive and Sexual Health
- Social Determinants
- Substance Abuse
- Tobacco

Source: U.S. Department of Health and Human Services. 2020 Topics & Objectives – Objectives A-Z; revised March 2013. http://www.healthypeople.gov/2020/topicsobjectives2020/default.aspx. Accessed August 19, 2013.

Table 18–7 *Healthy People 2020* Goals and Focus Areas

Mission

Healthy People 2020 strives to:

- Identify nationwide health improvement priorities.
- Increase public awareness and understanding of the determinants of health, disease, and disability and the opportunities for progress.
- Provide measurable objectives and goals that are applicable at the national, State, and local levels.
- Engage multiple sectors to take actions to strengthen policies and improve practices that are driven by the best available evidence and knowledge.
- Identify critical research, evaluation, and data collection needs.

Overarching Goals

- Attain high-quality, longer lives free of preventable disease, disability, injury, and premature death.
- Achieve health equity, eliminate disparities, and improve the health of all groups.
- Create social and physical environments that promote good health for all.
- Promote quality of life, healthy development, and healthy behaviors across all life stages.

Focus Areas

1. Access to health services[a]
2. Adolescent health[b]
3. Arthritis, osteoporosis, chronic back conditions[a]
4. Blood disorders and blood safety[b]
5. Cancer[a]
6. Chronic kidney disease
7. Dementias, including Alzheimer's disease[b]
8. Diabetes[a]
9. Disability and secondary conditions[a]
10. Early and middle childhood[b]
11. Educational and community-based programs[a]
12. Environmental health[a]
13. Family planning
14. Food safety
15. Genomics[b]
16. Global health[b]
17. Health communication and health information technology[a]
18. Healthcare-associated infections[b]
19. Health-related quality of life and well-being[b]
20. Hearing and other sensory or communication disorders
21. Heart disease and stroke[a]
22. Human immunodeficiency virus (HIV)
23. Immunization and infectious diseases[a]
24. Injury and violence prevention[a]
25. Lesbian, gay, bisexual, and transgender health[b]
26. Maternal, infant, and child health[a]
27. Medical product safety[a]
28. Mental health and mental disorders[a]
29. Nutrition and overweight[a]
30. Occupational safety and health[a]
31. Older adults[b]
32. Oral health[a]
33. Physical activity[a]
34. Preparedness[b]
35. Public health infrastructure[a]
36. Respiratory diseases
37. Sexually transmitted diseases[a]
38. Sleep health[b]
39. Social determinants of health[b]
40. Substance abuse[a]
41. Tobacco use[a]
42. Vision

[a]Objectives related to oral health are also included in these focus areas.

[b]Objectives were not in *Healthy People 2010*.

Source: US Department of Health and Human Services. *2020 Topics & Objectives–Objectives A-Z*; revised March 2013. http://www.healthypeople.gov/2020/topicsobjectives2020/default.aspx. Accessed August 19, 2013.

Table 18–8 Summary of *Healthy People 2020* Oral Health Objectives

Oral Health Objective Number	Oral Health Objective	Target Setting Method	Target
OH–1	Reduce children and adolescents who have dental caries experience in their primary or permanent teeth	• Children aged 3 to 5 with dental caries experience in primary teeth • Children aged 6 to 9 with dental caries experience in primary and permanent teeth • Adolescents aged 13 to 15 with dental caries experience in permanent teeth	10% improvement by 2020
OH–2	Reduce children and adolescents with untreated dental decay	• Children aged 3 to 5 with untreated dental decay in primary teeth • Children aged 6 to 9 with untreated dental decay in primary and permanent teeth • Adolescents aged 13 to 15 with untreated dental decay in permanent teeth	10% improvement by 2020
OH–3	Reduce adults with untreated dental decay	• Adults aged 35 to 44 years with untreated dental decay • Adults 65 to 74 years with untreated coronal caries • Adults aged 75 years and older with untreated root surface caries	10% improvement by 2020
OH–4	Reduce adults who have ever had a permanent tooth extracted because of dental caries or periodontal disease	• Adults aged 45 to 64 years who have ever had a permanent tooth extracted because of dental caries or periodontal disease • Adults aged 65 to 74 years who have lost all of their natural teeth	10% improvement by 2020
OH–5	Reduce adults with moderate or severe periodontitis	Adults aged 45 to 74 years with moderate or severe periodontitis	10% improvement by 2020
OH–6	Increase oral and pharyngeal cancers detected at the earliest stage	Increase oral and pharyngeal cancers detected at the localized stage (stage 1)	10% improvement by 2020
OH–7 *LHI	Increase children, adolescents, and adults who used the oral health care system in the past year	People aged 2 years and older	10% improvement by 2020
OH–8	Increase low-income children and adolescents who received any preventive dental service during the past year	Children and adolescents aged 2 to 18 at or below 200 percent of the federal poverty level	10% improvement by 2020
OH–9	Increase school-based health centers with an oral health component	• School-based health centers that include dental sealants • School-based health centers that include dental care • School-based health centers that include topical fluoride	10% improvement by 2020
OH–10	Increase local health departments and Federally Qualified Health Centers (FQHC) that have an oral health program	• Federally Qualified Health Centers (FQHC) that have an oral health program • Local health departments that have oral health prevention or care programs	10% improvement by 2020

(continued)

Oral Health Objective Number	Oral Health Objective	Target Setting Method	Target
OH–11	Increase patients who receive oral health services at Federally Qualified Health Centers (FQHC) each year	Patients at FQHC receiving oral health services	10% improvement by 2020
OH–12	Increase children and adolescents who have received dental sealants on their molar teeth	• Children aged 3 to 5 who have received dental sealants on one or more of their primary molar teeth • Children aged 6 to 9 who have received dental sealants on one or more of their permanent first molar teeth • Adolescents aged 13 to 15 who have received dental sealants on one or more of their permanent molar teeth	10% improvement by 2020
OH–13	Increase the US population served by community water systems with optimally fluoridated water	US population served by community water systems that receive optimally fluoridated water	10% improvement by 2020
OH–14	(Developmental) Increase adults who receive preventive interventions in dental offices	• Adults who received information focusing on reducing tobacco use • Adults who received an oral and pharyngeal cancer screening in the past year • Adults who were tested or referred for glycemic control from dentist or dental hygienist in the past year	10% improvement by 2020
OH–15	(Developmental) Increase the number of states and the District of Columbia that have a system for recording and referring infants and children with cleft lips and cleft palates to craniofacial anomaly rehabilitative teams	• Increase systems for recording cleft lips and cleft palates • Increase systems for referral for cleft lips and cleft palates to rehabilitative teams	10% improvement by 2020
OH–16	Increase the number of states and the District of Columbia that have an oral and craniofacial health surveillance system	From 32 states to 51 states having an oral and craniofacial health surveillance system	Total coverage by 2020
OH–17	Increase health agencies that have a dental public health program directed by a dental professional with public health training	• Increase health agencies that serve jurisdictions of 250,000 or more persons with a dental public health program directed by a dental professional with public health training • Increase the number of Indian Health Service areas and tribal health programs that serve jurisdictions of 30,000 or more persons with a dental public health program directed by a dental professional with public health training	10% improvement by 2020

*Leading Health Indicator (new to *Healthy People 2020*)

Source: U.S. Department of Health and Human Services. *About Healthy People*; revised December 2012. http://www.healthypeople.gov/2020/about/. Accessed August 19, 2013. U.S. Department of Health and Human Services. *2020 Topics & Objectives – Objectives A-Z*; revised March 2013. http://www.healthypeople.gov/2020/topicsobjectives2020/default.aspx. Accessed August 19, 2013.

EVOLUTION OF HEALTHY PEOPLE The Healthy People initiative is a collaborative and evolving program. It is data driven and measures progress in 10-year intervals. The Office of Disease Prevention and Health Promotion, the Assistant Secretary for Health, various federal agencies of the Department of Health and Human Services (HHS) as well as non-HHS agencies, and the National Center for Health Statistics are key players in Healthy People's strategically aligned effort.[28] Designed to reduce health disparities in the United States, the mission of the Healthy People program is to

- Identify nationwide health improvement priorities.
- Increase public awareness and understanding of the determinants of health, disease, and disability and the opportunities for progress.
- Provide measurable objectives and goals that are applicable at the national, state, and local levels.
- Engage multiple sectors to take actions to strengthen policies and improve practices that are driven by the best available evidence and knowledge.
- Identify critical research, evaluation, and data collection needs.[28]

Going into the next decade of the Healthy People initiative requires an understanding of which objectives from the previous decade were met and which objectives still need a concentrated effort.[28] *Healthy People 2010 Final Review* is a report that provides data on the state of the nation's health at the end of the year 2010. These data were used to establish the objectives for *Healthy People 2020*. The final data showed that out of the 733 objectives, 23 percent met their targeted outcomes and 48 percent moved toward the desired targets. The final review evaluated whether each objective within the individual focus areas moved away from target, moved toward target, or met or exceeded target. For example, one objective was the reduction of deaths from heart disease and stroke, which are the first and third leading causes of death in the United States. At the end of 2010 the target to reduce cholesterol was met and the target to reduce smoking levels had progressed toward achieving the desired target outcome. These results indicated that deaths from heart disease and stroke moved toward achieving the proposed objectives.[28] Another example relates to assessment of obesity rates. There was no improvement in obesity; as a matter of fact, obesity rates increased in all age groups during the last decade.

Significant progress was achieved in moving toward the targets set within the *Healthy People 2010* oral health objectives. However, disparities are still prevalent among racial and ethnic population groups, as well as by sex and education level. See Table 18-9 ■ for progress made in *Healthy People 2010* oral health objectives.[28]

The key conclusion of the *Healthy People 2010* initiative was that significant progress was made in oral health objectives. In addition, most moved toward, met, or exceeded their target. The exceptions were the objectives to reduce dental caries and reduce untreated dental caries, which moved away from the target in some age groups, notably young children. However, disparities in oral disease continue to need significant improvement. The current focus is on meeting the target objectives set by *Healthy People 2020*.[28] (See Table 18-8 ■.)

Table 18–9 Progress on Oral Health Objectives Reported in *Final Review Healthy People 2010*

Objective		Percent of Targeted Change Achieved[1]	2010 Target	Baseline	Final	Percent Change[2]
21.1	*Dental caries experience*	Moved away from target	11%	18%	24%	33.3%
	a. Primary teeth – children (2–4 yrs.)	Moved away from target	42%	52%	53%	1.9%
	b. Primary or permanent teeth – children (6–8 yrs.)	Moved toward target: 50%	51%	61%	56%	–8.2%
	c. Permanent teeth – Adolescents (15 yrs.)					
21.2	*Untreated dental decay*	Moved away from target	9%	16%	19%	18%
	a. Primary teeth- children (2–4 yrs.)	Moved away from target	21%	28%	29%	3.6%
	b. Primary or permanent teeth children (6–8 yrs.)	Moved toward target: 40%	15%	20%	18%	–10.0%
	c. Permanent teeth-Adolescents (15 yrs.)	Moved away from target	15%	27%	28%	3.7%
	d. Adults (35–44 yrs.)					
21.3	No permanent tooth loss due to caries or periodontal disease in adults (35–44 yrs.)	Moved toward target: 80%	40%	30%	38%	26.7%

(continued)

Objective		Percent of Targeted Change Achieved[1]	2010 Target	Baseline	Final	Percent Change[2]
21.4	Complete tooth loss in older adults (65–74 yrs.)	Moved toward target: 71.4%	22%	29%	24%	−17.2%
21.5	Destructive periodontal disease in adults (35–44 yrs.)	Moved toward target: 75.0%	14%	22%	16%	−27.3%
21.6	Early detection of oral and pharyngeal cancers	Moved away from target	51%	36%	33%	−8.3%
21.7	Annual examinations for oral and pharyngeal cancers in adults (age adjusted, 40+ yrs.)	Moved toward target: 71.4%	20%	13%	18%	38.5%
21.8	*Dental Sealants* a. Children (8 yrs.) b. Adolescents (14 yrs.)	Moved toward target: 33.3% Moved toward target: 17.1%	50% 50%	23% 15%	32% 21%	39.1% 40%
21.9	Population served by optimally fluoridated community water	Moved toward target: 76.9%	75%	62%	72%	16.1%
21.10	Annual dental visits (age adjusted, 2+ yrs.)	Moved away from target	56%	44%	43%	−2.3%
21.12	Annual preventive dental services for low-income children and adolescents (<19 yrs.)	Moved toward target	66%	25%	31%	24.0%
21.13	School-based health centers with oral health components a. Dental sealants b. Dental care	Moved toward target: 400% Moved toward target: 50.0%	15% 11.1%	12% 9%	24% 10%	100.0% 11.1%
21.14	Community-based health centers with oral health components	100.0%	75%	52%	75%	44.2%
21.15	Recording and referral of children and youth with cleft lip or palate (number of states and DC)	Moved toward target: 48.6%	51	16	33	106.3%
21.16	Oral and craniofacial State-based surveillance systems (number of states and DC)	Moved toward target: 84.3%	51	0	43	*
21.17a	State and local dental programs directed by dental professional with public health training	Moved toward target	41	39	54	38.5%
21.17b	Indian Health Service and Tribal dental programs directed by dental professional with public health training	Moved toward target: Target met at baseline and exceeded at final	9	9	10	11.1%

[1]Percent of targeted change achieved = final value-Baseline value/Healthy People 2010 target − Baseline value × 100.

[2]Percent change = Final value-Baseline value. Differences between percents (%) are measured in percentage points.

*Percentage cannot be calculated.

Source: National Center for Health Statistics (NCHS). *Healthy People 2010 Final Review: Overview and Selected Findings.* PHS Publication No. 2012-1038. Hyattsville, MD: NCHS; 2012. http://www.cdc.gov/nchs/data/hpdata2010/hp2010_final_review.pdf. Accessed August 20, 2013.

Surgeon General's Reports

The US Surgeon General regularly issues reports on various health conditions. *Oral Health in America: A Report of the Surgeon General,* issued in May 2000 by Surgeon General David Satcher, MD, PhD, was the first-ever comprehensive report on the status of the nation's oral health.[29,30] The report provided scientific information on the growth and development of oral, dental, and craniofacial tissues; described oral diseases and conditions; and underscored the critical relationship between oral health and general health throughout life. The report discussed the extensive toll resulting from the range of oral, dental, and craniofacial diseases and conditions that affect the US population.[29,30] See Box 18-4 ■ for a summary of its major findings.

The report referred to the mouth and face as a mirror of the health and disease conditions found in the rest of the body. It discussed more than twenty diseases and conditions that cause lesions of the oral mucosa. For example, the report described associations between oral infections and diabetes, heart disease/stroke, respiratory ailments, and adverse pregnancy outcomes, such as premature births and low birth-weight babies. It also addressed the effects of oral diseases on well-being and quality of life. Dental hygienists are aware of the impact of tooth pain and oral disfigurement on eating, sleeping, cultural significance, social functions, and economics.

Box 18–4 Major Findings from *Oral Health in America: A Report of the Surgeon General*

- Oral disease and disorders in and of themselves affect health and well-being throughout life.
- Safe and effective measures exist to prevent the most common dental diseases: dental caries and periodontal diseases.
- Lifestyle behaviors that affect general health, such as tobacco use, excessive alcohol use, and poor dietary choices, affect oral and craniofacial health as well.
- There are profound and consequential oral health disparities within the US population.
- More information is needed to improve America's oral health and eliminate health disparities.
- The mouth reflects general health and well-being.
- Oral diseases and conditions are associated with other health problems.
- Scientific research is the key to further reduction in the burden of disease and disorders that affect the face, mouth, and teeth.

Source: U.S. Department of Health and Human Services, Public Health Service, National Institutes of Health, National Institute of Dental and Craniofacial Research. *Oral Health in America: A Report of the Surgeon General, 2000.* http://silk.nih.gov/public/hck1ocv.@www.surgeon.fullrpt .pdf. Accessed August 21, 2013.

The Surgeon General's 2000 oral health report does not mention the past or future critical role of the dental hygiene profession in preventing and treating oral diseases in the United States. However, it does highlight fluoridation, school water fluoridation, dietary fluoride supplements, fluoride mouth rinse programs, fluoride varnishes, dental sealants, and community oral health programs as approaches to promote oral health and prevent oral disease. Water fluoridation was reported to have the single greatest impact on the prevention of oral diseases. The dental hygiene profession is an integral part of such dental public health initiatives.

The Surgeon General's 2000 oral health report discussed a framework for action including the following recommendations:

- Change perceptions regarding oral health and ideas so that oral health becomes an accepted component of general health.
- Accelerate the building of the science and evidence base, and apply science effectively to improve oral health.
- Build an effective health infrastructure that meets the oral health needs of all Americans and integrate oral health effectively into general health.
- Remove known barriers between people and oral health services.
- Use public-private partnerships to improve the oral health of those who still suffer disproportionately from oral disease.

The Surgeon General's office released a follow-up report, *A National Call to Action to Promote Oral Health (Call to Action),* in May 2003. It describes the ongoing effort to address the country's oral health needs in the twenty-first century. Reflecting the work of a partnership of public and private organizations, the *National Call to Action* builds on *Oral Health in America: A Report of the Surgeon General* and *Healthy People 2020.*[31] It was an invitation to expand plans, activities, and programs designed to promote oral health and prevent disease, especially to reduce the health disparities that affect members of racial and ethnic groups, poor people, many who are geographically isolated, and others who are vulnerable because of special oral health care needs.[32] The report consists of five actions (see Box 18-5 ■) to which individuals from research, clinical care, and the community are enlisted to work collaboratively to improve the oral health of society. The World Health Organization gives priority to preventable diseases that are linked to risk factors such as an unhealthy diet and tobacco; this includes oral health.[33] It should be noted that the current emphasis on evidence-based practice in dentistry and dental hygiene is in line with the third recommended action.[31] The findings and recommendations of these various reports continue to form the foundation and be an integral part of dental public health policies and strategies today.

Box 18–5 Five Action Recommendations in the *National Call to Action to Promote Oral Health*

1. Change perceptions of oral health so that it is viewed to be as important as and related to general health.
2. Overcome barriers to oral health by replicating effective programs and proven efforts to enhance health promotion and health literacy, improve access to care, and reduce disabilities.
3. Build the science base of oral health by enhancing oral health research and accelerating the effective transfer of science to public and private practice.
4. Increase oral health workforce diversity, capacity, and flexibility to ensure a sufficient workforce pool to meet oral health care needs.
5. Increase collaborations to enhance partnering between the private and public sectors of oral health care.

Source: Based on U.S. Department of Health and Human Services. *National Call to Action to Promote Oral Health.* Rockville, MD: U.S. Department of Health and Human Services, Public Health Service, National Institutes of Health, National Institute of Dental and Craniofacial Research. NIH Publication No. 03-5303; Spring 2003.

http://www.surgeongeneral.gov/library/calls/oralhealth/nationalcalltoaction.html. Accessed August 25, 2013.

Box 18–6 Organizing Principles for a New Oral Health Initiative

1. Establish high-level accountability
2. Emphasize disease prevention and oral health promotion
3. Improve oral health literacy and cultural competence
4. Reduce oral health disparities
5. Explore new models for payment and delivery of care
6. Enhance the role of non-dental health care professionals
7. Expand oral health research and improve data collection
8. Promote collaboration among private and public stakeholders
9. Measure progress toward short-term and long-term goals and objectives
10. Advance the goals and objectives of *Healthy People 2020*

Advancing Oral Health in America

The Institute of Medicine (IOM), the health arm of the National Academy of Sciences, in 2009 organized an effort to assess oral health status and the current oral health care system. Published in 2011, *Advancing Oral Health in America*[34] reported the IOM findings to agencies of the US Department of Health and Human Services (HHS). Even though there have been improvements in oral health, profound disparities remain across the United States. IOM created the Committee on an Oral Health Initiative, which seeks to establish ways the HHS can improve oral health and oral health care systems in the nation.[34] The committee established new recommendations to build and enhance the current systems in place. These recommendations are called a New Oral Health Initiative. (See Box 18-6 ■.)

Global Oral Health Database

The Global Oral Health Database managed by the World Health Organization (WHO) contains oral epidemiologic data from around the world.[32] It uses data systematically collected by the WHO from countries that use its recommended data collection methods and maintains these country-specific data sets.[15] Data are provided for dental caries, periodontal diseases, tobacco use, oral cancer, and other oral conditions and programs.[32,33] In many cases, these data apply to large groups from the most populous parts of a country to provide an epidemiologic estimate of health conditions rather than being fully representative.

Sources and references are provided for every data set presented in the relevant country pages. Links to these databases are available on the Companion Website created specifically to accompany this text book.

Concepts of Epidemiologic Studies

Certain concepts that are germane to epidemiologic studies include risk of disease, causes of disease, types of epidemiologic studies, and effectiveness and efficacy of treatment modalities. It is vital to comprehend these concepts and how they relate to and differ from each other in meaning. This understanding will help the dental hygiene practitioner apply the results of epidemiologic studies to evidence-based decision making.

Risk and Causality

To understand research, classify a study design, and be able to apply research results to dental hygiene practice, one must first understand the difference between risk and causality.[5,6,7] *Causality,* also referred to as *cause and effect* or *causation,* means that a particular exposure results in a particular outcome.[6] This could be exposure to a causative agent that results in a specific disease, exposure to a preventive agent that results in preventing the disease, or exposure to treatment that results in resolving or controlling the disease. Causality routinely is used in dental hygiene practice to make decisions about what prevention and treatment programs to implement with individual patients or a population. Some examples are provided in Box 18-7 ■. Experimental studies are used to establish causality without question.[13] However, in many cases in oral epidemiology, causality has been inferred from non-experimental, analytic (observational) studies that have identified risk. Levels of

Box 18–7 Examples of Causality in Dental Hygiene Practice

Plaque biofilm causes gingivitis:
- Plaque biofilm is causally related to gingivitis, established by randomized clinical trials in which the effect of plaque biofilm on the gingiva was observed after a period of no oral hygiene and compared with the effect of good oral hygiene.
- This is why oral hygiene is promoted with patients.

Sugar causes dental caries:
- Sugar is causally related to caries, established with experimental studies that compared caries rates in children who had high sugar diets with caries rates of similar children who had low sugar diets.
- This is why diet counseling is provided.

Causality of professional fluoride treatment in preventing dental caries:
- This is established by experimental studies that compared caries rates in groups of children that received fluoride treatments with similar groups of children that did not.
- This is why fluoride treatments are recommended.

Flossing is causally related to resolution (healing) of gingivitis:
- This is demonstrated by the reduction of papillary gingival bleeding in one group who practiced proper flossing along with brushing, compared with continual papillary gingival bleeding in another similar group that only brushed.
- This is why flossing is promoted.

Box 18–8 Levels of Evidence for Evidence-Based Practice

1. Systematic review with meta analysis
2. Systematic review without meta analysis
3. One or more randomized controlled clinical trials
4. Well-designed cohort studies
5. Well-designed case control studies
6. Cross-sectional studies without concurrent controls; uncontrolled experiments
7. Case series
8. Opinions of respected authorities, based on clinical experience; descriptive surveys; case reports; reports of expert committees
9. Non-human (animal) research

Sources: Howick J. *Levels of Evidence 1.* Oxford Center for Evidence-Based Medicine; 2009. http://www.cebm.net/?o=1025. Accessed August 31, 2013. *Evidence Based Medicine Tutorial.* Icahn School of Medicine at Mount Sinai, Levy Library; 2013. http://libguides.mssm.edu/hierarchy. Accessed August 31, 2013.

evidence for evidence-based practice are based on causation and control of bias. Studies that are higher on this hierarchy of evidence provide stronger indication of causality. Thus, experimental studies are ranked above non-experimental studies (cohort, case control, cross sectional, case series, and descriptive surveys). (See Box 18-8 ■.)

When conducting experimental studies to establish causation is not practical or ethical, observational studies may be used to infer it. For example, it would not be ethical to randomly expose young children to malnutrition for comparison to a control group of well nourished children for the purpose of establishing a causal link to the development of caries. In this case, we must establish risk by conducting analytic studies that associate an attribute or exposure with the disease or condition. For example, the nutritional history of young children with and without dental caries can be studied to associate malnutrition with caries.

Establishing risk is not the same as establishing causality, but risk can be used to infer or suggest causality. While causality means that a cause-and-effect relationship

has been established, risk is the possibility that a specified event will occur.[13] The purpose of analytic studies is to quantify the degree of risk in specific circumstances. Risk establishes an association or relationship between the exposure and the condition that is used to infer or suggest causality.

See Box 18-9 ■ for a description of the criteria that support inferring causality from observational studies. Not all of these criteria must be in place to support causality, but the more that are, the stronger the case for causality of a risk factor in relation to the disease or condition.[6,7,15,35] Some examples of inferred causality from analytic studies in oral epidemiology that are commonly accepted in dental hygiene practice are the causal relationships between malnutrition and dental caries, excess fluoride and fluorosis, tobacco use and oral cancer, and presence of plaque biofilm bacteria and periodontal diseases. Although none of these causal relationships has been confirmed with experimental studies, causality has been accepted because of the strong, consistent results of multiple observational studies that suggest it and the criteria for inferring causality have been met.[36]

As evidenced by the hierarchy of evidence in Box 18-8 ■, some types of analytic studies establish risk more strongly than others.[6,13] To understand why, it is important to first understand the three types of attributes—risk factors, risk indicators, and risk markers—associated with diseases and conditions and how they are established.[6,13] Risk factors and risk indicators can refer to attributes that result in disease as well as those that control or prevent disease. The difference between risk factors and risk indicators is the strength of risk suggested according to the type of study used to demonstrate the risk.[37]

Box 18–9 Criteria for Inferring Causality from Observational Studies

- **Strength of Association.** The stronger the association between exposure and outcome, the greater is the likelihood of causation.
- **Consistency of Association.** If the association holds in a large number of studies (replication studies), it is more likely to be causal.
- **Sensitivity of Association.** If those who have the disease were exposed to the suspected causative factor, the factor is more likely to be causal.
- **Specificity of Association.** If absence of exposure is associated with absence of the disease outcome, the exposure is more likely to be causal.
- **Time Relationship.** If the exposure precedes the outcome, causality is more likely. This condition is considered to be absolute.[a]
- **Dose-Response Relationship.** If the disease outcome increases as the degree of exposure increases, causality is more likely.
- **Plausibility.** If the association is congruent with current biological, medical, epidemiologic, and scientific knowledge, causality is more likely.
- **Analogy.** If the association is similar to other associations that have been shown to be causal, the transfer of knowledge can be used to support causality.

Source: Chattopadhyay, A. Associations and causation. In Chattopadhyay A. Oral Health Epidemiology: Principles and Practice, pp 49–61. Burlington, MA: Jones and Bartlett; 2011.

A *risk factor* is a modifiable attribute or exposure known to be associated with a health condition or disease.[6,13] Increased exposure increases the risk; reduced exposure reduces the risk. Three criteria must be met to establish an exposure as a risk factor:

- Exposure must precede the onset of disease or health condition.
- Exposure must covary with the frequency of the disease or health condition.
- Observed association must not be due to bias or error in sample selection, measurement, or data analysis.

Risk factors can be used to infer causality and are therefore considered important to prevent. If the risk factor meets the criteria in Box 18-9 ■, causality can be inferred. These criteria can be illustrated by examining the relationship between smoking and periodontitis. Smoking is modifiable in that people can quit smoking. Smoking has preceded the development of periodontal disease in the studies (temporality). Multiple long-term observational studies have demonstrated that the frequency of periodontal disease covaries with smoking status. In other words, smokers have been observed in multiple longitudinal studies confirming that they develop periodontal disease more frequently than nonsmokers. Additionally, it has been observed that smokers who have quit smoking develop periodontal disease less frequently than those who continue to smoke. These studies have been well controlled to prevent error and show a strong association of smoking with periodontitis. The biology of the association is plausible in that the physiological tissue changes that occur with smoking potentially increase the risk of disease. Therefore, although experimental studies cannot be conducted to confirm a causal relationship, the causation of smoking relative to periodontitis is accepted because of the strength of these observational studies and the number of criteria that are met.

A *risk indicator* is a modifiable attribute that has been shown to be associated with a disease in cross-sectional studies or limited longitudinal studies.[37] Risk indicators are suspected risk factors that have not been confirmed; in other words, they do not meet the three criteria to establish a risk factor that were described earlier in this chapter (exposure must precede the onset of disease or health condition, exposure must covary with the frequency of the disease or health condition, and observed association must not be due to bias or error in sample selection, measurement, or data analysis). For example, if only cross-sectional studies have been conducted, the temporal relationship of the exposure and outcome is not clear. Additionally, if studies have not been well controlled, observed associations can be due to bias and errors in study design. The difference between a risk factor and a risk indicator is the amount or quality of evidence from the observational studies that have been conducted to examine the risk. Therefore, a risk indicator does not provide the same level of evidence for risk; risk is only assumed in relation to developing the disease or condition, and causality cannot be inferred.

Without confirmation, there is no way to be sure that a risk indicator is truly a risk factor. Experience has shown that risk indicators suggested by cross-sectional studies can disappear when assessed in longitudinal studies.[37] Therefore, it is critical to understand the difference between risk factors and risk indicators to prevent making inappropriate recommendations to patients or conducting potentially ineffective preventive programs in a community setting.

A *risk marker,* also called a *risk predictor* or a *demographic risk factor,* is an attribute that is associated with the increased probability of disease but is not considered to have a causal role in its development.[37] Risk markers are also established by conducting cross-sectional studies. Risk markers such as age, gender, race, ethnicity, and SES are nonmodifiable. Therefore, they are not useful when considering prevention based on controlling risk.

The significance of discriminating between these attributes relates to the way they are applied to clinical decision making about preventive recommendations in dental hygiene practice.[13] Risk factors should be considered to help patients control disease because the risks have been established, such as those with tobacco, alcohol, and diet.

Risk indicators should be applied with care in practice decisions because the risk is assumed but not confirmed as is the case with some systemic conditions in relation to periodontitis.[37] Risk markers are not useful in controlling disease, but they point to an increased need to address confirmed, modifiable risk factors to reduce the risk of disease in individual members of an at-risk population. Risk markers also have application in making decisions about what groups to target with dental public health programs.[37] See Table 18-10 ■ for a summary of risk factors, risk indicators, and risk markers and Table 18-11 ■ for the types of studies that are used to identify them.

Table 18–10 Summary of Risk Attributes

Attribute	Modifiability	Studies	Application to Dental Hygiene Practice
Risk factor	Yes	Longitudinal	• Has an established risk role; can be used to infer causality • Should be an important consideration in making recommendations
Risk indicator	Yes	Cross-sectional Correlational Limited longitudinal	• Has a possible risk role; cannot be used to infer causality • Should be applied with care when making recommendations
Risk marker (demographic risk factor/risk predictor)	No	Cross-sectional Correlational	• Is not important in making individual recommendations to control the factor • Indicates greater need to control modifiable risk factors and risk indicators • Should be considered to identify target populations for dental public health programs

Table 18–11 Classification of Different Epidemiologic Studies and Risk

Type of Study	Number of Groups	Number of Measures	Classification	Used to Identify
Experimental	2 or more	2 or more	N/A	Causality
Cohort	1 (plus a comparison group)	2 or more over time	Longitudinal Prospective	Risk factor Incidence
Case–control	2	1	Longitudinal Retrospective	Risk factor
Cross-sectional	1	1	Cross-sectional	Risk indicator Demographic risk factor
Ecological	2	None (existing population data are used)	N/A	Potential associations; hypotheses for future research
Descriptive	1	1	N/A	Prevalence Incidence (if descriptive surveys are repeated over time)

Sources: Chattopadhyay A. *Oral Health Epidemiology: Principles and Practice.* Burlington, MA: Jones and Bartlett; 2011. Merrill RM. *Introduction to Epidemiology.* 5th ed. Burligton confirming ton, MA: Jones & Bartlett; 2010. Friis RH, Sellers TA. *Epidemiology for Public Health Practice.* 5th ed. Burlington, MA: Jones & Bartlett; 2013. Gerstman BB. *Epidemiology Kept Simple: Introduction to Traditional and Modern Epidemiology.* 2nd ed. Oxford, England: Wiley-Blackwell; 2013. Centers for Disease Control and Prevention. *Principles of Epidemiology in Public Health Practice.* 3rd ed; 2012. http://www.cdc.gov/osels/scientific_edu/ss1978/lesson1/Section11.html. Accessed August 15, 2013.

Types of Epidemiologic Studies

Epidemiology is the study of the occurrence of health and disease in populations and how this knowledge is applied to control disease. To understand the epidemiology of oral disease, one must first comprehend the various types of epidemiologic studies and concepts related to research methodology. Epidemiologic studies are used to answer research questions and test hypotheses. The *null hypothesis* of a study is a negative statement that proposes no relationship or difference between two variables. The *alternative hypothesis*, also called the *research hypothesis*, is a positive statement that proposes a relationship or difference between two variables. There are two major categories of epidemiologic research studies, experimental and non-experimental.[4,5,6,7,13] These are described and contrasted in Tables 18-11 ■ and 18-12 ■ and illustrated in Boxes 18-10 ■ through 18-14 ■.

EXPERIMENTAL STUDIES *Experimental studies* are interventional, which means the conditions of the study are manipulated to try to affect the outcome, with one or more variables manipulated. The purpose of an experimental study is to test a hypothesis related to a comparative question and establish a cause-and-effect relationship. The *experimental group*, the group that receives the experimental intervention, is compared to the *control group*, which is the group that does not receive the intervention. The control group can receive no treatment (*passive control*), the current or standard treatment (*active control*), or a fake treatment that simulates the experimental treatment (*placebo*). Variables in experimental studies are the *independent variable* (the variable manipulated) and the *dependent variable* (the variable measured to determine the effect of the independent variable). Study procedures are carefully organized to control the effect of *extraneous variables* (other variables that can influence the relationship between the variables of interest in the study) and other sources of error. Two types of experimental studies are clinical trials and field trials. *Clinical trials* are well controlled and alter the natural progression of a disease or condition. *Field trials* are carried out on people in the community who may or may not be patients.[4,5]

Clinical trials are classified as either efficacy or effectiveness trials.[37] The differences relate to the purpose of the trial. Understanding the difference is important to interpret the results correctly. The purpose of an *efficacy trial* is to test whether an agent or treatment regimen works. It is conducted on a population susceptible to the disease or condition being studied.[37] Susceptibility could be based on age, gender, race, SES, geographic location, or other factors identified in previous studies. Results can be generalized only to the susceptible population sampled for the study. Therefore, generalizing results of efficacy trials to the population at large produces an error in interpretation. These trials are conducted under very controlled conditions. They have requirements such as the use of a control group that is similar and in which procedures are duplicated, random allocation of the study participants to groups, and double-blind methods. In addition, controls are in place to assure the agent is used exactly as intended in terms of concentration, length and frequency of use, and application procedures. The term *application procedure* refers to instructions given to study participants, application by a person who will apply it correctly (self or professional), or professional supervision if self-applied.

An example of an efficacy trial is testing the ability of a new power toothbrush (whether it works or not) to reduce gingivitis by evaluating its use in a sample population that

Table 18–12 Contrast of Non-experimental and Experimental Research Studies

Non-experimental: Descriptive/Analytic	Experimental Studies
Non-interventional	Interventional
Variables are observed in their natural state	Variables are manipulated
Establish risk (analytic studies)	Establish causality
Variables are observed (descriptive studies) and/or associated or related (analytic studies)	Cause-and-effect relationship of variables is established
Answer status questions (descriptive) or relationship questions (analytic)	Answer difference questions
Lower level of evidence	Higher level of evidence

Sources: Chattopadhyay A. *Oral Health Epidemiology: Principles and Practice*. Burlington, MA: Jones and Bartlett; 2011. Merrill RM. *Introduction to Epidemiology*. 5th ed. Burlington, MA: Jones & Bartlett; 2010. Friis RH, Sellers TA. *Epidemiology for Public Health Practice*, 5th ed. Burlington, MA: Jones & Bartlett; 2013. Gerstman BB. *Epidemiology Kept Simple: Introduction to Traditional and Modern Epidemiology*. 2nd ed. Oxford, England: Wiley-Blackwell; 2013. Centers for Disease Control and Prevention. *Principles of Epidemiology in Public Health Practice*. 3rd ed; 2012. http://www.cdc.gov/osels/scientific_edu/ss1978/lesson1/Section11.html. Accessed August 15, 2013.

has high plaque biofilm, gingivitis, and bleeding scores. To ensure that it is operated correctly, the power toothbrush would be used by the study participants under close supervision after careful instruction by the researcher. These procedures are used in an efficacy trial because the test product must be given every chance to succeed.[37]

The purpose of an *effectiveness trial* is to test the way an agent or treatment regimen works in everyday conditions after its efficacy has been established.[37] This type of trial is conducted on a broad community population with varying degrees of the disease or condition under study. Results of effectiveness trials can be generalized to the population at large because they are conducted on a sample drawn from this broad population. Effectiveness trials also are conducted under controlled conditions, but there is less control of the application procedures than in efficacy trials so the agent can be used as it normally would be used in "real-life" situations. For example, professionals who apply the agent are given instructions but not supervised as they apply it. If it is self-applied, study participants receive professional instructions and then take the agent home to use.[37] This allows greater generalizability to the use of the product or treatment in the real world situation.

The previous example of an efficacy trial can be adapted to illustrate an effectiveness trial. The effectiveness of the same power toothbrush could be tested in a sample that represents the general population of varied ages, abilities, and oral health status. The toothbrush would be used at home without supervision after receiving standardized instruction from the researcher. This would be done after the efficacy trial determined that the power toothbrush reduces gingivitis under more controlled conditions in a sample that exhibits gingivitis.

NON-EXPERIMENTAL STUDIES *Non-experimental studies* in epidemiology show the occurrence of health and disease as they naturally occur in a population. In contrast to experimental studies, the variables in non-experimental studies are not manipulated but simply observed to detect how the outcome is affected; thus, non-experimental studies are referred to as *observational studies*. Three classifications of non-experimental studies are descriptive, analytic, and ecological. *Descriptive studies* are used to answer questions about the status or presence of a disease or condition in the population. Variables are simply measured and reported in descriptive studies.

Analytic studies, also referred to as *developmental studies,* are used to answer questions and test hypotheses about an association or relationship between health and disease and other elements related to risk. Analytic studies identify how health and disease are influenced by various risk factors, identify determinants of disease, and determine appropriate prevention and control measures. The variables of an analytic study are the *exposure* (the variable thought to affect the disease or condition being studied, similar to the independent variable of an experimental study) and the *outcome* (the disease or condition thought to be affected by the exposure, similar to the dependent variable in an experimental study). Three types of analytic research studies are *cohort, case control,* and *cross-sectional.*[4–7,12,37] An analytic study that uses correlation statistics to relate variables to each other is also referred to as a *correlational study*. It is important to remember that correlation does not imply causality.[14,36]

Ecological studies focus on the comparison of existing population-based data previously collected for another purpose rather than data collected from individuals in which the exposure and outcome are known for each individual.[37] As a result, studies of this type possess many methodological problems that severely limit causal inference. However, they are useful for generating hypotheses by identifying potential associations that can then be tested with more carefully designed analytic studies.

See Tables 18-11 ■, 18-12 ■, and 18-13 ■ for definitions, explanations, and examples of these types of non-experimental studies in contrast to experimental studies. Further examples of experimental and non-experimental studies are presented in Boxes 18-11 ■, 18-12 ■, 18-13 ■ and 18-14 ■.

Validity of Epidemiologic Studies

The validity and reliability of measurements was discussed earlier in this chapter. Here validity will be discussed in relation to conducting an epidemiologic research study. *Validity* is the accuracy of a study, which is affected by procedures and controls used while conducting the study.[38] Researchers are concerned with validity because they must ensure that research is meaningful. Validity is increased by controlling errors and bias when conducting a study. See Box 18-10 ■ for a summary of ways to increase validity in epidemiologic studies.

Internal Validity

Two types of validity are internal and external. *Internal validity* refers to the accuracy of the results of the study.[13] Internal validity is enhanced by controlling sources of error and extraneous variables when conducting the research, increasing subject retention, achieving compliance of study participants, enhancing data quality, and applying appropriate methods for statistical data analysis. To increase the accuracy of an experimental study, procedures followed during the study should be carefully controlled and supervised to standardize study conditions between the experimental and control groups.

Several procedures increase internal validity by controlling errors in the measurement of the variables.[38] For example, the validity and reliability of instruments and examiners must be ensured. The measurement instrument must be valid and reliable and provide consistent, reproducible results.[38] Measuring the dependent or outcome variable with established or pretested measures and using instruments that have documented reliability increase the internal validity of a study.

Box 18–10 Ways to Control Errors and Bias to Increase Validity of Epidemiologic Research Designs

- Have a researchable hypothesis
- Base the study on valid assumptions
- Operationally define variables clearly
- Use the appropriate population for the type of study
- Use a sample that represents the population
- Have an adequate sample size for the purpose of the study and to accommodate for loss of participants in longitudinal and experimental studies
- Control extraneous variables
- Use an appropriate type of control or comparison group when called for by the study design
- Control group differences by using randomization and stratification (experimental studies)
- Use participants as their own control when appropriate (experimental studies)
- Use blind and double-blind procedures when possible

- Use a pretest for comparison (experimental studies)
- Control for pretest sensitization (experimental studies)
- Use valid and reliable instruments and measures of the variables
- Control errors in measuring variables; control examiner error with standardization and calibration
- Carefully control and supervise procedures in relation to the purpose of the study
- Standardize study conditions in all groups (experimental studies)
- Use repeated measures when appropriate (experimental studies)
- Use several measures of the dependent variable when called for (experimental studies)
- Have a long enough trial to detect new disease or change (longitudinal and experimental studies)

Box 18–11 Application of Knowledge: Sample Epidemiologic Study #1

A dental hygienist managing a school sealant program seeks to identify what factors relate to parents' return of consent forms for their children to participate in the program, in order to improve future response rates. A study is conducted with a representative sample of the school population to determine the relationship of parents' SES, health literacy, dental history, and other factors to their return of consent forms.

What kind of study is this (cross-sectional, case control, cohort, or experimental)? Cross-sectional (non-experimental, observational): There is only one group, they are measured only one time, and the condition (return of consent forms) and risk factors (SES, health literacy, dental history, and other factors) are measured to see if they relate; it is also correlational since correlation statistics are used to determine these relationships

Is this study experimental or non-experimental? Non-experimental: There is no manipulation of a variable; variables are observed as they naturally occur

Does this study measure incidence or prevalence? Prevalence: the variables are measured in the population to determine their rates at a given point in time

How is this study ranked on the hierarchy of evidence? Cross-sectional studies are ranked low on the hierarchy of evidence; they have the lowest ranking of the analytic studies

Does this study identify a risk factor, risk indicator, or risk marker? Risk marker: cross-sectional studies identify risk indicators and risk markers; SES, dental IQ, and dental history are non-modifiable risk markers

Box 18–12 Application of Knowledge: Sample Epidemiologic Study #2

Management of a dental corporation is concerned about the high rate of exposure to blood-borne infection in employees of one of its clinics. Employees are observed over a period of time to identify what factors are contributing to the high exposure rate. Employees of another clinic who have a low rate of exposure to blood-borne infection are observed as a comparison group.

What type of study is this? (Cross-sectional, case control, cohort, or experimental) Cohort (non-experimental, observational): one group of clinic employees is observed, and the exposure variables (factors that can contribute to blood-borne infection exposure) are measured over time (longitudinal) to determine if they are creating a risk for the outcome (exposure to blood-borne infection); the second clinic with a low rate of outcome (exposure to blood-borne infection) is used as a comparison group

Is this study experimental or non-experimental? Non-experimental: variables are not manipulated but are observed and measured as they occur naturally

How is this study ranked on the hierarchy of evidence? Highest ranking of non-experimental studies; below experimental studies

Does this study identify a risk factor, risk indicator, or risk marker? Risk factor: cohort studies are longitudinal and therefore identify risk factors

Does this study establish causality or risk? Risk; experimental studies are required to establish causality; causality can be inferred from these risk factors if criteria to infer causality are met

Box 18–13 Application of Knowledge: Sample Epidemiologic Study #3

A study was conducted to compare the GUM® Soft-Pick® interproximal cleaner to traditional floss in terms of their ability to reduce gingival inflammation and bleeding in patients with large embrasure spaces. Volunteer patients were recruited from a dental school periodontal clinic. Patient criteria to be included in the sample were that patients had periodontal surgery within the last five years, had >5 mm of clinical attachment loss, and had localized moderate to severe gingivitis. Patients were randomized into two groups, one of which was instructed to use the GUM® Soft-Pick®, while the other group was instructed to use traditional floss one time daily. One examiner who was blind to group assignment and trained in the use of the index used the Sulcus Bleeding Index (SBI) with full mouth probing to record the presence or absence of bleeding in the gingival sulcus. Probe readings were recorded at baseline and at three- and six-month intervals.

Is this study experimental or non-experimental? Experimental: the independent variable (interdental cleaning agent) was manipulated, groups were randomly formed, sources of error were controlled, and effect on the dependent variable (bleeding) was measured

Is this classified as a clinical trial or a field trial? Clinical trial: the experimental study was carried out with patients in a dental school clinic

Do the procedures used in the study enhance the internal or external validity of the study? Internal validity: a baseline (pretest) was used, a standardized index was used that had documented reliability (SBI), the experimental group and control group were randomized, the examiner was blind to group assignment, and the examiner was calibrated; a convenience sample of volunteer patients reduced external validity so replication studies are indicated

Is this an efficacy or effectiveness trial? Efficacy: it was conducted on a population susceptible to the disease (had periodontal surgery within the last five years, had >5 mm of clinical attachment loss, had localized moderate to severe gingivitis, and had large embrasure spaces) to test whether the agent (GUM® Soft-Pick®) produced the desired results (reduction in bleeding)

Is this study used to identify risk or causality? Causality: it demonstrates that a particular exposure to a preventive agent (the GUM® Soft-Pick®) results in the outcome of preventing a disease or condition (reduced bleeding)

Source: Based on Yost KG, Mallatt ME, Liebman J. Interproximal gingivitis and plaque reduction by four interdental products. *J Clin Dent.* 2006;17(3):79–83.

Box 18–14 Application of Knowledge: Sample Epidemiologic Study #4

During the early stages of research on fluorosis, researchers compared a group of people with severe fluorosis to a group without fluorosis. They examined their history to determine what factor(s) related to the presence of fluorosis, and found that the common factor among those with fluorosis was the water. This led the researchers to begin looking for the common component of water that was linked to fluorosis.

What type of study is this? (Cross-sectional, case control, cohort, or experimental) Case control (non-experimental, observational): There were two naturally occurring groups (one with fluorosis and one without), they were measured only one time, it was retrospective (looking back at the history of the people in each group), and there was an attempt to relate factors (exposure) to fluorosis (outcome)

Is this study experimental or non-experimental? Non-experimental: variables were not manipulated but were observed and measured as they occurred naturally

How is this study ranked on the hierarchy of evidence? Lower than cohort studies and higher than cross-sectional studies

Does this study identify a risk factor, risk indicator, or risk marker? Risk factor: case-control studies are longitudinal and therefore identify risk factors, although they do not provide as strong an indication of risk as cohort studies because temporality may not be as certain

Does this study establish causality or risk? Risk; experimental studies are required to establish risk; causality can be inferred from a risk factor if criteria to infer causality are met

Table 18–13 Experimental and Non-experimental Research Designs

Type of Study	Description of Study	Example of Study
Experimental	One or more variables are manipulated and the effect is measured to test the effect of an agent, procedure, or program	A study to test the effect of using a power toothbrush versus a manual toothbrush on brushing frequency
Cohort	One population or subset with common characteristics is observed and measured over time; longitudinal; prospective	Observation of the effects of poor oral hygiene habits in children over a 10-year period
Case Control	Group with disease is compared to group without disease to establish functional relationships; retrospective	Assessment of the relationship of oral hygiene to gingivitis by comparing previous oral hygiene data in a group with gingivitis to a group without gingivitis
Cross-sectional	One group surveyed at one point in time; assessment of the relationship of variables to the disease or condition measured	Assessment of the relationship of oral hygiene habits to gingivitis in a population surveyed
Ecological	Compare previously recorded population data from two or more populations	Existing data from different populations are used to attempt to relate oral hygiene and gingivitis
Descriptive	Describes extent and distribution of disease or condition in a population or sample; measured at one point in time; can be repeated to determine change and trends	Description of oral hygiene habits in a population surveyed; survey can be repeated over time to measure changes in oral hygiene to establish a trend

Sources: Chattopadhyay A. *Oral Health Epidemiology: Principles and Practice.* Burlington, MA: Jones and Bartlett; 2011. Merrill RM. *Introduction to Epidemiology.* 5th ed. Burlington, MA: Jones & Bartlett; 2010. Friis RH, Sellers TA. *Epidemiology for Public Health Practice.* 5th ed. Burlington, MA: Jones & Bartlett; 2013. Gerstman BB. *Epidemiology Kept Simple: Introduction to Traditional and Modern Epidemiology.* 2nd ed. Oxford, England: Wiley-Blackwell; 2013. Centers for Disease Control and Prevention. *Principles of Epidemiology in Public Health Practice.* 3rd ed; 2012. http://www.cdc.gov/osels/scientific_edu/ss1978/lesson1/Section11.html. Accessed August 15, 2013.

Did You Know?

Double blind study designs can control the reliability of data by reducing experimenter bias and participant expectations.

The length of the study can also affect the internal validity. It must be long enough to detect new disease, extension of current disease, and resolution of disease. The ideal length varies with the disease being studied. The recommendation is 2 to 3 years for caries reduction trials, 8 to 21 days for plaque biofilm-inhibiting studies, 90 days for supragingival calculus prevention agents, longer for subgingival calculus prevention, and 6 months for gingivitis reduction trials.[13]

The sample size can affect internal validity in several ways. Humans have the right to participate or not in a study. This volunteer involvement can result in the loss of participants from longitudinal and experimental studies. The sample must be large enough to compensate for this loss; otherwise, resulting group sizes can be too small to produce valid results. Even when compensating with a larger sample, the fewer participants lost, the less susceptible the study is to invalid results.[6] Loss of participants from an experimental study can result in groups that are no longer equivalent, thus invalidating the study results.[6] When participants are lost, it is important also to test for equivalency of the final groups and to determine whether those who dropped from the study were similar to those who completed it.[6] Research reports should include the size of the sample in terms of the number approached to participate, the number who agreed to begin the study, and the number who completed it.[13]

Finally, internal validity is affected by the validity of the statistical procedures used, which depends in part on the sample size. Group sizes must be adequate; data must meet certain assumptions for the application of parametric inferential statistics. The use of multiple groups as required by factorial and Solomon designs necessitates the use of a larger sample than other designs to allow for adequate group sizes. Samples also must be larger when small differences are expected in the dependent variable

between the test and control group.[13] For example, early fluoride studies compared a group exposed to fluoride to a group not exposed, and large differences in caries rates were expected because other uses of fluorides were uncommon.[39] Today, because of the prevalence of fluoride exposure in our population, we expect smaller caries differences when comparing a group exposed to fluoride with a group not exposed. Therefore, larger groups (hence, larger samples) are needed today to obtain the statistical results required to reject the null hypothesis. Finally, the statistics used should meet the needs of the type of data, number of variables, and number of groups compared. (See Chapter 17.)

External Validity

The accuracy of inferring (generalizing) the results from the sample to the population at large is referred to as external validity.[13] It is affected by how well the sample represents the population. If it is a good representation, it is safe to generalize results to that population. If it is not representative, results from the sample cannot be inferred to the population. Therefore, selection of study participants is critical. Regardless of the type of study, the sample should be similar to the population in age, gender, SES, ethnicity, other demographic factors, and variables that relate to the area of study.[6]

The type of study determines the type and sample size required to increase external validity.[7] Use of a large, representative sample is critical for descriptive surveys.[6] Distribution of several hundred questionnaires would be the goal of a survey, depending on population size.[6] Generally at least 10 percent of the population is suggested for survey research. Also, when an interview or questionnaire is used to collect survey data, in order to increase external validity, the size of the sample approached must be adjusted to accommodate for the anticipated response rate.

Sampling must be precise for survey research. Because the intent is to infer the results to the population, the sample must represent it. Use of a nonrepresentative sample results in a discrepancy between the sample and the population in one or more important characteristics, and the results cannot be generalized. For example, if only dental hygiene students were surveyed when studying college students, the sample clearly would not represent the population. Dental hygiene students differ from other college students in terms of GPA, health interest, age, and other characteristics.

Even when precise sampling methods are used, sampling error can occur.[7] Sampling error can be calculated statistically when a probability sample is used. With a probability sample, which is a method of sampling that uses some form of random selection, the chance of each person being selected in the sample is known but is not necessarily equal.[7] The degree of sampling error for a probability sample can be calculated; thus, how well the results can be inferred to the population is known. The

chance of each person being selected for a non-probability sample is not known. In this case, the sampling error cannot be calculated, and problems with interpretation of the data can arise. Probability samples are used to conduct many large, national epidemiologic surveys, such as those described earlier in this chapter.[7]

A small sample can be used for a pilot study, which is a trial run in preparation for a major large research project.[40] Also, nearly all randomized clinical oral health trials are accomplished with smaller convenience samples, which are composed of subjects who are most readily available.[4] Replication studies are used to compensate for the use of unrepresentative samples in experimental research by confirming that similar results occur with different samples. Additional studies that test the same hypothesis using similar methods in different populations and obtaining similar results provides evidence that the observed effect is real and can be generalized to the population at large.[4]

The delimitations of the study sample to control the internal validity of efficacy trials (described earlier in this chapter) reduce the study's legitimacy when applied to the population at large because certain individuals are excluded in an efficacy trial. Also, controlling and supervising the use of a product or procedure limits the legitimacy in the uncontrolled circumstances of the real world. Thus, effectiveness trials are conducted after efficacy trials show positive results.[12] For example, if a fluoride varnish study shows its efficacy to reduce dental caries in a Head Start program in a low SES urban population of children recently emigrated from Mediterranean and Middle Eastern countries, these results do not generalize to all children. Replication studies would be needed to test the fluoride varnish in various groups of children representing different ages, dietary practices, ethnic backgrounds, and exposure to fluoridated water. If similar results occur in these different studies, it would be possible to generalize the results to the general population.[13]

Other procedures used when conducting research also affect external validity. For example, the dependent variable measure must have reference and meaning to the real world. Also, using more than one measure of the dependent variable improves the external validity of the study.[6,38] An example is assessing both bleeding and gingival appearance with a bleeding index and a gingival index as a measure of gingivitis. Pretest sensitization occurs when subjects have been pretested and as a result may act or react differently once an independent variable is studied. This too can decrease external validity, but the effect can be controlled by using posttest-only or Solomon research designs. Another issue of external validity is that some changes measured at posttest, such as improved plaque biofilm scores to measure success of oral health education, may not hold over time. When this is the case, it is recommended that the dependent variable be measured three times after introducing the independent variable.[6]

DENTAL HYGIENIST SPOTLIGHT ·······················

Public Health Column: Vicki Gianopoulos Pizanis, RDH, MS

This month's spotlight focuses on a dental hygienist who recently received the New Mexico Future Leader Award, Professor Vicki Gianopoulos Pizanis. Vicki has a true passion for dental hygiene. She has focused her career on teaching others about dental hygiene as a science and practice, and she treats patients in a variety of public health settings. With these aspirations in mind, she has ventured into an international venue while simultaneously building an interdisciplinary group of professionals to further help the underserved. She is focusing on integrating oral health into existing health-care systems, which has been a main focus of dental hygiene since its inception. I recently asked Vicki about her career, and here are her thoughts.

Why did you go into dental hygiene?

I have always been interested in working in a health-care field. I thought I wanted to go into optometry, so I began my undergraduate career as a biology major. As I went through school, I was inspired by my aunt, who is a dental hygienist. She is one of the most positive people with one of the greatest personalities that I know. I looked into the prerequisite requirements for dental hygiene and learned that I had already completed most of them. So I changed directions and applied to the dental hygiene program at UNM. I am thankful for my decision. This career has been amazing to me, with endless opportunities in education, clinical, research, and being an advocate for the profession. Now I can't see myself doing anything else.

How did you get into dental public health? Did you need additional education?

During my work toward an M.S. in dental hygiene, my first experience in public health was at a school-based health program at a local middle school. The program at the time was fairly new, so in addition to seeing patients, I did what I could to help improve the program. After receiving my MS degree in dental hygiene, I worked at a pediatric clinic in an underserved part of the city where patients were low income and primarily Spanish-speaking. I gained experience working with patients with developmental disabilities in another clinic we operate. I quickly learned the vast differences of the working environment in public health compared to a private practice setting. I enjoy how the work I do in public health is very patient-centered as opposed to profit-focused. The patients are very much in need and thankful for the services and education they receive. I also feel that I have more autonomy as a health-care provider in public health. I can schedule and treat patients the way I feel benefits them the most. I feel an MS in dental hygiene or public health prepared me for that working environment. Higher education teaches one how to think and problem solve, which are good skills to have in public health.

What are your current positions?

I teach a variety of courses in the dental hygiene program at the University of New Mexico. Clinically, I work in a UNM public health clinic one to two days a week. The experience is rewarding. I feel like I learn more every day.

Can you discuss any particularly interesting experiences you have had in your dental public health positions?

Yes, one particular experience comes to mind where I feel like I had a big impact on a patient. When working at one of the pediatric public health clinics, I treated a sweet young Vietnamese girl. At her first and every subsequent appointment she arrived with her make-up carefully applied, her hair fixed meticulously, and wearing a well-planned outfit. She was brought in by her grandmother who didn't speak any English. She was 14 years old, and this had been her first time to be seen by an oral health-care provider. When I looked into her mouth, she presented with severe gingival hyperplasia extending to the incisal third of her teeth. She had heavy, tenacious subgingival calculus with extremely inflamed soft tissue. I was surprised to see a young girl that took such good care of her appearance present with this extent of extreme oral infection. We worked together through education and multiple appointments. Within four weeks, her oral health drastically improved. She took every recommendation to heart, from her brushing and flossing technique to oral rinse suggestions. I could see how much she appreciated the transition in her mouth. It was rewarding to make such a difference to this young girl. Together, we were able to alleviate her pain and increase her self-confidence, and I trust that she will carry her oral health education with her for the rest of her life.

What type of advice would you give to a practicing hygienist who is thinking of doing something different?

Public health is unique and requires innovative thinking and problem-solving to reach out to the community. I believe that a hygienist who works in public

health has many opportunities for creative thinking and to make a positive difference in the needs of his or her community.

Do you have any additional experiences to share?

I had the opportunity to travel to South Africa with other dental hygiene educators in October 2009. The trip was organized by People to People in collaboration with the ADHA. The experience taught me how oral health care is practiced in a country with a very different model for the education and scope of practice for health-care providers. This was also the first time I had seen a population with such abundant health-care needs.

We provided oral health screenings in a community of very low-income people. Many of the patients walked several miles to have a health-care provider look at their mouths. This was very touching to me and motivated me to do more. I wanted to give others a similar opportunity to see, firsthand, the needs outside our country. From this experience, we started an international health program to take UNM dental hygiene students and community dental hygienists to rural areas outside of Granada, Nicaragua, to provide oral health care. In 2011, I organized 36 health-care providers and volunteers, and we treated 243 patients who otherwise would not have received care. For our second medical mission, we've opened this opportunity to the entire University of New Mexico community. In 2013, in addition to traveling with dental hygiene students, we will be taking students from nursing, physical therapy, and occupational therapy, as well as medical residents, to widen our scope of practice and provide interdisciplinary services.

Source: Christine Nathe writes the Public Health Column in *RDH* magazine published by Pennwell Publishing. For more public health spotlights please see RDH magazine online at http://www.rdhmag.com/index.html.

Summary

Evidence-based practice requires understanding epidemiologic research methods to be able to interpret their results and apply them to dental hygiene practice. Various epidemiologic methods are used to track oral disease and related conditions in the population. Surveillance systems in place in the United States help to determine what public health programs are needed and to track trends that can be used to evaluate the success of these programs. Non-experimental and experimental research designs are used to measure the presence and distribution of oral disease in the population, track progress of disease over time, determine population needs, and evaluate the success of programs, treatment regimens, and methods of preventing and controlling disease.

Self-Study Test Items

1. *Epidemiology* has been defined as the study of the nature, cause, control, and determinants of the frequency and distribution of
   a. Disease
   b. Disability
   c. Death
   d. All of the above

2. The agent of disease is the biologic or mechanical cause of the disease or condition. Examples of agents are the specific bacteria in relation to dental caries or brushing with a hard toothbrush in relation to abrasion.
   a. The first statement is true; the second statement is false.
   b. The first statement is false; the second statement is true.
   c. Both statements are true.
   d. Both statements are false.

3. The occurrence of an illness in excess of normal expectancy in a community or region, usually occurring suddenly and spreading rapidly, is termed a(n)
   a. Endemic
   b. Epidemic
   c. Pandemic
   d. All of the above

4. Which study attempts to relate outcome with exposure to a suspected risk factor using data that are available for the population?
   a. Case–control
   b. Case study
   c. Ecological
   d. Time series

5. What is a modifiable attribute or exposure that is known to be associated with a health condition?
   a. Risk ratio
   b. Risk factor
   c. Risk attribute
   d. Risk indicator

References

1. ADA Center for Evidence-Based Dentistry. *About EBD*; revised 2013. Retrieved from http://ebd.ada.org/about.aspx .on July 8, 2013.
2. Forrest JL, Miller SA, Miller G. Keeping current: Clinical decision support systems. *J Dent Hyg.* 2012;86(1):18–20.
3. Law K, Howick J. *OCEMB table of evidence glossary*. Center for Evidence Based Medicine (CEBM); revised July 2013. Retrieved from http://www.cebm.net/index.aspx?o=1116. on July 8, 2013.
4. Chattopadhyay A. *Oral Health Epidemiology: Principles and Practice.* Burlington, MA: Jones and Bartlett; 2011.

5. Merrill RM. *Introduction to Epidemiology*. 5th ed. Burlington, MA: Jones & Bartlett; 2010.

6. Friis RH, Sellers TA. *Epidemiology for Public Health Practice*. 5th ed. Burlington, MA: Jones & Bartlett; 2013.

7. Gerstman BB. *Epidemiology Kept Simple: Introduction to Traditional and Modern Epidemiology*. 2nd ed. Oxford, England: Wiley-Blackwell; 2013.

8. Centers for Disease Control and Prevention (CDC). *Principles of Epidemiology in Public Health Practice*. 3rd ed; 2012. Retrieved from http://www.cdc.gov/osels/scientific_edu/ss1978/lesson1/Section11.html. on August 15, 2013.

9. Centers for Disease Control and Prevention. *Lesson 1: Understanding the Epidemiologic Triangle Through Infectious Disease*; n.d. Retrieved from http://www.cdc.gov/bam/teachers/documents/epi_1_triangle.pdf. on August 15, 2013.

10. World Health Organization. *The Determinants of Health*. Health Impact Assessment (HIA); 2013. Retrieved from http://www.who.int/hia/evidence/doh/en/. on August 15, 2013.

11. Siegel JS. *The Demography and Epidemiology of Human Health and Aging*. North Bethesda, MA: Springer; 2012.

12. Glendor U, Anderson L. Public health aspects of oral diseases and disorders—dental trauma. In: Pine C, Harris R, eds. *Community Oral Health*. 2nd ed. Hanover Park, IL: Quintessence; 2007:203–214.

13. Scheutz F. Principles and methods of oral epidemiology. In: Pine C, Harris R, eds. *Community Oral Health*. 2nd ed. Hanover Park, IL: Quintessence; 2007:115–140.

14. Jewell NP. *Statistics for Epidemiology*. Boca Raton, Florida: Chapman & Hall/CRC; 2009.

15. Hebel JR, McCarter RJ. *A Study Guide to Epidemiology and Biostatistics*. 7th ed. Burlington, MA: Jones & Bartlett; 2012.

16. Roush SW. *Chapter 18: Surveillance Indicators*. 5th ed. Atlanta, GA: Centers for Disease Control and Prevention; 2011. Retrieved from http://www.cdc.gov/vaccines/pubs/surv-manual/chpt18-surv-indicators.html. on August 17, 2013.

17. National Cancer Institute, Surveillance Epidemiology and End Results. *About the SEER Program*; n.d. Retrieved from http://seer.cancer.gov/about/. on August 17, 2013.

18. National Institute of Dental and Craniofacial Research. *NIDCR Fast Facts*; 2013. Retrieved from http://www.nidcr.nih.gov/AboutUs/FastFacts.htm. on August 17, 2013.

19. U.S. Department of Health and Human Services. *National Health and Nutrition Examination Survey (NHANES)*. Healthy People 2020; 2013. Retrieved from http://healthypeople.gov/2020/data/datasource.aspx?id=91. on August 18, 2013.

20. Caldwell J, Kirby J. *Statistical Brief #383: Preventive Health Care Utilization by Adult Residents of MSAs and non-MSAs: Differences by Race/Ethnicity*. Agency for Healthcare Research and Quality, Medical Expenditure Panel Survey; August 2012. Retrieved from http://meps.ahrq.gov/mepsweb/data_files/publications/st383/stat383.shtml. on August 18, 2013.

21. Association of State and Territorial Dental Directors (ASTDD). *Guidance on Selecting a Sample for a School-Based Oral Health Survey*; 2013. Retrieved from http://www.astdd.org/docs/BSS_GUIDANCE_ON_SELECTING_A_SAMPLE_FOR_A_SCHOOL-BASED_ORAL_HEALTH_SURVEY_Jan_2013.pdf. on August 18, 2013.

22. Association of State & Territorial Dental Directors (ADTDD). *ADTDD Basic Screening Surveys*; 2013. Retrieved from http://www.astdd.org/basic-screening-survey-tool/. on August 19, 2013.

23. Association of State & Territorial Dental Directors (ADTDD). *The Basic screening Survey: A Tool for Oral Health Surveillance not Research*; February 2011. Retrieved from http://www.astdd.org/docs/BSS_What_is_Oral_Health_Surveillance_4.26.2011.pdf. on August 19, 2013

24. U.S. Department of Health and Human Services. *About Healthy People*; revised December 2012. Retrieved from http://www.healthypeople.gov/2020/about/. on August 19, 2013.

25. U.S. Department of Health and Human Services. *2020 Topics & Objectives — Objectives A-Z*; revised March 2013. Retrieved from http://www.healthypeople.gov/2020/topicsobjectives2020/default.aspx. on August 19, 2013.

26. U.S. Department of Health and Human Services. *Objective Development and Selection Process*; revised April 2011. Retrieved from http://healthypeople.gov/2020/about/objectiveDevelopment.aspx. on August 19, 2013.

27. U.S. Department of Health and Human Services. *2020 Topics & Objectives—Oral Health*. Healthy People. Gov; revised April 2013. Retrieved from http://healthypeople.gov/2020/topicsobjectives2020/overview.aspx?topicid=32. on August 19, 2013.

28. National Center for Health Statistics (NCHS). *Healthy People 2010 Final Review: Overview and Selected Findings*. PHS Publication No. 2012-1038. Hyattsville, MD: NCHS; 2012. Retrieved from http://www.cdc.gov/nchs/data/hpdata2010/hp2010_final_review.pdf. on August 20, 2013.

29. National Institute of Dental and Craniofacial Research. *Oral Health in America: A Report of the Surgeon General*; 2013. Retrieved from http://www.nidcr.nih.gov/DataStatistics/SurgeonGeneral/sgr/. on August 20, 2013.

30. U.S. Department of Health and Human Services. *Oral Health in America: A Report of the Surgeon General*. Rockville, MD: U.S. Department of Health and Human Services, National Institute of Dental and Craniofacial Research, National Institutes of Health; 2000. Retrieved from http://silk.nih.gov/public/hck1ocv.@www.surgeon.fullrpt.pdf. on August 25, 2013.

31. U.S. Department of Health and Human Services. *National Call to Action to Promote Oral Health*. Rockville, MD: U.S. Department of Health and Human Services, Public Health Service, National Institutes of Health, National Institute of Dental and Craniofacial Research. NIH Publication No. 03-5303; Spring 2003. Retrieved from http://www.surgeongeneral.gov/library/calls/oralhealth/nationalcalltoaction.html. on August 25, 2013.

32. World Health Organization. *Global Oral Health Database*; Oral Health; 2013. Retrieved from http://www.who.int/oral_health/databases/global/en/index.html. on August 25, 2013.

33. World Health Organization. *Strategies for Oral Disease Prevention and Health Promotion*. Oral Health; 2013. Retrieved from http://www.who.int/oral_health/strategies/en/. on August 25, 2013.

34. National Academy of Sciences, Institute of Medicine. *Advancing Oral Health in America*; 2011. Retrieved from http://www.iom.edu/~/media/Files/Report%20Files/2011/AdvancingOral-Health-in-America/Advancing%20Oral%20Health%202011%20Report%20Brief.pdf. on August 25, 2013.

35. Thompson NJ, Boyer EM. Validity of oral health screening in field conditions: Pilot study. *J Dent Hyg*. 2006;80(2):1–10. Retrieved from www.ingenta.com. on August 25, 2013.

36. Chattopadhyay A. Associations and causation. In: Chattopadhyay A. ed. *Oral Health Epidemiology: Principles and Practice*. Burlington, MA: Jones and Bartlett; 2011:49–61.

37. Burt BA, Eklund SA. Research designs in oral epidemiology. In: Burt BA, Eklund SA. *Dentistry, Dental Practice, and the Community*. 6th ed. St. Louis, MO: Elsevier; 2005:173–182.

38. Friis RH, Sellers TA. Data interpretation issues. In: Friis RH, Sellers TA. *Epidemiology for Public Health Practice*. 5th ed. Sudbury,MA: Jones & Bartlett; 2013:435–458.

39. Centers for Disease Control and Prevention. *National Oral Health Surveillance System Oral Health Indicators*. Revised August 2010. Retrieved from http://www.cdc.gov/nohss/. on August 26, 2013.

40. Leon AC, Davis LL, Kraemer HC. The role and interpretation of pilot studies in clinical research. *J Psychiatr Res.* 2011;45(5):626–629. Retrieved from http://www.ncbi.nlm.nih .gov/pmc/articles/PMC3081994/. on September 7, 2013.

Current Oral Epidemiological Findings

OBJECTIVES

After studying this chapter, the dental hygiene student should be able to:

- Describe the current epidemiological issues of disease and conditions
- Describe the current risk factors of diseases
- Describe prevention by dental care utilization

COMPETENCIES

After studying this chapter and participating in accompanying course activities, the dental hygiene student should be competent to do the following:

- Use critical thinking skills and comprehensive problem-solving to identify oral health care strategies that promote patient health and wellness
- Use evidence-based decision making to evaluate emerging technology and treatment modalities to integrate into patient dental hygiene care plans to achieve high-quality, cost-effective care
- Integrate accepted scientific theories and research into educational, preventive, and therapeutic oral health services
- Evaluate factors that can be used to promote patient adherence to disease prevention or health maintenance strategies
- Utilize methods that ensure the health and safety of the patient and the oral health professional in the delivery of care

KEY TERMS

Incidence *264*
Morbidity *274*
Mortality *274*
Prevalence *264*

As discussed in Chapter 18, the study of disease in human populations is called *epidemiology,* but it includes more than this. The science and tools of epidemiology are used to identify health, disease, and use of dental services. Oral diseases, risks, and preventive strategies are affected by many variables including societal forces and demographics. Therefore, the epidemiology of oral diseases constantly changes, and it is important for the dental hygienist to stay informed about current epidemiological findings of diseases and conditions and the rates of dental care utilization.

The Epidemiology of Oral Diseases and Conditions

The range of oral, dental, and craniofacial ideas and conditions that affect the populations is extensive. Just as there is no single measure of overall health or overall disease, there is no single measure of oral health or the burden of oral diseases and conditions.[1] See Boxes 19-1 and 19-2 ■ for findings from the landmark US Surgeon General's report on oral health and subsequent principles published for oral health initiatives.

The following sections present epidemiological data for the specific oral disease or condition named. When

> ## Box 19–1 Findings from the US Surgeon General's Report on Oral Diseases and Conditions
>
> - Microbial infections, including those caused by bacteria, viruses, and fungi, are the primary cause of the most prevalent oral diseases. Examples include dental caries, periodontal diseases, herpes labialis, and candidiasis.
> - The etiology and pathogenesis of diseases and disorders affecting the craniofacial structures are multifactorial and complex, involving interplay among genetic, environmental, and behavioral factors.
> - Many inherited and congenital conditions affect the craniofacial complex, often resulting in disfigurement and impairments that may involve many body organs and systems and affect millions of children worldwide.
> - Tobacco use, excessive alcohol use, and inappropriate dietary practices contribute to many diseases and disorders. In particular, tobacco use is a risk factor for oral cavity and pharyngeal cancers, periodontal diseases, candidiasis, and dental caries, among other diseases.
> - Some chronic diseases, such as Sjögren's syndrome, present with primary oral symptoms.
> - Oral-facial pain conditions are common and often have complex etiologies.

Source: US Department of Health and Human Services. *Oral health in America: A Report of the Surgeon General.* Rockville, MD: Department of Health and Human Services, National Institute of Dental and Craniofacial Research, National Institutes of Health; 2000.

> ## Box 19–2 Organizing Principles for a New Oral Health Initiative
>
> - Establish high-level accountability.
> - Emphasize disease prevention and oral health promotion.
> - Improve oral health literacy and cultural competence.
> - Reduce oral health disparities.
> - Explore new models for payment and delivery of care.
> - Enhance the role of non-dental health care professionals.
> - Expand oral health research and improve data collection.
> - Promote collaboration among private and public stakeholders.
> - Measure progress toward short-term and long-term goals and objectives.
> - Advance the goals and objectives of *Healthy People 2020.*

Source: National Research Council. *Advancing Oral Health in America.* Washington, DC: The National Academies Press; 2011. Retrieved from http://www.iom.edu/Reports/2011/Advancing-Oral-Health-in-America/Report-Brief.aspx?page=2 on October 26, 2015.

assessing data, it is important to understand the prevalence and incidence of diseases or conditions. For each oral disease or condition, risk factors are presented and specific preventive aspects are discussed.

Prevalence is the number of all existing cases of a disease in a population measured at a given point whereas **incidence** is the number of new cases of a disease in a population over a given period of time. Prevalence can be described as the proportion of disease status in a population, and incidence is the rate of occurrence of the disease within the population. So, prevalence defines how widespread the disease is in the population, and incidence provides the risk of contracting the disease.

Periodontal Diseases

Periodontal diseases can be defined as inflammatory diseases affecting the periodontium, which encompasses the tissues that surround and support the teeth. Periodontal diseases involve progressive loss of the gingival tissues and alveolar bone around the teeth and, if left untreated, can lead to tooth mobility and subsequent loss of teeth. A convergence of bacteria and an overly aggressive immune response against these bacteria cause periodontal diseases. Although bacterial infections cause periodontal diseases, a variety of factors affects its severity.

EPIDEMIOLOGY   As most dental hygienists could anecdotally predict, many individuals experience gingivitis. (See Figure 19-1 ■.) The third National Health and Nutrition Examination Survey (NHANES III) found that 50 percent of adults have gingivitis on at least three or four teeth.[2] Refer to Table 19-1 ■ for additional information

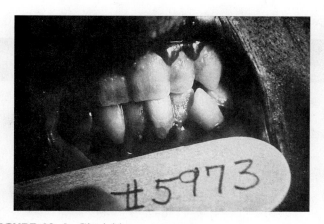

FIGURE 19–1 Gingivitis
Source: Centers for Disease Control.

about the prevalence of periodontal diseases for adults. The facts have been well documented that only 5 to 15 percent of any population suffers from severe generalized periodontitis and that older adults, African-American and Hispanic adults, current smokers, and those with lower incomes and less education are more likely to have periodontal disease.[2,3,4]

RISK FACTORS   The host response is important in severe periodontal disease. Risk factors for periodontal diseases are numerous (see Box 19-3 ■). Although the majority of the population does not have severe periodontal disease, most have a mild to moderate form. Risk factors can be summarized including smoking, genetic predisposition, (probably) psychological stress, diabetes, and several uncommon systemic diseases.[5]

Table 19–1 Prevalence of Periodontal Disease: Adults 20–64 Years of Age, 1999–2004

Characteristic	Periodontal Disease (percent)[a]	Moderate or Severe Periodontal Disease (percent)[b]
Age in Years		
20–34	3.84	NA
35–49	10.41	5.00
50–64	11.88	10.73
Gender		
Male	10.65	6.74
Female	6.40	3.46
Race and Ethnicity		
White, non-Hispanic	5.82	4.15
Black, non-Hispanic	16.81	8.30
Mexican American	13.76	6.43
Poverty Status (*income compared to federal poverty level*)		
Less than 100 percent	13.95	9.92
100 percent–199 percent	15.34	9.42
More than 200 percent	5.96	3.50
Education		
Less than high school	17.33	11.64
High school	9.34	5.65

(continued)

Table 19–1 Prevalence of Periodontal Disease: Adults 20–64 Years of Age, 1999–2004 (continued)

Characteristic	Periodontal Disease (percent)[a]	Moderate or Severe Periodontal Disease (percent)[b]
More than high school	5.78	3.11
Smoking History		
Current smoker	14.74	11.14
Former smoker	7.61	4.62
Never smoked	5.94	2.34
Overall	8.52	5.08

[a]Periodontal disease is defined as having at least one periodontal site with 3 millimeters or more of attachment loss and 4 millimeters or more of pocket depth.

[b]According to CDC-American Academy of Periodontology definitions: Moderate periodontal disease is defined as having at least two teeth with interproximal attachment loss of 4 millimeters or more *or* at least two teeth with 5 millimeters or more of pocket depth at interproximal sites. Severe periodontal disease is defined as having at least two teeth with interproximal attachment loss of 6 millimeters or more *and* at least one tooth with 5 millimeters or more of pocket depth at interproximal sites.

Source: The National Health and Nutrition Examination Survey (NHANES). Tables 1–4. http://www.nidcr.nih.gov/DataStatistics/FindDataByTopic/GumDisease/PeriodontaldiseaseAdults20to64.htm

DENTAL HYGIENIST SPOTLIGHT

Public Health Column: Lt. Comm. Angela Girgenti, RDH, BS

Lieutenant Commander Angela Girgenti of the US Public Health Service (USPHS) currently is a senior public health analyst with the Health Resources and Services Administration (HRSA), Office of Performance Review, Regional Division, Dallas, Texas. She is a graduate of the Texas Woman's University Dental Hygiene Program in Denton and is currently enrolled in the master's of public health program at the University of North Texas Health Science Center in Fort Worth. Lt. Comm. Girgenti, the recipient of two PHS commendation medals, has worked in a variety of public health settings and has spoken about and presented programs on numerous topics.

I asked for her comments on several professionally related topics.

Why did you decide to go into dental hygiene?

I started in dentistry as a volunteer for the Red Cross in Fort Ritchie, Maryland. I received free training as a dental assistant from the Red Cross and the Fort Ritchie Army dental clinic in exchange for 200 hours of volunteer work at the dental clinic. This was my first exposure to the field of dentistry, which heightened my interest in working in health care. After I completed the volunteer hours, I was hired as a dental assistant in a private practice where I continued to learn more about dentistry and dental hygiene. I

loved working with patients and knew a career in dental hygiene would suit me well. After returning to Texas, I enrolled at Texas Woman's University and was accepted into the school of dental hygiene.

How did you get into dental public health? Did you need additional education?

The opportunity to work in a public health setting began with an internship with the USPHS I completed between my junior and senior years of hygiene school. The internship allowed me to work at a federal prison, providing care to federal inmates under the supervision of the chief dental officer. This introduced me to the possibility of a full-time career in the uniformed services and public health. I learned about the various ways dental hygienists could work with underserved populations in the Federal Bureau of Prisons and in other federal agencies, such as the Indian Health Service. After graduation, I was offered a full-time position at the federal prison and received my commission as an officer in the USPHS.

What are your current positions?

Currently, I am a public health analyst for Health Resources and Services Administration in Dallas. HRSA, part of the US Department of Health and Human

Services, is the primary federal agency for improving access to health care services for people who are uninsured, isolated, or medically vulnerable. Information about HRSA and its programs can be found at www.hrsa.gov. I continue to serve HRSA as an officer in the USPHS. My role is to provide guidance to federal grantees and assist them in improving performance and increasing health care access to the underserved and uninsured. I also continue to provide dental hygiene services at the federal prison on a regular basis to stay clinically active and fulfill my desire to provide patient care.

Can you discuss any particularly interesting experiences you have had in your dental public health positions?

My career in the USPHS has been both extremely exciting and rewarding. I am grateful for the experience I gained as a new hygienist at the Bureau of Prisons. I learned to work with culturally diverse populations and underserved populations. Many of my patients never had the opportunity to have dental care; I was their first dental provider. This experience allowed me to grow as a clinician and health educator.

After Katrina, the USPHS deployed hundreds of officers to the Gulf Coast to assist in stabilizing the region. I was sent to Baton Rouge temporarily and served in an administrative role on the Emergency Response Team of the Secretary of Health and Human Services. This was my first deployment as a commissioned officer, and I learned a great deal about the operations of federal, state, and local governments in times of disaster. I felt fortunate to serve the Gulf Coast residents in this capacity and was impressed by the dedication of my fellow officers.

One of the most unique experiences of my career was in 2007 when I was deployed on the Navy hospital ship the *USNS Comfort*. Four teams of USPHS officers were invited to participate in the US Training and Humanitarian Assistance Mission to Latin and South America. I spent an entire month onboard the ship and provided direct care to residents of Nicaragua, El Salvador, and Peru. I was amazed by the overwhelming crowds that gathered to receive care. I was also touched by the kindness and hospitality we were shown in each country. Most of all, I was proud of those I served alongside on the *USNS Comfort* and how well they represented our country.

What type of advice would you give to a practicing hygienist who is thinking of doing something different?

Continuing my education has proven to be a success. Looking back, most of my opportunities came from internships, other school activities, and volunteering. I am currently finishing my master's degree in public health, which was essential in obtaining my current position at HRSA. Also, having a variety of mentors is extremely helpful. Along the way, I have had wonderful mentors who helped me succeed and encouraged me to continually grow. For those who are looking for a change, don't be afraid to embrace new opportunities and have confidence in your abilities. Hygienists are excellent teachers, problem solvers, and promoters of change. Our skills are not strictly clinical. Last, volunteering is an excellent way to network and meet other professionals. The need for dental care in this country is overwhelming, and volunteering in alternative settings can help increase access to care for those who need it most and positively impact your career.

Source: Christine Nathe writes the Public Health Column in *RDH* magazine published by Pennwell Publishing. For more public health spotlights please see RDH magazine online at http://www.rdhmag.com/index.html.

Box 19–3 Risk Factors for Periodontal Diseases

- **Age:** Risk increases with age
- **Gender:** Diseases are more prevalent in males than females
- **Socioeconomic Status:** Lower socioeconomic status increases risk
- **Genetics:** Research continues
- **Plaque:** Plaque and gingivitis increase risk
- **Tobacco:** Smokers have an increased risk
- **Systemic Conditions:** Diabetes and other systemic stressors increase risk

Increase in probing depth over a period of years is the strongest predictor of future periodontal disease activity.

Did You Know?

Dental hygienists focus attention on periodontal diseases for good reason. Most individuals experience some stage of periodontal infection during their lifetime.

Tooth Loss

By maintaining a healthy dentition and receiving regular dental hygiene care, most people have the ability to keep their teeth throughout their lives. The prevalence of both partial and total tooth loss in adults has decreased from the early 1970s through the latest (1999–2004) National Health and Nutrition Examination Survey. In spite of this improvement, significant disparities remain in some population groups.[6]

EPIDEMIOLOGY See Table 19-2 and Figure 19-2 ■ for information about tooth loss for adults age 20 to 64 years and other selected population groups. The same populations that suffer from severe generalized periodontitis have fewer remaining teeth than other populations.

RISK FACTORS Risk factors for tooth loss include dental caries. In addition, tooth loss can be caused by periodontal diseases associated with the risk indicators of age, male gender, smoking, lack of professional maintenance, inadequate oral hygiene, diabetes mellitus, hypertension, rheumatoid arthritis, and anterior tooth type. Trauma can

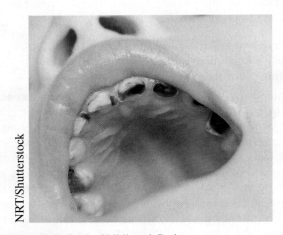

FIGURE 19–2 Early Childhood Caries

also lead to tooth loss. Maintaining a healthy dentition and wearing athletic mouth guards during sporting events are the best ways to avoid tooth loss.

Dental Caries

Dental caries, commonly referred to as *tooth decay,* is one of the most common of all diseases, second only to the common cold. It usually occurs in children and young adults, but any person can experience it. It is a common cause of tooth loss in young people. Bacterial plaque converts all foods, especially sugar and starches, into acids that subsequently dissolve the enamel surface of the tooth, called *demineralization.* If left untreated, demineralization progresses to form a "cavity." Most recent efforts have focused on the remineralization of demineralized tooth surface, as opposed to restoring the subsequent cavity.

Did You Know?

Many individuals believe that if one of their parents lost all of their teeth, they are destined for the same fate, but as noted, only a very small percentage of the US population experiences total tooth loss.

EPIDEMIOLOGY Dental caries remains the most prevalent chronic disease in both children and adults even though it is largely preventable. Although caries has significantly

Table 19–2 Tooth Loss for Adults Ages 20 to 64 Years, by State

State	Yes %	No %	State	Yes %	No %
Alabama	54.7	45.3	Idaho	38.1	61.9
Alaska	45.1	54.9	Illinois	45.5	54.5
American Samoa	–	–	Indiana	45.1	54.9
Arizona	33.8	66.2	Iowa	42.3	57.7
Arkansas	50.4	49.6	Kansas	42.7	57.3
California	33.6	66.4	Kentucky	52.1	47.9
Colorado	35.4	64.6	Louisiana	44.7	55.3
Connecticut	38.3	61.7	Maine	46.9	53.1
Delaware	42.4	57.6	Maryland	40.9	59.1
DC	45.3	54.7	Massachusetts	43.9	56.1
Florida	41.5	58.5	Michigan	39.2	60.8
Georgia	49.2	50.8	Minnesota	36.6	63.4
Guam	N/A	N/A	Mississippi	58.2	41.8
Hawaii	30.7	69.3	Missouri	53.5	46.5

(continued)

State	Yes %	No %	State	Yes %	No %
Montana	41.3	58.7	Puerto Rico	57.1	42.9
Nebraska	38.6	61.4	Rhode Island	43.7	56.3
Nevada	42.1	57.9	South Carolina	52.0	48.0
New Hampshire	43.4	56.6	South Dakota	44.0	56.0
New Jersey	43.4	56.6	Tennessee	53.3	46.7
New Mexico	41.2	58.8	Texas	39.4	60.6
New York	44.1	55.9	Utah	31.2	68.8
North Carolina	49.8	50.2	Vermont	43.8	56.2
North Dakota	45.3	54.7	Virgin Islands	50.9	49.1
Ohio	46.4	53.6	Virginia	40.2	59.8
Oklahoma	54.0	46.0	Washington	35.6	64.4
Oregon	37.2	62.8	West Virginia	65.6	34.4
Palau	–	–	Wisconsin	40.0	60.0
Pennsylvania	48.9	51.1	Wyoming	40.7	59.3

Source: National Oral Health Surveillance System. Retrieved From http://apps.nccd.cdc.gov/nohss/Listv.asp?qkey=7&Dataset=2 on February 17, 2014.

decreased for most Americans over the past decades, disparities remain among some population groups. In addition, this downward trend has recently reversed for young children, who can be afflicted with early childhood caries. All populations can suffer from occlusal and interproximal carious lesions. (See Table 19-3 ■ for untreated dental decay and urgent need for dental care in children and Figure 19-2 ■ for early childhood caries.)

Did You Know?

Early childhood caries, also known as *baby bottle caries* and *nursing bottle decay*, is a syndrome characterized by severe decay in the teeth of infants or young children. Frequent and prolonged drinking from a bottle (especially at bedtime) increases the risk of this disease, which first affects the maxillary primary anterior teeth.

Table 19–3 **Percentage of Third Grade Students with Untreated Tooth Decay**

Sort list by: State Percent with Untreated Tooth Decay

State	School Year	Percent with Untreated Tooth Decay		Response Rate[1] (%)	Percent eligible for the National School Lunch Program[2]		
					Sample		
					Schools[3]	Students[4]	State
Alabama	2005–2007	% CI N	**27.6** (25.5–29.7) 9301	73	51	NR	56
Alaska	2007–2008	% CI N	**26.2**[5] (23.2–29.3) 826	48	42	NR	46
Arizona	2009–2010	% CI N	**40.4** (36.8–44.1) 3150	37	51	NR	48

(*continued*)

Table 19–3 Percentage of Third Grade Students with Untreated Tooth Decay (continued)

State	School Year		Percent with Untreated Tooth Decay	Response Rate[1] (%)	Percent eligible for the National School Lunch Program[2]		
					Sample		
					Schools[3]	Students[4]	State
Arkansas	2009–2010	%	29.0[5]	53	55	NR	65
		CI	(27.1–30.0)				
		N	4239				
California	2004–2005	%	28.7	52	64	NR	57
		CI	(27.0–30.4)				
		N	10444				
Colorado	2006–2007	%	24.5	79	40	NR	41
		CI	(23.0–26.1)				
		N	3012				
Connecticut	2006–2007	%	17.8	81	37	NR	35
		CI	(14.8–20.8)				
		N	8755				
Delaware	2001–2002	%	29.9	43	37	41	40
		CI	(25.3–34.4)				
		N	1032				
Georgia	2010–2011	%	18.7	52	62	60	61
		CI	(16.2–21.5)				
		N	3359				
Idaho	2008–2009	%	22.5	87	37	NR	45
		CI	(20.3–24.6)				
		N	4634				
Illinois	2008–2009	%	29.1	52	57	NR	NR
		CI	(25.4–32.7)				
		N	3696				
Iowa	2008–2009	%	21.9[5]	65	38	NR	34
		CI	(19.2–24.6)				
		N	1206				
Kansas	2003–2004	%	27.6[5]	32	NR	NR	NR
		CI	(24.9–30.4)				
		N	3375				
Kentucky	2000–2001	%	34.6	64	52	NR	NR
		CI	(31.9–37.4)				
		N	3244				
Louisiana	2007–2009	%	41.9	42	61	NR	65
		CI	(37.8–45.9)				
		N	2642				
Maine	1998–1999	%	20.4[5]	51	NR	31	32
		CI	(18.3–22.6)				
		N	1297				
Maryland	2000–2001	%	25.9	50	NR	28	36
		CI	(21.6–30.2)				
		N	2482				

(continued)

State	School Year	Percent with Untreated Tooth Decay		Response Rate[1] (%)	Percent eligible for the National School Lunch Program[2]		
					Sample		
					Schools[3]	Students[4]	State
Massachusetts	2006–2007	%	**17.3**[5]	46	NR	28	32
		CI	(14.0–20.7)				
		N	2211				
Michigan	2009–2010	%	**27.1**	33	41	48	43
		CI	(23.4–30.9)				
		N	2056				
Minnesota	2009–2010	%	**18.1**[5]	58	38	NR	42
		CI	(14.9–21.4)				
		N	1766				
Mississippi	2009–2010	%	**30.6**	55	74	73	72
		CI	(28.5–32.7)				
		N	1928				
Missouri	2004–2005	%	**27.0**	49	45	NR	46
		CI	(26.0–28.0)				
		N	3535				
Montana	2005–2006	%	**28.9**[5]	90	41	NR	35
		CI	(26.1–31.9)				
		N	957				
Nebraska	2004–2005	%	**17.0**	92	34	NR	34
		CI	(13.6–20.4)				
		N	2057				
Nevada	2008–2009	%	**28.1**	41	41	NR	40
		CI	(24.3–31.8)				
		N	1786				
New Hampshire	2008–2009	%	**12.0**	64	24	NR	22
		CI	(9.6–14.3)				
		N	3015				
New Mexico	1999–2000	%	**37.0**[5]	47	NR	NR	NR
		CI	(32.3–41.6)				
		N	2136				
New York	2001–2003	%	**33.1**	38	NR	48	51
		CI	(29.6–36.6)				
		N	10895				
North Dakota	2009–2010	%	**20.7**	90	36	NR	36
		CI	(18.6–22.7)				
		N	1499				
Ohio	2009–2010	%	**18.6**	50	41	44	45
		CI	(17.1–20.3)				
		N	16839				
Oklahoma	2009–2010	%	**22.6**[5]	42	61	NR	61
		CI	(19.3–25.8)				
		N	751				
Oregon	2006–2007	%	**35.4**	76	47	NR	47
		CI	(31.4–39.4)				
		N	1259				

(*continued*)

Table 19–3 Percentage of Third Grade Students with Untreated Tooth Decay (continued)

| State | School Year | Percent with Untreated Tooth Decay | | Response Rate[1] (%) | Percent eligible for the National School Lunch Program[2] | | |
| | | | | | Sample | | |
					Schools[3]	Students[4]	State
Pennsylvania	1998–1999	%	**27.3**	NR	NR	NR	NR
		CI	(23.9–30.6)				
		N	1767				
Rhode Island	2007–2008	%	**28.2**[5]	66	46	NR	42
		CI	(22.5–33.9)				
		N	1303				
South Carolina	2007–2008	%	**22.6**[5]	38	56	56	51
		CI	(21.0–24.3)				
		N	2657				
South Dakota	2009–2010	%	**29.1**	54	45	42	32
		CI	(25.0–33.2)				
		N	570				
Texas	2007–2008	%	**42.7**	51	NR	NR	NR
		CI	(38.6–46.7)				
		N	3864				
Utah	2000–2001	%	**23.0**[5]	51	NR	NR	NR
		CI	(21.0–25.0)				
		N	800				
Vermont	2002–2003	%	**16.2**	68	31	NR	31
		CI	(12.9–19.5)				
		N	409				
Virginia	2008–2009	%	**15.4**[5]	52	38	29	34
		CI	(15.2–15.7)				
		N	7838				
Washington	2009–2010	%	**14.9**	80	46	51	45
		CI	(13.6–16.3)				
		N	2875				
West Virginia	2010–2011	%	**17.1**[5]	35	51	NR	55
		CI	(13.6–20.6)				
		N	449				
Wisconsin	2007–2008	%	**20.1**	89	36	NR	37
		CI	(18.9–21.3)				
		N	4413				

% Percentage

CI 95% Confidence Interval

N Number of students in sample

NR Not Reported

[1]Survey response rates differ among states. Differential nonresponse can bias the estimates. Response rates, the percent of selected children who actually participated, are presented to help the reader judge the potential for bias.

[2]Untreated tooth decay may be associated with income. Eligibility for the National School Lunch Program is presented to help the reader assess whether the survey sample is representative of all 3rd graders in the state.

[3]The percent eligible for the National School Lunch Program among students attending schools that participated in the survey.

[4]The percent eligible for the National School Lunch Program among students who participated in the survey.

[5]The percent with untreated tooth decay reported by this state has not been adjusted for nonresponse.

Source: http://apps.nccd.cdc.gov/nohss/IndicatorV.asp?Indicator=3

Adults experience dental decay, and because many of them have exposed root surface(s), they experience root caries. Approximately 85 percent of adults in the United States has at least one tooth with decay (untreated or treated.) (See Table 19-4 ■.) Root caries affects approximately 50 percent of adults seventy-five years and older.

Table 19–4 Percent of Adults with Caries in Permanent Teeth

Prevalence of caries in permanent teeth (DMFT) among adults 20 to 64 years of age, by selected characteristics: United States, National Health and Nutrition Examination Survey, 1999–2004

Characteristic	Percent with Caries, Missing, or Filled Permanent Teeth
Age	
20 to 34 years	85.58
35 to 49 years	94.30
50 to 64 years	95.62
Sex	
Male	90.57
Female	92.66
Race and Ethnicity	
White, non-Hispanic	93.49
Black, non-Hispanic	87.51
Mexican American	82.97
Poverty Status *(Income compared to Federal Poverty Level)*	
Less than 100%	88.69
100% to 199%	88.91
Greater than 200%	93.05
Education	
Less than High School	85.93
High School	92.38
More than High School	92.91
Smoking History	
Current Smoker	91.48
Former Smoker	92.83
Never Smoked	91.19
Overall	91.63

Data Source: The National Health and Nutrition Examination Survey (NHANES) has been an important source of information on oral health and dental care in the United States since the early 1970s. Tables 1 through 4 present the latest NHANES (collected between 1999 and 2004) data regarding dental caries in adults.

Source: https://www.nidcr.nih.gov/DataStatistics/FindDataByTopic/DentalCaries/DentalCariesAdults20to64.htm

RISK FACTORS   Risk factors for dental caries include susceptibility of teeth and age. The use of dental sealants and fluoride decreases the risk for dental caries. Specifically, dental sealants create a barrier to protect fissures and pits from demineralization. Fluoride protects teeth from demineralization and actually can aid in the remineralization of demineralized tooth surfaces. See specific risk factors in Box 19-4 ■.

Oral and Pharyngeal Cancer

Oral and pharyngeal cancers occur in the oral cavity, lips, and/or pharyngeal tissues. An individual can have oral cancer, but certain risk factors seem to increase the likelihood of developing it. As with any cancer, treatments for oral and pharyngeal cancers are most effective when the cancer is diagnosed at an early stage.

EPIDEMIOLOGY   More than 45,750 Americans will be diagnosed with oral or pharyngeal cancer this year,[7] and it will cause more than 8,650 deaths, killing roughly one person per hour, twenty-four hours per day.[7] Of those 45,750 newly diagnosed individuals, only slightly more than half will be alive in five years, a percentage that has not significantly improved in decades.[7] **Mortality,** defined as the ratio of the number of deaths from a given disease or health problem to the total number of cases reported, from oral cancer is nearly twice as high in some minorities (especially African-American males) as it is in Caucasians. Methods used to treat oral cancers, such as surgery, radiation, and chemotherapy, cause **morbidity,** which is defined as the ratio of "sick" (affected) individuals to well individuals in a community, and are disfiguring and costly.[8] See Figures 19-3 ■ and 19-4 ■ for oral cancer information.

Box 19–4 Risk Factors for Dental Caries

Teeth Most Susceptible
- Molars (high incidence)
- Mandibular molars (attacked first)
- Higher incidence in pits and fissures

Socioeconomic Status
- Most powerful determinant

Age—Early Childhood Caries
- Low socioeconomic status
- Diet

Gender
- Incidence of decayed, missing, filled teeth (DMF index) higher for females than for males

Race/Ethnicity
- Heritage (Mexican-Americans, Native Americans, immigrants to the United States)

Environment
- Low socioeconomic status
- Family lifestyles and behaviors

Genetics
- Intrafamilial transmission of *S. mutans* (ie, mother's transmission of pathogen to baby)

Diet
- Frequency and total intake of sugar
- Type of sugar

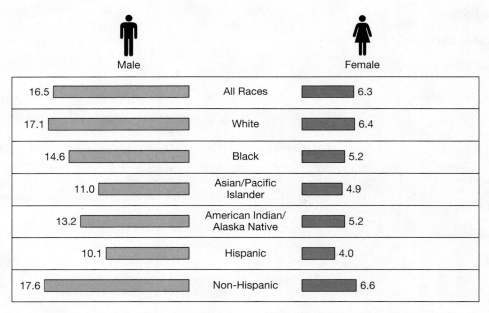

FIGURE 19–3 Oral Cavity and Pharynx Cancer: Number of New Cases per 100,000 Persons by Race/Ethnicity

Source: http://seer.cancer.gov/statfacts/html/oralcav.html

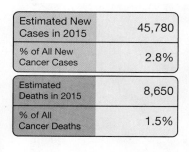

Estimated New Cases in 2015	45,780
% of All New Cancer Cases	2.8%
Estimated Deaths in 2015	8,650
% of All Cancer Deaths	1.5%

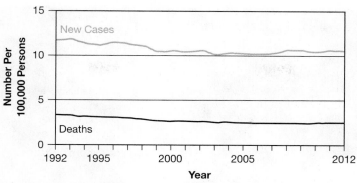

Percent Surviving 5 Years

63.2%

2005–2011

FIGURE 19–4 Oral Cavity and Pharynx Cancer

Source: http://seer.cancer.gov/statfacts/html/oralcav.html

Most oral cancers start in squamous cells and form in any of three main areas: lips, oral cavity and the oropharynx. (See Figure 19-5 ■.) Oral cancer is more common in men than in women, but the number of women in the United States diagnosed with tongue cancer has increased significantly over the past twenty years. In Western countries, including the United States, the most common areas for oral cancer are the tongue and the floor of the mouth. In parts of the world where chewing tobacco or betel nuts is common, oral cancer often forms in the retromolar area and buccal mucosa.[9] The human papillomavirus has also been linked to oral cancer.[10,11] Refer to Box 19-5 ■ for signs and symptoms of oral cancer.

RISK FACTORS Approximately 75 percent of oral cavity and pharyngeal cancers are attributed to the use of

Box 19–5 Signs and Symptoms of Oral Cancer

- Mouth sore that fails to heal or that bleeds easily
- White or red patch in the mouth that will not go away
- Lump, thickening, or soreness in the mouth, throat, or tongue
- Difficulty chewing or swallowing food.

smoked and smokeless tobacco. These cancers affect the mouth, tongue, lips, throat, parts of the nose, and larynx. Those who chew tobacco are at high risk for gingival and buccal mucosa lesions that can lead to cancer. Alcohol consumption is another risk factor. Combinations of tobacco and alcohol are believed to be substantially higher risk factors than consumption of either substance alone. Other risk factors for these cancers are viral infections, immunodeficiencies, poor nutrition, exposure to ultraviolet light (a major cause of lip cancer), and certain occupational hazards, such as exposure to specific chemicals.[8]

Not engaging in the high-risk behaviors listed earlier is critical in preventing oral cancers. Early detection is key to increasing the survival rate for these cancers.

Mucosal Infections and Diseases

Large-scale population-based screening studies have identified the most common oral lesions as candidiasis, recurrent herpes labialis, recurrent aphthous stomatitis, mucocele, fibroma, mandibular and palatal tori, pyogenic granuloma, erythema migrans, hairy tongue, lichen planus, and leukoplakia.[12,13,14]

EPIDEMIOLOGY Primary oral infection with the herpes simplex virus (HSV) typically occurs at a young age, is asymptomatic, and is not associated with significant morbidity.[12] After primary oral infection, HSV may persist in a latent state in the trigeminal ganglion and later reactivate as the more common herpes labialis, commonly referred to as cold sores.

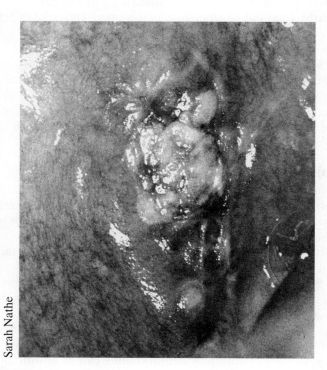

Sarah Nathe

FIGURE 19–5 Oral Cancer

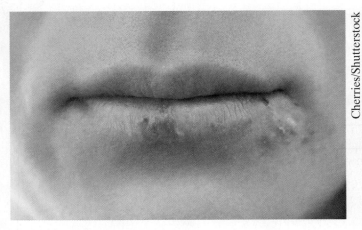

FIGURE 19–6 Herpetic Lesion

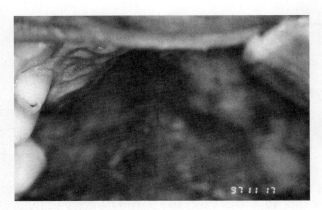

FIGURE 19–7 Oral Candidiasis

RISK FACTORS Common triggers for reactivation include ultraviolet light, trauma, fatigue, stress, and menstruation. These lesions affect approximately 15 to 45 percent of the US population.[12,15] Infection with the oral herpes simplex virus has been related to socioeconomic factors; 75 to 90 percent of individuals from lower socioeconomic populations develop antibodies by the end of the first decade of life.[16] (See Figure 19-6 ■.)

EPIDEMIOLOGY Recurrent aphthous stomatitis, commonly referred to as canker sores, is an oral ulcerative condition that is usually painful. Recurrent aphthous stomatitis has a prevalence ranging from 5 to 21 percent.[17] Recurrent aphthous stomatitis is characterized by recurring, painful, solitary, or multiple ulcers, typically covered by a white-to-yellow pseudomembrane and surrounded by an erythematous halo.[12]

RISK FACTORS Although various host and environmental factors have been implicated, the precise pathogenesis remains unknown. Smoking is associated with a lower prevalence, but other associations, such as nutritional deficiencies (eg, vitamin B_{12}, folate, iron), remain unclear.[17]

EPIDEMIOLOGY Candidiasis, sometimes referred to as thrush, is a fungal infection of any of the *Candida* species, of which *Candida albicans* is the most common. As many as 60 percent of healthy adults carry *Candida* species as a component of their normal oral flora.[12] (See Figure 19-7 ■.)

RISK FACTORS However, certain local and systemic factors may favor overgrowth: use of dentures or a steroid inhaler, xerostomia, endocrine disorders, human immunodeficiency virus (HIV) infection, leukemia, malnutrition, and reduced immunity based on age, radiation therapy, systemic chemotherapy, and use of broad-spectrum antibiotics or corticosteroids.[18,19,20,21,22]

Cleft Lip/Palate

Cleft lip and cleft palate are variations of a congenital deformity caused by abnormal facial development during gestation. Cleft lip is formed in the top of the lip as either a small gap or an indentation in the lip continuing into the nose. It can occur as unilateral or bilateral and is due to the failure of the maxillary and medial nasal processes to fuse. Cleft palate is a condition in which the two plates of the skull that form the hard palate are not completely joined. The soft palate in these cases also is cleft. In most cases, cleft lip is also present. Both deformities can be successfully treated with surgery soon after birth.

EPIDEMIOLOGY Cleft lip and cleft palate are among the most common classes of congenital malformation. (See Figure 19-8 ■). In the United States, the prevalence for cleft lip with or without cleft palate is 2.2 to 11.7 per 10,000 births. Cleft palate alone results in a prevalence rate of 5.5 to 6.6 per 10,000 births.[23]

RISK FACTORS Cleft lip and cleft palate are thought to be caused by a combination of genes and other factors. Smoking during pregnancy increases the chance of their occurrence, as can certain medications, changes in nutrition, and other factors.[24] Cleft lips/palates are more common in Native Americans than any other ethnic group.[25]

Injury

Many injuries to the dentition are complex and costly. Losing incisor teeth or even fracturing teeth causes tremendous change to the dentition. Even more important is the fact that blows to the oral cavity can result in concussion due to the excessive physical force exerted during the arches occlusion.

EPIDEMIOLOGY The leading causes of head and face injuries that result in emergency room visits are falls, assaults, sports injuries, and motor vehicle collisions.[1] The majority of dental trauma occurs to the anterior teeth.[26] Regardless of the patient's age, dental trauma can be emotional and painful. Cost of the repairs can also be a substantial

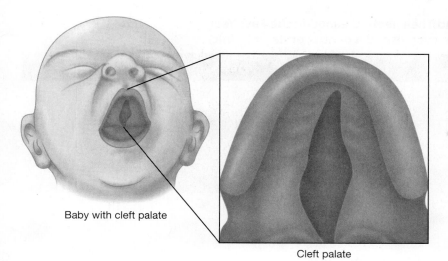

Baby with cleft palate

Cleft palate

FIGURE 19–8 Cleft Lip and Palate

Source: United States Department of Health and Human Services, Centers for Disease Control and Prevention, National Center for Chronic Disease Prevention and Health Promotion, Division of Oral Health. October 27, 2008. http://apps.nccd.cdc.gov/nohss/ListV .asp?qkey=6&DataSet=2 Accessed January 5, 2009.

economic burden. Individuals of all ages can be especially troubled psychologically because of unsightly fractures,[27,28] especially when the front teeth are adversely affected. Another burden is the amount of time involved in the healing process and in receiving treatment. Dental trauma's effects include tooth death, root resorption, tooth loss, and altered potential to develop permanent teeth.[29]

RISK FACTORS   Interestingly, 36 percent of all unintentional injuries to children and adults occurs during sports activities.[30] Prevention is a significant consideration because 20 million children age six to sixteen years are playing out-of-school sports, and 25 million youths are participating in competitive sports.[31] Although many orofacial injuries can be prevented during participation in athletic activities by using protective devices such as athletic mouth guards, many individuals do not use them. An athletic mouth guard, sometimes referred to as a mouth protector, is a removable oral appliance that protects the hard and soft tissues of the oral cavity and brain during contact sports. Mouth guards protect by absorbing energy during an impact, thus decreasing the likelihood of trauma.[32]

Toothaches

A toothache is a type of morbidity that causes pain. This pain can substantially impact the quality of life.

EPIDEMIOLOGY   Oral facial pain can greatly reduce quality of life.[1] Toothache pain can be caused by infection to the pulpal tissues or periodontium, dental caries infections, periodontal infections, trauma, mucosal sores, and temporomandibular joint (TMJ) disorder. In a six-month period, 22 percent of adults experience at least one type of oral facial pain.[33] Adults living in poverty are more likely to report toothaches than adults living above the poverty level.[34]

RISK FACTORS   Undoubtedly the major risk factor for toothache is untreated disease. Many times dental disease,

whether it be carious lesions or periodontal infection, initially does not produce pain, so infection goes unnoticed. Many people may believe a stain on a tooth or bleeding gums are natural, the latter possibly caused by brushing too vigorously, rather than recognizing a problem. When pain does begin and is not treated, it can become severe.

Many individuals who have difficulty accessing dental care postpone seeking it until symptoms, such as severe toothache and facial abscess, become so debilitating that they seek care in hospital emergency and operating rooms. This is not cost effective and—most important—does not address dental disease management because few hospitals deliver comprehensive dental services.

Did You Know?

By preventing infection, dental hygiene is one solution to decreasing the painful toothaches many individuals experience.

Prevention by Dental Care Utilization

Dental Visits

Many individuals in the United States do not seek regular dental care. See Tables 19-5 ■ and 19-6 ■ for the percentages of adults over the age of eighteen who have had their teeth cleaned or visited a dental provider in a one-year period. Remember that these data do not necessarily reveal regular, consistent assessment and preventive care but identify dental care received only during the time period. Although most oral diseases are preventable, untreated dental disease remains prevalent throughout the United States. Disparities in oral health are most evident among populations with low income and educational levels, special needs, and those who live in communities without access to oral health services. Oral diseases have been associated with a number of

Table 19–5 Adults Aged 18+ Who Have Had Their Teeth Cleaned in the Past Year (among adults with natural teeth who have ever visited a dentist or dental clinic)

State	Yes %	No %	State	Yes %	No %
Alabama	64.0	36.0	Montana	62.2	37.8
Alaska	62.3	37.7	Nebraska	70.1	29.9
American Samoa	—	—	Nevada	62.4	37.6
Arizona	66.2	33.8	New Hampshire	77.1	22.9
Arkansas	62.1	37.9	New Jersey	74.9	25.1
California	68.8	31.2	New Mexico	64.3	35.7
Colorado	66.6	33.4	New York	73.1	26.9
Connecticut	79.9	20.1	North Carolina	68.3	31.7
Delaware	76.3	23.7	North Dakota	71.4	28.6
DC	71.3	28.7	Ohio	71.9	28.1
Florida	67.4	32.6	Oklahoma	56.6	43.4
Georgia	70.0	30.0	Oregon	70.1	29.9
Guam	63.3	36.7	Palau	—	—
Hawaii	73.4	26.6	Pennsylvania	70.9	29.1
Idaho	67.4	32.6	Puerto Rico	76.2	23.8
Illinois	66.3	33.7	Rhode Island	78.8	21.2
Indiana	68.1	31.9	South Carolina	66.5	33.5
Iowa	74.1	25.9	South Dakota	70.8	29.2
Kansas	70.7	29.3	Tennessee	65.5	34.5
Kentucky	62.5	37.5	Texas	60.2	39.8
Louisiana	69.0	31.0	Utah	70.1	29.9
Maine	72.1	27.9	Vermont	75.7	24.3
Maryland	71.0	29.0	Virgin Islands	56.1	43.9
Massachusetts	79.3	20.7	Virginia	75.4	24.6
Michigan	75.0	25.0	Washington	71.6	28.4
Minnesota	74.3	25.7	West Virginia	61.6	38.4
Mississippi	57.2	42.8	Wisconsin	72.2	27.8
Missouri	61.6	38.4	Wyoming	65.7	34.3

Source: United States Department of Health and Human Services, Centers for Disease Control and Prevention, National Center for Chronic Disease Prevention and Health Promotion, Division of Oral Health. Retrieved from http://apps.nccd.cdc.gov/nohss/ListV.asp?qkey=6&DataSet=2 on February 17, 2014.

Table 19–6 Preventive Modalities

State	Yes %	No %	State	Yes %	No %
Alabama	63.4	36.6	Montana	64.6	35.4
Alaska	65.3	34.7	Nebraska	70.4	29.6
American Samoa	—	—	Nevada	61.5	38.5
Arizona	66.4	33.6	New Hampshire	75.9	24.1
Arkansas	61.5	38.5	New Jersey	73.8	26.2
California	67.6	32.4	New Mexico	64.0	36.0
Colorado	67.2	32.8	New York	72.5	27.5
Connecticut	78.6	21.4	North Carolina	67.2	32.8
Delaware	75.3	24.7	North Dakota	72.9	27.1
DC	70.5	29.5	Ohio	71.2	28.8
Florida	67.3	32.7	Oklahoma	56.7	43.3
Georgia	70.0	30.0	Oregon	70.4	29.6
Guam	62.6	37.4	Palau	—	—
Hawaii	73.4	26.6	Pennsylvania	69.9	30.1
Idaho	68.0	32.0	Puerto Rico	73.0	27.0
Illinois	67.6	32.4	Rhode Island	77.7	22.3
Indiana	66.5	33.5	South Carolina	65.7	34.3
Iowa	72.4	27.6	South Dakota	72.1	27.9
Kansas	70.5	29.5	Tennessee	64.4	35.6
Kentucky	63.9	36.1	Texas	59.8	40.2
Louisiana	67.7	32.3	Utah	71.5	28.5
Maine	70.2	29.8	Vermont	74.4	25.6
Maryland	71.4	28.6	Virgin Islands	60.0	40.0
Massachusetts	77.8	22.2	Virginia	74.0	26.0
Michigan	74.6	25.4	Washington	72.6	27.4
Minnesota	74.5	25.5	West Virginia	59.9	40.1
Mississippi	57.5	42.5	Wisconsin	72.4	27.6
Missouri	61.1	38.9	Wyoming	66.7	33.3

Source: United States Department of Health and Human Services, Centers for Disease Control and Prevention, National Center for Chronic Disease Prevention and Health Promotion, Division of Oral Health. Retrieved from http://apps.nccd.cdc.gov/nohss/ListV.asp?qkey=5&DataSet=2on February 17, 2014.

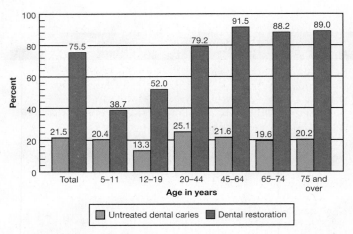

FIGURE 19–9 Prevalence of untreated dental caries and existing dental restorations in teeth, by age: United States, 2005–2008

Source: CDC/NCHS, National Health and Nutrition Examination Survey, 2005–2008. http://www.cdc.gov/nchs/data/databriefs/db96.htm

systemic conditions and chronic diseases such as diabetes, cardiovascular disease, and preterm low birth-weight babies, underscoring the importance of oral health services for all individuals.[1]

Dental sealants are highly effective in preventing dental caries that occur on the surfaces of teeth that have pits and fissures and increasingly have been used as a preventive modality. (See Figure 19-9 ■.) Fully retained sealants are 100 percent effective.[35,36] In examining the effectiveness of school-based or school-linked dental sealant programs, the *Guide to Community Preventive Services* documented a 60 percent decrease in tooth decay on the chewing surfaces of posterior teeth up to five years after sealant application.[37] School-based sealant programs also are cost efficient.[38] In 2002, the Task Force on Community Preventive Services strongly recommended school-based or school-linked sealant programs to prevent and control dental caries.[37]

Community water fluoridation prevents tooth decay mainly through direct contact with teeth throughout life and when consumed by children during the tooth-forming years. The most inexpensive way to deliver the benefits of fluoride to all residents of a community is through water fluoridation. All water naturally contains some fluoride; when a community fluoridates its water, it adjusts the level in the water to an optimal level for preventing tooth decay.[39]

Nearly 70 percent of US residents whose water comes from public systems now have fluoridated water. The objectives of *Healthy People 2020,* which sets health goals for the nation for the year 2020, is 80 percent. Currently, more than 184 million people in the United States are served by public water supplies containing enough fluoride to protect teeth. (See Figure 19-10 ■.) Water fluoridation is a low-cost way to bring the benefits of fluoride to all residents of a community.[39]

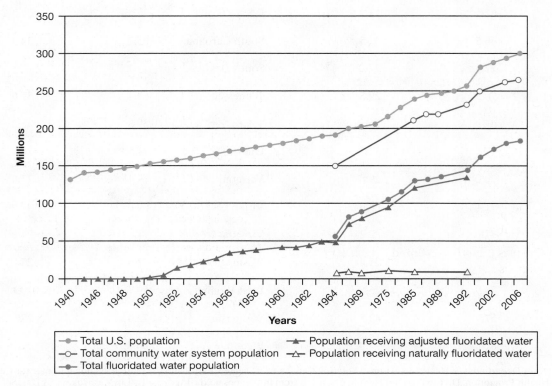

FIGURE 19–10 Fluoridation Growth

Source: http://www.cdc.gov/Nohss/FSGrowth.htm

Summary

Although the fact that many oral health disparities are based on gender, race/ethnicity, age, and SES has been established, more information is needed in the field of oral epidemiology. Various oral diseases and conditions including periodontal diseases and dental caries are widespread in the United States and are major issues regarding the nation's health. These findings reflect the minor value that society in general places on oral health care. The dental hygienist must be aware of the epidemiology of all oral diseases, conditions, and manifestations and have a clear understanding of the need for and ways to provide dental care in the United States.

Self-Study Test Items

1. Tobacco use, excessive alcohol use, and inappropriate dietary practices contribute to a number of diseases and disorders. In particular, tobacco use is a risk factor for oral cavity and pharyngeal cancers, periodontal diseases, candidiasis, and dental caries among other diseases.
   a. The first statement is true; the second statement is false.
   b. The first statement is false; the second statement is true.
   c. Both statements are true.
   d. Both statements are false.

2. Which gender do periodontal diseases affect the most?
   a. Males
   b. Females
   c. Neither
   d. Teen and elderly females

3. In which teeth are early childhood caries most evident?
   a. Permanent molars
   b. Permanent anteriors
   c. Primary anteriors
   d. Primary molars

4. Early detection frequently affects the outcome of
   a. Oral cancer treatment
   b. Cleft lip rates
   c. Cleft lip and palate rates
   d. None of the above

5. When toothaches are not prevented, which services might individuals seek?
   a. Medical
   b. Dental hygiene
   c. General dentistry
   d. Cosmetic dentistry

References

1. US Department of Health and Human Services. *Oral Health in America: A Report of the Surgeon General*. Rockville, MD: US Department of Health and Human Services, National Institute of Dental and Craniofacial research, National Institutes of Health; 2000.
2. Oliver RC, Brown LJ, Loe H. Periodontal diseases in the United States population. *J Periodontol.* 1998;69:269–278.
3. US Public Health Service, National Institute of Dental Research. *Oral Health of United Sates Adults: National Findings*. Bethesda, MD: National Institute of Dental Research; 1987. NIH Publication No. 87-2868.
4. *Third National Health and Nutrition Examination Survey, 1988–1994*. Hyattsville, MD: Centers for Disease Control; 1997. Public Use Data File No. 7-0627.
5. Epidemiology of Periodontal Diseases: Position Paper. American Association of Periodontology Academy Report. *J Periodontol.* 2005;76:1406–1419.
6. *National Health and Nutrition Examination Survey, 1999–2004*. Hyattsville, MD: Centers for Disease Control; 2005.
7. Oral Cancer Facts. Retrieved from http://www.oralcancerfoundation.org/facts/. on September 8, 2015.
8. Oral Cancer. Retrieved from http://www.cdc.gov/OralHealth/topics/cancer.htm. on September 8, 2015.
9. What Is Oral Cancer? Retrieved from http://www.nidcr.nih.gov/OralHealth/Topics/OralCancer/. on September 8, 2015.
10. Haddad RI. *Human Papilloma Virus Infection and Oropharyngeal Cancer*. Alexandria, VA: American Society of Clinical Oncology; 2007.
11. D'Souza G, Kreimer AR, Viscidi R, et al. Case–Control Study of Human Papillomavirus and Oropharyngeal Cancer. *N Engl J Med.* 2007;356(19):1944–1956.
12. Gonsalves W, Chi AC, Neville BW. Common Oral Lesions: Part I. Superficial Mucosal Lesions. *Am Fam Physician.* 2007;75:501–507.
13. Shulman JD, Beach MM, Rivera-Hidalgo F. The prevalence of oral mucosal lesions in U.S. adults: Data from the Third National Health and Nutrition Examination Survey, 1988–1994. *J Am Dent Assoc.* 2004;135:1279–1286.
14. Bouquot JE. Common oral lesions found during a mass screening examination. *J Am Dent Assoc.* 1986;112:50–57.
15. Herpes simplex virus. In: Neville B, Damm DD, Allen CM, Bouquot J. *Oral and Maxillofacial Pathology*. Philadelphia, PA: Saunders; 2002:213–220.
16. Whitley RJ. Prospects for vaccination against herpes simplex virus. *Pediatr Ann.* 1993a;22:726,729–732.
17. Rivera-Hidalgo F, Shulman JD, Beach MM. The association of tobacco and other factors with recurrent aphthous stomatitis in a U.S. adult population. *Oral Dis.* 2004;10:335–345.
18. Fotos PG, Vincent SD, Hellstein JW. Oral candidosis. Clinical, historical, and therapeutic features of 100 cases. *Oral Surg Oral Med Oral Pathol.* 1992;74:41–49.
19. Candidiasis. In: Neville B, Damm DD, Allen CM, Bouquot J. *Oral and Maxillofacial Pathology*. Philadelphia, PA: Saunders; 2002:189–197.
20. Epstein JB, Gorsky M, Caldwell J. Fluconazole mouthrinses for oral candidiasis in postirradiation, transplant, and other patients. *Oral Surg Oral Med Oral Pathol Oral Radiol Endod.* 2002;93:671–675.
21. Ghannoum MA, Abu-Elteen KH. Pathogenicity determinants of Candida. *Mycoses.* 1990;33:265–282.
22. Abu-Elteen KH, Abu-Elteen RM. The prevalence of *Candida albicans* populations in the mouths of complete denture wearers. *New Microbiol.* 1998;21:41–48.

23. Forrester MB, Merz RD. Descriptive epidemiology of oral clefts in a multiethic population, Hawaii, 1986–2000. *Cleft Palate-Craniofacial Journal.* 2004;41(6):622–628.

24. Cleft Lip and Palate Fact Sheet. Retrieved from http://www.cdc.gov/ncbddd/bd/cleft.htm. on. on September 8, 2015.

25. Lowry RB, Thunem NY, Uh SH. Birth prevalence of cleft lip and palate in British Columbia between 1952 and 1986: Stability of rates. *Can Med Assoc J.* 1989;140(10):1167–1170.

26. Cuttrell G. Dental trauma. In: Harris NO, Garcia-Godoy F, Nathe CN, eds. *Primary Preventive Dentistry.* 8th ed. Upper Saddle River, NJ: Pearson; 2014.

27. Slack GL, Jones JM. Psychological effect of fractured incisors. *Br Dent J.* 1955;99:386–388.

28. Cortes MI, Marcenes W, Shelham A. Impact of traumatic injuries to the permanent teeth on the oral health-related quality of life in 12- to 14-year old children. *Community Dent Oral Epidemiol.* 2002;30:193–198.

29. Douglass AB, Douglass JM. Common dental emergencies. *Am Fam Phys.* 2003;67(3):515.

30. Bijur PE, Trumbel A, Harel Y, Overpeck MD, Jones D, Scheidt PC. Sports and recreation injuries in US children and adolescents. *Arch Pediatr Adolesc Med.* 1995:149:1009–1016.

31. National Youth Sports Foundation. *Fact Sheet.* Needham, MA: National Youth Sports Foundation; 1994.

32. Nathe CN. Athletic Mouthguard. In: Harris NO, Garcia-Godoy F, Nathe CN. *Primary Preventive Dentistry.* 7th ed. Upper Saddle River, NJ: Pearson; 2008.

33. Lipton JA, Ship JA, Larach-Robinson D. Estimated prevalence and distribution of reported orofacial pain in the United States. *J Am Dent Assoc.* 1993;4(10):113–121.

34. Vargas CM, Macek MD, Marcus SE. Sociodemographic correlates of tooth pain among adults: United States 1989. *Pain.* 2000;85(1–2):87–92.

35. National Institutes of Health. Consensus development conference statement on dental sealants in the prevention of tooth decay. *J Am Dent Assoc.* 1984;108:233–236.

36. Llodra JC, Bravo M, Delgado-Rodriguez M, Baca P, Galvez R. Factors influencing the effectiveness of sealants—A meta analysis. *Community Dent Oral Epidemiol.* 1993;21:261–268.

37. Task Force on Community Preventive Services. Recommendations on selected interventions to prevent dental caries, oral and pharyngeal cancers, and sport-related craniofacial injuries. *Am J Prev Med.* 2002;23(suppl 1):16–20.

38. Griffin SO, Griffin PM, Gooch BF, Barker LK. Comparing the costs of three sealant delivery strategies. *J Dent Res.* 2002;81:641–645.

39. 2012 Water Fluoridation Statistics. Retrieved from http://www.cdc.gov/fluoridation/statistics/index.htm. on September 8, 2015.

Visit www.pearsonhighered.com/healthprofessionsresources to access the student resources that accompany this book. Simply select Dental Hygiene from the choice of disciplines. Find this book and you will find the complimentary study tools created for this specific title.

20

Evaluation of Scientific Literature and Dental Products

OBJECTIVES

After studying this chapter, the dental hygiene student should be able to:

- Describe how to evaluate dental care products
- Defend the dental hygienists' value in advocating the use of effective dental care products and treatment modalities
- Educate the public in evaluating dental care products
- Effectively critique dental research reported in dental and lay publications

COMPETENCIES

After studying the chapter and participating in accompanying course activities, the dental hygiene student should be competent to do the following:

- Use critical thinking skills and comprehensive problem-solving to identify oral health care strategies that promote patient health and wellness
- Use evidence-based decision making to evaluate emerging technology and treatment modalities to integrate into patient dental hygiene care plans to achieve high-quality, cost-effective care
- Assume responsibility for professional actions and care based on accepted scientific theories, research, and the accepted standard of care
- Integrate accepted scientific theories and research into educational, preventive, and therapeutic oral health services
- Evaluate factors that can be used to promote patient adherence to disease prevention or health maintenance strategies
- Utilize methods that ensure the health and safety of the patient and the oral health professional in the delivery of care

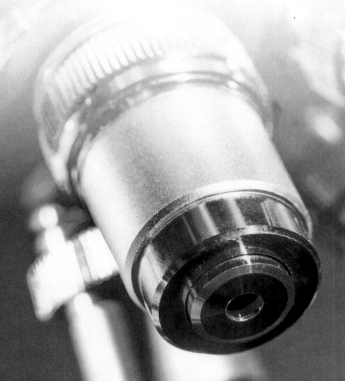

KEY TERMS

Abstract *289*
Peer reviewed *285*
PubMed *285*
Refereed *290*
Regulation *284*
Sample size *289*
Statistical significance *290*

Dental hygienists are recognized as advocates in health care today because of the valuable information they provide patients concerning dental hygiene treatment philosophies, oral health behavioral education, and dental care products.[1] The recent branding campaign conducted for the American Dental Hygienists' Association (ADHA) indicated that most patients seek advice first and foremost from their dental hygienist regarding dental care products.[2] Dental hygienists working in any aspect of health care are required to understand and effectively critique published research reports.

A few decades ago, supermarkets and drug stores had only a small portion of shelves available for dental care products; now they generally dedicate an entire aisle to oral health. This increased availability underscores the need for professionals who are able to provide consumers with valuable information about these products. For these reasons, the dental hygienist must have a background in research to be able to recognize effective and ineffective dental care products, product ingredients, and treatment modalities.

Regulation of Dental Care Products

Currently, dental products are under the **regulation,** that is, the rule or order, of the Food and Drug Administration (FDA), which is organizationally housed within the Department of Health and Human Services.[3] See Figure 20-1 ■ for information concerning the regulation of dental care products. The FDA's responsibility is to ensure that food, cosmetics, and radiation-emitting products are safe and that medicines and medical devices are safe and effective. The organization has the authority to encourage a company that violates its enforceable laws to voluntarily correct the problem or to recall a faulty product from the market. If a company cannot or will not correct a public health problem, the FDA can bring legal sanctions to bear and impose criminal penalties, including imprisonment, if warranted.

Did You Know?

Regulation of dental care products governs the control and guidelines of the products for safety and efficacy.

Periodically, the FDA provides dental professionals information concerning various oral health products through the *FDA Medical Bulletin*. It also publishes monographs concerning therapeutic products. FDA approval of drug products is mandated by law; without FDA approval, a manufacturer may not legally market a product.[4,5]

The American Dental Association (ADA) offers guidelines for testing and advertising products through its ADA Seal of Acceptance Program.[4] Although the program is strictly voluntary, and not government regulated, many companies participate in it. The ADA's Council on Scientific Affairs and staff scientists review oral care products and declare them safe, effective, and worthy of the ADA seal, which is generally awarded for a three-year period. A manufacturer that applies for the seal must meet specific guidelines and, upon its expiration, reapply to continue using it. In some instances, the ADA may conduct or request additional product testing.[5,6]

The ADA reviews all advertising claims for a product bearing the seal. A product with the ADA Seal featured in an advertisement may promote dentists as the preventive experts, since the organization represents dentists, as opposed to dental hygienists. However, the ADA Seal has been an excellent marketing tool for dentistry and to some extent, dental hygiene.

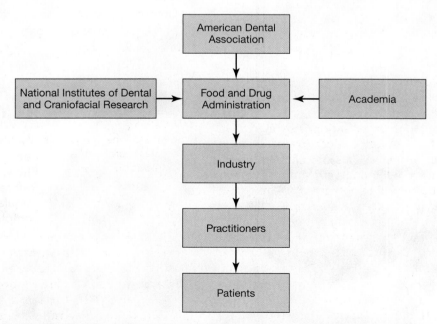

FIGURE 20–1 Regulation of Dental Care Products

As a health care professional, the dental hygienist should recommend a product or treatment modality based on documented evidence rather than a product seal, which may not always be a reliable gauge of safety or effectiveness. For example, toothbrush manufacturers sued the ADA for failing to adequately warn people about the possible dangers of brushing. Specifically, the lawsuit sought damages on behalf of anyone who suffers from toothbrush abrasion.[7] The ADA is not a government entity but represents the interests of the dental profession. The dental professional consequently must base recommendations on scientific literature and reported product findings. This is a good rule to follow regardless of the organization involved. Dental hygienists must be able to understand advertisement mechanisms and effectively critique published research so that the public receives accurate information.

Did You Know?

The ADA Seal is not mandatory for any dental care product and does not imply the superiority of that product to other products on the market.

Research Sources for Dental Care Products

Sales representatives are definitely knowledgeable about the products they carry and frequently about competitors' products, but it is important to remember that sales representatives may have bias toward their products. However, this contact can be especially helpful in gathering clinical reports and published articles that are **peer reviewed** that is, have been reviewed for content and accuracy by other dental health researchers. (See Box 20-1.)

Dental hygiene and dental schools can be great sources of information. Faculty members could be researching certain products or techniques and may have access to scientific information not available to clinical providers. Many faculty members have contacts around the world and can be a great resource.

Another way to gather information is by attending courses or seminars for continuing education, which most states require. Although some courses may not provide the desired information, collegial contacts and distributed resources can often be helpful in obtaining it. Companies generally make articles pertinent to their products easily accessible. (See Box 20-2 ■.)

The Internet provides a great deal of information regarding dental health care. Most Internet sites are not peer reviewed, however, so information gleaned from them should be used with caution. One reliable source is **PubMed,** http://www.ncbi.nlm.nih.gov/pubmed/, a Web site from the US National Library of Medicine (NLM) that includes more than 17 million citations from

Box 20–1 What is the Peer Review Process?

In academic publishing, the goal of *peer review* is to *assess the quality* of articles submitted for publication in a scholarly journal. Before an article is deemed appropriate to be published in a peer-reviewed journal, it must undergo the following process:

- The author of the article must submit it to the journal editor who forwards the article to experts in the field. Because the reviewers specialize in the same scholarly area as the author, they are considered the author's peers (hence "peer review").
- These impartial reviewers are charged with carefully evaluating the quality of the submitted manuscript.
- The peer reviewers check the manuscript for accuracy and assess the validity of the research methodology and procedures. If appropriate, they suggest revisions. If they find the article lacking in scholarly validity and rigor, they reject it.

Because a peer-reviewed journal will not publish articles that fail to meet the standards established for a given discipline, peer-reviewed articles that are accepted for publication exemplify the best research practices in a field.

Source: Evaluating Information Systems. NYC: Lloyd Sealy Library, The City University of New York. March 25, 2013. Retrieved from URL: http://guides.lib.jjay.cuny.edu/evaluatingsources on January 23, 2014.

Box 20–2 Sources of Information on Dental Care Products

- Colleagues
- Continuing education courses/professional meetings
- Dental hygienists and dental schools
- Lay magazines
- Library
- Internet
- Patients
- Professional magazines, journals, and newsletters
- Sales representatives
- Television

MEDLINE (the National Library's medical literature analysis and retrieval system online) and life science journals for biomedical articles back to the 1950s.[8] Furthermore, PubMed brings together authoritative information from NLM, the National Institutes of Health (NIH), and other government agencies and health-related organizations.

Box 20–3 Questions to Ask When Assessing Scientific Information Found on the Internet

- Who is/are the author(s) of the material? What are the author's (or authors') affiliations, qualifications, and biases?
- Is the source peer reviewed or edited?
- Is the site authored by an organization? What are its affiliations, qualifications, and biases?
- What is the domain name? (ie, .gov, .edu, .org, .net, .com, .mil)
- Does the author list sources or citations?
- Can the information be verified elsewhere?
- Does the site reflect a particular bias or viewpoint?
- Are obvious errors in spelling or grammar present?
- Why and for whom was this Web site created?
- Is there advertising on this Web site?
- When was the site first presented and last updated? Has it been revised?
- When was this Web site reviewed by a professional organization?
- Are the links current, good, and helpful? Are any links dead?
- Is the Web site comprehensive?
- Is the site easy to read?
- Is the color easy on the eyes?
- Are the site and the material well organized?

Source: Data from Beatty CF. Presentation at: 12th Annual Dental Public Health Educator's Workshop. University of New Mexico, Division of Dental Hygiene; October 3, 2013; Albuquerque, NM.

Internet sites are usually reliable if they originate from well-established, reputable professional organizations, government agencies, accredited universities, and community foundations and agencies. The information found on sites hosted by companies selling their products should be verified. A dental hygienist should research Web sites to determine the accuracy of their information. Some simple questions, such as those in Box 20-3 ■, can be asked to help make decisions on information quality.

Did You Know?

It is always important to thoroughly research products. Reading information from the top Googled companies is not enough.

Patients often alert the dental hygienist to products and therapies available, but their information may have been obtained at the local supermarket or from a magazine advertisement. Therefore, it is important for the dental hygienist to keep up-to-date on advertisers' claims and advise patients as to their accuracy.

Evaluation of Advertisements

The dental hygienist should be able to effectively critique both published studies and lay magazine advertisements and infomercials in order to be a good consumer advocate. This role is becoming increasingly important with the proliferation of advertising in print, electronic, and nontraditional formats, such as brand placement in movies. The dental hygienist needs to be aware of what advertisements may be implying or promoting to the public.

One example of an influential advertisement claim is that a mouthwash is the number one choice of hospitals. This advertisement has been notably effective, yet it says nothing about the product's effectiveness or method of efficacy. What does that claim mean to dental hygienists? They generally recommend a product that meets the needs of individual patients or groups. A patient who has questions about mouthwash selection is not likely to contact a local hospital but would more likely ask the dental hygienist and/or dentist during a dental visit.

In addition, it is important to realize the influence advertisements have on patients. For instance, many patients now think they should buy toothpastes with tartar control. Does an advertised tartar control remove plaque more effectively or prevent the accumulation of calculus? Probably not, but advertising causes many patients to believe it.

Making information about dental products available to patients is another way to help them assess the validity of manufacturers' claims. The dental hygienist should be familiar with common ingredients used in dental care products, such as those in Tables 20-1 ■ and 20-2 ■.

Table 20–1 Toothpaste Constituents

Ingredient	Percentage
Abrasives	20–40%
Water	20–40
Humectants	20–40
Foaming agent (soap or detergent)	1–2
Binding agent	Up to 2
Flavoring agent	Up to 2
Sweetening agent	Up to 2
Therapeutic agent	Up to 5
Coloring or preservative	<1

Source: Zayan M. Dentifrices, Mouthrinses, and Chewing Gums. In: Harris, NO, Garcia-Godoy, F, Nathe CN, eds. *Primary Preventive Dentistry.* 8th ed. Upper Saddle River, NJ: Pearson; 2014.

Table 20–2 Some Agents Added to Chewing Gums

Agent	Purpose/Claim	US Example(s)
Aspirin	Relieve pain	Aspergum
Caffeine	Increase alertness	Stay Alert
Calcium carbonate	Neutralize stomach acid	Chooz
Casein phosphopeptide–amorphous calcium phosphate	Remineralize and strengthen teeth	Trident Advantage
Chlorhexidine	Prevents plaque, gingivitis	None
Dimenhydrinate	Prevents motion sickness	None
Fluoride	Prevents caries	None
Sodium bicarbonate	Freshens breath	Dental Care
	Whitens teeth	Trident Advantage
	Reduces plaque	
Xylitol	Prevents caries	Trident
		BreathRx
		Theragum

Source: Zayan M. Dentifrices, Mouthrinses, and Chewing Gums. In: Nathe C, ed. *Primary Preventive Dentistry.* 8th ed. Upper Saddle River, NJ: Prentice Hall; 2014.

Evaluation of Scientific Literature

Dental hygienists rely on scientific literature such as published research reports, literature reviews, and commentaries to gather information about products and treatment modalities, but for the information to be useful, the dental hygienist must be able to assess the credibility of such data. In the past decade, many periodicals that include literature reviews have been published; their articles examine pertinent studies conducted on a particular topic and provide current theories and paradigms for dental hygiene practice. These literature reviews should contain an introduction stating the significance of the topic, a main body describing advantages and disadvantages of the study results, and a summary. These reviews can be valuable in helping the dental hygienist stay current with ever-changing technological advances but normally are merely summaries of the current literature available on a particular topic, and not the report of actual research.[9] Literature reviews come in various types, with systematic review and meta-analysis being the highest level of reviewed evidence and narrative reviews providing information in a structured manner based on the organizational structure defined by the publishing journal.

The need for dental hygienists to be savvy, consumer-oriented professionals has never been greater and underscores the need to critically review scientific literature to be able to assess evidence found in it when making decisions. Evidence-based practice requires being able to critique information appropriately. Specifically, it entails the use of multiple resources. Basing practice on available evidence includes using information derived from a body of knowledge as opposed to a single study. A study's effectiveness also depends on its characteristics, basically a hierarchy of evidence (see Table 20-3 ■) and methods based on causation and control of evidence.

Knowing the components of a well-written study is the first step in assessing a study's quality. See Box 20-3 ■ for the current *Journal of Dental Hygiene* guidelines for reporting original research.

Did You Know?

When "abstracting" the key concepts from a published study, it is necessary to identify its purpose; the problem investigated; the methodology, materials, and equipment used; the results obtained; and the conclusions drawn.

Table 20–3 Levels of Evidence

Level	Evidence
1	Systemic reviews, meta-analysis, and randomized controlled trials
2	Case–control studies
3	Case series
4	Traditional narrative reviews (no critical appraisal)
5	Studies that do not involve human subjects

Source: Beatty CF. Presentation at: 12th Annual Dental Public Health Educator's Workshop. University of New Mexico, Division of Dental Hygiene; October 3, 2013; Albuquerque, NM.

Knowing how to assess each part of a study equips the dental hygienist with the tools to evaluate a study's quality. See Box 20-5 ■ for details of specific areas of research reports that the dental hygienist should consider. Some of these aspects are discussed in the following sections.

Title

The title should accurately describe the purpose of the study. The main concept of the study should be clearly communicated so that the reader can decide whether the report is of interest. The authors are listed after the title. The authors' affiliation should be stated and dental hygienists should focus on articles written by authors whose work is frequently cited. This helps ascertain their expertise in the topic. The publication date is important. More recent research generally takes into account previous findings and confirms and changes current theories. Sometimes, landmark studies may be indicated for review. Although published years ago, they can be important to modern-day research and treatment.

Box 20–5 Questions to Ask When Judging a Research Report

- When was the work published?
- Where was it published?
- Are the authors' qualifications appropriate?
- Is the purpose clearly stated?
- Is the experimental design clearly described?
- Have the possible influences on the findings been identified and controls instituted?
- Has the sample been appropriately selected?
- Has the reliability of the scoring been assessed?
- Is the experimental therapy compared appropriately to the control therapy?
- Is the investigation of sufficient duration?
- Is the statistical analysis appropriate to answer the research questions or hypotheses?
- Have the research questions or hypotheses been answered?
- Do the interpretations and conclusion logically follow the experimental findings?

Source: McCann A, Schneiderman E. Interpreting and evaluating a research report. *Dent Hyg News.* 1997;5:5–10.

Box 20–4 *Journal of Dental Hygiene* Guidelines for Original Research Reports

Reports of basic, clinical, and applied studies that provide new information, applications, or theoretical developments typically include an abstract, introduction, review of the literature, methods and materials, results, discussion, and summary or conclusion.

- **Abstract:** Approximately 250 words in length. Use the headings "Purpose" (purpose), "Methods" (design, subjects, procedures, measurements), "Results" (summary of findings), and "Conclusion."
- **Introduction:** Briefly orient the reader to the given subject with an overview of the research problem studied with enough detail to ensure clarity.
- **Review of the Literature:** Cite a variety of relevant, current studies. Compare findings, clearly indicating all sources of concepts and data. When a source is quoted, use quotation marks. Note the current status of the topic, and if further study is needed, provide a sound case for it. Define the variables, the hypotheses or research objectives, and how this study relates to previous research.

- **Methods and Materials:** Describe the research instruments, equipment, procedures, and method of data analysis. Specify the measurements and statistical tests used as well as their significance. Furthermore, assure the reader that all pertinent federal and state regulations concerning the protection of the rights and welfare of all human and animal subjects have been adhered to.
- **Results:** Summarize all relevant data including statistics and data characteristics.
- **Discussion:** Evaluate and interpret the findings. Compare them with those of other related studies. Discuss study limitations and the study's implications to dental hygiene practice, education, and research and recommendations/plans for further study.
- **Conclusion:** State the conclusions, theories, or implications that may be drawn from the study. Discuss how they relate to the dental hygiene practice, profession, education, and research. Include overall health promotion and disease prevention, clinical and primary care for individuals and groups, and basic and applied science.

Abstract

The **abstract** is a study section that basically outlines its content by concisely stating its purpose, intent (why the study is so significant), previous findings, methodology, results, and suggestions for future studies in no more than 250 words. The abstract gives an overview of the entire project so that readers can decide whether the article is of interest to them.

Introduction

The introduction should provide a clear, concise statement of purpose for the research study. Its importance cannot be stressed enough. To illustrate how it can affect study results and uses, consider the following scenario. Suppose a company is promoting information that its plaque-removing, brushing prerinse product removes excess plaque when compared with brushing without the rinse. The study on which the promotion is based may have clearly delineated that rinsing and brushing together does in fact remove more plaque than just brushing without rinsing. Common sense would lead us to believe in the validity of this statement. To dental hygienists, however, it is evident that this study was designed to promote the product, not necessarily to support its claims with a scientific base.

Literature Review

The literature review should include a brief, detailed outline of previous research, clinical care standards, landmark studies, and commentaries that address specific issues and controversies that impact the current study. It is important to have current information, although the use of landmark studies or historical benchmarks sometimes is appropriate to help explain phenomena and provide a historical context for current studies results regarding diseases or treatments. The research also should be from a reputable journal; although

information in lay or dental hygiene magazines may be appropriate for identifying practice trends or controversies, it generally should not be included in a literature review.

Methodology

This research report section describes the methods and materials used for the study. Many of these are discussed in detail in Chapter 18 of this textbook. Important considerations when evaluating the quality of a study's methodology follow:

Sample Selection. Randomization ensures that subjects in the study are selected by chance.

Sample Size. The size of the sample needs to be large enough to be representative of the population. For clinical trials data on at least 30 subjects is important.

Ethical Considerations. The study must be free of plagiarism, copyright, or patent infringement; falsifying or fabricating data; misrepresenting data; and conflict of interest. Participation must be voluntary. Carefully, review this section, to make sure that ethical considerations have been employed in the study.

Research Design. A double-blind study requires neither the researcher nor the subjects participating in it to know who receives placebos, but this is not always possible.

Product Usage. Uses of the researched product need to be defined, including patient education protocols and the number and specific times the product was used. The study duration should be at least six months. The longer the study period, the more valid are its results.

Endpoints. Endpoints are the defined criteria that are used to determine whether treatment is effective. An endpoint for a study of flossing modalities could be focused on the reduction of interproximal bleeding or the reduction of interproximal plaque biofilm.

DENTAL HYGIENIST SPOTLIGHT ·····················

Pubilc Health Column: Michele Hair

A dental hygienist who has a diverse background in public health, Michele Hair was the Golden Scaler award recipient in the Wayne County Community College Dental Hygiene Program in 1988 and went on to receive her bachelor's degree in dental hygiene from the University of Detroit. She is currently working with Head Start and Early Head Start as an oral health coordinator. She finds her career in dental public health to be fulfilling.

Why did you decide to go into dental hygiene?

I always enjoyed going to the dentist as a child; however, I had never "been" to a dental hygienist because my dentist did not have a dental hygienist working at his office. I wanted to become a hygienist because one had come to my elementary school. I

loved getting fluoride treatments (which I guess was odd), and I think I knew then that this is what I wanted to do. I did well in science classes in high school, so I wanted to have a career that focused on science.

How did you get into dental public health? Did you need additional education?

I worked in public health during a student rotation at the Detroit Institute for Children, which treated special needs children. In 1993, I applied for a summer job working for the Colorado migrant health program as a dental hygienist providing fluoride treatments, sealants, and education to children attending the migrant school. This was when I realized that I was passionate about this type of dental hygiene.

I went on to work as the supervisor/coordinator of the migrant health program in Denver the following year. In this position, I supervised dental professionals located throughout Colorado. Then I created a full-time dental hygiene position in Colorado Springs at the Community Health Center (now Peak Vista).

What are your current positions?

Currently, I am the oral health program coordinator for Head Start and Early Head Start children enrolled through Community Partnership for Child Development (CPCD) in Colorado Springs. Head Start and Early Head Start are programs of the US Department of Health and Human Services that provide comprehensive education, health, nutrition, and parent involvement services to low-income children aged zero to five and their families. Head Start was created in 1965 and is the longest-running program to address systemic poverty in the United States.

I am responsible for developing and implementing the oral health program serving approximately 1135 Head Start and Early Head Start children. I provide clinical assessment and preventive therapies to children and give presentations on the oral health issues concerning pregnant women, infants, and young children to the dental and medical community. I also coordinate dental volunteers who provide dental education to parents during parent center meetings.

Can you discuss any particularly interesting experiences you have had in your dental public health positions?

There are so many rewards to working for CPCD. Head Start has clear goals that are set by the federal government but with the opportunity for each program to be creative in meeting those goals. The comprehensive program that CPCD offers to children and families provides a well-rounded approach to success. I also appreciate the fact that CPCD works with the community as a whole, not only the children and families that it serves through its programs.

What advice would you give someone in choosing a career in public health?

If you are interested in public health, my advice would be to pursue opportunities that allow you to work in it. Contacting your local and state health departments may lead you to areas that have public health opportunities. Everyone has gifts and talents, so if you enjoy clinical hygiene work, then work in that area where you make a difference. If you enjoy public health, you might have to do something other than dental public health initially, but it could lead later to a dental public health opportunity. Don't give up! Again, I feel that public health is not more or less valuable than clinical hygiene. What is important is what excites you.

Source: Christine Nathe writes the Public Health Column in *RDH* magazine published by Pennwell Publishing. For more public health spotlights please see RDH magazine online at http://www.rdhmag.com/index.html.

Quality of Examiners. The examiners should be calibrated and the same one used throughout the study. *Statistical Significance.* The result is unlikely to have occurred by chance. In the scientific community, a $p \leq .05$ is considered the cutoff point for **statistical significance,** meaning that an obtained result could happen by chance only five times or less in 100 instances.

Results and Discussion

The results and discussion section discusses the study and the study findings. In this section, the researcher compares the findings with those of related studies; discusses study limitations, implications for dental hygiene practice, education, and research; and suggests needs for further study.

Conclusion and Recommendation

This section states the study's conclusion and addresses its implications. The conclusion discusses theories that relate to dental hygiene practice, the profession, education, and research and suggests recommendations for further studies.

Data Sources and Publications

Biomedical informatics is a young and growing science of managing information for health care, research, education, and administration by applying, integrating, and evaluating information technology. Biomedical informatics (BMI) is the interdisciplinary field that studies and pursues the effective uses of biomedical data, information, and knowledge for scientific inquiry, problem solving, and decision making, motivated by efforts to improve human health.[10] Dental hygienists can use a variety of sources to obtain information, data, research results, and technology.

Pertinent information may be published in peer-reviewed (**refereed**) publications. To be accepted for publication, several other researchers review the report and agree with its content. See Box 20-6 ■ for a list of peer-reviewed publications germane to the dental hygiene science. Reviewers at one time were generally not told who conducted the study, so peer review was sometimes referred to as *blind review;* however, this practice is not as common today. Studies that contain valid research results are occasionally published in nonpeer-reviewed publications. Another great source for information are the Cochrane reviews, available on the

Box 20–6 Peer-Reviewed Dental Hygiene Periodicals

- *Journal of Dental Hygiene*
- *International Journal of Dental Hygiene*
  - *International Journal of Evidence-Based Practice for the Dental Hygienist*
- *Dimensions in Dental Hygiene*
- *Dental Health*
- *Canadian Journal of Dental Hygiene*
- *Journal of Oral Hygiene and Health*

Internet. And, it is important to remember, that although peer-reviewed journals are an excellent source of information for dental hygienists, magazines such as *RDH* and online forums such as hygienetown.com, which discuss new modalities and trends, are valuable as well.

Summary

Dental hygienists should be able to understand and evaluate published research reports and educate consumers regarding dental care products. Clearly understanding the principles of research methods will enhance dental hygienists' decision-making skills when treating patients and recommending dental care products. Practicing professionals must always be consumer advocates and stay current with contemporary products and modalities.

Self-Study Test Items

1. The ADA Seal of Approval program is regulated by the FDA. It is mandatory for all over-the-counter dental care products.
   a. The first statement is true; the second statement is false.
   b. The first statement is false; the second statement is true.
   c. Both the statements are true.
   d. Both the statements are false.

2. PubMed is a service of the US National Library of Medicine (NLM). It includes more than 17 million citations from MEDLINE and other life science journals for biomedical articles back to the 1950s.
   a. The first statement is true; the second statement is false.
   b. The first statement is false; the second statement is true.

c. Both the statements are true.
d. Both the statements are false.

3. Which of the following is/are part of a research report's methods and materials section?
   a. Research design
   b. Ethical considerations
   c. Sample size
   d. All of the above

4. Which of the following terms defines the review of manuscripts by experts for content and accuracy before they can be included in refereed journals?
   a. Critique
   b. Double blind
   c. Primary evaluation
   d. Peer reviewed

5. *Statistical significance* means that the result was not caused by
   a. Control
   b. Chance
   c. Placebo effect
   d. Sugar pill

References

1. *Roles of the Dental Hygienist. Bylaws American Dental Hygienists' Association.* Chicago, IL: American Dental Hygienists' Association; 2014.
2. ADHA Branding Campaign [video]. Presented at: New Mexico Dental Hygienists' Scientific Session; October 15, 2007; Albuquerque, NM.
3. US Department of Health and Human Services: What We Do. Retrieved from http://www.fda.gov/aboutfda/whatwedo/default.htm on September 8, 2015.
4. How drugs are developed and approved. US Food and Drug Administration. Retrieved from http://www.fda.gov/drugs/developmentapprovalprocess/howdrugsaredevelopedandapproved/default.htm on September 8, 2015.
5. Rippere J. FDA regulation of OTC oral health care drug products. *Journal of Public Health Dentistry.* 1992;52:329–332.
6. Whall C. The how and why of the ADA's evaluation program for dental therapeutic products. *Journal of Public Health Dentistry.* 1992;52:338–342.
7. Toothbrush abrasion spurs suit. *Albuquerque Journal,* 1998.
8. About Medline Plus. http://www.nlm.nih.gov/medlineplus/aboutmedlineplus.html. Accessed September 8, 2015.
9. McCann A, Schneiderman E. Interpreting and evaluating a research report. *Dent Hyg News.* 1997;5:5–10.
10. Definition of Biomedical Informatics. American Medical Informatics Association. Retrieved from http://www.amia.org/biomedical-informatics-core-competencies on September 8, 201523,.

Visit www.pearsonhighered.com/healthprofessionsresources to access the student resources that accompany this book. Simply select Dental Hygiene from the choice of disciplines. Find this book and you will find the complimentary study tools created for this specific title.

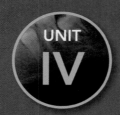

Practical Strategies for Dental Public Health

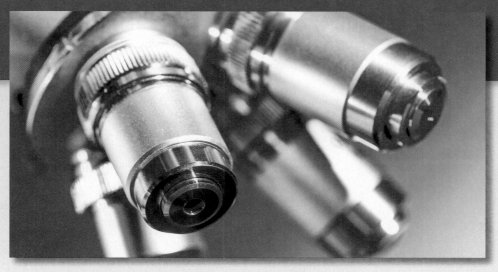

Science photo/Shutterstock

The dental hygiene profession is responsible for expanding the public's opportunities to receive quality dental hygiene care. This final unit discusses the current careers available in dental public health and explains how a practitioner can work in a governmental position. This unit also presents information on how a dental hygienist could effectively create a dental hygiene position in an organizational setting or a private dental hygiene practice. This

entrepreneurial endeavor will undoubtedly increase the underserved populations' access to dental hygiene care.

The final chapter serves as a review of dental public health principles germane to dental hygiene. Test-taking strategies and an overview of the topics and sample test items on National Dental Hygiene Examination Boards are presented to assist students preparing for examinations.

21

Careers in Dental Public Health

Karen Portillo, RDH, MS

OBJECTIVES

After studying this chapter, the dental hygiene student should be able to:

- Describe dental public health careers
- Identify various governmental careers in dental public health
- Define dental hygiene positions in a variety of settings

COMPETENCIES

After studying this chapter and participating in accompanying course activities, the dental hygiene student should be competent to do the following:

- Promote the values of the dental hygiene profession through service-based activities, positive community affiliations, and active involvement in local organizations.
- Promote positive values of overall health and wellness to the public and organizations within and outside the profession.
- Provide screening, referral and educational services that allow patients to access the resources of the health care system.
- Provide community oral health services in a variety of settings.
- Facilitate patient access to oral health services by influencing individuals or organizations for the provision of oral health care.
- Advocate for effective oral health care for underserved populations.
- Pursue career opportunities within health care, industry, education, research, and other roles as they evolve for the dental hygienist.

KEY TERMS

Civil service employment 298
COSTEP program 299
Independent contractor 298
National Health Service
  Corps 297
United States Public Health
  Service Commissioned
  Corps 295
US Public Health Service
  (PHS) 295

Science photo/Shutterstock

As discussed previously in Chapter 1, a dental hygienist has several professional roles to fulfill. The professional roles include administrator, entrepreneur, clinician, corporate, researcher, educator, and public health. In many ways, all of these roles affect the public's health. The past dental hygiene roles depicted public health encircling all the roles because, as a dental hygienist, opportunities present themselves that require the dental hygienist to fill the public health roles in some capacity. This same sentiment should be realized, even with the additional roles added. At all times, dental hygiene can influence the public's health. For this reason, public health is a fundamental part of all of the professional roles of a dental hygienist.

Chapter 3 focused on dental care delivery in the United States. The focus of this discussion will be how the dental hygienist roles actually can be integrated into the delivery of dental care. An important characteristic of most dental hygienists who work in public health is an advanced educational level. Although a dental hygienist can enter into public health with an entry-level certificate, associate, or baccalaureate degree like many career fields, advancing educational level will provide the dental hygienist with additional skills and knowledge needed in these roles. These roles tend to involve leadership skills, which are necessary when advocating for change. These skills also open more doors and career opportunities for the dental hygienist.

Many students may ask what type of skills the dental hygienist should possess to be employed in the field of public health. Public health is centered on people, people who live in a certain region who might be underserved, people who represent a certain special population and cannot advocate for themselves, or people in a community who have a need that is not being met. A dental hygienist in public health should be willing to think and work outside traditional parameters to be able to address the needs of the population.

Public health settings are often referred to as "alternative practice" settings. This requires the dental hygienist to be able to provide dental hygiene care outside of a "traditional" private dental practice setting. Alternative practice settings allow the dental hygienist to bring care to populations who need the services, thereby addressing certain barriers such as transportation. Alternative practice settings could be in a community-based clinic that might be located in an underserved area, a school-based location in which portable dental equipment is brought in to treat the children, a long-term care facility, an acute care hospital or clinic, a cancer center, or even a mobile van to provide care to outreach areas. The alternative practice setting can be as creative as the dental hygienist can envision to increase care to a population.

This chapter will examine several areas in which a dental hygienist can seek opportunities, such as at the federal/national level, the state level, and local levels.

Federal/National Public Health Career Opportunities

A plethora of positions exists in dental public health from clinical dental hygiene to administrative posts in governmental agencies. See Figure 21-1 for acronyms for a variety of government agencies affecting public health. Examples of employment for dental hygienists by the federal government include the following:

- Contract with Navy to provide clinical and educational services to military personnel in a military dental clinic
- Work with the National Institutes of Dental and Craniofacial Research as a lead researcher in a study on the relationship of periodontal diseases to systemic conditions/diseases
- Hold an administrative position with the Centers for Disease Control and Prevention, overseeing the agency's agenda on community water fluoridation
- Initiate dental hygiene services as an entrepreneur

US Public Health Service

The **US Public Health Service (PHS)** is a part of the US Department of Health and Human Services with eleven agencies dedicated to improving and advancing the health of this country's people. It offers career opportunities in dental public health among other areas. As a major division of the Department of Health and Human Services, the PHS encompasses all federal civil service employees including the personnel of the PHS Commissioned Corps. See Box 21-1 ■ for the mission and core values of the PHS.[1] As one of the seven uniformed services in the United States, the **United States Public Health Service Commissioned Corps** provides highly trained and mobile health professionals who conduct programs to promote the health of the nation, understand and prevent disease and injury, ensure safe and effective drugs and medical devices, deliver health services to federal beneficiaries, and provide health expertise in time of war or other national or international emergency. As one of the seven uniformed services of the United States, the PHS Commissioned Corps is a specialized career system designed to attract, develop, and retain health professionals who may be assigned to federal, state, or local agencies or international organizations to accomplish its mission.

The PHS Commissioned Corps, with approximately 6000 officers, is led by the Surgeon General. See Figure 21-2 ■ for a PHS officer in uniform.

Did You Know?

The first Surgeon General was appointed in 1871 to head the Marine Hospital Service (MHS), itself established in 1798 to minister to sick and injured merchant seamen. It was reorganized as the US Public Health Service in 1912.

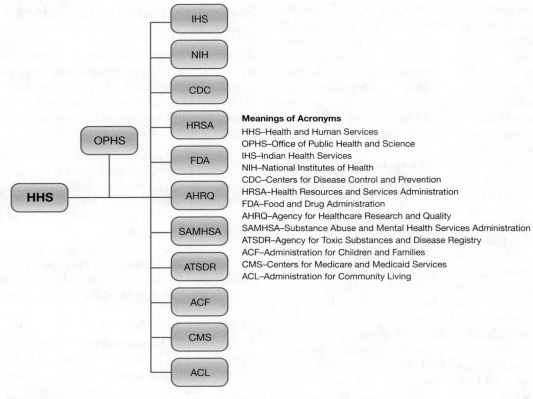

Meanings of Acronyms
HHS–Health and Human Services
OPHS–Office of Public Health and Science
IHS–Indian Health Services
NIH–National Institutes of Health
CDC–Centers for Disease Control and Prevention
HRSA–Health Resources and Services Administration
FDA–Food and Drug Administration
AHRQ–Agency for Healthcare Research and Quality
SAMHSA–Substance Abuse and Mental Health Services Administration
ATSDR–Agency for Toxic Substances and Disease Registry
ACF–Administration for Children and Families
CMS–Centers for Medicare and Medicaid Services
ACL–Administration for Community Living

FIGURE 21–1 Health and Human Services Organizational Chart

Source: www.hhs.gov/about/orgchart/index.html#text ies

Box 21–1 Mission and Core Values of US Public Health Service Agencies/Programs

The mission of the US Public Health Service Commissioned Corps is to protect, promote, and advance the health and safety of our nation. As America's uniformed service of public health professionals, the Commissioned Corps achieves its mission through:

• Rapid and effective response to public health needs
• Leadership and excellence in public health practices
• Advancement of public health science

Retrieved from http://www.usphs.gov/aboutus/mission.aspx on February 19, 2015.

Dental hygienists serve as health services officers (HSOs), a category that represents approximately 10 percent of all PHS commissioned officers. The majority of HSOs are assigned to the agencies listed in Box 21-2 ■. Eligibility requirements for obtaining a commissioned officer position with the PHS include the following:

• US native or naturalized citizen
• Less than 44 years of age (this may be adjusted upward for current/prior active duty service)

• Meet current medical and security requirements
• Must have a qualified degree from an accredited program, usually approved in American university and colleges and graduate from a dental hygiene program that is accredited by the Commission on Dental Accreditation and be at a baccalaureate level.
• Have a current, unrestricted valid dental hygiene license to practice in one of the states, Puerto Rico, Virgin Islands, or Guam.

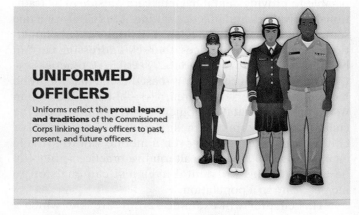

FIGURE 21.2 US PHS Officers in Uniform

Source: www.usphs.gov/images/aboutus/USPHS_Infographic_082614_web-01.png

Did You Know?

US PHS dental hygienists have career ladder opportunities that often are not available in the private sector.

Civil Service Positions

The US Civil Service includes all appointed positions in the executive, judicial, and legislative branches of the federal government other than military positions. The civil service offers a number of opportunities to dental hygienists in many government agencies and institutions, including federal prisons, Veterans Affairs (VA) hospitals, and military bases.[2,34] A candidate must apply to a specific vacancy announcement, which may be used to fill a single vacancy or multiple vacancies over a period of time. Vacancies can change every two weeks or so; the candidate should visit the USAJOBS Web site frequently. Vacancy announcements on the Web site provide information on specific duties, qualification requirements, ranking factors, and application forms and procedures. Required application materials and instructions regarding submission of the application vary from announcement to announcement. Dental hygiene positions require copies of transcripts, licenses, and/or certifications. In addition, almost all civil service positions in the US Department of State require at least a secret security clearance. Evaluation procedures vary and are specified in each announcement. In all cases, the evaluation is based on the application material submitted.

National Health Service Corps

The **National Health Service Corps** (NHSC) is a part of the Health Resources and Services Administration (HRSA), a PHS agency. According to its mission statement, the NHSC "is committed to improving the health of the nation's underserved by uniting communities in need with caring health professionals and supporting communities' efforts to build better systems of care"[3] and works closely with state programs for underserved areas. (See Box 21-3 ∎.) Working with other HRSA bureaus and programs, the NHSC recruits primary care clinicians to provide comprehensive team-based health care that bridges geographic, financial, cultural, and language barriers.

Dental hygienists may work as clinicians with the NHSC, and those with qualifying educational loans may be eligible to compete for repayment of those loans if they choose to serve in a community of greatest need. In addition to loan repayment, these clinicians receive a competitive salary, some tax relief benefits, and a chance to have a significant impact on a community.

Veterans Affairs

The Department of Veterans Affairs (VA) was created to treat veterans' ongoing disabilities incurred during military service.[4] Comprehensive care is delivered primarily at medical centers and outpatient clinics located nationwide. They offer a full range of primary, acute, chronic, and inpatient and outpatient health care services.

VA dental services are an integral part of this health care system. Dental services are offered in each medical center and in most of the major outpatient clinics. The VA

employs dentists, dental hygienists, dental assistants and other support personnel. Dental hygienists are employed as civil service employees.

Service on Military Bases

Dental hygienists may practice in any military branch dental clinic as a civil service employee, independent contractor, professional dental management company employee, or active duty military personnel. In this setting, the dental hygienist usually works with a variety of dentists and specialists and frequently works with other health care providers.[5] These opportunities vary from base to base.

Did You Know?

Dental hygienists who work for the federal government often have the opportunity to expand their scope of practice based on the most permissive state's practice act. For example, if a dental hygienist is licensed in a state that does not permit the provision of local anesthesia, that dental hygienist could, after taking a course on local anesthesia, provide local anesthesia in a federal employment setting because other states permit that practice.

Federal Prisons

It is the mission of the US Bureau of Prisons to protect society by confining offenders in the controlled environments of prisons and community-based facilities that are safe, humane, cost-efficient, and appropriately secure and that provide work and other self-improvement opportunities to assist offenders in becoming law-abiding citizens.[6] The Health Services Division coordinates the Bureau of Prisons' medical, dental, and mental health services to federal inmates. Dental hygienists provide routine and advanced prophylactic and therapeutic dental care to the inmate population and plan and direct the preventive dental health program. Qualified applicants must be currently licensed to practice as dental hygienists in a state or territory of the United States or the District of Columbia and must possess specialized experience performing oral prophylactic care and provide oral health education services to patients. They must also have experience performing advanced oral prophylactic, therapeutic, and preventive procedures in cases of periodontal diseases or inflammation or on patients with other medical or dental problems; placing temporary fillings; and finishing amalgam restorations. Dental hygienists can be hired as civil service employees, independent contractors, US PHS officers, or employees of a professional dental management firm.

Independent Contractors

Dental hygienists who are **independent contractors,** also known as consultants, freelancers, self-employed, entrepreneurs, and business owners, work for themselves. They earn their livelihoods from their own independent businesses instead of working for employers. Dental hygienists may provide clinical, consultative, and educational services. Independent contracting dental hygienists usually earn more than those who work for employers but receive no employer-paid benefits.

There is no single, clear-cut test for classifying workers as employees or independent contractors. Various government agencies use different legal tests for granting independent contractor positions including the following:

- Internal Revenue Service
- US Labor Department
- National Labor Relations Board
- State unemployment compensation insurance agencies
- State workers' compensation insurance agencies
- State tax departments

Each of these agencies is involved with worker classification for different reasons, and each has different policies and practices. Each agency normally makes classification decisions independently, which means that one agency might classify a person as an independent contractor but another would not. If opportunities exist, dental hygienists can work as independent contractors for the Bureau of Prisons, the military, and various community dental clinics.

Dental Staffing Agency Employee

A number of professional management firms act as agencies to find health care personnel for federal dental and medical facilities throughout the United States.[7] These companies hire a dental hygienist as an employee and then place the dental hygienist in a dental clinic that is government-operated. Although the dental hygienist works in a government dental clinic, the dental hygienist is still an employee of the professional management firm. The government agency pays the company a set fee for supplying a dental hygiene employee, and the firm then pays the dental hygienist. These professional firms usually provide a variety of benefits for their dental hygiene employees.

DPS, Inc., is a professional management firm that has administered health care service contracts with the Air Force, Army, Coast Guard, Navy, and Bureau of Prisons. The firm finds employment for dentists, dental hygienists, dental assistants, and dental lab technicians at federal facilities.

Health Systems Opportunities

Dental hygienists are now becoming employable in a variety of health systems organizations. Cancer centers, ambulatory clinics, acute care hospitals, and nursing facilities are integrating dental care in their health care offerings. Dental hygienists graduating in this decade will have more opportunities and will need to utilize entrepreneurial skills to develop these types of positions, which are discussed in further detail in Chapter 22.

Student Dental Public Health Opportunities

In 1948, the PHS established a summer employment program for medical students and in 1955 added other health disciplines to the program.[1] Finally, in 1956 the Commissioned Officer Student Training and Extern Program (COSTEP) was formally established. COSTEP enables students to enhance their educational background and provides hands-on experience to those with a commitment to future employment. It also introduces them to health disciplines for potential PHS careers. Students assigned to the Federal Bureau of Prisons receive hands-on training in correctional medicine, policies, and procedures.

The **COSTEP program** was established to attract qualified students in accredited health care programs into the Commissioned Corps and service in the PHS. Effective the first day of formal studies for the last academic year, selected students are called to "active duty for training." They will be paid the salary of an ensign for that year. Please see the Companion Website for more information on this opportunity.

DENTAL HYGIENIST SPOTLIGHT ···

Public Health Column: Jennifer Brown, RDH

This spotlight focuses on a dental hygienist who works in a particularly interesting setting—a cancer center. Jennifer Brown practices in Colorado and has received two clinical excellence awards, one from the Colorado Dental Hygienists' Association. Her career exemplifies an important role that dental hygienists should be playing in our national health care systems. Additionally, this career is a great example of how important it is for dental hygienists to work with an interdisciplinary team.

Why did you decide to go into dental hygiene?

I was fortunate to grow up in a dental office. My mom was a dental assistant and also worked at the front desk. As a child, I remember doing all of my science fair projects on tooth decay and root canal therapy. When it was time to go to college I was advised by many to pursue a degree in business and/or finance, and at first I went in that direction. However, it was not long before I realized I was pursuing the wrong profession, and when the opportunity arose to work in a dental office, I jumped on it! I worked my way up from "office gopher" to assisting, and I quickly realized dental hygiene was where I needed to be.

What is your current position?

I currently work at the Dorcy Cancer Center in Pueblo, Colorado. I serve as a hygienist on the CARES Team (Cancer Assessment Resources/Research Education and Survivorship). We are a team of health care professionals (dental hygienist, speech pathologist, nutritionist, and physical therapist) who assist head-and-neck cancer patients through their radiation treatment. Our goal is to meet each individual's unique and complex needs.

First, we assess each patient before they begin treatment, and we continue to meet with them weekly to address complications that arise from treatment. We also follow up with them for one year post radiation treatment. I'm personally responsible for all correspondence with the patient's dentist and oral surgeon, coordinating their dental needs before radiation treatment begins. Also, if needed, I fabricate fluoride trays, mouth guards, and stents to meet their individual treatment needs. I spend a lot of time researching evidence-based theories in order to implement the best dental care for each patient. I also try to reach out to other dental professionals. I have another dental hygienist teammate, Cindy Purdy, who reaches out to the dental community. She travels frequently to attend dental conventions, and she advises me of new products. I also practice three days a week in a private practice setting. I'm currently developing a cancer patient care protocol for private practices to meet the needs of patients who are receiving chemotherapy and/or radiation therapy.

How did you get into dental public health?

One of my long-term patients presented in my chair with a letter from an "oncology dental hygienist" that informed us of his recent radiation treatment for head-and-neck cancer, and his special dental needs and concerns for lifelong treatment. I contacted the hospital about the duties of an oncology hygienist, and after being put in touch with her, I learned more about the position and informed her of my interest in her work.

Debra Flesher-Bratt, RDH, who started the hygiene position at Dorcy Cancer Center, has held the position for several years at two hospitals in Colorado. When she resigned from her position at Dorcy, she told the staff about my desire to have the position, and almost one year later, here I am. It's been an intense learning curve, but I love this position and my interest in this work grows with each patient. I recently attended an Oral Oncology Symposium at MD Anderson Cancer Center, and I look forward to

continuing my education through work experience and other symposiums across the country.

Can you discuss any particularly interesting experiences you've had in your dental public health positions?

Every week and every new diagnosis brings a new learning experience and a chance to think outside the box to meet the needs of patients. I meet with each patient once a week, and in between visits the gears are continuously turning in my head as to how to personalize their treatment. As with all dental hygiene, each patient responds to instruction and treatment differently. At times, my biggest challenge is encouraging their compliance, knowing that what we're recommending will serve them in the later weeks of treatment. Until they experience the intense and severe complications radiation treatment brings, it's a struggle to explain the need for preventive care.

Depending on the patient's diagnosis and proposed treatment, they all present in the dental chair with a different story and oral care needs. Many of my patients have ignored their dental health for years and must deal with their dental needs immediately, and many need full-mouth extractions. We strive to preserve their dental function, but we often have to make difficult decisions to avoid severe dental complications in the future. Head-and-neck radiation treatment has acute and chronic side effects, and I am responsible for educating my patients, seeing them through treatment, and showing them how to maintain their oral health for life.

What type of advice would you give to practicing hygienists who are thinking of doing something different?

This position has changed my career. It has fueled a newfound passion in me for my patients, both at the cancer center and in private practice. I'm excited to help people in a new and challenging way. There is a profound need in the health care world for the influence of dental hygiene. Perhaps crossing into the hospital setting will help us break down the barriers and misconceptions and show that oral health greatly serves in overall health. The health care setting is very different from the typical dental office, and it has been a challenge to integrate dental services into a hospital setting. It's a balancing act to provide the best patient care and meet corporate and government standards.

Do you have anything else you'd like to share?

Please be aware of the rising epidemic of HPV-positive oropharyngeal cancers. The face of oral cancer is changing and cannot be ignored. Insist that proper oral cancer screenings and oral cancer awareness have a big presence in your office. I have witnessed the early signs and symptoms ignored by both patient and physician. Be prepared to meet the unique and complex needs of oral cancer patients, as we are their first line of defense and the best suited to treat and minimize their complications. Many of these cancer patients will not be well informed regarding their dental needs, because there aren't many programs like the CARES Team at Dorcy Cancer Center.

Jennifer's career highlights the importance of dental hygiene in comprehensive health care. Dental hygienists such as Jennifer, Cindy, and Debra are pioneers who have integrated dental hygiene into a comprehensive health care system, and programs like this need to be replicated throughout the country. As a profession, it's refreshing to know that dental hygiene continues to advance, thus helping those in need of our services!

Source: Christine Nathe writes the Public Health Column in *RDH* magazine published by Pennwell Publishing. For more public health spotlights please see RDH magazine online at http://www.rdhmag.com/index.html.

State Opportunities

Many state health departments employ dental hygienists to work as clinicians, educators, administrators, or researchers. Additionally, some states contract with private companies and/or independent dental hygiene contractors to provide clinical care and consulting. In many states, a dental hygienist with additional education and experience can be employed as the state dental director or often titled the oral health program manager for the state.

Local Opportunities

Dental hygienists have the opportunity to work in several different capacities on a local level. There are school-based dental sealant programs, preschool varnish programs such as those conducted in Head Start early educational programs, and oral cancer screening programs in long-term care facilities. The need for dental hygienists throughout various areas in a community is huge, and the sky is the limit to what programs a dental hygienist can start to meet the needs of the community. If a dental hygienist is interested in starting an oral health program, one of the first steps is to conduct a needs assessment to determine what the need is and ensure that other programs are not in existence to address the same problem. Work with stakeholders to gain support and funding for your program. There are many resources to help a dental hygienist address the needs in his/her community; the first step is making the decision to do it!

International Opportunities

Dental hygienists have the opportunity to work in many different countries. In fact, only 25 countries educate dental hygienists, so there are ample opportunities for dental hygienists to initiate dental public health programs and dental hygiene educational programs in most of the world. The student Web site lists many opportunities for the dental hygienist overseas, including opportunities with the US Peace Corps.

Summary

As dental hygienists, there are several professional roles to fulfill, and all encompass roles affecting public health. After reading this chapter and learning about how various dental hygienists work in diverse aspects and levels in public health, it should become apparent why public health encompasses all the roles of the dental hygienist. As dental hygienists, we have many skills and a substantial amount of knowledge to provide to our communities, and the field of public health is a perfect arena to present opportunities for dental hygienists to fill all the professional roles in dental hygiene.

Self-Study Test Items

1. Dental hygienists initially are eligible to be a US PHS Commissioned Officer with which of the following credentials?
   a. Certificate in dental hygiene
   b. Associate's degree in dental hygiene
   c. Bachelor's degree in dental hygiene
   d. Master's degree in dental hygiene

2. Civil service agencies fall under the State Department. Many times hygienists are employed at VA hospitals as a civil service employee.
   a. The first statement is true; the second statement is false.
   b. The first statement is false; the second statement is true.
   c. Both statements are true.
   d. Both statements are false.

3. Students are eligible for the COSTEP program during their dental hygiene education. The COSTEP program is part of the US Department of Defense health care system.
   a. The first statement is true; the second statement is false.
   b. The first statement is false; the second statement is true.
   c. Both statements are true.
   d. Both statements are false.

4. Dental hygienists can work on military bases in the United States as
   a. Military officers
   b. PHS Officers
   c. Contract employees
   d. None of the above

5. Which of the following is a goal of the US Public Health Services?
   a. Prevent and control disease
   b. Identify health hazards in the environment
   c. Help provide health care to Native Americans
   d. All of the above

References

Much of the information provided came from the following Web sites. These Web sites are recommended as a resource to students interested in further exploring specific career opportunities.

1. www.usphs.gov: US Public Health Service
2. www.state.gov: Civil Service
3. http://nhsc.hrsa.gov/National Health Service Corps
4. www.va.gov Veterans Affairs
5. www.defenselink.gov Military Base Dental Clinics or Active Duty Opportunities
6. www.bop.gov Prison Dental Hygiene
7. www.dpsjobs.com Private Employment within Government-Operated Clinics

Visit www.pearsonhighered.com/healthprofessionsresources to access the student resources that accompany this book. Simply select Dental Hygiene from the choice of disciplines. Find this book and you will find the complimentary study tools created for this specific title.

Strategies for Creating Dental Hygiene Positions in Dental Public Health Settings

OBJECTIVES

After studying this chapter, the dental hygiene student should be able to:

- List the populations most in need of dental hygiene care.
- Describe the paradigm for creating a dental hygiene position.
- Develop protocol for a newly developed dental hygiene position.

KEY TERMS

Blueprint *307*
Legislative initiatives *303*
Marketing *304*
Practice management *307*
Proposal *307*
Public relations *304*

COMPETENCIES

After studying the chapter and participating in accompanying course activities, the dental hygiene student will be competent to do the following:

- Promote the values of the dental hygiene profession through service-based activities, positive community affiliations, and active involvement in local organizations.
- Promote positive values of overall health and wellness to the public and organizations within and outside the profession.
- Provide screening, referral and educational services that allow patients to access the resources of the health care system.
- Provide community oral health services in a variety of settings.
- Facilitate patient access to oral health services by influencing individuals or organizations for the provision of oral health care.
- Evaluate reimbursement mechanisms and their impact on the patient's access to oral health care.
- Evaluate the outcomes of community-based programs, and plan for future activities.
- Advocate for effective oral health care for underserved populations.
- Pursue career opportunities within health care, industry, education, research, and other roles as they evolve for the dental hygienist.
- Develop practice management and marketing strategies to be used in the delivery of oral health care.

Although dental hygiene initially began as a profession focused on public health initiatives, the professional has long been positioned primarily in the private dental office. In this setting, dental hygienists frequently have little control over the delivery of dental hygiene care, but this is changing because society is demanding a more appropriate delivery system for dental hygiene services.[1]

Not all individuals in our society are able to visit a dentist's office for a variety of reasons such as a disability, chronic illness, lack of funds, or rural location. Refer to Box 22-1 ■ for a list of populations that frequently need dental hygiene services. For these populations, access to dental hygiene services has been virtually unattainable. These populations could receive dental hygiene care brought directly to them in their homes; facilities or nearby dental clinics could increase access. This situation is especially significant because those who have the least access to dental hygiene services are the ones who would likely benefit most from care that emphasizes prevention.[2]

Stakeholders, including individuals who work for government agencies, various health care providers, social service workers, and dental hygienists, have shown significant interest in establishing dental hygiene programs in settings other than private dental offices. In some of these settings, the dental hygienist may be required to establish a distinct dental hygiene business.

Although most states have a difficult time containing health care costs while delivering quality care to all members of the population, access to preventive health care should undoubtedly improve overall costs while increasing autonomy for the dental hygiene practitioner. Moreover, the presence of educated dental hygiene professionals should improve the quality and accountability of care. Few would argue that the practitioner specifically educated in dental hygiene sciences best provides the optimum level of dental hygiene care.[3] This chapter focuses on the strategies for implementing dental hygiene positions within the health care delivery systems.

Legislative Perspective

Some states do not allow the public the opportunity to subscribe to dental hygiene services in any way other than from a private dental practice. In fact, a few states require that dental hygienists work only in a private dental setting and be directly supervised by a dentist. Proposals to change or enact laws called **legislative initiatives** may be necessary to increase the accessibility of dental hygienists to the entire population. Please see Chapter 6 for more information on legislative initiatives.

Did You Know?

Legislative initiatives are what led to so many states permitting dental hygienists to practice outside of a private dental practice.

The majority of states allow the dental hygienist to work in a variety of settings without a dentist present. By providing dental hygiene care in alternative settings, dental hygienists are able to interact with those population segments currently underserved.

Proposed Plan for Action

The process for establishing a dental hygiene position should follow the dental public health program planning paradigm discussed in Chapter 12. It is important to identify the various aspects that an alternative delivery of dental hygiene care would entail and to establish the parameters for setting up a dental hygiene position. Alternative positions could be developed in nursing facilities, school-based clinics, primary care clinics, hospitals, health centers, cancer centers, or hospice agencies to name a few.

Assessment

During the assessment phase, the dental hygienist proposing the new position should conduct a needs assessment of the population, facilities, funding, and infrastructure. Information to be obtained may include the number, ages, and medical needs of individuals within the population, specific dental needs of the population, administrative support, facility space, staff support, reimbursement mechanisms, and values of dental hygiene care. Assessment mechanisms, which will also serve as evaluation mechanisms, including the use of dental indexes, dental records, surveys, and/or interviews, should be implemented. Involving entities within the organization during the assessment phase can help identify current unmet dental needs and demands.

The assessment should identify whether dental hygienists in the specific state can be reimbursed directly by Medicaid, CHIPS, and/or dental insurance companies. If not, ask the following questions to determine how this avenue of reimbursement can be achieved: Does it require legislation or a rule change? Is the organization amenable to hiring a dental hygienist as an employee and completing all collection services?

Box 22–1 Populations Needing Dental Hygiene Care

- People who are homebound
- People who live in institutions
- Populations with disabilities
- Residents of rural areas
- Prison inmates
- Populations with financial barriers

As a dental hygienist, never underestimate the importance of understanding which organizations will value dental hygiene services. Many individuals still do not know what a dental hygienist is, and many do not value preventive dental care. For these reasons, the dental hygienist must be clear in defining what services will be marketed.

Dental Hygiene Diagnosis

At this stage, the dental hygienist should develop a comprehensive dental hygiene diagnosis for the target population. For example, consider a dental hygiene diagnosis directed at a population employed by a major company (4000 employees). The company survey revealed that only 25 percent of the employees were currently seeking dental treatment (dental demand), either preventive or restorative, and that more than 500 days were lost to sick days due to toothaches (dental need). In addition, the company's on-site registered nurse calculated that 25 percent of visits made to her were for dental problems (dental need). A diagnosis of the population would therefore state that the population has tremendous dental needs (toothaches) but has a low dental demand because 75 percent were not seeking dental care.

Planning

The planning stage requires the prioritization of goals and objectives and the development of strategies and a program blueprint. This stage would address issues such as support of staff, space availability, reimbursement mechanisms, patient management systems, and dental health promotional activities. During the planning stage, **public relations,** the practice of managing the dispersion of information between an organization and its public, should also be made. Meeting with administrators and/or other interested parties contributes to effective and efficient planning. See Table 22-1 ■ for a detailed business plan of action for dental hygienists starting their own business.

Did You Know?

With a dental hygiene program, public relations can be defined as the process of strengthening ties with the population by promoting the value of a program through education.

Practice promotion occurs when the practice effectively markets its service. **Marketing** is an organized approach to selecting, servicing, and informing markets of a product or service as distinct from an impromptu approach to selling a service. The purpose of marketing a dental hygiene practice is to have patients select the practice for their dental hygiene care. The four Ps of marketing include products/service, price, plan for distribution, and promotion. See Table 22-2 ■ for more information on marketing strategies for a dental hygiene practice.[4]

Implementation

Implementation refers to carrying out a plan and involves the actual program operation and generally includes

Table 22–1 American Dental Hygienists' Association's Business Plan

Business Plan	What It Really Means
Service development	Continually refining what you are providing/selling to meet the changing needs of your potential clients
Marketing	Continually taking action to become more aware of your clients' needs and informing your potential clients why to use your service
Sales	Talking face-to-face with your potential clients and getting them to retain your services
Operations	Doing the work of the business, everything from answering the telephone to working directly with patients
Personnel	Managing the people who work with you
Finance	Measuring the financial results of your business, comparing them with your desired results, and using this comparison to identify critical business issues
Management	Making sure the preceding six areas are working in concert to meet your goals for the business

Source: http://members.adha.org/script/content/fetch.cfm?file=ADHA_marketing_workbook.pdf. Accessed July 2, 2009.

Table 22–2 Marketing a Dental Hygiene Practice

Service Line	Funding Mechanisms
• Quality dental hygiene services • Possible comprehensive dental services • Or referral mechanism for comprehensive dental services • Services will decrease infection and pain and should improve overall health	• Public or private dental insurance • Private donations/subsidies • Public grant opportunities
Infrastructure	**Advertisement**
• Specify practice setting, location, and hours • Workforce, to include providers and staff support • Collaboration within health system	• Promote quality image of program • Promote dental health as part of overall health • Continue to engage partners and stakeholders to promote program

Source: Adapted from Kotler P. *Marketing for Nonprofit Organizations.* Upper Saddle River, NJ: Prentice Hall; 1982.

revisions as needed. During implementation, the dental hygienist should manage the program, which can entail collaborating and sometimes supervising people. See Box 22-2 ■ for specific management skills needed. Evaluation during this process helps focus on the plan.

Evaluation

During evaluation, which should be continuous, the program's intended outcomes are measured and possibly revised. Measurement is performed by using dental indexes, records, and surveys. Moreover, other entities within the organization can be helpful at providing information concerning continuing unmet needs.

Providing administrators with written documented and oral reports concerning the measurement of the program's outcomes and revisions is vital. These reports emphasize the importance of the dental hygiene program and maintain its visibility. Additionally, reports can be a testament to its value. Ongoing communication and reporting to patients and other health care providers are equally necessary so that needed revisions can be made.

Box 22–2 Skills Involved in Managing Programs

- Leadership
  - Coordinating effective change
  - Motivating personnel
  - Making logical, effective decisions
- Management
  - Coordinating all operations
  - Providing comprehensive resource management
  - Implementing personnel evaluation and supervision
  - Using effective problem solving
  - Using effective conflict resolution
- Planning
  - Performing long-term strategic planning
  - Performing short-term strategic planning
  - Formulating policies and procedures
  - Determining evaluation measurements
  - Planning for effective and logical decision-making practices by all

DENTAL HYGIENIST SPOTLIGHT

Public Health Column: C. Austin Risbeck, RDH

C. Austin Risbeck, RDH, is experiencing a fulfilling career that combines private practice and public health opportunities. Although he works in a progressive private practice, he has formed his own company to promote public health and has won several awards related to it. He has spoken throughout the country and published numerous articles in various dental hygiene periodicals. Mr. Risbeck has decided to respond to a number of challenges in dental hygiene, and the public is certainly benefiting.

Why did you decide to go into dental hygiene?

At the age of nineteen, I joined the Army to become a dental assistant. After a few years as a dental assistant, my next step up the military career ladder was dental hygiene school. At the time, I thought it was a

way to get promoted. I had no idea what my future as a dental hygienist would entail.

How did you get into dental public health? Did you need additional education?

During National Dental Hygiene Month in 2000, the ADHA theme was "Want Some Life-Saving Advice? Ask Your Dental Hygienist," stressing the importance of oral health to total health. I was not prepared to educate my patients about the oral-systemic connection, so I ordered a copy of *Oral Health in America: A Report of the Surgeon General*. This publication opened my eyes to the ongoing research regarding the connection between chronic oral infections and other health problems including heart disease, diabetes, and adverse pregnancy outcomes. One major theme in this publication is "Lifestyle behaviors that affect general health such as tobacco use, excessive alcohol use, and poor dietary choices affect oral and craniofacial health as well." As a health care provider, I assumed the responsibility of promoting healthy lifestyles by incorporating tobacco cessation and nutritional counseling into my clinical practice. I want my patients to benefit from the research regarding the connection between periodontal disease and systemic conditions. I emphasize the importance of maintaining periodontal health.

We don't need additional education to improve and promote oral health. We need to work together with other health care providers to broaden the public's understanding of the importance of oral health and its relevance to systemic health. However, I am planning to pursue a master's degree in public health soon.

What are your current positions?

I serve as a member of the ADHA Council on Public Health, ADHA Tobacco Cessation Task Force, and California Dental Hygienists' Association (CDHA) Public Health Council, as a California Tobacco Cessation liaison, and I am a consultant to the Smoking Cessation Leadership Center and a continuing education provider. I am owner of a consulting firm that provides tobacco cessation, nutrition resources, and other educational information to local, state, and national organizations. I currently work at The Center for Aesthetic Dentistry in San Francisco as a clinical dental hygienist three days a week and as a consultant from home the rest of the week. This includes weekend work sometimes, but it's worth it! My firm provided the resources and helped with the design of the ADHA's "Ask. Advise. Refer." Web site. In 2004 and 2005, I designed several Web pages as part of CDHA's public health Web site to provide dental hygienists the resources to help their patients quit using tobacco, eat better, and manage their diabetes and to help hygienists include oral cancer, diet, and blood pressure screening as part of their dental hygiene appointments.

Can you discuss any particularly interesting experiences you've had in your dental public health positions?

In April 2004, I attended and provided a poster for the second national Steps to a HealthierUS Prevention Summit in Baltimore, Maryland. This national summit created by former Secretary of the Department of Health and Human Services Tommy Thompson focused on chronic disease prevention and health promotion. It featured presentations on obesity, diabetes, heart disease, stroke, and cancer as well as lifestyle choices including tobacco use, nutrition, and physical activity. The Steps to a HealthierUS program aims to help Americans live longer and healthier lives by reducing the burdens of diabetes, overweight, and obesity and through tobacco cessation, healthy eating, and physical activity.

As the only dental hygienist at this national summit with more than 1400 participants, I was asked by two participants, "What is a dental hygienist doing at a prevention summit?" and "Why does a dental hygienist need to know about nutrition?" I loved these questions. I answered that dental hygienists are now involved in treating tobacco use and dependence and have long been involved in nutritional counseling and blood pressure screening. By providing these services and obtaining a comprehensive health history, dental hygienists can establish the presence or risk of chronic disease and refer those who are at risk to an appropriate medical provider.

I gathered my information from many sources that suggest:

- "Dental hygienists have more interaction time with their patients than other health care providers, and their patients visit them two to four times per year as they perceive themselves as healthy."
- "Dental hygienists can expand their role to help other health professionals with the responsibility of achieving and maintaining the total health of the public."
- "Dental hygienists can expand health promotion and chronic disease prevention efforts by incorporating tobacco cessation, nutritional counseling, and blood pressure screening into their practices."
- "Many diabetics, or those at risk for diabetes, do not regularly visit a primary care provider but may seek the services of a dental hygienist."

- "Dental hygienists are well positioned to deliver prevention messages, communicate the need for metabolic control, and facilitate multidisciplinary diabetes care."
- "By all of us working together and sharing our expertise and experiences, we can all improve quality of life and reduce the burden of chronic diseases in America."

These two participants replied that they had no idea. At the Steps to a HealthierUS Summit, Secretary Thompson released Prevention: A Blueprint for Action. This US Department of Health and Human Services' Steps to a HealthierUS Initiative outlines simple steps that people can take to promote healthy lifestyles. I brought this blueprint to the CDHA leadership, who implemented an effective weight-reducing initiative and continued to promote a smoking cessation initiative called The New California Gold Rush. CDHA is committed to informing and educating individuals about the importance of healthy eating, regular physical activity, disease screening, and avoiding risky behaviors such as tobacco use to promote health and prevent chronic disease.

What advice would you give a practicing hygienist who is thinking of doing something different?

Dental hygienists are teachers and educators. An exciting way to teach colleagues and the public is by publishing articles in scientific and peer-reviewed journals and taking continuing education courses.

Source: Christine Nathe writes the Public Health Column in *RDH* magazine published by Pennwell Publishing. For more public health spotlights please see RDH magazine online at http://www.rdhmag.com/index.html.

Documentation and Practice Management

During the planning stage, issues involving the effective ongoing operation of a dental hygiene practice—known as **practice management,** which is the process of planning, organizing, and managing resources to bring about the successful completion of specific project goals and objectives—should be defined and then further refined during the implementation and evaluation stages. These issues can include tracking patients, scheduling appointments, promoting practice, and collecting fees. Documentation including electronic or written patient records are extremely important in dental hygiene treatment. Information in these records should be comprehensive and include patient contact information (address, phone numbers, and other pertinent information); health history; dental hygiene assessments, diagnoses, planning, implementation, and evaluative documentation; and financial records. Maintaining accurate records is imperative and serves to enhance the operation.

Did You Know?

Practice management deals with issues involving a program's effective ongoing operation.

Effective appointment scheduling improves practice operations by decreasing patients' wait time and increasing productivity. Appointment scheduling could become more complicated in health care settings if patients have made arrangements for health care treatment a number of times during the day. Therefore, it could be beneficial to integrate appointment scheduling procedures within the institution.

Proposal Development and Presentation

Refer to Box 22-3 ■ for an example of a **proposal**—a written description of a planned program or project—for example, a dental hygiene position in a nursing facility, intended to motivate an entity such as the administrators or other decision makers to adopt a program or project, such as to open a dental hygiene position. The proposal should always include an introduction stating the dental hygiene program's purpose and a statement of the significance of the suggested dental hygiene position.

A program's **blueprint**—a skeletal framework developed before implementing a program—should include a detailed budget and financing section. Specific teaching strategies will help the dental hygienist effectively present the proposal. The reader should be able to read a paragraph or two and understand the program's basic premise. The conclusion should summarize the important points and convince the reader on the need for this specific program.

Generally, ten to fifteen minutes are allowed for this presentation. Using a proposal handout and possibly a PowerPoint presentation can greatly enhance the attractiveness of the position. To sell the service, dental hygienists must be prepared and organized in addition to using effective and appropriate media. See Chapter 9 for more tips on effective presentation strategies.

Dental Hygiene Consultation and Policies

Contracts between a dental hygienist and nursing facility for the dental hygienist's services can be developed according to facility policies and procedures. Many times a dental hygienist can be hired as staff of the facility, or the

Box 22–3 Proposal to Fones Nursing Facility for the Establishment of a Dental Hygiene Program

Introduction

This proposal addresses the recognition of the oral health care needs of elderly people, the institution of a preventive dental program, and the addition of a contract dental hygienist. Dental hygienists have the scientific background and clinical skills to initiate dental programs in long-term care facilities; therefore, it is the intention of this proposal to clarify the procedures necessary to establish a dental hygiene position.

Significance

The relationship that exists between oral health and systemic health has been verified and well documented. Additionally, certain physiological changes occur in the oral cavities of elderly people, including loss of teeth, recession of gums, and teeth that are becoming brittle and more prone to chipping and cracking. Due to the loss of muscle tone about the face and mouth, other conditions such as cheilosis (cracking in the corners of the mouth), flaccid tongue, and epulis fissuratum (growths due to ill-fitting dentures) occur. As a result of aging or certain medication, xerostomia, or drying of the oral tissues, also can exist, causing discomfort, difficulty in speaking, loss of taste sensations, high incidence of gum-line cavities, and discomfort in denture wearers, to mention only a few problems.

In addition, dentures may cause serious conditions if they do not fit properly and can be a factor in oral cancer, which comes from the continual irritation of the soft tissue. The importance of examining the soft tissues of the face, neck, lips, and the structures inside the mouth cannot be adequately stressed. The incidence of oral cancer increases with age and detection and prompt treatment make a difference in the prognosis of cancer.

Dental Hygiene Program

As a member of the health team and in collaboration with the dentist, the dental hygienist performs necessary procedures for total patient care. These services include counseling and instructing patients, conducting regularly scheduled in-service programs for the nursing staff, and providing preventive clinical services such as intra- and extraoral examinations, scaling (teeth cleaning), nonsurgical periodontal therapy, radiographs, fluoride treatments to desensitize exposed roots, denture care, denture labeling, and referral either to the patients' private dentist or to the facility's dental consultant. Moreover, the dental hygienist formulates a recall system by which annual and admission exams are regularly performed to meet federal and state health requirements.

A dental hygienist registered in New Mexico may be licensed to work in collaboration with a dentist. Therefore, employing a dental hygienist in a nursing home is legally permissible in New Mexico. Many dental hygienists are employed in nursing homes in different states. A contract dental hygienist may be reimbursed through Medicaid or fees charged directly to the patient for services provided, thus decreasing cost to the nursing home.

Conclusion

The quality of care provided to the residents of an institution is a priority of both the administration and staff. However, dental care often is not a priority and sometimes neglected. The dental hygienist contracted to work would improve and expand the quality of care, which would be beneficial to the staff, administration, and, most importantly, the residents of a nursing facility. This contract position, which provides necessary preventive dental care, can become an integral part of existing interdisciplinary comprehensive services.

Source: Modified from Dental Advisory Role, Suzann C. Chenery, RDH, BS, Ashlar of Newtown, CT; 1990.

facility could choose to contract with the dental hygienist for these services. Box 22-4 ■ is a sample policy statement for providing dental hygiene services. It can serve as an example for the dental hygienist in developing specific institutional policy. Finally, a beneficial addition to the dental hygiene program is the use of dental hygiene

Box 22–4 Policy for Dental Hygiene Services

Dental hygiene services are available to residents on specified dates and times.

Residents must consent to these services. Services provided by the dental hygienist include:

- Obtaining medical clearance from resident's physician prior to treatment
- Consultation and coordination with facility dentist or the resident's private dentist to obtain comprehensive dental care
- Document all examinations and treatment rendered
- Coordinate communications between the nursing staff, the facility dentist, and resident physicians
- Initiate and reevaluate the dental recall system
- Provision of all dental hygiene services as defined in the state practice act

Source: Modified from Dental Hygiene Services, Suzann C. Chenery, RDH, BS, Ashlar of Newtown, CT; 1990.

students, which can bring motivation and a learning initiative to the program. Colleges and universities will have their own agreements that can be adapted per facility.

Summary

When deciding whether to start a dental hygiene practice in a public health setting, dental hygienists should consider their clinical skills as well as communication skills, motivation skills, knowledge of health and wellness, assessment and treatment-planning skills, and an interdisciplinary team approach to providing care. Dental hygienists can adapt these skills to working with the public in a wide variety of settings.

Author's Note

For dental hygienists interested in entrepreneurial skills please see ADHA's career resource center at http://careers.adha.org/jobseekers/resources/. Another great resource is the ADHA Careers in Public Health Presentation available at http://www.adha.org/resources-docs/7781_Careers_in_Public_Health_Presentation.pdf.

Self-Study Test Items

1. Members of the public, government agencies, and other health care professionals, as well as the dental hygiene profession itself, are showing significant interest in establishing dental hygiene programs in settings other than private dental offices. Many states have expanded the dental hygienists' scope of practice.
   a. The first statement is true; the second statement is false.
   b. The first statement is false; the second statement is true.
   c. Both statements are true.
   d. Both statements are false.

2. What may be necessary to increase dental hygienists' accessibility to the underserved public?
   a. Marketing promotion
   b. Blueprint development
   c. Legislative initiatives
   d. None of the above

3. During which phase should a target population's needs be determined?
   a. Assessment
   b. Dental hygiene diagnosis
   c. Planning
   d. Implementation

4. Continually refining the product is which part of the business plan?
   a. Service development
   b. Marketing
   c. Sales
   d. Operations

5. Which phase involves prioritizing goals and objectives?
   a. Assessment
   b. Dental hygiene diagnosis
   c. Planning
   d. Implementation

References

1. Nathe C. National Dental Public Health Educator's Workshop *Dental*. Albuquerque, NM: University of New Mexico; 2014.
2. *A Resource Guide for Dental Hygienists in Non-traditional Settings*. Nepean, Canada: Ontario Dental Hygienists' Association; 1998.
3. Nathe C. Dental hygienists: a needed reality [editorial]. *Contact International*. 1998;12:3.
4. Kotler P. *Marketing for Nonprofit Organizations*. Upper Saddle River, NJ: Prentice Hall; 1982.

Visit www.pearsonhighered.com/healthprofessionsresources to access the student resources that accompany this book. Simply select Dental Hygiene from the choice of disciplines. Find this book and you will find the complimentary study tools created for this specific title.

23

Dental Public Health Review

Meg Zayan, RDH, MPH, EdD

OBJECTIVES

After studying the chapter, the dental hygiene student should be able to:

- Describe the National Board Dental Hygiene Examination dental public health format
- Identify topics that may appear on this examination
- Identify strategies for studying for the dental public health section of boards
- Review sample test items

COMPETENCIES

After studying the chapter and participating in accompanying course activities, the dental hygiene student should be competent to do the following:

- Apply a professional code of ethics in all endeavors
- Use critical thinking skills and comprehensive problem-solving to identify oral health care strategies that promote patient health and wellness
- Use evidence-based decision making to evaluate emerging technology and treatment modalities to integrate into patient dental hygiene care plans to achieve high-quality, cost-effective care
- Assume responsibility for professional actions and care based on accepted scientific theories, research, and the accepted standard of care
- Continuously perform self-assessment for lifelong learning and professional growth

(continued)

KEY TERMS

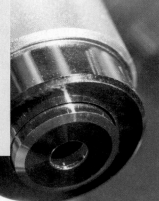

Science photo/Shutterstock

- Integrate accepted scientific theories and research into educational, preventive, and therapeutic oral health services
- Promote the values of the dental hygiene profession through service-based activities, positive community affiliations, and active involvement in local organizations
- Apply quality assurance mechanisms to ensure continuous commitment to accepted standards of care
- Communicate effectively with diverse individuals and groups, serving all persons without discrimination by acknowledging and appreciating diversity
- Record accurate, consistent and complete documentation of oral health services provided
- Initiate a collaborative approach with all patients when developing individualized care plans that are specialized, comprehensive, culturally sensitive, and acceptable to all parties involved in care planning
- Initiate consultations and collaborations with all relevant health care providers to facilitate optimal treatments
- Promote positive values of overall health and wellness to the public and organizations within and outside the profession
- Respect the goals, values, beliefs, and preferences of all patients
- Identify individual and population risk factors, and develop strategies that promote health-related quality of life
- Evaluate factors that can be used to promote patient adherence to disease prevention or health maintenance strategies
- Utilize methods that ensure the health and safety of the patient and the oral health professional in the delivery of care

- Assess the oral health needs and services of the community to determine action plans and availability of resources to meet the health care needs
- Provide screening, referral and educational services that allow patients to access the resources of the health care system
- Provide community oral health services in a variety of settings
- Facilitate patient access to oral health services by influencing individuals or organizations for the provision of oral health care
- Evaluate reimbursement mechanisms and their impact on the patient's access to oral health care.
- Evaluate the outcomes of community-based programs, and plan for future activities
- Advocate for effective oral health care for underserved populations
- Determine the outcomes of dental hygiene interventions using indices, instruments, examination techniques, and patient self-reports as specified in patient goals
- Compare actual outcomes to expected outcomes, reevaluating goals, diagnoses, and services when expected outcomes are not achieved
- Pursue career opportunities within health care, industry, education, research, and other roles as they evolve for the dental hygienist
- Develop practice management and marketing strategies to be used in the delivery of oral health care
- Access professional and social networks to pursue professional goals

Specific dental hygiene **licensure requirements,** which are the requirements dental hygienists must meet to obtain a dental hygiene license to practice in each state, vary among states, but all states have four types: (1) an **educational requirement,** which is the requirement of how much instruction and what type of degree a dental hygienist must receive, (2) a **written examination requirement,** which is the written examination a dental hygienist must pass before becoming eligible for a dental hygiene license, (3) **jurisprudence requirement,** which is the required reading and possible examination of state laws governing dental hygiene practice, and (4) a **clinical examination requirement,** which is the clinical board requirement, which is mandatory in all states. The **National Board Dental Hygiene Examination,** which is the examination given by the American Dental Association to fulfill the written examination requirement, is intended to fulfill or partially fulfill the written examination requirements, but acceptance of a national board score is completely at the discretion of the states. Alabama is the only state that does not require a dental hygiene candidate to pass the National Board Dental Hygiene Examination.

This chapter reviews the community health/research principles section of the National Dental Hygiene Board

Examination given by the American Dental Association's **Joint Commission on National Dental Examinations,** the agency responsible for the development and administration of the National Board Dental Examinations.[1] The commission includes representatives of dental and dental hygiene schools, dental and dental hygiene practice, state dental examining boards, and the public. After completing a course in dental public health and during the crucial period of studying for boards, students can use this chapter as a study guide.

Did You Know?

Students can get up-to-date information regarding the content and format of the national examination for dental hygienists by going onto the American Dental Association Web site at www.ada.org.

Study Guide

The board exam is comprehensive and consists of approximately 350 multiple-choice test items. It has two components. The discipline-based component includes 200 items addressing the scientific basis for dental hygiene practice (anatomic sciences, physiology, biochemistry, nutrition, microbiology, immunology, pathology, and pharmacology); provision of clinical dental hygiene clinical services (patient assessments, radiology, dental hygiene care, periodontology, dental biomaterials, and professional responsibility); and community health/research principles (dental public health science).

The second component includes 150 case-based items that refer to patient cases. See Box 23-1 ■ (for the composition

Box 23–1 Compilation of Examination Specifics

Community Health Research Principles (24)
a. Promoting Health and Preventing Disease Within Groups (6)
b. Participating in Community Programs (10)
   1. Assessing populations and defining objectives
   2. Designing, implementing, and evaluating programs
c. Analyzing Scientific Information, Understanding Statistical Concepts, and Applying Research Results (8)

of items in the community dental health/research principles category for the exam. This section of the exam is written using a **testlet** format that introduces a case study involving an issue pertinent to dental public health. The testlets are written in paragraph form followed by a series of multiple-choice questions. (See Table 23-1 ■) The target populations often mentioned in these testlets may involve persons in programs such as Head Start; preschool/elementary/middle/high school; substance abuse; geriatric (nursing homes, senior day cares, senior centers); people who are physically or mentally challenged; teen pregnancy; veterans; immigrants; ethnic groups; prisoners; migrant farmers; sport teams; caregivers; forensic; and special needs. The best preparation methods include the suggestions in Box 23-2 ■.

Test-Taking Strategies

First and foremost when taking an exam, prepare in advance and use your time wisely. Attempt to answer all questions

Table 23–1 Sample Item Format

For national board use, a multiple-choice item must have at least three and not more than five possible answers. Only one of the possible answers listed is correct.

Format	Definition
Completion	Requires correctly finishing a statement regarding a concept or idea
Question	Communicates a problem or set of circumstances
Negative	Includes a word such as *except* or *not* in capital letters and/or italics in the stem
Paired true-false	Varies only in the stem, which consists of two sentences on the same topic
Cause-and-effect	Varies only in the stem, which consists of a statement and reason written as a single sentence and connected by *because*
Testlet	Begins with a case study or problem associated with a group of test items; used exclusively for the Community Health/Research Principles and case-based sections.

Source: American Dental Association. *National Board Dental Hygiene Examination. 2015 Guide.* Chicago, IL: American Dental Association; 2015.

Box 23–2 Suggestions for Exam Preparation

- Be prepared, which will increase your confidence.
- Organize your notes from dental hygiene school and prerequisite classes.
- Outline notes in a manner that works well for you.
- When reviewing notes, look up in text books or Internet any information that is still unclear.
- Review key concepts from professors.
- Review previous board examination questions.
- Study with groups and by yourself.

even if you hope to go back to a question later. Look for logical clues and a word or concept repeated in both the question and the answer. Also look at the length of the responses; often the correct response is the longest. Eliminate potential answers involving contradictory answers.

Specific types of test items can be answered more effectively when you understand the test item model. Multiple-choice test items evaluate knowledge and understanding of specific concepts. These items are composed of a stem, which poses a problem and a list of possible answers to that problem. The stem may be a question, a statement, or an incomplete sentence. Only one of the possible answers is correct; the other answers are called *distractors*.

Did You Know?

The ADHA offers a National Board Review course online as a benefit to dental hygiene students. Please see www .adha.org for more information.

Key Concepts

The community dental activities section on the exam generally covers key concepts such as the following.

Promoting Health and Preventing Disease Within Groups

- The overall goal of dental public health programs is to reduce oral disease.
- The major aspect of dental public health programs is promotion and prevention. These are accomplished through activities to enhance positive behavior, education, and clinical services.
- *Dental health education* is defined as the teaching of oral health behaviors whereas *dental health promotion* is defined as informing and motivating individuals to adopt healthy behaviors.
- In areas where dental public health programs are indicated, the demand for dental care is low but the need is high. It is the intent of public health programs

to achieve a higher demand for dental care and to decrease the need.

- Dental public health dental hygienists should concentrate on teaching those individuals who work closely with the target population including teachers, caregivers, nurse assistants, and more.
- State dental health departments' primary purpose is to serve as a consultant regarding state dental issues for public and private health care.
- When teaching a population to adopt positive dental health behaviors, the values they may hold concerning oral health need to be changed.
- Behavior change will not be attained until value adoption is complete; providing dental health education to a population does not ensure behavior change.
- When distributing educational materials, be careful to critique them beforehand to make sure they are not blatantly promoting a dental care product, and, most importantly, that they have factual information that is not misleading.
- Community water fluoridation has proven to be cost effective although opponents may feel that fluoridation itself violates human rights and/or personal freedom.
- Advocates of community water fluoridation may find developing long-term strategies for adoption to be beneficial.

Participating in Community Programs, Assessing Populations and Defining Objectives, and Designing, Implementing, and Evaluating Programs

- Assessment of populations and defining objectives are important factors in such programs.
- Establishing community programs involves designing, implementing, and evaluating programs.
- Planning consists of determining consumer needs, which a dental professional can diagnose as compared with consumer demands, which can be defined as the frequency of dental visits or attempted dental visits.
- Program planning should include the dental hygiene process of care including assessment, dental hygiene diagnosis, planning, implementation, evaluation and documentation. Many public health paradigms place the diagnosis stage in the planning stage.
- Prioritizing is a necessary component during the dental hygiene diagnosis and planning stages of program development.
- Program planning should include developing measurable objectives so that the program can be effectively evaluated and measured.
- To increase participation in a program, having personal contact with the target population is beneficial.
- Dental hygienists should include the target population or its representatives when planning a dental public health program.

- Dental hygienists working with programs that target specific populations should include those populations' leaders during planning to obtain their support.
- When initiating a dental public health program, dental hygienists should contact the head administrator for approval and support.
- A dental sealant program should be planned to target children in the second through sixth grades to ensure they have fully erupted molars for placement of the sealants.
- Always have support from the target group. If a program involves parents, their support is crucial.

Analyzing Scientific Information, Understanding Statistical Concepts, and Applying Research Results

- *Prevalence* is the number of existing cases of a specific disease or condition in a population at a specific point in time.
- *Incidence* is the expression of the new number of cases of a disease or condition in a population at a specific point in time.
- *Mortality* is the ratio of the number of deaths from a specific disease to the total number of cases of that disease.
- *Morbidity* is the ratio of sick to well persons in a population.
- *Reliability* is the consistency or degree to which an instrument will produce the same results in the same population every time the characteristic is measured.
- *Validity* is the degree to which the research study measured what it was supposed to measure (internal) and that the study can be generalized to the entire population (external).
- A *pilot study* is a trial of a research study so its variables can best be controlled during the long-term study.
- The *dependent variable* is the measure as a result of the manipulation of the independent variable.
- *Independent variable* is the manipulated measure expected to be changed under the investigator's control.
- *Measures of central tendency,* including the mean, median, and mode, measure what is typical in the sample group.
- *Measures of dispersion,* including range, variance, and standard deviation, are used to describe the variability of scores in a distribution. If a relation has a normal distribution, it is a *normal bell curve.* If a relationship has a few extreme scores, it is *skewed.*
- *Correlation* is the determination of the strength of the linear relationship between two variables. The closer the number is to 1, the stronger is the relationship.
- Research studies utilize different approaches to sample the population.

Sample Questions

This section provides sample testlet questions that may be asked on the national examination. It is intended to familiarize you with necessary information about these items. Answers to the questions appear upside down at the bottom of each page.

Testlet 1 (Questions 1–5)

The Indian Health Service approached a state department of dental public health about establishing a caries prevention program in a Native American elementary school. The school consists of grades 1–6 with twenty-five to thirty students per grade. The community is not fluoridated, and local dentists are concerned about the high incidence of dental caries recognized during the past six years. The elementary school receives state and federal funding for health care services including nursing, dental, and nutritional care. Of these children, 30 percent receive Medicaid funding. The school employs a nurse full-time as well as a dental hygienist and nutritionist two days per week. A dentist volunteers his time one day per week. The Indian Health Service is asking for assistance in determining the needs of the schoolchildren and supporting the implementation of a program to reduce dental caries. It is asking for the program to include educational, therapeutic, and referral services.

1. What is the first step in developing a dental health prevention program for this school?
   a. Contacting the state's department of public health
   b. Identifying the students who will participate in the pilot study
   c. Meeting with the parents to identify the students' oral hygiene habits
   d. Selecting a data collection instrument to assess caries rate
   e. Obtaining informed consent from the parents of the students

2. Possible negative reactions and conflict could be avoided by obtaining which of the following:
   a. Permission from the board of dentistry
   b. Permission from the state department of education
   c. Support of the school nurse and teachers
   d. Support from the local dental hygiene association
   e. Permission from the governor

3. If it is determined that the school vending machines contain highly sugared snacks and the removal of these machines is approved, which of the following does this action exemplify?
   a. Health prevention
   b. Disease progression
   c. Health promotion
   d. Health services

4. In this nonfluoridated community, which of the following preventive dental health programs would have the maximum cost benefit for controlling caries in these elementary schoolchildren?
   a. Pit and fissure sealant program
   b. Fluoride mouth rinse program
   c. Restorative care program
   d. Parent-teacher education program

5. The primary purpose of referring indicated children to a dentist for treatment is to
   a. Provide a follow-up activity to the program
   b. Ensure that parents are aware of their children's dental needs
   c. Increase the probability that dental disease will be reduced
   d. Create an environment in which dentists are treating more patients

Testlet 2 (Questions 6–10)

The board of education approached a public health dental hygienist about establishing a dental health education curriculum for the students enrolled in a public school system. The board was concerned that the only dental health education students received was during Children's Dental Health Month when volunteer dental hygienists provided education to grades K, 3, 7, and 12. The classroom teachers were interested in implementing dental health education in the student's health classes but were looking for guidance with lesson plan content and activities. The school system consists of 3500 students, grades K–12. Health care facilities, including a nurse who is available twice a week, are available at each school.

6. The primary purpose of the public health dental hygienist is to
   a. Provide dental hygiene services to the public school students
   b. Provide age-appropriate dental health knowledge and preventive techniques to improve oral health
   c. Encourage more volunteer dental hygienists to visit all classes during Children's Dental Health Month
   d. Lobby the board of education to hire a dental hygienist to work on days when the nurse is not present at the public school

7. To fully understand the oral hygiene knowledge of the public school students, the dental hygienist should
   a. Perform DMFS on all students
   b. Conduct a caries-activity test
   c. Perform clinical examinations and radiographs
   d. Conduct a discussion group with all teachers
   e. Conduct an oral hygiene questionnaire for all students and teachers

8. When the classroom teachers discuss the importance of good oral hygiene habits and the prevention of dental disease during their health classes, which of the following is (are) the *best* technique(s) for teaching this material?
   a. Lecture and question–answer session
   b. Distribution of brochures and class activities
   c. Lecture only
   d. Lecture with slides and posters
   e. Lecture with slides, posters, and class activities

9. If more funding than currently allocated is needed, which of the following strategies is the most effective in obtaining additional financial support?
   a. Partnering with other community agencies to develop a collaborative request to local foundations
   b. Approaching local businesses and industries requesting program funds
   c. Engaging community churches to conduct fundraising efforts
   d. Sending high school students door-to-door in the affluent parts of the community to solicit funds

10. After the program has been developed, the *most* effective role for the public health dental hygienist would be as a (an)
    a. Major provider for classroom instruction
    b. Consultant for the parents
    c. Clinical chair-side instructor
    d. Evaluator of the program's success

Testlet 3 (Questions 11–15)

A dental hygienist employed by a dental clinic in a federal correctional institution is planning to implement a plaque control program for female prisoners. She has worked at the prison for three years and has noticed a high prevalence of gingival and periodontal disease. The prison warden has given her permission to develop a pilot program with funding for additional supplies and increased working hours. One of the first steps the dental hygienist performed was to distribute a survey to the seventy-five female prisoners involved in the pilot program. The questionnaire data indicated that 65 percent brush daily, 10 percent floss on a regular basis, and 80 percent of emergency dental cases are due to toothaches.

11. The primary purpose of implementing a pilot program is to
    a. Solicit more funding to implement the full program
    b. Encourage other federal prisons to implement similar programs into their dental clinics
    c. Perform the planned program on a small population to ascertain its success before performing it on a larger population
    d. Develop measurable objectives so that the program can be effectively evaluated

12. To further ascertain the dental needs of the prisoners, which of the following should be utilized?
    a. Pre-index scores for plaque and gingival and periodontal conditions
    b. A survey regarding prisoners' dental knowledge, values, and attitudes
    c. The level of prisoners' demand for dental care
    d. Financial resources in planning treatment for the dental clinic
    e. Access to care regarding clinic hours, payment, and prisoner schedules

13. The overall goal of this plaque control program is to
    a. Reduce the amount of gingival and periodontal diseases
    b. Increase the number of prisoners seeking dental treatment
    c. Increase the amount of practicing dentists in the clinic
    d. Decrease overall expenses of dental care in the clinic

14. The statistics regarding brushing, flossing, and emergency dental care visits imply that
    a. The need for dental care is lower than the demand for dental care
    b. The need for dental care is higher than the demand for dental care
    c. The need and the demand for dental care are equal

15. If additional funding is needed, which of the following governments should be helpful?
    a. Federal government
    b. State government
    c. Local government
    d. A partnership between state and local governments

Testlet 4 (Questions 16–20)

Several community dental hygienists conducted a five-year study on dental caries incidence rates in permanent teeth of school-age children. The study compared incidence rates of dental caries in students who received sealants and routine professional fluoride treatments to those for students who received professional fluoride treatments only. The study was conducted at a public school district whose population was 5000 students in grades K–12. At the beginning of the study, no schools in the district had fluoridated water, and fewer than 20 percent of the children attending these public schools had sealants.

To decrease the number of subjects involved in the study, a sample was taken from the 5000 students; however, students who did not have their permanent first molars could not participate. When those students without permanent first molars were eliminated, the remaining students were randomly selected from each grade level and classroom. The sample size then consisted of 2000 students K–12. The sample was then further divided into two groups: Group 1 received sealants at the start of the study and fluoride treatments every six months for five years. Group 2 received only fluoride treatments every six months for five years.

In addition, dental caries and plaque accumulation indexes were performed on both groups. A mean plaque index score of 2.6 (based on a 3.0 scale) was recorded for both Group 1 and Group 2, and at the end of the five years, the plaque index for Group 1 was 2.0 and for Group 2 was 2.3. There was high interrater reliability among the community dental hygienists.

16. What type of research study did the dental hygienists conduct?
    a. Historical
    b. Experimental
    c. Cross-sectional
    d. Descriptive

17. The mean plaque index score for both groups at the beginning of the study revealed that the students had
    a. No plaque
    b. Slight plaque
    c. Moderate plaque
    d. Severe plaque
    e. Cannot be determined

18. The type of sampling performed for this study suggests
    a. Random
    b. Systematic
    c. Stratified
    d. Convenience

19. The dependent variable that is investigated in this study is
    a. Dental caries
    b. Fluoride treatments
    c. Occlusal sealants
    d. Gingivitis

20. The best way to gather information about the students' knowledge of dental health care is by
    a. Interviewing each student regarding oral hygiene habits
    b. Utilizing a plaque and calculus index
    c. Performing a DMFT survey
    d. Conducting a questionnaire

Testlet 5 (Questions 21–25)

Three state public health dental hygienists are identifying oral health needs of persons residing in state-subsidized drug and alcohol rehabilitation centers. One study compared oral lesions in persons who smoke cigarettes to those who do not smoke. This study was performed in three state rehabilitation centers, and patient selection was done in alphabetical order by choosing every third individual from the patient list. The two dental hygienists who worked jointly for one day at each of the three sites calibrated the index.

21. The type of research utilized in this study is
    a. Historical
    b. Descriptive
    c. Experimental
    d. Ex post facto

22. The research design is an example of what type of epidemiologic study?
    a. Cross-sectional
    b. Prospective cohort
    c. Case–control
    d. Longitudinal

23. Which of the following is characteristic of the type of sampling used in these data?
    a. Stratified
    b. Simple random
    c. Convenience
    d. Systematic

24. The dental hygienists established the research hypothesis as "there is no significant correlation between cigarette smoking and oral lesions." This is an example of what type of hypothesis?
    a. Positive
    b. Correlational
    c. Null

25. When the dental hygienists select the most effective index to measure oral lesions, which of the following is a necessary criterion?
    a. Predictability of outcome
    b. Ease in calibration
    c. Flexibility in measurement

Testlet 6 (Questions 26–30)

A dental hygienist was asked to plan an in-service program to present to a group of nursing assistants in a 200-bed nursing home. Its overall purpose was to improve the residents' oral hygiene status by teaching proper toothbrushing. Using a written questionnaire, the dental hygienist first surveyed the nursing assistants concerning their understanding of dental health concepts. Following compilation and evaluation of the answers, the dental hygienist planned the program including writing goals and objectives to be met.

26. Which of the following private practice activities do these activities parallel?
    a. History taking and diagnosis
    b. Diagnosis and treatment planning
    c. History taking, diagnosis, and treatment planning
    d. History taking, diagnosis, and evaluation
    e. History taking, treatment planning, implementation, and evaluation

27. Before initiating the in-service training program, the dental hygienist should confer with whom?
    a. Nursing home residents
    b. Residents' family members
    c. Nursing home administrator and consulting dentist
    d. Local dental hygienist association board members

28. Utilizing the cognitive learning model, the intended outcome for this program is
    a. Knowledge
    b. Behavioral change
    c. Attitude

29. In writing a behavioral objective, the verb should indicate what the learner is expected to do. Which of the following is the best learner performance verb?
    a. To believe
    b. To know
    c. To demonstrate
    d. To understand
    e. To feel

30. The more specific are the objectives, the more effective the intent will be communicated to the nursing assistants. In-service evaluation is more effective without objectives.
    a. The first statement is true; the second statement is false.
    b. The first statement is false; the second statement is true.
    c. Both statements are true.
    d. Both statements are false.

Testlet 7 (Questions 31–35)

A high school class of twelve physically challenged students, fourteen to nineteen years of age, shows a need for improved oral hygiene. The high school nurse has asked the district dental hygienist to assess their needs and to work with the nurse to implement a dental public health program for these students. The dental hygienist plans to set up a portable dental unit to orally screen the students and to implement an evaluative tool to understand the dental health knowledge of the group. In addition, the

dental hygienist plans to provide oral hygiene instruction each month during the remainder of the school year, and the nurse will follow up with the instructions once a week. The Patient Hygiene Performance (PHP) scores during the initial assessment of the class were 2.5, 2.75, 1.5, 3.0, 2.5, 2.0, 2.5, 2.75, 2.5, 2.5, 2.0, and 3.0. The mean OHI-S score of the twelve individuals was 4.8.

31. A complete dental assessment of the class should include all of the following *except* one. Which one is the *exception*?
    a. Plaque and gingival scores
    b. Dental hygiene treatment needs
    c. Individual dexterity skills
    d. Familial income and education level
    e. Level of physical disabilities

32. Based on the severity of the physical disabilities, the dental hygienist may need to make accommodations for all of the following *except* one. Which one is the *exception*?
    a. Oral hygiene instruction
    b. Transportation to area dentists if needed
    c. Utilization of the portable dental chair
    d. Selection of dental indices

33. Which of the following represents the mean PHP score?
    a. 2.45
    b. 2.0
    c. 2.75
    d. 2.25
    e. 2.95

34. Which of the following PHP scores represents the mode?
    a. 1.5
    b. 2.0
    c. 2.5
    d. 2.75
    e. 3.0

35. When performing a correlation test between the debris and calculus scores of this class, the correlation coefficient was +.94. The relationship between gingival disease and plaque accumulation according to this test is statistically
    a. Strong
    b. Moderate
    c. Weak
    d. Not correlated

Testlet 8 (Questions 36–40)

A dental product company became concerned with the number of dental staff personnel and patients with sensitivity to its low-cost latex gloves. Its research department investigated the need to eliminate all latex from its products. It sent a questionnaire to 250 dental offices throughout the United States that had large accounts with the company. Although most mailings were randomly selected, the department ensured that any dental office that had reported sensitivity receive the questionnaire. Its overall purpose was to determine the degree of people experiencing sensitivity, the possible causes of the latex sensitivity, and ways to prevent it. The questionnaire requested data on the dermatological signs and symptoms, medical gloves used, foods commonly eaten, other personal hygiene products used, medical care received, and health history.

36. What is the primary focus of this research questionnaire?
    a. Assessment and evaluation
    b. Service and education
    c. Therapy and promotion
    d. Referral and treatment

37. What type of research study is being conducted?
    a. Experimental
    b. Ex post facto
    c. Historical
    d. Descriptive

38. This study's overall effectiveness can be best measured by
    a. Its length
    b. Its cost
    c. The number of participants involved
    d. The degree to which the study met its objectives

39. If the research department of this dental product company concludes that a high prevalence of latex sensitivity has been reported, this should be interpreted as follows:
    a. A high number of new cases of latex sensitivity have been reported during the year.
    b. A high number of dental staff personnel and patients are sensitive to latex gloves.
    c. Many dental staff personnel are choosing alternative solutions to latex gloves.
    d. Patients are refusing to have dental office personnel wear gloves from this company.

40. What is the best action for this dental product company based on the high prevalence rate and low cost of latex gloves?
    a. Continue making only latex gloves and target sales to those not sensitive to latex
    b. Find a nonlatex product regardless of price and recall all latex gloves
    c. Continue making latex gloves and offer an alternative type of glove
    d. Change nothing at this time and have the research department continue sending out questionnaires

Testlet 9 (Questions 41–45)

A public health educator received a request to develop an employee worksite training at a company whose workers have a high rate of diabetes and obesity. Ninety two percent (92%) of the employees are residents of the community where the company is located. Based on your knowledge of disease trends for this area, you also suspect a high rate of

periodontal disease and dental caries. As part of your planning process, you consult the *Healthy People 2020* document and decide on ways to engage the adult learner. When trying to schedule a common meeting time for all employees to attend, you are finding it difficult to meet everyone's requests.

41. When prioritizing the employee health needs, problems that should be addressed first are those that are
    a. Changeable and important
    b. Not changeable and important
    c. High risk and relevant
    d. Low risk and relevant

42. Which federal government agency is primarily responsible for *Healthy People 2020*?
    a. Centers for Disease Control
    b. Office of Disease Prevention and Health Promotion
    c. US Consumer Product Safety Commission
    d. National Institutes of Health

43. Due to the difficulty in finding one common meeting time for all employees to attend the training, which of the following is the best option?
    a. Conduct a series of seminars at the company, with make-up sessions for those who cannot make the meetings
    b. Create an interactive distance learning module that employees can complete as they have time
    c. Create a pamphlet with tips on ways to eat healthy that can be distributed to employees
    d. Create a cookbook with healthy recipes for the employees to use

44. The public health educator plans to reach outside the company and raise more public awareness using resources such as a press release, letters to the newspaper, and interactive Web resources. This type of advocacy is referred to as
    a. Clinical advocacy
    b. Policy advocacy
    c. Media advocacy
    d. Legislative advocacy

45. Due to the success of the training with this company, three other companies request worksite training. Company One is a large company where employee health is relatively good. Company Two is a smaller company that has high health care costs and high absenteeism among employees. Company Three wants a training seminar on any health topic in order to fulfill policy requirements for employee training. Based on the urgency of the need for education and the potential impact on the organization, which company should be top priority for training?
    a. Company One
    b. Company Two
    c. Company Three

Reference

1. http://www.ada.org/en/jcnde/examinations/national-board-dental-hygiene-examination/

Table Clinic Presentation

A *table clinic* is a presentation on a tabletop booth setting that uses both verbal communication and visual aids to disseminate a review of the literature on a specific topic (Figure A-1 ■). The presentation may include slides, graphs, and/or pictures displayed on the poster board. The length of a typical table clinic presentation is five to seven minutes. The topic chosen may be a technique, theory, service, trend, or career opportunity in the practice of dental hygiene. See Box A-1 ■ for tips on preparing a table clinic.

Research

Students can share information regarding research. It is inevitable that as health care professionals, dental hygienists will be questioned about oral care products and specific techniques. The information gathered during a table clinic is a perfect way to formulate recommendations about issues that may arise.

After choosing a topic, select a theme. Brainstorm for ideas. When researching the topic, use all available resources. The internet, practicing providers and school libraries are great places to gather information. Make sure to include research on pubmed to get up to date information. Include journals, newspapers, and videos; contacting companies directly is a fantastic way to get information. Remember to keep a list of all of resources because this will be needed to share information ina handout that includes the main concepts of the topic. In addition, other professionals may ask where the information was obtained.

Visual Display

Next, is the preparation of the poster board. The purpose of the visual media is to inform, clarify, and/or review specific material. Begin by looking at arts and crafts stores or stores that cater to teachers. Items such as foam board, stick-on lettering, artwork, and crepe or construction paper can usually be found in these stores. Next, have pictures or graphs enlarged, copied, or colored at a copy center. Generally, a trifold or bifold display board can be purchased at office supply stores. The poster/foam board should be neat, organized, easy to read from a distance, and eye catching and should stimulate the audience's curiosity.

Presentation

When the visual component is completed, it is time to begin the verbal section. Generally, two speakers will make the presentation, so plan the presentation accordingly. Next, write the presentation on note cards, and then practice, practice, practice. Present it to friends and family members. Be sure to practice voice projection and control, eye contact, and body language. Also practice using the

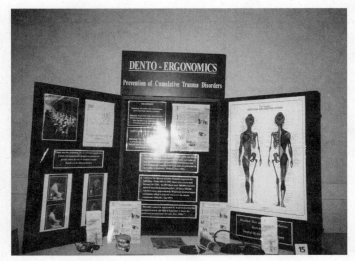

FIGURE A–1 Table Clinic

Box A–1 Tips on Preparing Your Table Clinic

- **Getting Started:** Choose a topic that is interesting to you
- **Research:** Determine a theme for your presentation and work to develop it
- **Research:** Do thorough research of your topic and have documentation of your findings available
- **Research:** Be prepared for questions and discussion.
- **Visual Aids:** Use visual aids effectively to reinforce what you are saying
- **Presentation:** Limit your presentation to approximately 7 minutes
- **Presentation:** Practice your communication skills: voice projection, body language, and eye contact in front of friends and family. Ask for constructive criticism
- **Handouts:** Prepare handouts to outline, summarize, or supplement your presentation

visual aids, which are reinforcing what is being presented. It is best to have the speech memorized, which should not be difficult. Remember to limit it to only five to seven minutes. Videoing the practice is a great way to help make improvements. In addition to preparing for the speech, also be prepared for questions and controversial feedback. The best way to promote confidence about the topic is to be well versed in other areas that closely relate.

Handouts

In addition to the display, handouts should be available. The information in a handout is used to outline, summarize, and/or supplement your presentation. It should include the table clinic's title and date of presentation, the name of the presenter(s), dental hygiene affiliation, and references. The audience should be able to use the handout as a reference guide concerning your topic and, if needed, a way to contact the presenter later.

American Dental Hygienists' Association (ADHA) Guidelines

Every year at the ADHA annual session, students from around the country compete in the table clinic presentations (see Box A-2 ■). More information on ADHA current guidelines is available at (800) 243-ADHA or www .adha.com. The basic guidelines developed by ADHA for table clinic presentations are summarized in Box A-1. These guidelines change slightly every year, so it is a good idea to contact ADHA for current guidelines.

Summary

By preparing a table clinic, you have the opportunity not only to expand you knowledge of a specific topic but also to inform others. A table clinic is also an excellent way to meet other health care professionals and possibly make new employment contacts. Often the sponsors of the table clinics present awards to the best-prepared and presented table clinic. Have fun and be creative!

Box A–2 ADHA Rules and Regulations

- Handouts must be available and should include the clinic title, date, bibliography, and your dental hygiene affiliation.
- Only one 3 ft. × 6 ft. table is permitted for each table clinic.
- All clinics are conducted at individual tables; no more than two clinicians are permitted to be present at one time.
- Advertising matter, commercial promotion, and solicitation of sales of any type are prohibited.
- Drugs should be identified by their generic or chemical formula rather than the commercial trade name.
- Any trade name on instruments must be covered.
- You must supply all equipment, except for the table, cloth cover, identification sign, and two chairs. You may order electrical outlets, audiovisual equipment, and so on directly from the supplier. Each accepted table clinic presenter receives an order form. The charges for this equipment are your responsibility.
- You are not permitted to use patients or live models for treatment or demonstration.
- Sound devices of any kind are not permitted.
- You must have completed setup of your table clinic 30 minutes prior to commencement of judging.
- You must remain at your clinic at all times because judging times may overlap with the public viewing time.
- Charts or diagrams must be constrained to the tabletop. Easels and materials on the floor or in the aisles are not allowed.

Source: ADHA Guidelines. Chicago: ADHA; 2008.

Poster Session Preparation

A poster session presents information about an original dental hygiene research study. Basically, a poster session disseminates the study's results whereas a table clinic disseminates a literature review on a specific topic. Poster sessions actually incorporate visual media that reflect an area of dental hygiene research.

Refer to Box B-1 ■ for an outline of the format to use for the poster session. The research should have been conducted in the order the box indicates.

As with all professional endeavors, organization is the key. Faculty members should serve as mentors during research, and it is recommended that all research conducted have numerous reviews before, during, and after the process to ensure success in presenting the information. The ADHA has set criteria for preparing a poster session (Box B-2 ■).

Please see www.adha.org for the rules and regulations for research poster sessions at the American Dental Hygienists' Association annual sessions.

Box B–1 Poster Session Format

- Purpose of study or hypothesis tested
- Statement of the problem and significance of the study
- Brief overview of methodology
- Statistical tests employed
- Study results including statistical data analysis
- Conclusion

Box B–2 Poster Session Criteria

- Clearly define the purpose for the research study
- State the problem and significance of the study
- dentify and outline the research methodology
- Describe the results including statistical data analysis
- Clearly state how the results support the conclusions or findings
- Be prepared for questions and discussions

Dental Terms and Phrases Translated into Spanish and Vietnamese with Spanish Pronunciation Guide

English	Spanish	Vietnamese
dentist	dentista	Nha sĩ
tooth	diente	Răng
throat	garganta	Cuống họng
neck	cuello	Cổ
mouth	boca	Miệng
head	cabeza	Đầu
face	cara	Mặt
ear	oido	Tai
nose	nariz	Muỗi
tongue	lengua	Lưỡi
tonsils	amigdalas	Hạch
denture	dentadura	Hàm răng
toothbrush	cepillar(v), cepillo(n)	Bàn chãy đánh răng
show me	enseneme	Chỉcho tôi
relax	relajese	Bình tỉnh, thông thả
don't move	no se muera	Đừng nhúc nhích
look straight ahead	vea derecho	Nhìn thẳng phía trước
swallow	trague	Nuốc vào
open your mouth	abra la boca	Mở miệng ra
stick out your tongue	saque la lengua	Lè lưỡi ra
close	cerra	Đóng lại
spit	escupir	Nhổ ra
abscess	abceso	Ung, nhọt
asthma	astma	Bệnh suyễn
bleeding	sangrado	Nhay máu
cold	frio	Lạnh
diabetes	diabetes	Bệnh tiểu đường
edema	edema	Chứng phù thủng
fracture	fractura	Chỗ nứt, chỗ gãy
headache	cefalea	Nhức đầu
high blood pressure	presion alta	Chứng cao huyết áp
hot	caliente	Nóng
infection	infeccion	Nhiễm trùng
injured	herido	Bị thương
pregnant	embarazada	Mang thai
stitches	puntadas	Khâu, vá
swelling	inflamacion	Bị sưng
trauma	trauma	Chấn thương
wound	herida	Vết thương
mild	suave	Nhẹ, êm
moderate	moderado	Vừa phải
severe	severo	Nghiêm khắc

(continued)

earache	dolor de oido	Bệnh đau tai
sore throat	dolor de garganta	Đau họng
difficulty swallowing	dificultad al tragar	Khó khăn khi nuốt
toothache	dolor de muela	Nhức răng
neck pain	dolor de cuello	Đau cổ
sensitive	sensible	Nhạy cảm
disease	enfermedad	Bệnh tật
medications	medicamentos	Bốc toa thuốc (dùng thước)
antibiotics	antibioticos	Kháng sinh
pain pills	calmantes	Thuốc đau nhức
narcotics	narcoticos	Thuốc mê
penicillin	penicilina	Thuốc trụ sinh
right	derecho (m.) derecha (f.)	Phải
left	izquierdo (m.) izquierda (f.)	Trái

English	**Spanish**	**Pronunciation**
Good day! How are you?	Buenos dias! Como esta?	Boo-eh-nus dee-ass. Kum-muh estah?
Does it hurt?	Le duele?	Leh doo-eh-leh?
When does it hurt?	Cuando le duele?	Kwan-doh leh doo-eh-leh?

All of the time?
Todo el tiempo¿
(toh-doh el tee-m-poh)

Where does it hurt?
Donde le duele¿
(dun-deh leh doo-eh-leh)

Does the cold water or air hurt you?
Le molesta el agua o el aire frio¿
(leh muh-les-tah el ah-goo-ah oh el i-reh free-oh)

Does it hurt when you bite?
Le duele cuando muerde¿
(leh doo-eh-leh kwan-doh moo-erdeh)

Open your mouth.
Abra la boca.
(ahbra lah bokah)

Close your mouth a little.
Cierre la boca un poco.
(see-ehreh lah bokah oon poh-koh)

Bite slowly.
Muerda despacio.
(moo-erdah des-pah-see-oh)

Bite again.
Muerda otra vez.
(moo-erdah oh-trah vez)

Spit out, please.
Escupa, por favor.
(ess-coo-pah por favor)

Turn your head to the right.
—to the left.
Volte la cabeza a la derecha.
—a la izquierda.
(vol-teh lah ka-beh-zah ah lah deh-reh-chah
—ah lah eez-kee-erdah)

Do not eat or drink for 30 minutes.
No coma ni beba por 30 minutos.
(noh koh-mah nee beh-bah por trentah mee-nuh-tohs)

Do not chew on this side for 24 hours.
No mastique en este lado por 24 horas.
(no mahs-teekeh en esteh lahdoh por ven-tee kwah-troh
o-rahs)

Do not brush tonight.
No se cepille esta noche.
(no seh seh-peeyeh ess-tah no-cheh)

Do not rinse tonight.
No se enjuage esta noche.
(noh seh en-huah-ghe ess-tah no-cheh)

Standards for Dental Hygienists in Dental Public Health Education

Commission on Dental Accreditation, Dental Public Health Standards

Dental hygiene students may attend programs that have been accredited by the Commission on Dental Accreditation, which is part of the American Dental Association. The Commission is composed of twenty members including a representative from the American Dental Hygienists' Association. The Commission has been accrediting dental hygiene educational programs since 1953.

The Accreditation Standards for Dental Hygiene Education Programs includes mandatory curriculum content. Dental hygiene students must prove competency in dental public health. Specifically, dental hygiene graduates must include and advocate for the evaluation of current literature to prepare for lifelong learning in dental hygiene practice. Faculty should integrate these principles of lifelong learning throughout the curriculum.

Moreover, content in community dental health and public health dentistry must be included in the curriculum to provide students background in the procedures of assessing, planning, implementing, and evaluating community oral health programs. Curriculum must also include experience in oral health education and preventive counseling for groups. The dental hygiene faculty must implement a mechanism for planning, supervising, and evaluating community field experiences.

Curricular requirements for community health instruction can be found in the Accreditation Standards for Dental Hygiene Education Programs, Commission on Dental Accreditation. Chicago, IL: American Dental Association; 2015. Please see http://www.ada.org/~/media/CODA/Files/2016_dh.ashx for these standards.

Joint Commission on National Dental Examinations: National Board Dental Hygiene Examination

Prospective dental hygienists in all states except Alabama are required to take and pass the National Board Dental Hygiene Examination. The information included on this examination includes the following topics under the section entitled Community Health/Research Principles.

- Promoting Health and Preventing Disease within Groups
- Participating in Community Programs
  1. Assessing Populations and Defining Objectives
  2. Designing, Implementing, and Evaluating Programs
- Analyzing Scientific Information, Utilizing Statistical Concepts, and Applying Research Results

Refer to Chapter 23 for a more complete discussion of the National Board Dental Hygiene Examination.

Guide to Scientific Writing

The following guidelines to writing can be used when writing scientifically based papers for table clinic presentations and poster presentations.[1]

Title Page

The title page should include the title of the manuscript in boldface; each author's name, credentials, rank or title, and organizational affiliation; and the primary author's mailing address and telephone, e-mail, and fax numbers. In addition, if an organization funded the investigation, its name should be noted on the bottom of the title page.

Length

Manuscripts should be six to ten pages in length excluding references, tables, figures, and photographs.

Presentation

All manuscripts must be written in the English language. Manuscripts must include an abstract and the following:

- Original research, including an introduction, methods and materials, results, and discussion and conclusion
- Case studies, including an introduction and case as described in the dental hygiene process of care; assessment, dental hygiene diagnosis, treatment planning, implementation, and evaluations; and summary
- Literature reviews containing an introduction, the significance of the topic, main body, and conclusions
- Position papers, which are written to reflect a position taken on a specific issue, including an introduction, the significance of the issue, main body, and summary

References

All references should be numbered in the order they are cited. The following style of citation should be used:

Periodical: Fones, AC and Newman, I: The inception of the professional dental hygienist. *J Dent Hyg* 2008;78:395–402.

Textbook: Nathe, CN: Dental Public Health and Research. 3rd edition. Upper Saddle River, NJ: Pearson. 2010:10–12.

Tables, Figures, and Photographs

All tables, figures, and photographs should be at the end of the manuscript, not inserted into it. Written permission for the use of copyrighted material must be included with the manuscript and is the author's responsibility.

Acknowledgments

The authors may acknowledge one to two individuals for their assistance in manuscript preparation.

Authors

Primary authors of all manuscripts must be dental hygienists or dental hygiene students; secondary authors may represent any discipline.

Content

Manuscripts may be original research, case studies, literature reviews, or position papers.

Reference

1. http://www.adha.org/jdh/guidelines.htm

Answers to Self-Study Test Items

Chapter 1

1. What is an example of primary public health prevention?
   a. Disease prevention
   b. Periodontal debridement
   c. Fluoride treatments
   d. Restorative materials

   ANSWER: a

2. Public health is credited with the dramatic increase in the average life span because of which of the following?
   a. Vaccinations
   b. Safety policies
   c. Family planning
   d. All of the above

   ANSWER: d

3. What is an example of secondary public health prevention?
   a. Prevention of disease
   b. Fluoride treatments
   c. Restorations
   d. Patient education

   ANSWER: b

4. What is the main health care research institution in the United States?
   a. Centers for Disease Control and Prevention
   b. Food and Drug Administration
   c. National Institutes of Health
   d. Johns Hopkins University

   ANSWER: c

5. How has malpractice directly impacted dental care delivery and quality?
   a. Enabled patients to sue
   b. Decreased the number of dental providers because of the fear of malpractice suits
   c. Decreased quality of care
   d. Increased the number of suits against dental providers

   ANSWER: a

Chapter 2

1. What is referred to as a constituent member in the ADHA organization?
   a. National organizations
   b. State organizations
   c. Local organizations
   d. Student organizations

   ANSWER: b

2. When is school fluoridation recommended?
   a. When an independent water source is available
   b. For children who have caries
   c. For children who have brown discolored areas on enamel
   d. None of the above

   ANSWER: a

3. Demineralization, enhancement of remineralization, and inhibition of bacterial activity are examples of what?
   a. Water fluoridation
   b. Topical fluoridation
   c. Systemic fluoridation
   d. Fluoride supplements

   ANSWER: b

4. Which type of fluoride increases children's risk of developing dental fluorosis?
   a. Supplements
   b. Systemic
   c. Topical
   d. Both a and b

   ANSWER: d

5. When are sealants most effective?
   a. When applied without etchant
   b. When an assistant is utilized
   c. In the presence of saliva
   d. When material is cured for one minute

   ANSWER: b

Chapter 3

1. What has been recognized as a major unmet need in the United States?
   a. Health insurance
   b. Oral Health
   c. Access to health care
   d. Geriatric awareness
   ANSWER: b

2. What branch of the federal government has a direct impact on dental care delivery?
   a. Legislative
   b. Executive
   c. Judicial
   d. All of the above
   ANSWER: b

3. Who or what directs the US Public Health Service?
   a. US Surgeon General
   b. Centers for Disease Control and Prevention
   c. Johns Hopkins University
   d. Dental Public Health Committee
   ANSWER: a

4. Which organization provides a system of health surveillance to monitor and prevent outbreak of diseases and maintain national health statistics?
   a. National Institutes of Health
   b. Centers for Disease Control and Prevention
   c. Food and Drug Administration
   d. Indian Health Service
   ANSWER: b

5. Which organization is responsible for the Head Start Program?
   a. Administration on Aging
   b. Centers for Medicare and Medicaid Services
   c. Administration for Children and Families
   d. Indian Health Services
   ANSWER: c

Chapter 4

1. Which European country has a history of establishing the profession of dental hygiene?
   a. England
   b. Italy
   c. Germany
   d. Portugal
   ANSWER: a

2. Which of the following is a reason for the lack of access to dental hygiene services worldwide?
   a. Insufficient funding
   b. Lack of social and cultural awareness
   c. Legal restraints
   d. All of above
   ANSWER: d

3. How many countries in the European Union report no or virtually no hygienists?
   a. 3
   b. 7
   c. 10
   d. 17
   ANSWER: b

4. In industrialized nations where do dental hygienists mainly practice?
   a. Public health clinics
   b. Educational institutions
   c. Government positions
   d. Private dental clinics
   ANSWER: d

5. What organization is a nonprofit group that unites dental hygiene associations from around the world in their common cause of promoting access to quality preventive oral services and to raise public awareness of the prevention of dental disease?
   a. American Dental Hygiene Association
   b. European Dental Hygienists' Federation
   c. International Federation of Dental Hygienists
   d. European Federation of Periodontology
   ANSWER: c

Chapter 5

1. Which of the following does financing of dental treatment involve?
   a. Private sector
   b. Dental practitioner
   c. Public sector
   d. Both a and c
   ANSWER: d

2. What payment is based on an office visit and is always the same regardless of the services rendered?
   a. Encounter
   b. Fee-for-service plan
   c. Capitation
   d. Barter system
   ANSWER: a

3. What term refers to a portion of the cost of each service that the patient pays—in other words, the part of the payment not covered by the third party?
   a. Insurance payment
   b. Copayment
   c. Deductible
   d. Exchange

   ANSWER: b

4. What is defined as the number given to a specific procedure as designated in the *Codes on Dental Procedures and Nomenclature* published by ADA?
   a. Premium number
   b. Procedure number
   c. Contract number
   d. Benefit number

   ANSWER: b

5. What form is sent to the patient and provider explaining the payment or denial for procedures rendered?
   a. Explanation of benefits
   b. Managed care
   c. Exclusive provider arrangement
   d. Dental claim

   ANSWER: a

Chapter 6

1. State agencies such as state dental boards fall within which type of law?
   a. Common
   b. Statutory
   c. Constitutional
   d. Administrative

   ANSWER: d

2. Which branch of government makes laws for the state?
   a. Legislative
   b. Executive
   c. Administrative
   d. Judicial

   ANSWER: a

3. Laws which explain what services dental hygienists can provide are found in
   a. Medicaid rules.
   b. state law.
   c. federal Law.
   d. health care regulations.

   ANSWER: b

4. Judges do not make laws, but they interpret them.
   a. The first statement is true; the second statement is false.
   b. The first statement is false; the second statement is true.
   c. Both statements are true.
   d. Both statements are false.

   ANSWER: c

5. Because federal laws regulate dental hygiene practice, federal senators are involved with state regulation.
   a. The first statement is true; the second statement is false.
   b. The first statement is false; the second statement is true.
   c. Both statements are true.
   d. Both statements are false.

   ANSWER: d

Chapter 7

1. Which of the following is an individual or group who causes a social, cultural, or behavioral change, be it intentional or unintentional?
   a. Mentor
   b. Change agent
   c. Lobbying
   d. Grants writer

   ANSWER: b

2. Which of the following is *not* a way in which social advocates initiate change in dental public health?
   a. By delivering dental care
   b. By helping to sustain dental public health programs
   c. By determining the type of dental treatment rendered
   d. By determining who receives dental care

   ANSWER: c

3. What is necessary to create change?
   a. Influencing individuals who govern policy
   b. Increasing an organization's financial status
   c. Redesigning the public health facility
   d. All of the above

   ANSWER: a

4. What are the roles identified for the dental hygiene change agent?
   a. Catalyst
   b. Solution giver
   c. Resource linker
   d. All of the above

   ANSWER: d

5. Making basic changes without losing the essential components is termed?
   a. Modification
   b. Competency
   c. Application
   d. Networking

   ANSWER: a

Chapter 8

1. Empowerment models that focus on patient autonomy and collaborative relationships are paternalist regimens. These regimens are led by patients whose knowledge of health and disease increases the likelihood that healthy behaviors are attained.
   a. The first statement is true; the second statement is false.
   b. The first statement is false; the second statement is true.
   c. Both statements are true.
   d. Both statements are false.

   ANSWER: d

2. Which of the following aspects is part of the multidimensional model of health?
   a. Spirituality
   b. Knowledge
   c. Behavior
   d. Values

   ANSWER: a

3. The local dental hygiene association worked on policy change that banned sugary beverages from school vending machines. This is an example of
   a. healthy behavior.
   b. health action.
   c. health education.
   d. health promotion.

   ANSWER: d

4. For behavior change to occur, an individual must reach what milestone?
   a. Value the change
   b. Understand the healthy behavior
   c. Understand unhealthy behavior
   d. Understand why a behavior was chosen

   ANSWER: a

5. A patient who receives praise for having healthy gums during two routine dental hygiene appointments will be more likely to maintain good home care to ensure that the praise will continue at subsequent appointments. This theory is called
   a. classical conditioning.
   b. operant conditioning.
   c. modeling.
   d. empowerment.

   ANSWER: a

Chapter 9

1. The best way to ensure an effective presentation is to
   a. decrease the number of participants.
   b. utilize audiovisual aids.
   c. have at least ten objectives for each presentation.
   d. be prepared.

   ANSWER: d

2. "Following the presentation, the audience will be able to compare ten healthy and unhealthy snack choices" is an example of a(n)
   a. goal.
   b. lesson plan.
   c. objective.
   d. healthy behavior.

   ANSWER: c

3. Lecturing is always an effective way to teach dental health education. Lecture always includes the problem-based method of learning.
   a. The first statement is true; the second statement is false.
   b. The first statement is false; the second statement is true.
   c. Both statements are true.
   d. Both statements are false.

   ANSWER: d

4. Which verb pertains to the psychomotor domain?
   a. Demonstrating
   b. Comparing
   c. Advocating
   d. Defending

   ANSWER: a

5. When used as an objective, the verb *understand*
   a. is easily measured.
   b. is open to misinterpretation.
   c. always requires skill.
   d. is frequently used.

   ANSWER: b

Chapter 10

1. A group from a local church youth group could be considered a
   a. target population.
   b. target population profile.
   c. faith-based initiative.
   d. community agency.

   ANSWER: a

2. It is important not to frighten child patients. It is better not to tell the truth if a procedure could involve some discomfort.
   a. The first statement is true; the second statement is false.
   b. The first statement is false; the second statement is true.
   c. Both statements are true.
   d. Both statements are false.

   ANSWER: a

3. Faith-based initiatives funded by the federal government do not generally include health care.
   a. The first statement is true; the second statement is false.
   b. The first statement is false; the second statement is true.
   c. Both statements are true.
   d. Both statements are false.

   ANSWER: a

4. Social workers and dental hygienists can work together during programs for target populations
   a. to provide dental hygiene care.
   b. to assess dental health.
   c. to ensure social services for the population.
   d. to implement periodontal treatment.

   ANSWER: c

5. Inconvenient office hours of a dental practice can become a
   a. target population profile technique.
   b. faith-based issue.
   c. barrier to care.
   d. long-term strategic plan.

   ANSWER: c

Chapter 11

1. The fact that only a small number of minorities work in the oral health care professions may be considered a barrier to oral health care. A study of the racial and ethnic composition of the health care workforce reveals that the dental workforce is the least diverse of all the health professions.
   a. The first statement is true; the second statement is false.
   b. The first statement is false; the second statement is true.
   c. Both statements are true.
   d. Both statements are false.

   ANSWER: c

2. Which of the following could prevent a patient from seeking care or reduce effectiveness of care?
   a. Unhealthy behaviors
   b. Severe pain
   c. Language barrier
   d. None of the above

   ANSWER: c

3. A country in which people strive to acculturate into a new society and make valiant attempts to change their cultural patterns to those of their host society is colloquially called
   a. a melting pot.
   b. a salad bowl.
   c. jello.
   d. amalgam.

   ANSWER: a

4. Which of the following is/are guidelines to effective communication?
   a. Assess one's own cultural beliefs and values
   b. Recognize those cultural influences affecting communication
   c. Understand a patient's belief system
   d. All of the above

   ANSWER: d

5. Cross-cultural dental hygiene is the effective integration of the population's socioethnocultural background into the process of care. Recognizing how your culture influences your values, behaviors, beliefs, and decision making is part of cross-cultural dental hygiene.
   a. The first statement is true; the second statement is false.
   b. The first statement is false; the second statement is true.
   c. Both statements are true.
   d. Both statements are false.

   ANSWER: c

Chapter 12

1. Which of the following is part of the planning phase of program planning?
   a. Identify methods to measure goals
   b. Assess the population's dental needs
   c. Begin program operation
   d. Revise program as needed

   ANSWER: a

2. Dr. Fones's original paradigm for the school dental hygienist focused on
   a. restoration.
   b. utilization of a case manager.
   c. prevention of disease.
   d. all of the above.

   ANSWER: c

3. Which school program is particularly advantageous for middle school athletes?
   a. Sealant program
   b. School fluoridation
   c. Case management
   d. Athletic mouth guard program

   ANSWER: d

4. During which stage of the program paradigm planning should the target population's needs be identified?
   a. Assessment
   b. Dental hygiene diagnosis
   c. Planning
   d. Evaluation

   ANSWER: a

5. A dental hygienist employed in a nursing home could provide routine preventive care. In addition, the dental hygienists could have a collaborative relationship with a dentist, so that restorative and urgent care is provided as need.
   a. The first statement is true; the second statement is false.
   b. The first statement is false; the second statement is true.
   c. Both statements are true.
   d. Both statements are false.

   ANSWER: c

Chapter 13

1. Program goals should be evaluated based on
   a. measurement tools.
   b. baseline data.
   c. national guidelines.
   d. state surveillance records.

   ANSWER: b

2. During which phase of program planning should evaluation be started?
   a. Assessment
   b. Dental hygiene diagnosis
   c. Planning
   d. Evaluation

   ANSWER: c

3. Which type of evaluation refers to the internal evaluation of a program?
   a. Formative
   b. Summative
   c. Quantitative
   d. Qualitative

   ANSWER: a

4. Which type of evaluation is a basic screening?
   a. Nonclinical
   b. Clinical
   c. Provider driven
   d. Educational

   ANSWER: b

5. An index that measures a conditioin that will not change, such as dental caries, is termed a(n)
   a. clinical index.
   b. nonclinical index.
   c. irreversible index.
   d. reversible index.

   ANSWER: c

Chapter 14

1. Evidence-based decisions come from research, practice, and
   a. science.
   b. patient preferences.
   c. disciplines.
   d. none of the above.

   ANSWER: b

2. Dental public health has been an important component in the creation of a body of research that impacts dental hygiene practice. Every dental hygienist, whether or not directly involved in research, should be familiar with basic research design.
   a. The first statement is true; the second statement is false.
   b. The first statement is false; the second statement is true.
   c. Both statements are true.
   d. Both statements are false.

   ANSWER: c

3. An occupational dental hygienists provides care based upon
   a. dentists' recommendations.
   b. evidence-based knowledge.
   c. sales representatives advice.
   d. internet search and clinical knowledge.

   ANSWER: a

4. In clinical practice the dental hygienists completes a health history on a patient. In research, the dental hygienists would complete a parallel function called:
   a. Research proposal.
   b. Informed consent.
   c. Literature review.
   d. Reference check.

   ANSWER: c

5. Dental hygiene research began two decades ago, after the MSDH programs were created.
   a. The first statement is true; the second statement is false.
   b. The first statement is false; the second statement is true.
   c. Both statements are true.
   d. Both statements are false.

   ANSWER: b

Chapter 15

1. A dental hygiene researcher's first obligation to the patient is to do no harm which is termed
   a. nomaleficence.
   b. beneficence.
   c. autonomy.
   d. veracity.

2. Which principle is based on respect for others and the belief that patients have the power to make decisions about things that may affect their health.
   a. Autonomy
   b. Beneficence
   c. Justice
   d. Nonmaleficence

3. Informed consent is an ongoing process that is initially obtained at the first step of the research process. It should be discussed in a group setting.
   a. The first statement is true; the second statement is false.
   b. The first statement is false; the second statement is true.
   c. Both statements are true.
   d. Both statements are false.

4. Private institutions design and carry out the bulk of medical research in the United States. Their funding for research may come from federal government grants, from the institution itself, from private companies, or through philanthropy.
   a. The first statement is true; the second statement is false.
   b. The first statement is false; the second statement is true.
   c. Both statements are true.
   d. Both statements are false.

5. Research misconduct includes intentional plagiarism, and falsifying data. For this reason, research bias, or disagreement about the meaning of the results does not constitute misconduct.
   a. Both the statement and reason are correct and related.
   b. Both the statement and reason are correct but NOT related.
   c. The statement is correct, but the reason is NOT.
   d. The statement is NOT correct, but the reason is correct.
   e. NEITHER the statement NOR the reason is correct.

Chapter 16

1. Which of the following is a descriptive approach to research?
   a. Case study approach
   b. Experimental approach
   c. Retrospective approach
   d. Prospective approach

   ANSWER: a

2. Which studies combine descriptive and historical research to establish patterns from the past and present to predict future occurrences?
   a. Document analysis studies
   b. Correlational studies
   c. Trend studies
   d. Prospective studies

   ANSWER: c

3. In a split mouth study, one side of the mouth is used for the test treatment. The other side of the mouth is used for the control treatment.
   a. The first statement is true; the second statement is false.
   b. The first statement is false; the second statement is true.
   c. Both statements are true.
   d. Both statements are false.

   ANSWER: c

4. A quasi-experimental study is designed as an experimental study but lacks inherent control. However, results from a quasi-experimental study may be used when planning further studies.
   a. The first statement is true; the second statement is false.
   b. The first statement is false; the second statement is true.
   c. Both statements are true.
   d. Both statements are false.

   ANSWER: c

5. Studying the relationship between obesity and oral health is an example of which type of study?
   a. Experimental
   b. Quasi-experimental
   c. Correlational
   d. Analytic

   ANSWER: c

Chapter 17

1. Which variable is made up of distinct and separate units or categories but is counted only in whole numbers?
   a. Quantitative
   b. Qualitative
   c. Continuous
   d. Discrete

   ANSWER: d

2. Which scale of measurement contains all of the characteristics of the preceding scales and has an absolute zero point determined by nature?
   a. Interval
   b. Ordinal
   c. Ratio
   d. Numerical

   ANSWER: c

3. Which type of correlational relationship would the following statement indicate: as the consumption of fluoridated water increases, the caries rate decreases.
   a. Positive
   b. Inverse
   c. Strong
   d. Weak

   ANSWER: b

4. The research hypothesis, also called the *alternative* or *positive hypothesis,* is the logical opposite of the null hypothesis. The research hypothesis can indicate a direction of difference.
   a. The first statement is true; the second statement is false.
   b. The first statement is false; the second statement is true.
   c. Both statements are true.
   d. Both statements are false.

   ANSWER: c

5. The chi-square test (χ^2) is the most commonly used nonparametric statistic. It is used to determine whether a significant difference exists between frequency counts of nominal (categorical or dichotomous) data by comparing the observed frequencies to expected frequencies.
   a. The first statement is true; the second statement is false.
   b. The first statement is false; the second statement is true.
   c. Both statements are true.
   d. Both statements are false.

   ANSWER: c

Chapter 18

1. *Epidemiology* has been defined as the study of the nature, cause, control, and determinants of the frequency and distribution of
   a. disease.
   b. disability.
   c. death.
   d. all of the above.

   ANSWER: d

2. The agent of disease is the biologic or mechanical cause of the disease or condition. Examples of agents are the specific bacteria in relation to dental caries or brushing with a hard toothbrush in relation to abrasion.
   a. The first statement is true; the second statement is false.
   b. The first statement is false; the second statement is true.
   c. Both statements are true.
   d. Both statements are false.

   ANSWER: c

3. The occurrence of an illness in excess of normal expectancy in a community or region, usually occurring suddenly and spreading rapidly, is termed a(n)
   a. endemic.
   b. epidemic.
   c. pandemic.
   d. all of the above.

   ANSWER: b

4. Which study attempts to relate outcome with exposure to a suspected risk factor using data that are available for the population?
   a. Case–control
   b. Case study
   c. Ecological
   d. Time Series

   ANSWER: c

5. What is a modifiable attribute or exposure that is known to be associated with a health condition?
   a. Risk ratio
   b. Risk factor
   c. Risk attribute
   d. Risk indicator

   ANSWER: b

Chapter 19

1. Tobacco use, excessive alcohol use, and inappropriate dietary practices contribute to a number of diseases and disorders. In particular, tobacco use is a risk factor for oral cavity and pharyngeal cancers, periodontal diseases, candidiasis, and dental caries, among other diseases.
   a. The first statement is true; the second statement is false.
   b. The first statement is false; the second statement is true.
   c. Both statements are true.
   d. Both statements are false.

   ANSWER: c

2. Which gender does periodontal diseases affect the most?
   a. Males
   b. Females
   c. Both are affected the same
   d. Teen and elderly females

   ANSWER: a

3. In which teeth are early childhood caries most evident?
   a. Permanent molars
   b. Permanent anteriors
   c. Primary anteriors
   d. Primary molars

   ANSWER: c

4. Early detection frequently affects the outcome of
   a. oral cancer treatment.
   b. cleft lip rates.
   c. cleft lip and palate rates.
   d. None of the above

   ANSWER: a

5. When toothaches are not prevented, which services might individuals seek?
   a. Medical
   b. Dental hygiene
   c. General dentistry
   d. Cosmetic dentistry

   ANSWER: a

Chapter 20

1. The ADA Seal of Approval program is regulated by the FDA. It is mandatory for all over-the-counter dental care products.
   a. The first statement is true; the second statement is false.
   b. The first statement is false; the second statement is true.
   c. Both the statements are true.
   d. Both the statements are false.

   ANSWER: d

2. PubMed is a service of the US National Library of Medicine (NLM). It includes more than 17 million citations from MEDLINE and other life science journals for biomedical articles back to the 1950s.
   a. The first statement is true; the second statement is false.
   b. The first statement is false; the second statement is true.
   c. Both the statements are true.
   d. Both the statements are false.

   ANSWER: c

3. Which of the following is/are part of a research report's methods and materials section?
   a. Research design
   b. Ethical considerations
   c. Sample size
   d. All of the above

   ANSWER: d

4. Which of the following terms defines the review of manuscripts for content and accuracy before they can be included in refereed journals?
   a. Critique
   b. Double blind
   c. Primary evaluation
   d. Peer reviewed

   ANSWER: d

5. *Statistical significance* means that the result was not caused by
   a. control.
   b. chance.
   c. placebo effect.
   d. sugar pill.

   ANSWER: b

Chapter 21

1. Dental hygienists initially are eligible to be a US PHS Commissioned Officer with which of the following credentials?
   a. Certificate in dental hygiene
   b. Associate's degree in dental hygiene
   c. Bachelor's degree in dental hygiene
   d. Master's degree in dental hygiene
   ANSWER: c

2. Civil service employment falls under the state department. Many times hygienists are employed at a VA Hospital as a civil service employee.
   a. The first statement is true; the second statement is false.
   b. The first statement is false; the second statement is true.
   c. Both statements are true.
   d. Both statements are false.
   ANSWER: c

3. Students are eligible for the COSTEP program during their dental hygiene education. The COSTEP program is part of the US Department of Defense health care system.
   a. The first statement is true; the second statement is false.
   b. The first statement is false; the second statement is true.
   c. Both statements are true.
   d. Both statements are false.
   ANSWER: a

4. Dental hygienists can work on military bases in the United States as
   a. military officers.
   b. PHS officers.
   c. contract employees.
   d. None of the above
   ANSWER: c

5. Which of the following are goals of the US Public Health Services?
   a. Prevent and control disease
   b. Identify health hazards in the environment
   c. Help provide health care to Native Americans
   d. All of the above
   ANSWER: d

Chapter 22

1. Members of the public, government agencies, and other health care professionals, as well as the dental hygiene profession itself, is showing significant interest in establishing dental hygiene programs in settings other than private dental offices. Many states have expanded the dental hygienists' scope of practice.
   a. The first statement is true; the second statement is false.
   b. The first statement is false; the second statement is true.
   c. Both statements are true.
   d. Both statements are false.
   ANSWER: c

2. What may be necessary to increase dental hygienists' accessibility to the underserved public?
   a. Marketing promotion
   b. Blueprint development
   c. Legislative initiatives
   d. None of the above
   ANSWER: c

3. During which phase should a target population's needs be determined?
   a. Assessment
   b. Dental hygiene diagnosis
   c. Planning
   d. Implementation
   ANSWER: a

4. Continually refining the product is which part of the business plan?
   a. Service development
   b. Marketing
   c. Sales
   d. Operations
   ANSWER: a

5. Which phase involves prioritizing goals and objectives?
   a. Assessment
   b. Dental hygiene diagnosis
   c. Planning
   d. Implementation
   ANSWER: c

Dentist Professional who provides clinical and educational dental services to the public.

Dentistry Art and science of restorative oral health.

Dependent variable In clinical study, variable that is being tested.

Descriptive approach Variety of methods, including surveys, case studies, developmental studies, document or content analysis, trend studies, and correlational studies used in research.

Descriptive statistics Procedures that are used to summarize, organize, and describe quantitative data.

Determinants of health Factors that interact to create specific health conditions, including physical, biological, behavioral, social, cultural, and spiritual.

Developmental disability Disability that occurs during uterine development.

Discrete (categorical) variable Variable made up of distinct and separate units or categories and counted only in whole numbers; also referred to as *mutually exclusive*.

Discipline A unique scientific body of knowledge

Disease rate Number of disease cases or deaths among a population or target group during a given time period expressed as a ratio.

Double-blind study Type of most experimental research in which neither the subjects nor the investigators know who is in the control (or placebo) group and who is in the other (independent variable) group that receives the experimental treatment.

E

Early and periodic screening, diagnosis and treatment (EPSDT) Service for persons under twenty-one years of age for medical, dental, and vision care paid for by Medicaid.

Early childhood caries Dental caries that affect children, sometimes referred to as *nursing bottle decay* or *baby bottle decay*.

Early Head Start Federal program that promotes the economic and social well-being of pregnant women and their children up to age three.

Educational requirement The requirement of how much instruction and what type of degree a dental hygienist must receive.

Educator Dental hygiene role which focuses on teaching about and promotes dental health issues to various target populations.

Empower To coordinate change or cause others to take action or make a change.

Encounter fee plan Plan that basically pays for each care encounter regardless of the service provider.

Endemic Relatively low but constant level of occurrence of a disease or health condition in a population.

Entrepeneur Dental hygiene role which focuses on developing new dental initiatives

Epidemic Disease or condition occurring among many individuals in a community or region at the same time and usually spreading rapidly.

Epidemiology Study of the nature, cause, control, and determinants of the frequency and distribution of disease, disability, and death in human populations.

Epidemiology triangle Factors—host, agent, environment—organized by epidemiologists to demonstrate the interaction and interrelatedness of these factors over time in bringing about a disease or condition.

Ethics Guiding principles for individuals or groups based on what is right and what is wrong.

Ethnocentrism Belief that one's own culture or traditions are better than other cultures.

Etiology Theory of causation for a disease or condition.

Eurocentric Reflecting a tendency to interpret the world in terms of western and especially European or Anglo-American values and experiences.

Evaluation Part of the dental hygiene process of care that encompasses evaluation of a dental public health program.

Evidence-based practice Inclusion of experience, research, clinical practice, and patient preference when providing dental hygiene care.

Exclusive provider arrangement (EPA) Contract between dental care providers and an employer (which eliminates the third party) stating the negotiated fees for services offered to the employer's employees.

Executive branch Government entity that executes, or carries out, the laws passed by the legislature.

Experimental approach Research study also known as a *clinical trial* that studies an experimental treatment or intervention.

Explanation of benefits Form sent to the patient and provider explaining the approval or denial of payment for procedures rendered.

F

Facilitator Person who conducts meetings, brings diverse ideas together, and helps a group work to reach goals.

Faith-based initiative Community-based actions that are valued and essential partners to assist Americans in need.

Federal National; of or pertaining to the United States of America.

Fédération Dentaire Internationale (FDI) Organization that represents the international community of dentists.

Fee-for-service plan Charge based on a fee scale for all covered services; bills the patient for services rendered by a dental hygienist, dentist, or denturist; most common payment method used in the United States.

Fee slip Form a dental practice uses to detail the services rendered a patient.

Fluoridation *See* community water fluoridation.

Field of Study A subdiscipline of a scientific body of knowledge

Fluoride Salt of hydrofluoric acid.

Fluoride varnish Varnish of fluoride applied to teeth to prevent dental caries; particularly effective in the prevention of early childhood caries.

Fluorosis Form of enamel hypomineralization due to excessive ingestion of fluoride during the development of the teeth.

Formative evaluation Internal examination of a program's process usually conducted while planning the program.

Frontier Geographic area even more sparsely populated than a rural area.

G

Government Method or system of controlling people.

Government branches Three sections of the US government: legislative, executive, and judicial.

Grantmanship Art of obtaining grants for funding projects.

Graph Diagram showing the variation of a variable in comparison with one or more other variables; also called a *chart*.

Grass roots Local efforts to affect change and help guide policy-making decisions.

Group *See* target population.

H

Habit Act of behavior change that becomes automatic, such as daily flossing.

Head Start Federal program that promotes the economic and social well-being of families and children from three to five years of age.

Health education Instruction regarding health behaviors that bring an individual to a state of health awareness.

Health Maintenance Organizations (HMOs) Organizations that provide comprehensive health care to enrolled individuals and families in a specified region by participating physicians and financed by fixed periodic payments.

Health promotion Process that informs and motivates people to adopt healthy behavior to enhance their health and prevent disease.

Healthy behavior Action that helps prevent illness and promote health.

Healthy People 2020 Report released by federal government stating the goals and objectives necessary to improve the health and quality of life for individuals and communities.

Historical approach Research designed to determine the meaning of past events by reviewing records and literature and conducting interviews.

Hypothesis Question that is developed to be answered by a study.

I

Implementation Part of the dental hygiene process of care that includes the actual operation of a program.

Incidence Number of new cases of a disease in a population over a given period of time.

Independent contractor Person who works for himself or herself and can perform contracted work for a governmental agency or another business.

Independent practice Practice of dental hygiene without the supervision of a dentist, although the dental hygienist refers all dental needs to a dentist; sometimes called *unsupervised practice* or *collaborative practice*.

Independent variable In a clinical study, the variable that is being manipulated.

Index *See* dental index.

Inferential statistics Data generally presented by describing and summarizing them to make inferences or generalizations about a population based on data taken from a sample of that population.

Informed consent Ethical consideration that requires educating a subject in a research study to be educated about the study's purpose, duration, experimental procedures, alternatives, risks, and benefits.

Institutional review board (IRB) Entity charged with reviewing the ethical implications of every research study.

International Federation of Dental Hygienists (IFDH) Organization representing the international community of dental hygienists.

Interpretation Explanation of results that is used in a research report.

Interval scale of measurement Device with equal distance between any two adjacent units of measurement but without a meaningful zero point.

J

Joint Commission on National Dental Examinations Organization whose purpose is to assist state boards in determining qualification of the dental hygienist who seeks licensure to practice dental hygiene by being in charge of the community health/research principles section of the National Dental Hygiene Board Examination.

Judicial branch Government section composed of courts that interpret the laws the legislature passes but do not make them.

Jurisprudence requirement The required reading and possible examination of state laws governing dental hygiene practice.

L

Learning domain Category that includes a way to differentiate the individual types of learning.

Legislative branch *See* legislature.

Legislative initiative Proposal to change or enact laws.

Legislators Collective term used to describe senators and representatives/congressmen.

Legislature Section of a government that makes the laws.

Lesson plan Written document used in planning a presentation.

Licensure requirement The requirements dental hygienists must meet to obtain a dental hygiene license to practice in each state.

Literature review Examination of all pertinent reports and studies to determine what is currently known about a specific topic or issue.

Lobbying Attempting to influence or sway others to take or support a desired position or action; the "art of the sell."

Long-term care facility Facility that provides live-in care for patients with medical complications.

M

Malpractice Dental hygiene professional's negligence by act or omission when the care provided is not within the accepted standards of practice and negatively affects the patient's well-being.

Managed care Integration of health care delivery and financing.

Manager Developer and coordinator of dental public health programs; sometimes referred to as *administrator*.

Manpower Available personnel to do a job; referred to as *labor force*.

Manpower shortage Inadequate availability of personnel to perform a job.

Marketing Organized approach to selecting and servicing markets and informing the public of a service as distinct from an impromptu approach to selling a service.

Mean Average of scores.

Measurement Act or process of using a particular method to gauge or evaluate something.

Measures of central tendency Measures used to describe the central tendency of data within a research study.

Measures of dispersion Identification of how much variation is present in a group of data and description of the distribution of data within a research study.

Median Midpoint of scores.

Medicaid (Title XIX) Federal program that traditionally distributes funds to states for medical and dental care provided to certain groups, including aged, blind, and disabled people; those with low incomes; and certain members of families with dependent children.

Medicare (Title XVIII) Federal medical insurance program for people age 65 or older, people under age 65 with certain disabilities, and people of all ages with End-Stage Renal Disease (permanent kidney failure requiring dialysis or a kidney transplant).

Mentor Role model who actively works with an individual to enhance that person's professional knowledge and abilities.

Metropolitan Large population nucleus consisting of a city and surrounding suburban areas.

Modality Clinical or educational dental hygiene treatment.

Mode Score that occurs most often.

Morbidity Ratio of "sick" (affected) individuals to well individuals in a community.

Mortality Ratio of the number of deaths from a given disease or health problem to the total number of cases reported.

Motivation Will of the individual to act.

Multifactorial Approach that assumes that a disease or condition has multiple causes.

N

National Board Dental Hygiene Examination The examination given by the American Dental Association to fulfill the written examination requirement.

National Health Service Corps (NHSC) Part of the Health Resources and Services Administration, a PHS agency "committed to improving the health of the nation's underserved by uniting communities in need with caring health professionals and supporting communities' efforts to build better systems of care."

Need Normative, professional judgment as to the amount and kind of health care services required to attain or maintain health.

Networking Sharing resources or services to cultivate productive relationships.

Nominal scale of measurement Organizes data into mutually exclusive categories that have no rank order or value.

Nonclinical evaluation Study or appraisal employing questionnaires, individual or group interviews, telephone interviews, focus groups, direct observations, document analysis, and survey rather than being based on, relating to, or conducted in a clinic.

Nonparametric statistics Quantification that should be used for hypothesis testing when variables are discrete, sample size is small, population distributions are not normal, or group variances are not equal.

Normal distribution Curve in which the majority of subjects will fall under the large part of the middle with a few low and high outliers; a bell curve, representing the mean, median, and mode.

Null hypothesis Initial negative statement of belief about the value of a population parameter, for example, that two groups do not differ on as to a variable.

Nursing home *See* long-term care facility.

O

Oral epidemiology Study of the amount, distribution, determinant, and control of oral disease and oral health conditions among given populations.

Ordinal scale of measurement Scale that organizes data into mutually exclusive categories that are rank ordered based on some criterion but the difference between ranks is not necessarily equal.

Outreach workers Dental hygienists working "outside" the dental practice to bring patients in need of restorative dental care to private dental practices while providing preventive services outside the dental practice, such as in a school setting.

P

P.A.N.D.A. Acronym for Prevent Abuse and Neglect through Dental Awareness; educational program aimed at helping dental providers recognize and report child abuse.

Paradigm Outstandingly clear or typical example or framework that explains or illustrates a concept or theory.

Parameter Numerical characteristic of the population.

Parametric statistics Quantity of a sample computed from a sample to test a hypothesis when the data meet certain assumptions.

Partnership Intense form of collaboration, state, or condition of associating or participating with others regularly in pursuit of a joint interest.

Peer reviewed Published articles that have been reviewed for content and accuracy by peers.

Pilot study Version of a proposed study that is carried out on a small, sometimes intentionally chosen sample.

Placebo Independent variable used with a research control group that is not the factor being studied but a nontreatment, sometimes referred to as a "sugar pill" but more likely to be either a standard drug of choice for a disease or a standard treatment procedure against which the experimental one is being compared.

Planning Part of the dental hygiene process of care that includes the development of a program.

Policy Written description of rules, regulations, and stipulations to govern individual actions and procedures.

Policy Development The act of developing policies to solve health issues

Poster session Method utilized to disseminate original research findings.

Practice Act Statute that defines the practice of dental hygiene or dentistry.

Practice management Process of planning, organizing, and managing resources to bring about the successful completion of specific project goals and objectives.

Preceptorship The on-the-job training of dental hygienists, sometimes referred to as alternative education.

Preexisting condition Medical condition that exists prior to a person's coverage by an insurance entity.

Preferred Provider Organizations (PPOs) Organizations practitioners contract with to provide dental care services for lower than average fees in order to attract patient subscribers who are seeking lower costs.

Premium Amount a group or an individual pays to the insurance entity for coverage.

Prepaid group practice Large group of dental providers contracted to provide services to groups of patients.

Prevalence Number of all existing cases of a disease in a population measured at a given point.

Prevention program Program designed to prevent disease in a target population.

Primary prevention Employment of strategies and agents to forestall the onset of disease, reverse its progress, or arrest its process before treatment becomes necessary.

Procedure number Identification given to a specific procedure as designated in the *Codes on Dental Procedures and Nomenclature* published by the ADA.

Program planning Process of developing a dental public health program that includes the stages of assessment, diagnosis, implementation, and evaluation.

Promulgate To put a law into practice as done by state dental boards.

Proposal Written description of a planned program or project intended to motivate an entity to adopt it.

Provider Legally licensed dental hygienist or dentist operating within a scope of pactice.

Psychomotor domain Name of a category that describes actions.

Public health Dental hygiene role focusing on the public health science and practice

Public health goals Goals that guide all public health activities.

Public health officer *See* US Public Health Service Officer.

Public health services Services that help attain goals of public health.

Public relations Practice of managing the dispersion of information between an organization and its public.

PubMed Web site that includes more than 17 million citations from MEDLINE and life science journals for biomedical articles back to the 50s.

p-value Probability that the findings of a study are due to chance.

Q

Qualitative evaluation Answering the why and how of a dental public health program or research project.

Quantitative evaluation A numerical evaluation of a dental public health program or research project.

Quasi-experimental approach Research design that lacks inherent control.

R

Range Number determined by subtracting the highest score from the lowest score.

Ratio scale of measurement Scale containing all characteristics of the preceding scales and an absolute zero point determined by nature.

Refereed Description of publications that includes peer-reviewed articles.

Regulation Rules of order imposed by an executive authority or government agency governing practice.

Reliability Consistency or degree to which an instrument will produce the same results on repeated trials within the same population every time the characteristic is measured.

Representative Elected member of the US or individual state house of representatives.

Request for proposal Request for proposal (RFP) by groups or agencies; also called *request for applications, notice of funding availability*, or *program announcement*.

Research approach Type of research used to obtain information; all types involve observation, description, measurement, analysis, and interpretation of occurring phenomena.

Research design Overall plan for conducting a study.

Researcher Dental hygiene role which focuses on research germane to the study of health and disease.

Research proposal Protocol or detailed plan for a study.

Retrospective (ex post facto) approach Research that looks backward (ex post facto, or after the fact) to investigate a group of people with a particular disease, usually via medical records.

Risk factor Characteristic of an individual or population that may increase the likelihood of experiencing a given health problem.

Rural Geographic area that is sparsely populated.

S

Sample Subgroup of a target population.

Sample size Referring to an adequate number of subjects within a research study.

Sampling technique Technique used when selecting a sample from a population to study.

Scales of measurement Classification of data as (1) nominal (or categorical), (2) ordinal, (3) interval, and (4) ratio.

Scientific method Body of techniques using observation, reason, and experimentation to gather evidence that is empirical and measurable.

Secondary Prevention Routine treatment methods to terminate a disease process and/or restore tissues to as near normal as possible and can be termed restorative care.

Self-regulation Governing of dental hygiene practice by dental hygienists.

Senator Elected member of the US or individual state senate.

Single procedure Specific process designated by a specific code.

Skew Tail of a distribution formed by a few extreme scores.

Skewed distribution Description of distribution of asymmetrical scores causing the curve to be distorted, or skewed.

Social worker Professional who works to help individuals or the community enhance their capacity for social functioning.

Sociocultural theory Theory proposed by Lev Vygotsky that an individual's social interaction as a child leads to continuous changes in thought and behavior that can vary greatly from culture to culture.

Socioeconomic status (SES) Individual's comparative social and economic standing within a community.

Sound natural teeth Either primary or permanent teeth that have adequate hard and soft tissue support.

Stakeholder Individual in an organization who has a vested interest in a specific topic, issue, or initiative.

Standard deviation Measure of dispersion.

Statistical decision Determination made about the null hypothesis based on the results of the inferential statistics.

Statistical significance Research study whose results show the quality of being statistically important.

Statute Law enacted by a government's legislature.

Statutory law Legislature-enacted, written law, which serves to promote justice.

Subculture Group of people with a culture that differentiates them from the larger culture to which they belong.

Summative evaluation Examination of a program's merit after it has been implemented.

Supply Amount of dental care services available.

Surgeon general Appointed administrator of the US Public Health Service.

Surveillance Ongoing observation, persistent watching over, scrutiny, constant monitoring, and assessment of changes in populations related to disease, conditions, injuries, disabilities, or death trends.

T

Table clinic Method utilized to disseminate past research studies and literature reviews of a specific topic.

Target population Clearly identified segment of the population.

Target population profile Comprehensive overview of the target population that includes specific descriptions.

Teaching strategy Plan or method used in instruction.

Tertiary prevention Strategy to replace lost tissues through rehabilitation.

Testlet Format that introduces a case study involving an issue pertinent to dental public health in the community dental health/research principles category for the Board Examination.

Therapeutic services Services the dental hygienist provides that benefit the patient; can include periodontal debridement, polishing, fluoride application, local anesthesia, dental sealants, education, and behavior modification interventions.

Three-party system Program in which a dental provider renders the service for which the patient's sponsor (insurance company or employer) pays.

Tobacco cessation program Program to encourage patients to quit using tobacco.

Transcultural communication skill Ability to interpret and transmit information to someone from a different culture.

TRICARE Health care program serving active-duty service members, National Guard and Reserve members, retirees, their families, survivors, and certain former spouses worldwide; formerly known as Civilian Health and Medical Program of the Uniformed Services (CHAMPUS).

Two-party system Program in which a dental provider renders the service for which the patient pays.

Type I error Error that occurs when the null hypothesis is rejected but is actually true; also called an alpha error.

Type II error Error that occurs when the null hypothesis is accepted but is actually false and should have been rejected; also called a beta error.

U

US Public Health Service Commissioned Corps Unit of highly trained and mobile health professionals who conduct programs to promote the health of the nation, understand and prevent disease and injury, ensure safe and effective drugs and medical devices, deliver health services to federal beneficiaries, and provide health expertise in time of war or other national or international emergency.

Urban Concentrated human settlement, usually consisting of at least 2500 people.

Usual, customary, and reasonable (UCR) fee Average dentist fee per service in the immediate local region.

Utilization Number of dental care services actually consumed, not just desired.

V

Validity Degree to which a research study measured what it was supposed to measure (internal) and that can be generalized to the entire population (external).

Values Ideas and beliefs a person possesses that influence behavior, giving meaning to life.

Variables Quantity whose value may change over the course of a research study.

Variance Squared deviation of each score from the mean's sum.

W

Washout period Period of time in research with no treatment; in drug trials, period allowed for all of any administered drug to be eliminated from the body.

Water fluoridation *See* community water fluoridation.

Workforce Workers whose members deliver health care to the public.

World Health Organization (WHO) Body that addresses unmet oral health needs of global populations in its commitment to improve oral health as an integral part of general health.

Written examination requirement The written examination a dental hygienist must pass before becoming eligible for a dental hygiene license.

X

Xylitol Sugar substitute found in berries, fruit, vegetables, mushrooms, and birch wood that has shown promising results in reducing dental decay and ear infections.

Z

Zone of proximal development Difference between a child's actual level of development displayed by unassisted performance and the child's potential level as indicated by assisted performance.

Index